Ondrej Bradac
Editor

Normal Pressure Hydrocephalus

Pathophysiology, Diagnosis, Treatment and Outcome

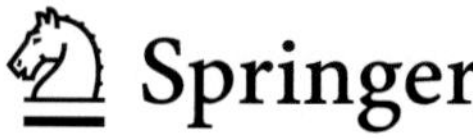

Editor
Ondrej Bradac
Department of Neurosurgery, 2nd Medical
School, Motol University Hospital
Charles University
Prague, Czech Republic

ISBN 978-3-031-36524-9   ISBN 978-3-031-36522-5 (eBook)
https://doi.org/10.1007/978-3-031-36522-5

This Springer imprint is published by the registered company Springer Nature Switzerland AG
The registered company address is: Gewerbestrasse 11, 6330 Cham, Switzerland

Normal Pressure Hydrocephalus

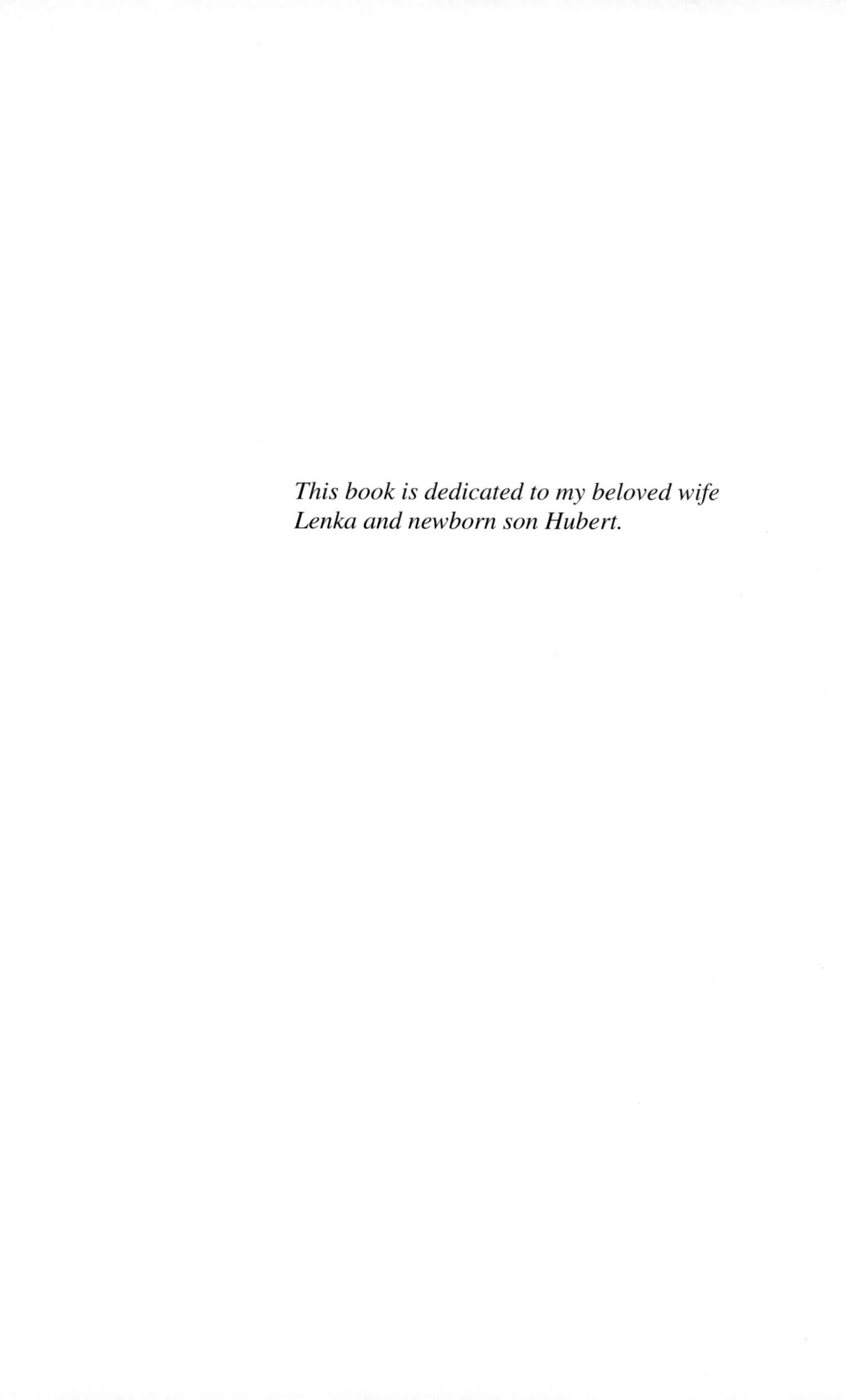

*This book is dedicated to my beloved wife
Lenka and newborn son Hubert.*

Foreword by Prof. Vladimír Beneš

The book on normal pressure hydrocephalus (NPH) has been demanded in the neuro-surgical literature for a long time. This book, edited by Ondrej Bradac, is so far the most comprehensive work on NPH where all aspects of the disease are covered. Part One—History and Background has two extremely important chapters, namely physiology and pathophysiology of cerebrospinal fluid circulation. This part of the book gives the real background of problematics. Separate and dedicated chapter describes NPH's history. History is paramount in general; there is no future without history.

Part Two, Diagnostics of NPH, gives the overview from clinical symptomatology to the most sophisticated radiological studies, and it is concluded by the chapter on machine learning as related to NPH. Again, this part is the essential one as it serves also as an introduction to Part Three which deals with the treatment and outcome. All the recent possibilities and techniques introduced in NPH treatment are covered along with the complications and outcome.

Many of the chapters were written by respected scientists in the area of NPH, neurologists, neurosurgeons, and radiologists. Careful selection of authors ensures the high quality of the text. Also the personality of Ondrej Bradac guarantees top-quality text. Ondrej Bradac is not only a professor of neurosurgery but also a doctor of natural sciences in mathematics. His long-lasting experience and interest in NPH ensure that the chapters are perfectly linked and in logical order.

Since the NPH is the only reversible cause of dementia, the relevance and importance of the book are without any doubt. The book should be studied by not only neurosurgeons but also by neurologists interested in dementia, all neuroscientists working in dementia problematics, neurorehabilitation specialists, and in general by all healthcare professionals in the field. Its importance is especially highlighted in lieu of recent Alzheimer's pandemics.

March 2023

Prof. Vladimír Beneš, MD, Ph.D.
Department of Neurosurgery
and Neurooncology
1st Faculty of Medicine
Military University Hospital
Charles University
Prague, Czech Republic

Foreword by Prof. David Netuka

Professor Bradac assembled an outstanding group of true experts in the field of normal pressure hydrocephalus. Since Salomón Hakim first described NPH in 1957, numerous articles and books have been published on this important topic. However, there is still a need for further research. This book is unique in that it presents all clinically relevant data in a comprehensive manner. The first part of the book covers the history and background of NPH, while acknowledging that much is still unknown about its pathophysiology. Nonetheless, this specific chapter presents all available data on the topic.

In the diagnostics part, the chapter on NPH imaging is particularly noteworthy, as it includes differential diagnosis of neurodegenerative disorders.

In the treatment and outcome part, the potential value of endoscopy is well discussed. Prognosis and outcome are crucial for patient counselling, and this chapter should be read with special attention.

The authors should be congratulated for producing an excellent book that sets a new benchmark for NPH literature. Every neurosurgeon with an interest in hydrocephalus should own this book. Let us hope that this book will have an impact on the future care of patients with suspected NPH.

March 2023

Prof. David Netuka, MD, Ph.D.
Department of Neurosurgery
and Neurooncology
1st Faculty of Medicine
Military University Hospital
Charles University
Prague, Czech Republic

Foreword by Assoc. Prof. Vladimír Beneš Jr.

You are about to embark on a remarkable journey into the heart of normal pressure hydrocephalus. Ondrej Bradac has managed to persuade renowned experts to contribute to this topic, and the following pages are the fruit of more than two years of their work on them. A thorough and complex discussion covers the whole topic and is a must-read for all neurosurgeons, neurologists, and other specialists in the field of neurodegeneration who deal with these patients on a daily basis. It brings a step-by-step description of clinical and radiological diagnostic procedures, differential diagnostic deliberations, strengths, and limitations of therapy as well as its complications and long-term expectations. Trainees, residents, and fully educated neurosurgeons will likely be grateful to Ondrej Bradac and his colleagues for years to come for this elegant book. No stone was left unturned, and the combination of clear text, comprehensive tables, precise illustrations, and numerous literature sources makes this work a reference book on normal pressure hydrocephalus for the following generations.

March 2023

Assoc. Prof. Vladimír Beneš Jr., MD, Ph.D.
Department of Neurosurgery
2nd Faculty of Medicine
Motol University Hospital
Charles University
Prague, Czech Republic

Acknowledgements

First of all, I wish to express my gratitude to the international group of authors who had written the chapters of this book and to all those without whose help the book would have never been written.

I feel obliged to express my respect and special thanks to all three authors of forewords, namely Prof. Vladimír Beneš Senior, Prof. David Netuka, and Associated Prof. Vladimír Beneš Junior—all of them influenced my professional career during various stages and helped this book to happen.

Special thank belongs to Miss Adéla Bubeníková who, besides of authorship of many chapters, helped with the organization of chapters and typesetting. Her performance and enthusiasm were the most seminal for successful finish of this book.

Furthermore, I have to thank Miss Helen Whitley and Miss Awista Zazay for their valuable help with English proof reading.

Last, but not least, I am deeply indebted to Miss Kateřina Nebřenská, Mrs. Lenka Bernardová, and Miss Tereza Drbohlavová for their valuable support in organizing patient care and scientific studies. Similarly as all research team members who permanently contribute to not only scientific work, but also take care of these fragile patients on a daily basis.

This book was supported by the Ministry of Health of the Czech Republic institutional grant no. NU23-04-00551.

Contents

"""

Contents   xvii

History and Background

Introduction

Petr Skalický and Ondřej Bradáč

Abstract In this chapter, we explore the challenges behind diagnosing normal pressure hydrocephalus (NPH), characterized by ventricular fluid accumulation in the brain leading to gait disturbances, cognitive decline, and urinary incontinence. The difficulty in distinguishing NPH from other neurological disorders necessitates comprehensive evaluations. Shunt surgery is the main treatment option, but selecting appropriate candidates and predicting responsiveness remain challenging. Integrating machine learning algorithms into MRI-based diagnosis shows promise in improving accuracy by identifying subtle biomarkers specific to NPH, potentially reducing misdiagnoses, and enabling earlier intervention for better patient outcomes. Continued research in this area will likely lead to more effective NPH management through the fusion of advanced technologies and clinical expertise.

Keywords Normal pressure hydrocephalus · Intracranial pressure · Ventriculoperitoneal shunt · Cerebrospinal fluid · Shunt surgery

Abbreviations

CSF	Cerebrospinal fluid
ICP	Intracranial pressure
iNPH	Idiopathic normal pressure hydrocephalus
NPH	Normal pressure hydrocephalus
sNPH	Secondary normal pressure hydrocephalus
VP	Ventriculoperitoneal

P. Skalický · O. Bradáč (✉)
Department of Neurosurgery, 2nd Medical Faculty, Charles University and Motol University Hospital, Prague, Czech Republic
e-mail: ondrej.bradac2@fnmotol.cz

O. Bradáč
Department of Neurosurgery and Neurooncology, 1st Medical Faculty, Charles University and Military University Hospital, Prague, Czech Republic

Normal pressure hydrocephalus (NPH) has been an important part of the differential diagnosis of dementia for more than 50 years. In 1965, Hakim and Adams described three patients who had ventriculomegaly on pneumoencephalography but did not have elevated intracranial pressure (ICP) [1]. They defined the clinical syndrome—the triad of symptoms: gait impairment (magnetic, shuffling, and broad-based gait), urinary incontinence (urgent pattern), and cognitive deterioration—accompanying this diagnosis [2]. This complete triad occurs in approximately 50% of patients [3]. Diagnosis of iNPH is based on clinical signs in combination with imaging methods (MRI, CT) and functional tests [4]. In practice, guidelines are often used to stratify iNPH into (1) possible iNPH, (2) probable iNPH, and (3) definite iNPH according to the probability of the disease [5–10].

NPH is divided into primary or idiopathic (iNPH) and secondary (sNPH). iNPH is a disease of the elderly with increasing incidence in the population over 65 years. In iNPH, the cause of hydrocephalus remains unclear despite more than 50 years of research in this field. Some concepts and mechanisms of the theoretical pathophysiological pathways and different aetiologies of iNPH will be presented in this book. sNPH can occur at any age following a previous insult such as meningitis, subarachnoid haemorrhage, tumours or traumatic brain injury [4].

The course of NPH can be reversed to some extent by shunt implantation, and therefore, this diagnosis should be known to anyone involved in patients with dementia [11]. The most commonly used treatment is the implantation of a ventriculoperitoneal (VP) shunt—a system that drains cerebrospinal fluid from the lateral ventricles of the brain to the abdominal cavity [12]. Shunt implantation leads to an improvement in clinical symptoms in 75% of patients [13]. The complication rate of VP shunts is between 13 and 38%, with 26–38% of cases with a fixed valve and 9–16% of cases with an adjustable valve requiring revision [13]. Good results can be maintained for many years in some patients, depending on the occurrence of comorbidities [14]. Prognosis and outcomes of the treatment will be discussed in the book and some follow-up and diagnostic hints, and tips will be given to help achieve the best possible outcomes in patients properly selected for shunting.

1 Why a Book About NPH?

There are several reasons why a book about NPH is needed. First of all, there are currently around 50 million people with dementia in the world, and this number is expected to triple by 2050 in line with population ageing [15]. Although the reported prevalence of iNPH due to under diagnosis is inaccurate, 1.3% prevalence of iNPH is expected for people aged 65 and over [16]. The annual incidence set in 2016 in Germany is 1.36/100,000 [17]. The socio-economic and healthcare burden is tremendous, but treatment options may reduce the impact of increasing care requirements on health systems [18–20]. NPH cases remain underdiagnosed. One of the main reasons is a difficult differential diagnosis in the context of neurodegenerative or cerebrovascular diseases such as the risk factors, age, and some of the clinical symptoms or imaging signs may be related to Alzheimer's disease, Parkinson's disease, Lewy body disease, vascular dementia, or other diseases [21]. As these disorders are prevalent in the elderly some of the NPH patients may suffer from neurodegenerative comorbidity [22]. One of the most important points is to consider NPH whether a patient presents with gait impairment, mental deterioration, and urinary incontinence. As comorbidities influence the outcome, the decision to treat should be individualized; however, any age-related risks are minimal and should not be a rejection of surgery [23]. NPH patients are at increased risk of falls [24], which may be reduced by shunt surgery [25]. A recent article suggests that screening for iNPH in the elderly presenting after falls can possibly identify iNPH patients in the earlier stage when these patients may benefit more from surgical treatment [26]. Practical aspects of the differential diagnosis, functional tests, imaging signs, or other modalities used in the NPH diagnostic work-up will get major attention in the book. Both hospital and outpatient care of NPH patients is demanding, and treatment and follow-up of the patients will be increasingly needed in the future. Neurosurgeons, neurologists, and other clinicians working with dementia patients must be aware of NPH diagnosis. The book provides a comprehensive view of the disease with the theoretical background and practical aspects.

Research is focussed on pathophysiological mechanisms, identification of patients responding to shunt therapy, identification and treatment of comorbidities, improvement of shunt systems, and non-invasive examinations. There is an increasing need for better shunt candidate selection and advances in the efficiency and effectiveness of the treatment. Nonsurgical treatment for hydrocephalus in animal models has been studied for many years, but no significant results have been obtained at the clinical translation stage [27].

With this book, we would like to contribute to the scientific literature of normal pressure hydrocephalus and provide a complex view of the disease with conclusions from the most up-to-date research.

References

1. Hakim S, Adams RD. The special clinical problem of symptomatic hydrocephalus with normal cerebrospinal fluid pressure. Observations on cerebrospinal fluid hydrodynamics. J Neurol Sci. 1965;2(4):307–27. https://doi.org/10.1016/0022-510X(65)90016-X.
2. Adams RD, et al. Symptomatic occult hydrocephalus with normal cerebrospinal-fluid pressure. New Eng J Med. 1965;273(3):117–26. https://doi.org/10.1056/NEJM196507152730301.
3. Hashimoto M, et al. Diagnosis of idiopathic normal pressure hydrocephalus is supported by MRI-based scheme: a prospective cohort study. Cerebrospinal Fluid Res. 2010;7. https://doi.org/10.1186/1743-8454-7-18.
4. Skalický P, et al. Normal pressure hydrocephalus—an overview of pathophysiological mechanisms and diagnostic procedures. Neurosurg Rev. 2019. https://doi.org/10.1007/s10143-019-01201-5.

5. Nakajima M, et al. Guidelines for management of idiopathic normal pressure hydrocephalus (third edition): endorsed by the japanese society of normal pressure hydrocephalus. Neurol Med Chir. 2021;61(2):63–97. https://doi.org/10.2176/nmc.st.2020-0292.
6. Marmarou A, et al. INPH guidelines, part I: development of guidelines for idiopathic normal-pressure hydrocephalus: Introduction. Neurosurgery. 2005;57(3 SUPPL.):S2-1–S2-3. https://doi.org/10.1227/01.NEU.0000168188.25559.0E.
7. Relktin N, et al. INPH guidelines, part II: diagnosing idio-pathic normal-pressure hydrocephalus. Neurosurgery. 2005;57(3 SUPPL.):S2-4–S2-16. https://doi.org/10.1227/01.NEU.0000168185.29659.C5.
8. Bergsneider M, et al. INPH guidelines, part IV: surgical management of idiopathic normal-pressure hydrocephalus. Neurosurgery. 2005;57(3 SUPPL.):S2-29–S2-39. https://doi.org/10.1227/01.NEU.0000168186.45363.4D.
9. Klinge P, et al. INPH guidelines, part V: outcome of shunting in idiopathic normal-pressure hydrocephalus and the value of outcome assessment in shunted patients. Neurosurgery. 2005;57(3 SUPPL.):S2-40–S2-52. https://doi.org/10.1227/01.NEU.0000168187.01077.2F.
10. Halperin JJ, et al. Practice guideline: idiopathic normal pressure hydrocephalus: response to shunting and predictors of response. Neurology. 2015;85(23):2063–71. https://doi.org/10.1212/WNL.0000000000002193.
11. Relkin N, et al. Diagnosing Idiopathic normal-pressure hydrocephalus. Neurosurgery. 2005;57(suppl_3):S2-4–S2-16. https://doi.org/10.1227/01.NEU.0000168185.29659.C5
12. AbdelRazek MA, Venna N. Ventriculoperitoneal-shunt placement for normal-pressure hydro cephalus. New Eng J Med. 2017;377(26): e35. https://doi.org/10.1056/NEJMicm1701226.
13. Giordan E, et al. Outcomes and complications of different surgical treatments for idiopathic normal pressure hydrocephalus: a systematic review and meta-analysis. J Neurosurg. 2018:1–13. https://doi.org/10.3171/2018.5.JNS1875.
14. Grasso G, et al. Long-term efficacy of shunt therapy in idiopathic normal pressure hydrocephalus. World Neurosurg. 2019;129:e458–63. https://doi.org/10.1016/j.wneu.2019.05.183.
15. Patterson C. International, World Alzheimer report 2018. 2018, Alzheimer's Disease International.
16. Martín-Láez R, et al. Epidemiology of idiopathic normal pressure hydrocephalus: a systematic review of the literature. World Neurosurg. 2015;84(6):2002–9. https://doi.org/10.1016/j.wneu.2015.07.005.
17. Lemcke J, et al. Nationwide incidence of normal pressure hydrocephalus (NPH) assessed by insurance claim data in Germany. Open Neurol J. 2016;10:15–24. https://doi.org/10.2174/1874205X01610010015.
18. Tinelli M, Guldemond N, Kehler U. Idiopathic normal-pressure hydrocephalus: the cost-effectiveness of delivering timely and adequate treatment in Germany. Eur J Neurol. 2021;28:681–90. https://doi.org/10.1111/ene.14581.
19. Kameda M, Yamada S, Atsuchi M, et al. Cost-effectiveness analysis of shunt surgery for idiopathic normal pressure hydrocephalus based on the SINPHONI and SINPHONI-2 trials. Acta Neurochir. 2017;159:995–1003. https://doi.org/10.1007/s00701-017-3115-2.
20. Tullberg M, Persson J, Petersen J, et al. Shunt surgery in idiopathic normal pressure hydrocephalus is cost-effective—a cost utility analysis. Acta Neurochir. 2018;160:509–18. https://doi.org/10.1007/s00701-017-3394-7.
21. Kiefer M, Unterberg A. The differential diagnosis and treatment of normal-pressure hydrocephalus. Dtsch Arztebl Int. 2012;109(1–2):15–26. https://doi.org/10.3238/arztebl.2012.0015.
22. Allali G, et al. Brain comorbidities in normal pressure hydrocephalus. Eur J Neurol. 2018;25(3):542–8. https://doi.org/10.1111/ene.13543.
23. Nakajima M, et al. Background risk factors associated with shunt intervention for possible idiopathic normal pressure hydrocephalus: a nationwide hospital-based survey in Japan. J Alzheimers Dis. 2019;68(2):735–44. https://doi.org/10.3233/JAD-180955.
24. Davis A, Luciano M, Moghekar A, et al. Assessing the predictive value of common gait measure for predicting falls in patients presenting with suspected normal pressure hydrocephalus. BMC Neurol. 2021;21:60. https://doi.org/10.1186/s12883-021-02068-0.

25. Larsson J, Israelsson H, Eklund A, Lundin-Olsson L, Malm J. Falls and fear of falling in shunted idiopathic normal pressure hydrocephalus—the idiopathic normal pressure hydrocephalus comorbidity and risk factors associated with hydrocephalus study. Neurosurgery. 2021;89(1):122–28. https://doi.org/10.1093/neuros/nyab094.
26. Oike R, Inoue Y, Matsuzawa K, Sorimachi T. Screening for idiopathic normal pressure hydrocephalus in the elderly after falls [published online ahead of print, 2021 Apr 24]. Clin Neurol Neurosurg. 2021;205:106635. https://doi.org/10.1016/j.clineuro.2021.106635.
27. Wang C, Wang X, Tan C, et al. Novel therapeutics for hydrocephalus: insights from animal models. CNS Neurosci Ther. 2021;27:1012–22. https://doi.org/10.1111/cns.13695.

History

Petr Skalický, Adéla Bubeníková, Aleš Vlasák, and Ondřej Bradáč

Abstract The first report of hydrocephalus with normal pressure is dated back to 1956, when Foltz and Ward published a case report of a patient with normal pressure communicating hydrocephalus after subarachnoid haemorrhage. However, there were no further investigations of the causes and consequences in this case. The first scholar and clinician who studied this specific type of hydrocephalus was Salomón Hakim a few years later. He and his counterpart Raymond Adams worked on a detailed description of the disease's manifestation, subsequently setting the cornerstones of the diagnosis and treatment options for patients suffering from, as currently officially recognised, normal pressure hydrocephalus (NPH). Since then, there has been a growing body of literature reports paying more attention to the disease—to its pathogenesis, pathophysiology, challenging diagnosis, and the demand for improving treatment efficacy. NPH was in the second half of the 20th century described as a new form of reversible dementia, a disorder that had long been considered terminal and irreversible. The famous story of Hakim's "discovery" of NPH initiated a new era dedicated to improving the diagnosis of the disease, more efficient treatment targeting in relation to significant technical improvement in cerebrospinal fluid drainage procedures, and therefore improving the overall prognosis of NPH patients. This chapter describes the historical findings of hydrocephalus over centuries that led to the uncovering of NPH, the discovery of NPH itself, together with fundamental breakthroughs in the past decades that have enabled us to study NPH more in detail, as further introduced in individual chapters throughout this book.

Keywords Hydrocephalus history · Salomón Hakim · Normal pressure hydrocephalus · Cerebrospinal fluid

P. Skalický · A. Bubeníková · A. Vlasák · O. Bradáč (✉)
Department of Neurosurgery, 2nd Medical Faculty, Charles University and Motol University Hospital, Prague, Czech Republic
e-mail: ondrej.bradac2@fnmotol.cz

A. Bubeníková · O. Bradáč
Department of Neurosurgery and Neurooncology, 1st Medical Faculty, Charles University and Military University Hospital, Prague, Czech Republic

O. Bradac (ed.), *Normal Pressure Hydrocephalus*,
https://doi.org/10.1007/978-3-031-36522-5_2

Abbreviations

CSF   Cerebrospinal fluid
DESH   Disproportionately enlarged subarachnoid space hydrocephalus
ELD   External lumbar drain
ICP   Intracranial pressure
iNPH   Idiopathic normal pressure hydrocephalus
LIT   Lumbar infusion test
NPH   Normal pressure hydrocephalus

1 Introduction

Although hydrocephalus has been known for a long time, the NPH unit (first referred to as symptomatic occult hydrocephalus) has only been known since the middle of the last century. The case of communicating hydrocephalus with normal pressure after subarachnoid haemorrhage was introduced by Foltz and Ward in 1956 [1]. However, the case was only described without further investigation of the causes and consequences. Later, Salomón Hakim paid more attention to this issue. He first noticed the manifestations of NPH in patients in 1957 at the San Juan de Dios Hospital in Bogotá, Colombia. He presented his findings and first case studies to the world for the first time in 1964 [2]. This was followed by the most famous works together with Dr. Raymond Adams published in The New England Journal of Medicine [3] and The Journal of the Neurological Sciences [4] in 1965. Hakim based his pathophysiological considerations on Pascal's law. The pressure is equal to the force divided by the area on which it acts and is simultaneously the same in all directions at a specific point in a resting fluid. He demonstrated the theory on an inflating balloon. In the first phase, when the balloon is inflated, both the pressure and the force acting on the rubber of the balloon increase, but after reaching the maximum, the pressure drops to a certain, later stable level, while the force still increases with increasing volume. Thus, the pressure in both the small and large space is equal, but the force in the larger space has increased in proportion to its increased surface [3].

Dr. Hakim cannot be denied the main credit for the discovery of NPH. Originally sceptical, Dr. Adams was only convinced by the case of Hakim's American patient, who wanted to return to the USA before performing drainage and shunt surgery. Hakim decided to accompany the patient, and after a meeting and discussions with Dr. Adams in Boston, the patient underwent shunt surgery with significant clinical improvement [2]. In their key work, they described together the case reports of three patients with improvement of symptoms after shunt surgery, the classic triad of symptoms, and basic pathophysiological hypotheses [3]. The article immediately received much attention, as NPH was a treatable cause of dementia. Over the following years, many pathophysiological theories emerged, examining a number of invasive examinations to predict shunt response from radionuclide cisternography, lumboventricular perfusion, to currently used methods in clinical practice—tap test, lumbar infusion test, and external (extended) lumbar drainage. MRI and CT imaging replaced the original pneumoencephalogram. New types of shunt systems were introduced also with regard to other aetiologies of hydrocephalus. Even Salomón Hakim and later his eldest son Carlos Hakim worked on developing their own valves [2]. Over the years, thousands of works have been created that deal with or touch on the topic of NPH. Unfortunately, there are still a large number of unknowns. There are a lack of unambiguous preoperative non-invasive techniques for predicting the shunt response, invasive examinations may not sufficiently explain the need for shunt surgery, and the high incidence of comorbidities and overlap with other diagnoses in these patients further limits prediction methods.

2 Hydrocephalus History

The first to describe hydrocephalus as a nosological unit was probably Hippocrates in the 5th century BC. However, his concept of "water over the brain" was more of a collection of fluid surrounding the brain than a typical accumulation of cerebrospinal fluid within the ventricular system as we understand it today [5]. A similar concept was adopted by Galen in the 2nd century BC. Galen believed that hydrocephalus was a subcutaneous fluid collection on the head due to improper handling by the midwife during parturition [6]. He distinguished several types of hydrocephalus— both extracranial and intracranial. This concept lasted almost 2000 years until the development of anatomy and physiology.

During the 16th century, several physicians correctly described individual cases of patients with hydrocephalus. Andreas van Wessel (Vesalius) described a case of a 2-year-old with an extremely enlarged ventricular system [7], and Jacob Spon and George Wheler described on their way to Italy and Greece as a curiosity a patient with an abnormally enlarged skull apparently after hydrocephalus in childhood [8]. Important contributions to our understanding of the anatomical properties of the ventricular system were made by Leonardo Da Vinci, mainly thanks to his famous anatomical drawings (Fig. 1).

Subsequently, during the post-Renaissance era of the 17th and 18th century, many European anatomists and physiologists came up with new theories. For example, Thomas Willis expressed the idea that cerebrospinal fluid is produced in choroid plexuses and must flow into the venous system [9]. Antonio Pacchioni described the arachnoid granulations, but mistakenly considered them a place of secretion of CSF instead of resorption [10]. And finally, Albrecht von Haller discovered the foramina of Luschka and presented the modern theory of CSF circulation.

In the 18th century, other authors continued the research they had started. We must remember above all Francois Magendie and Hubert von Luschka [11]. From the clinical point of view, it was Robert Whytt, the English physician, who correctly described hydrocephalus in patients with tuberculosis meningitis [12].

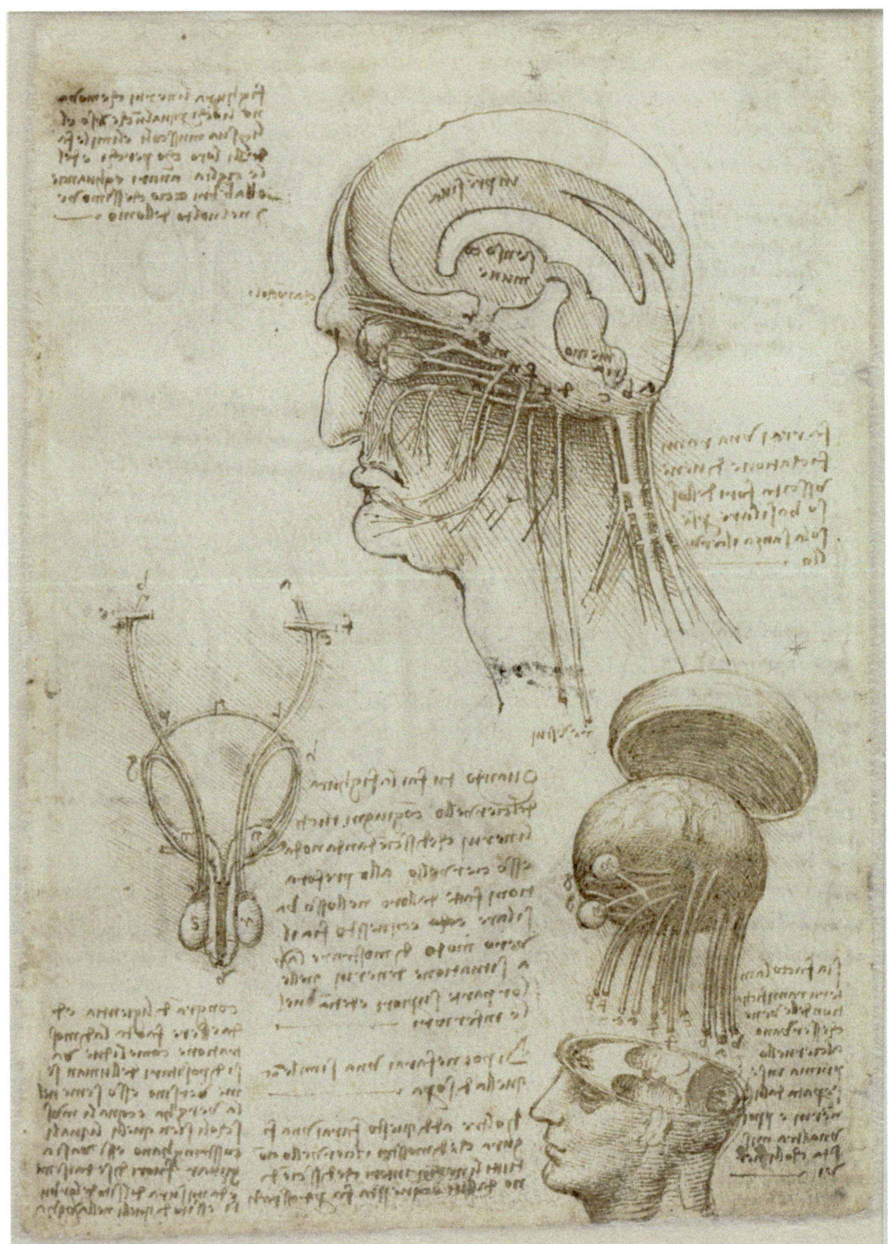

Fig. 1 Leonardo Da Vinci's studies of the human head, brain, and cranial nerves. Depiction of the cerebral ventricles and cranial nerves. The drawing on the left depicts the male reproductive tract. https://commons.wikimedia.org/wiki/File:Leonardo_Da_Vinci%27s_Brain_Physiology.jpg. In the public domain

In the next two centuries, a number of anatomists and physiologists participated in the description of the ventricular system and cerebrospinal fluid circulation in the CNS. This process was completed by Lewis Weed in the early 20th century. He correctly localised the production of cerebrospinal fluid into the choroid plexuses and mapped the circulation of the fluid through the central nervous system [13].

The key step in the description of the disease was the pivotal work of Australian pathologist, Dorothy Stuart Russell, "Observations on the Pathology of Hydrocephalus" [14], which had a major impact on the search for healing modalities for hydrocephalus.

3 Hakim's Discovery of NPH

At the time of Hakim's discovery, the literature available in this field was very weak. Three papers from the 20th century dealt with symptoms associated with adult hydrocephalus before later works by Hakim and Adams were published [1, 15, 16]. Riddoch's work from 1936 was related to the tumours of the third ventricle [15]. McHugh presented cases with occult hydrocephalus, based on a congenital obstruction, and reviewed neurological problems that may develop later in life after the asymptomatic period. Some cases even remained clinically silent, and hydrocephalus was described in autopsy findings. Few cases presented with normal pressure hydrocephalus like gait pattern [16]. Involvement of neuronal fibres taking course to the legs and stretch and damage with dilatation of ventricles was discussed [17]. Foltz et al. [1] in 1956 presented a case of communicating hydrocephalus from subarachnoid haemorrhage. However, no deeper investigations of the case have been made.

Salomón Hakim was born to a family of Lebanese immigrants in 1922 in the port town of Barranquilla in Colombia. His parents emigrated from Lebanon in 1921 through Cuba first to Barranquilla where Salomón Hakim was born and then to Ibague where Jorge Hakim (Salomón's father) founded a fabric shop. He had a passion for physics and liked to do experiments with electricity as a child. He would lock himself in his bedroom and make electric circuits for hours. At the age of 12, he started building radios. He enrolled in medical school in 1944 and subsequently became a neurosurgeon. His love for physics continued with examinations of digestion electrical output, the effect of current on uterine contraction, and the use of electrolysis in calcium formation. He left Colombia for two fellowships in the United States (Boston) in 1950 and 1954. However, he made his groundbreaking discovery in his native Colombia. He earned a PhD in neuropathology. During his fellowship research, he performed brain autopsies on patients who had neurodegenerative conditions such as Alzheimer's disease and noted that in many of the cases the ventricles were enlarged with no or minimal brain atrophy [2].

In 1957 while working in San Juan de Dios Hospital in Bogotá, Colombia, he faced for the first time a clinical condition that he had originally named "symptomatic occult hydrocephalus". A 16-year-old male patient who suffered severe craniocerebral trauma after being hit by a car while playing with a ball on the street and later developed a subdural haematoma that was drained. After the surgery, no clinical improvement was seen and the patient underwent pneumoencephalography which to Hakim's surprise showed ventriculomegaly. Lumbar puncture showed normal intracranial pressure (150 mm Hg). The patient improved after 15 ml of CSF was collected by lumbar puncture. This finding was confirmed by repeated punctures and the patient finally underwent ventriculoatrial shunt surgery and recovered completely, being able to go to school at 3 months of follow-up [18]. His original explanation of this phenomenon was related to Pascal's law. Even though the intracranial pressure may be normal in enlarged ventricles, the increased surface of the dilated ventricles leads to an abnormally large force—named by Hakim as the hydraulic press effect (Fig. 2) [4]. A second case soon presented in February 1958, a professional trombone player, who for the past year was unable to play the instrument. His legs were stiff, he had trouble turning and could not climb stairs with an unsteady balance. He also had other symptoms from the triad—urinary impairment and cognitive decline. The patient was apathetic and careless in his appearance. Pneumoencephalogram showed ventriculomegaly and his symptoms improved after spinal CSF drainage. Six weeks later, shunt was implanted and clinical symptoms remarkably improved [19]. Although there was scepticism by the contemporary clinicians, another publication was made in 1965 with Hakim's colleagues from Massachusetts describing the improvement of the clinical symptoms after shunt surgery in a patient that was accompanied by Hakim from Colombia to the USA, where Hakim convinced Dr. Raymond Adams that shunt surgery was indicated. The typical triad of symptoms—gait impairment, mental deterioration, and urinary incontinence, was described [3]. Some of the world-renowned neurologists, however, did not respond so positively. For example, H. Houston Merritt doubted NPH as the diagnosis. In a twist of fate, he later developed symptoms of NPH and died of complications of shunt surgery in Boston in 1979. The condition of NPH is still regarded with ambiguity by too many even after huge progress in NPH diagnostics, pathophysiology and treatment has been made. The lack of definitive diagnostic tests, the imprecision and variability of various invasive tests, high degree of clinical overlap with other diseases of the elderly are the factors that fuel the unfounded scepticism [2].

Dr. Salomón Hakim delivered > 85 lectures in more than 30 countries and became a professor in the Universidad Nacional de Colombia. He was an inventor and made numerous advancements in the valve technology of shunt systems. In 1966, unidirectional valve with spring-loaded pressure control which set the standards for all the future ball-in-cone valves for hydrocephalus treatment was developed (Fig. 3). A legacy continued by his son—Carlos Hakim. Professor Salomón Hakim passed away from a haemorrhagic stroke in 2011. Due to his nature, his ability to stand up for his opinions, and his interest in the possibility of reversing conditions that were previously unthinkable, Hakim was able to benefit thousands of patients within a context that still ranks dementia as incurable [2].

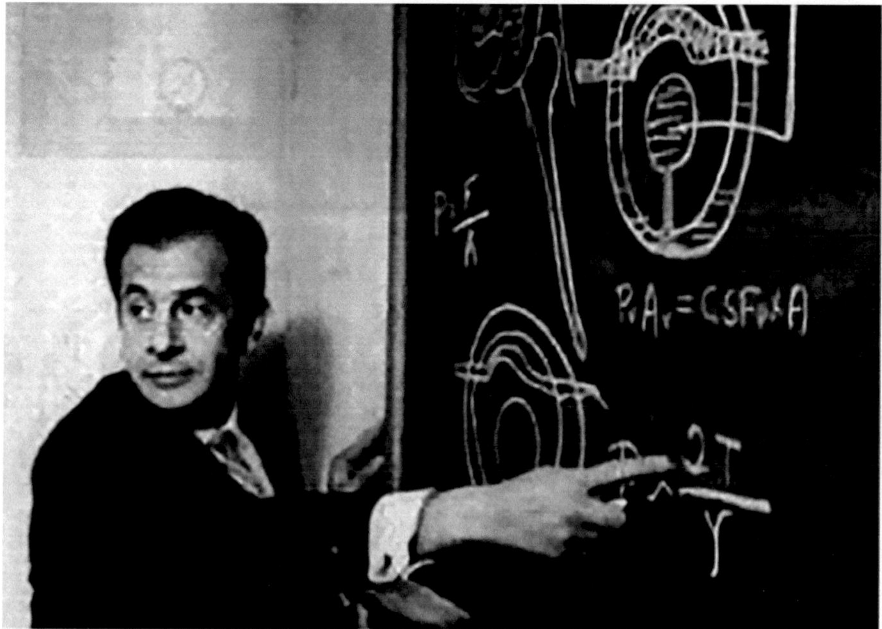

Fig. 2 Dr. Salomón Hakim describes the physical properties of normal pressure hydrocephalus in a photograph that appeared in Life en Español in 1968. The figure is distributed under the terms of the Creative Commons licensed under CC-BY-4.0 Attribution Licence, which permits unrestricted use, distribution, and reproduction in any medium, provided the original work is properly credited

4 Fundamental Discoveries in the Last Decades

4.1 *Pathophysiology*

Understanding NPH pathophysiology has been historically closely linked to known concepts of human physiology and available technical equipment. Although the first case of communicating hydrocephalus with normal ICP values was reported by Foltz and Ward in 1956 [1], the cornerstones of NPH pathophysiology, clinical manifestation, diagnosis, and treatment were explicitly introduced by Hakim and his colleagues in 1965 [3, 4]. Scholars such as Hoff and Barber in 1974 [20] or Raimondi in 1994 [21] further expanded Hakim's research and clarified the abnormal circulation of cerebrospinal fluid (CSF) in the context of hydrocephalus. The original theory assumed that NPH pathogenesis results from impaired CSF circulation, while ventricular dilatation is caused by increased intraventricular pressure exceeding the elastic tension of the surrounding brain parenchyma. The subsequent ventriculomegaly is considered to be a mechanism responsible for decreasing the pressure to normal values. Although the pressure is not abnormally raised, the forces acting on the ventricular walls are growing while simultaneously increasing ventricular

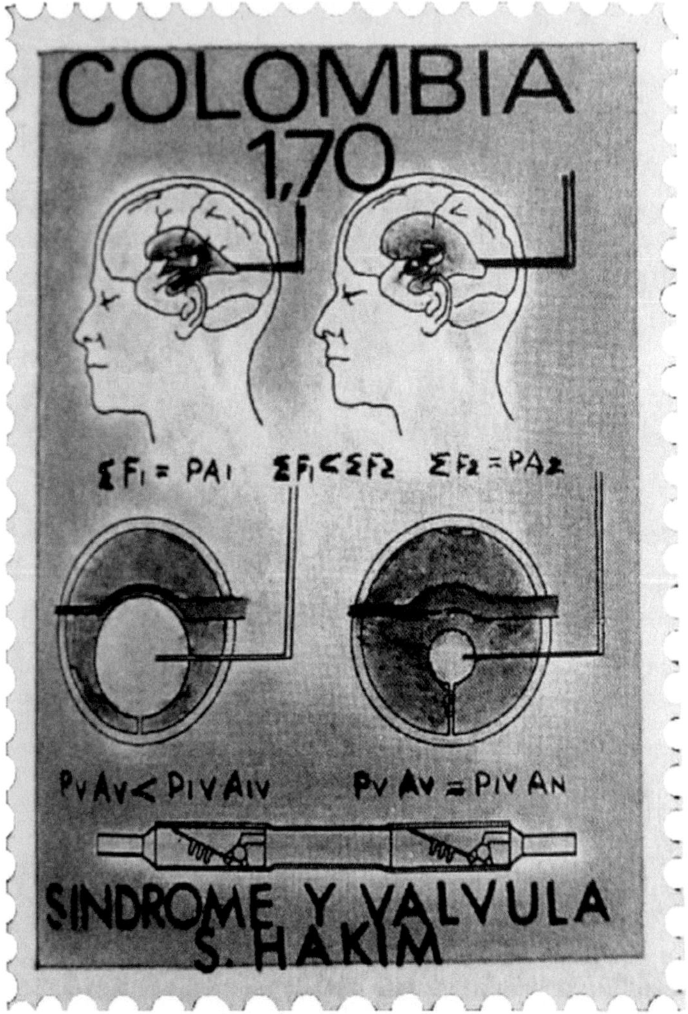

Fig. 3 Colombian stamp dedicated to Hakim's discovery of NPH and the invention of his own unidirectional pressure valve in 1966. https://commons.wikimedia.org/wiki/File:S%C3%ADndrome_y_V%C3%A1lvula_-_Salom%C3%B3n_Hakim_-_Estampilla_conmemorativa_Colombia.jpg. In the public domain

surface area, leading to their further expansion. Due to the advances in investigation methods for CSF circulation and factors contributing to disease development, the research on NPH notably accelerated at the beginning of the 21st century. The initial theory has been clarified, and further investigations defined additional factors involved in disease pathogenesis. It started to be certain that abnormal CSF hydrodynamics are not a single mechanism involved in the pathophysiology that influences the typical disease manifestation. For example, ventricular dilatation was shown to characteristically contribute to an increased volume of interstitial fluid in periventricular space, subsequently resulting in reduced brain compliance and potential ischaemic processes [22]. Hemodynamic factors, such as the reduced arterial pulsatility, elevated venous pressure, or changes in arterial elasticity, have been verified to contribute to NPH pathogenesis [23–25]. Not only the compression, resulting from the ventricular enlargement, causes changes in intraaxonal metabolism, but also alterations of haemodynamics contribute to the progression of neurological deficits—in NPH, characteristically urinary incontinence and gait disturbances [26, 27]. Recently, a new concept of the so-called glymphatic system has been investigated in NPH. Its impairment is believed to be associated with the osmotic disbalances, disrupted CSF drainage and CSF accumulation in subarachnoid spaces and intracerebral ventricles [28, 29]. Additionally, metabolic changes and neuroinflammatory factors have been recently studied in the context of hydrocephalus and neurodegenerative disorders. It was stated that these neuropathological changes are present in NPH patients and therefore may be useful markers of the disease prospectively [30–32].

Although NPH typically occurs in sporadic form, familiar forms of the disease have been encountered in associations with several genetic mutations. The first-ever cases of inheritable genetic predispositions for NPH are dated to the 1980s of the last century. Portenoy et al. [33] reported two elderly siblings, both having NPH and manifesting with the complete Hakim's triad. Until 2016, genetic aspects were not studied in more detail, although a few studies have reported familiar forms of NPH that linked among family members [34, 35]. So far, a few genetic mutations have been identified in association with the disease onset [36–38]. Further advances in our understanding of NPH genetics have been disclosed in recent years and their convenient results will be the issue of future investigations.

4.2 Diagnosis

Since there is still a lack of disease-specific diagnostic measures able to differentiate NPH from neurodegenerative comorbidities, it is challenging to clearly define the individual diagnosis. The first methods of non-invasive NPH evaluation were initially set upon pneumoencephalogram and later upon CT. The role of several radiologic markers has been studied in the past decades and some have been implemented to standard clinical practice. In 1942, Evans [39] introduced an imaging parameter concept that has borne his name since then. The so-called Evans' index is used to evaluate the extent of ventriculomegaly, and its value above 0.3 is considered as a marker of ventricular dilation, present not only in NPH but also in other types of hydrocephalus. The index itself is the ratio of the maximal internal diameter of the skull to the width of the frontal horns of the lateral ventricles at the same level, using the projections of axial CT and MRI scans. Benson et al. [40] introduced the concept of the callosal angle as a potential imaging marker of NPH on pneumoencephalogram in 1970. Three years later, Sjaastad and Nordvik [41] deepened this knowledge by studying the role of callosal angle in patients with ventriculomegaly. This marker is measured in the posterior commissure plane, perpendicular to the anterior commissure–posterior commissure plane on coronal projections. The callosal angle is characteristically narrower in NPH patients when compared to healthy individuals, due to the ventricular dilatation and widening of the Sylvian fissures. International guidelines by Relkin et al. [42] defined a value of 40° or greater as appropriate for NPH. Further MRI studies [43] stated that a callosal angle of less than 90° can distinguish NPH, Alzheimer's disease, and healthy controls. Since then, this marker is typically used with Evans' index in the diagnosis of NPH [43]. The first description of disproportionately enlarged subarachnoid space hydrocephalus (DESH) was introduced by Kitagaki et al. in 1998 [44]. It is composed of acute callosal angle, dilatation of Sylvian fissures, ventriculomegaly, high tight convexity, and focal sulci dilatation [45]. Recent Japanese guidelines [46] recommend using Evans' ratio for the evaluation of the ventricular size, callosal angle of less than 90°, and additional evaluation of DESH on MRI in accordance with gait impairment in order to predict shunt responsiveness and diagnose iNPH. These basic parameters can be easily measured on both CT and MRI. More detailed metabolic alterations in periventricular areas need detailed investigation on MRI machines [47, 48]. This topic is introduced more in detail in a specific chapter of this book.

Besides imaging studies, several invasive tests are currently used to predict shunt responsiveness in NPH patients. The CSF tap test simulates the physiological response to the shunt system. Hakim and Adams [4] described the first three patients who underwent this procedure. Following the performance of a lumbar puncture and removal of 15 ml of CSF, the clinical status of all three patients improved. The rationale of the CSF tap test has not dramatically changed since Hakim and Adams' descriptions, except that nowadays the recommendation is to remove between 30 and 50 ml of CSF and thereafter evaluate the clinical symptoms of individual patients. The lumbar infusion test (LIT) was described in a study by Katzman and Hussey in 1970 [49]. LIT is performed with the patient in a horizontal position, while ICP is measured during the infusion of CSF replacement, typically with Ringer's solution. One or two needles are inserted between L3–L4 or L4–L5 in the subarachnoid space of the lumbar region. The needle or needles are used as an infusion pump and are connected to pressure recording. The aim of the LIT is to evaluate changes in pressure curves and values during the test and thus to determine parameters of CSF behaviour. In a study by Katzman et al. [49], it turned out that a plateau pressure of more than 22 mmHg during the infusion may serve as a determinant of whether these patients should or should not undergo shunt implantation. Several years later, in 1977, Ekstedt et al. [50] used the constant pressure infusion test to measure the CSF outflow. Børgesen in 1979 [51] studied the value of the conductance to CSF outflow and proposed that it may be a useful determinant of positive shunt responsiveness. Interestingly, Boon et al. [52] analogously measured the resistance to CSF outflow, also known as Rout. They found out that patients with Rout values above 18 mmHg presented with improvement rates above 90% after shunting. Nowadays, a Rout value above 12 mmHg/ml/min is accepted as a positive test result [53]. A study from 2005 [54] defined CSF pressure pulsatility, i.e., a measure of mean CSF pressure amplitudes during the lumbar infusion, and suggested this as a more reliable predictor of shunt response than Rout itself.

Of all functional tests in NPH diagnosis, the most significant role is that of external lumbar drainage (ELD [55]. During ELD, which typically lasts up to five days, the clinical symptoms of each patient are evaluated, aiming to better predict shunt response. The first report of ELD insertion dates from 1744, performed by Claude-Nicholas Le Cat. Unfortunately, it was difficult to improve ELD functioning without technical improvement which were introduced at the turn of the 20th century. One of the biggest milestones in ELD history is a detailed analysis of ICP monitoring using ELD in patients with brain tumours in 1960, performed by Nils Lundberg [56]. Since then, ELD has been clinically used for a range of purposes; current practice tries to minimise the risk of infection and mechanical complications.

Another invasive test used for NPH, introduced in the 1960s for the first time, is intracranial pressure (ICP) monitoring. This plays an important role in managing a range of diseases and traumatic injuries of the central nervous system. The diagnostic role of ICP monitoring (through lumbar, intraventricular, epidural, or parenchymal devices) was studied intensively during the 1990s, but up-to-date findings of this invasive test remain controversial [57–59]. Values of ICP are not raised in NPH patients, but recent research from 2010 [60] found a correlation between ICP amplitude and shunt response.

In recent years, the need to distinguish NPH from other neurodegenerative comorbidities has been the reason for investigating CSF composition and studying different abnormalities in each disease. A range of CSF biomarkers have been reported as specific to NPH, but consensus on their clinical application has still not been reached, due to the higher number of statistically non-significant results and a number of neurodegeneration-related comorbidities that present with a similar CSF profile.

4.3 Shunt Systems

The beginnings of treatment interventions date back to the end of the nineteenth century. In 1891, Quincke demonstrated the clinical benefit of repeated lumbar punctures [61]. Over the following years, various methods of continuous external drainage have been gradually introduced into the treatment—ventricular, subdural, subarachnoid, or subgaleal. Hydrocephalus has also been studied and treated by Harvey Williams Cushing, the "father" of neurosurgery [62]. He was the first to perform lumboperitoneal drainage using a silver cannula. A truly revolutionary contribution to this issue was made by Cushing's former pupil and later opponent Walter Edward Dandy, who introduced resection of the choroidal plexus as a method to reduce cerebrospinal fluid production [63]. He was also the first to perform the third ventriculostomy [64].

Presumably the first precursor of the modern shunt system was developed by Arne Torkildsen in 1939 for non-communicating hydrocephalus [65]. Working with this, simplified catheter was associated with a higher risk of mechanical complications, predominantly catheter obstruction, and therefore the benefit of the treatment was very low. Eventually, the real breakthrough in treatment was the introduction of the ventriculojugular shunt by Frank Nulsen and Eugen Spitz in 1949 [66]. They were greatly assisted by the technician John W. Holter, whose son was born with severe spina bifida associated with hydrocephalus. Holter's son was treated by Nulsen and Spitz in Children's Hospital in Philadelphia. Unfortunately, Holter's son did not survive the disease, but the collaboration of the technician with neurosurgeons eventually led to the serial production of the first biocompatible valve in 1956 [67]. A one-way flow-regulating valve with 12-Fr soft rubber catheter was initially used. Polyether was used in ventricular catheters, but this material has been proposed to be unsuitable for these purposes, mainly due to the high rate of complications related to the device itself. Therefore, polydimethylsiloxane subsequently started to serve as an elastic biomaterial for shunt systems [68]. Robert Rudenz implanted silicone ventriculoatrial shunts in 1957 [69], and a year after, Richard Ames used the same material in ventriculoperitoneal shunt tubing for the first time. Ames continued to use the same material for an additional 9 years and finally reported 120 ventriculoperitoneal shunt implantations with promising results in hydrocephalus treatment [70]. Later, Hakim introduced a so-called J-shaped catheter consisting of a curved tip with a few holes inside. Unfortunately, the functionality of this shunt type was unsatisfactory. There were several other studies that contributed to the improvement of shunt systems, using materials such as polyhydroxyethylmethacrylate, polytetrafluoroethylene, or polyvinylpyrrolidone for shunt catheters. Nowadays, the vast majority of shunt systems are made of silicone polymer tubing and a range of valve devices are available in ongoing clinical practice. A summary of fundamental historical discoveries is given in Fig. 4.

5 Conclusion

Although there were historically a few reports describing patients suffering from hydrocephalus without abnormal pressure values, Salomón Hakim was the first to identify the syndrome and to give detailed descriptions of its pathogenesis, clinical manifestation, and treatment options. The discovery of NPH itself was a breakthrough in the understanding of neurodegeneration, which had long been considered irreversible. Hakim's work, supported by his former colleagues, initiated an international focus on the disease, and since then thousands of publications dedicated to the topic have become available globally. As we know now, the pathophysiology of NPH is a complex system of interacting pathways in which many factors contribute to the progression of the disease. We are becoming more familiar with the likely determinants of NPH pathogenesis thanks to a significant body of research about the pathophysiology of NPH, to new concepts extending our understanding of CSF physiology, and to inventions at the molecular level (inflammatory pathways, metabolic and osmotic disbalances, glymphatic pathway, etc.). Nonetheless, any single underlying causality remains unclear. Along with the invention of modern imaging techniques

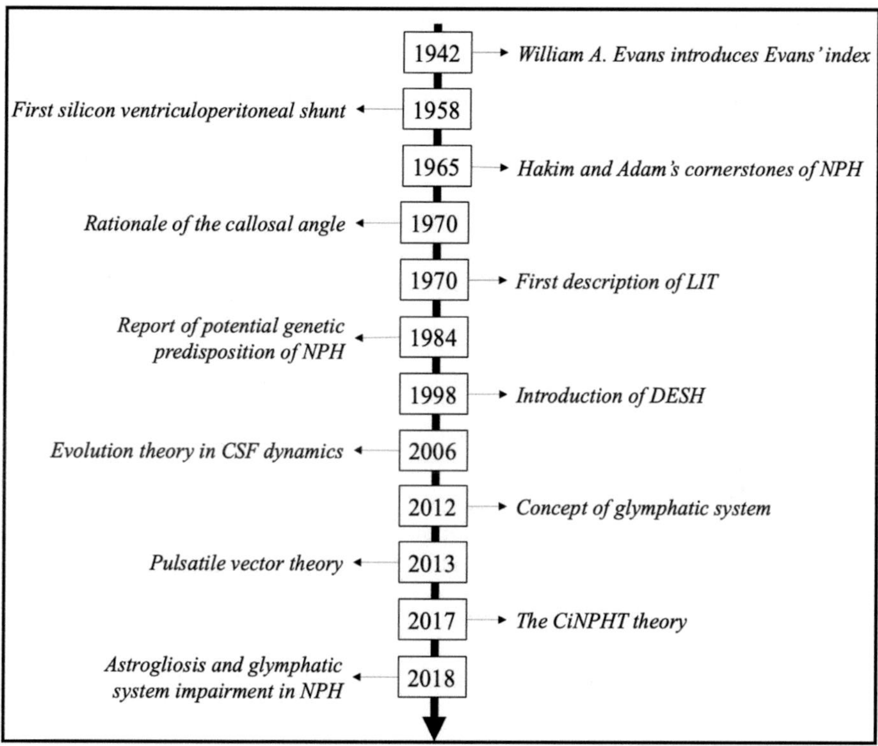

Fig. 4 Summary of historical discoveries related to NPH

(CT, later MRI), it has been possible to describe a range of radiological parameters that can be used to differentiate NPH patients, non-NPH patients, and patients with other neurodegenerative comorbidities. This allows more efficiently tailored therapy management. Technical improvements over the years, mainly involving new shunt systems with advanced pressure valves, have minimised surgery-related complications and simultaneously improved prognosis for NPH patients. The significant occurrence of comorbidities makes diagnosis a challenge, and it is hard to predict NPH patients' response to shunt surgery. Still, the improvement in our knowledge of the disease is enormous when compared to what was known in the second half of the twentieth century. Current unknowns are an incentive for improved studies of this disease prospectively.

6   Key Points

- Dr. Salomón Hakim has a major stake in the discovery of normal pressure hydrocephalus with a first observed case in 1957.
- Normal pressure hydrocephalus was originally referred to as symptomatic occult hydrocephalus.
- The original explanation of NPH was related to Pascal's law. Even though intracranial pressure may be normal in enlarged ventricles, the increased surface of the dilated ventricles leads to an abnormally large force—the hydraulic press effect.
- Hydrocephalus was first described by Hippocrates in the fifth century BC, although the concept of hydrocephalus was more of a collection of fluid surrounding the brain than an accumulation of CSF within the cerebral ventricular system.
- Although the first insertion of ELD was described at the end of the eighteenth century, it was challenging to improve ELD function without technical improvement which came at the turn of the twentieth century.
- The development of presumably the first "modern shunt system" precursor was introduced by Arne Torkildsen in 1939 and it served for the treatment of noncommunicating hydrocephalus.

Funding   This chapter was supported by the Ministry of Health of the Czech Republic institutional grant no. NU23-04-00551.

References

1. Foltz EL, Ward AA. Communicating hydrocephalus from subarachnoid bleeding. J Neurosurg. 1956;13:546–66. https://doi.org/10.3171/jns.1956.13.6.0546.
2. Wallenstein, MB, McKhann GM. II. Salomón Hakim and the discovery of normal-pressure hydrocephalus. Neurosurgery. 2010;67:155–59. https://doi.org/10.1227/01.NEU.0000370058.12120.0E.
3. Adams RD, et al. Symptomatic occult hydrocephalus with normal cerebrospinal-fluid pressure. New Eng J Med. 1965;273:117–26. https://doi.org/10.1056/NEJM196507152730301.
4. Hakim S., Adams R.D. The special clinical problem of symptomatic hydrocephalus with normal cerebrospinal fluid pressure. Observations on cerebrospinal fluid hydrodynamics. J Neurol Sci. 1965;2:307–27. https://doi.org/10.1016/0022-510x(65)90016-x.
5. Lifshutz J.I., Johnson WD. History of hydrocephalus and its treatments. Neurosurg Focus FOC. 2001;11(2):1–5. https://doi.org/10.3171/foc.2001.11.2.2.
6. Grunert P, Charalampaki P, Ayyad A. Concept and treatment of hydrocephalus in the Greco-Roman and early Arabic medicine. Minim Invasive Neurosurg. 2007;50(5):253–64. https://doi.org/10.1055/s-2007-991178.
7. Torack RM. Historical aspects of normal and abnormal brain fluids. I Cerebrospinal fluid Arch Neurol. 1982;39(4):197–201. https://doi.org/10.1001/archneur.1982.00510160003001.
8. Spon J, Wheler G. Voyage d'Italie, de Dalmatie, de Grece, et du Levant: fait aux années 1675 & 1676. Chez Rutgert Alberts; 1724

9. Pozeg ZI, Flamm ES. Vesalius and the 1543 Epitome of his De humani corporis fabrica librorum: a uniquely illuminated copy. Pap Bibliogr Soc Am. 2009;103(2):199–220. https://doi.org/10.1086/pbsa.103.2.24293987.

10. Brunori A, Vagnozzi R, Giuffrè R. Antonio Pacchioni (1665–1726): early studies of the dura mater. J Neurosurg. 1993;78(3):515–8. https://doi.org/10.3171/jns.1993.78.3.0515.

11. Torack RM. Historical aspects of normal and abnormal brain fluids. I Cerebrospinal fluid Arch Neurol. 1982;39(4):197–201. https://doi.org/10.1001/archneur.1982.00510160003001.

12. Breathnach CS. Robert Whytt (1714–1766): from dropsy in the brain to tuberculous meningitis. Ir J Med Sci. 2014;183(3):493–9. https://doi.org/10.1007/s11845-014-1106-3.

13. Weed L. Studies on cerebrospinal fluid; 1922.

14. Rusell DS. Observations on the pathology of hydrocephalus; 1949.

15. Riddoch G. Progressive dementia without headache or changes in the optic discs, due to tumours of the third ventricle. Brain. 1936;59:225–33. https://doi.org/10.1093/brain/59.2.225.

16. McHugh PR. Occult hydrocephalus. QJM: Int J Med. 1964;33:297–308. https://doi.org/10.1093/oxfordjournals.qjmed.a067021.

17. Yakovlev PI. Paraplegias of hydrocephalics; a clinical note and interpretation. Am J Ment Defic. 1947;51:561–76.

18. Hakim S. Some observation on CSF pressure. Hydrocephalic syndrome in adult with. Javeriana University School of Medicine; 1964.

19. Hoff J, Barber R. Transcerebral mantle pressure in normal pressure hydrocephalus. Arch Neurol. 1974;31:101–05. https://doi.org/10.1001/archneur.1974.00490380049005.

20. Raimondi AJ. A unifying theory for the definition and classification of hydrocephalus. Childs Nerv Syst. 1994;10:2–12. https://doi.org/10.1007/BF00313578.

21. Ammar A, et al. Idiopathic normal-pressure hydrocephalus syndrome: Is it understood? The comprehensive idiopathic normal-pressure hydrocephalus theory (CiNPHT). In: Hydrocephalus: What do we know? And what do we still not know?; 2017, p. 67–82. https://doi.org/10.1007/978-3-319-61304-8_5.

22. Chrysikopoulos H. Idiopathic normal pressure hydrocephalus: thoughts on etiology and pathophysiology. Med Hypotheses. 2009;73:718–24. https://doi.org/10.1016/j.mehy.2009.04.044.

23. Israelsson H, et al. Vascular risk factors in INPH: a prospective case-control study (the INPH-CRasH study). Neurology. 2017;88:577–85. https://doi.org/10.1212/WNL.0000000000003583.

24. Hamilton RB, et al. Opposing CSF hydrodynamic trends found in the cerebral aqueduct and prepontine cistern following shunt treatment in patients with normal pressure hydrocephalus. Fluids Barriers CNS. 2019;16:2. https://doi.org/10.1186/s12987-019-0122-0.

25. Castañeyra-Ruiz L, et al. Cerebrospinal fluid levels of tumor necrosis factor alpha and aquaporin 1 in patients with mild cognitive impairment and idiopathic normal pressure hydrocephalus. Clin Neurol Neurosurg. 2016;146:76–81. https://doi.org/10.1016/j.clineuro.2016.04.025.

26. Thompson PD. Frontal lobe ataxia. Handb Clin Neurol. 2012;103:619–22. Elsevier.

27. Ringstad G, et al. Brain-wide glymphatic enhancement and clearance in humans assessed with MRI. JCI Insight. 2018;3. https://doi.org/10.1172/jci.insight.121537.

28. Bae YJ, et al. Altered glymphatic system in idiopathic normal pressure hydrocephalus. Parkinsonism Relat Disord. 2021;82:56–60. https://doi.org/10.1016/j.parkreldis.2020.11.009.

29. Sosvorova L, et al. The Impact of selected cytokines in the follow-up of normal pressure hydrocephalus. Physiol Res. 2015;64:S283–90.

30. Sosvorova L, et al. Steroid hormones and homocysteine in the outcome of patients with normal pressure hydrocephalus. Physiol Res. 2015;64:S227–36.

31. Sosvorova L, et al. Steroid hormones in prediction of normal pressure hydrocephalus. J Steroid Biochem Mol Biol. 2015;152:124–32. https://doi.org/10.1016/j.jsbmb.2015.05.004.

32. Bräutigam K, et al. Pathogenesis of idiopathic normal pressure hydrocephalus: a review of knowledge. J Clin Neurosci. 2019;61:10–13. https://doi.org/10.1016/j.jocn.2018.10.147.

33. R. K. Portenoy, et al. Familial Occurrence of Idiopathic Normal-Pressure Hydrocephalus. Archives of Neurology 1984, 41:335–37 https://doi.org/10.1001/archneur.1984.04050150117029.

34. Cusimano MD, et al. Normal-pressure hydrocephalus: Is there a genetic predisposition? Can J Neurol Sci. 2011;38:274–81. https://doi.org/10.1017/S031716710001146X.

35. Takahashi Y, et al. Familial normal pressure hydrocephalus (NPH) with an autosomal-dominant inheritance: a novel subgroup of NPH. J Neurol Sci. 2011;308:149–51. https://doi.org/10.1016/j.jns.2011.06.018.

36. Yang HW, et al. Deletions in CWH43 cause idiopathic normal pressure hydrocephalus. EMBO Mol Med. 2021;13. https://doi.org/10.15252/emmm.202013249.

37. Sato H, et al. A segmental copy number loss of the SFMBT1 gene is a genetic risk for shunt-responsive, Idiopathic Normal Pressure Hydrocephalus (iNPH): a case-control study. PLoS One. 2016;11:e0166615. https://doi.org/10.1371/journal.pone.0166615.

38. Coutton C, et al. Mutations in CFAP43 and CFAP44 cause male infertility and flagellum defects in Trypanosoma and human. Nature Commun. 2018;9:686 https://doi.org/10.1038/s41467-017-02792-7.

39. Evans WA. An encephalographic ratio for estimating ventricular enlargment and cerebral atrophy. AMA Arch Neurol Psychiatry. 1942;47:931. https://doi.org/10.1001/archneurpsyc.1942.02290060069004.

40. Benson DF, et al. Diagnosis of normal-pressure hydrocephalus. New Eng J Med. 1970;283:609–15. https://doi.org/10.1056/NEJM197009172831201.

41. Sjaastad O., Nordvik A. The corpus callosal angle in the diagnosis of cerebral ventricular enlargement. Acta Neurol Scand. 2009;49:396–406. https://doi.org/10.1111/j.1600-0404.1973.tb01312.x.

42. Relkin N, et al. Diagnosing idiopathic normal-pressure hydrocephalus. Neurosurgery. 2005;57:S2-4–S2-16. https://doi.org/10.1227/01.NEU.0000168185.29659.C5.

43. Ishii K, et al. Automatic volumetry of the cerebrospinal fluid space in idiopathic normal pressure hydrocephalus. Dement Geriatr Cogn Dis Extra. 2013;3:489–96. https://doi.org/10.1159/000357329.

44. Kitagaki H, et al. CSF spaces in idiopathic normal pressure hydrocephalus: morphology and volumetry. Am J Neuroradiol. 1998;19:1277–84.

45. Shinoda N, et al. Utility of MRI-based disproportionately enlarged subarachnoid space hydrocephalus scoring for predicting prognosis after surgery for idiopathic normal pressure hydrocephalus: clinical research. J Neurosurg. 2017;127:1436–42. https://doi.org/10.3171/2016.9.JNS161080.

46. Nakajima, et al. Guidelines for management of idiopathic normal pressure hydrocephalus (third edition): endorsed by the Japanese society of normal pressure hydrocephalus. Neurol Med Chir. 2021;61:63–97. https://doi.org/10.2176/nmc.st.2020-0292.

47. Tang Y-M, et al. White matter microstructural damage associated with gait abnormalities in idiopathic normal pressure hydrocephalus. Front Aging Neurosci. 2021;13:660621. https://doi.org/10.3389/fnagi.2021.660621.

48. Kristensen B, et al. Regional cerebral blood flow, white matter abnormalities, and cerebrospinal fluid hydrodynamics in patients with idiopathic adult hydrocephalus syndrome. J Neurol Neurosurg Psychiatr. 1996;60:282–88. https://doi.org/10.1136/jnnp.60.3.282.

49. Katzman R, Hussey F. A simple constant-infusion manometric test for measurement of CSF absorption. I. Rationale and method. Neurology. 1970;20:534–44. https://doi.org/10.1212/wnl.20.6.534.

50. Ekstedt J. CSF hydrodynamic studies in man. 1. Method of constant pressure CSF infusion. J Neurol Neurosurg Psychiatr. 1977;40:105–19. https://doi.org/10.1136/jnnp.40.2.105.

51. Børgesen SE, et al. Cerebrospinal fluid conductance and compliance of the craniospinal space in normal-pressure hydrocephalus. J Neurosurg. 1979:521–25. https://doi.org/10.3171/jns.1979.51.4.0521.

52. Boon AJW, et al. Dutch normal-pressure hydrocephalus study: randomized comparison of low- and medium-pressure shunts. J Neurosurg. 1998:490–95. https://doi.org/10.3171/jns.1998.88.3.0490.

53. Kim DJ, et al. Thresholds of resistance to CSF outflow in predicting shunt responsiveness. Neurol Res. 2015;37:332–40. https://doi.org/10.1179/1743132814Y.0000000454.

54. Eide PK, Sorteberg W. Preoperative spinal hydrodynamics versus clinical change 1 year after shunt treatment in idiopathic normal pressure hydrocephalus patients. Br J Neurosurg. 2005;19:475–83. https://doi.org/10.1080/02688690500495125.

55. Walchenbach R, et al. The value of temporary external lumbar CSF drainage in predicting the outcome of shunting on normal pressure hydrocephalus. J Neurol Neurosurg Psychiatr. 2002;72:503–06. https://doi.org/10.1136/jnnp.72.4.503.

56. Srinivasan VM, et al. The history of external ventricular drainage: historical vignette. J Neurosurg. 2014;120:228–36. https://doi.org/10.3171/2013.6.JNS121577.

57. Sahuquillo J, et al. Reappraisal of the intracranial pressure and cerebrospinal fluid dynamics in patients with the so-called "normal pressure hydrocephalus" syndrome. Acta Neurochir. 1991;112:50–61. https://doi.org/10.1007/BF01402454.

58. Raftopoulos C, et al. Cognitive recovery in idiopathic normal pressure hydrocephalus: a prospective study. Neurosurgery. 1994;35:397–404; discussion 404–405. https://doi.org/10.1227/00006123-199409000-00006.

59. Saldarriaga-Cantillo A, et al. Normal pressure hydrocephalus: diagnostic delay. Biomedica. 2020;40:656–63. https://doi.org/10.7705/biomedica.5382.

60. Eide PK, Stanisic M. Cerebral microdialysis and intracranial pressure monitoring in patients with idiopathic normal-pressure hydrocephalus: association with clinical response to extended lumbar drainage and shunt surgery. J Neurosurg. 2010;112:414–24. https://doi.org/10.3171/2009.5.JNS09122.

61. Quincke H. Berliner klinische Wochenschrift: Die Lumbalpunction des Hydrocephalus. August Hirschwald; 1891.

62. Chesler DA, Pendleton C, Ahn ES, Quinones-Hinojosa A. Harvey Cushing's early management of hydrocephalus: an historical picture of the conundrum of hydrocephalus until modern shunts after WWII. Clin Neurol Neurosurg. 2013;115(6):699–701. https://doi.org/10.1016/j.clineuro.2012.08.018.

63. Dandy WE. Extirpation of the choroid plexus of the lateral ventricles in communicating hydrocephalus. Ann Surg. 1918;68(6):569–79. https://doi.org/10.1097/00000658-191812000-00001.

64. Dandy WE. An operative procedure for hydrocephalus. Bull Johns Hopkins Hosp. 1922;33:189–90.

65. Torkildsen A. A new palliative operation in cases of inoperable occlusion of the Sylvian aqueduct. Acta Psychiatr Scand. 1939;14:221–21. https://doi.org/10.1111/j.1600-0447.1939.tb06636.x.

66. Nulsen FE, Spitz EB. Treatment of hydrocephalus by direct shunt from ventricle to jugular vain. Surg Forum. 1951:399–403.

67. Boockvar JA, Loudon W, Sutton LN. Development of the Spitz—Holter valve in Philadelphia. J Neurosurg. 2001;95(1):145–7.

68. Colas A, Curtis J. Silicone biomaterials: history and chemistry. In: Ratner B, Hoffman A, Schoen E, editors. Biomaterials science: an introduction to materials in medicine. 2nd ed. Philadelphia: Elsevier; 2004. p. 80–5.

69. Pudenz RH, et al. Ventriculo-auriculostomy. A technique for shunting cerebrospinal fluid into the right auricle: preliminary report. J Neurosurg. 1957;14:171–79. https://doi.org/10.3171/jns.1957.14.2.0171.

70. Ames RH. Ventriculo-Peritoneal shunts in the management of hydrocephalus. J Neurosurg. 1967;27:525–29. https://doi.org/10.3171/jns.1967.27.6.0525.

Modern Hydrocephalus Classification Systems

Levi Coelho Maia Barros, Victor Lomachinsky, and Petr Libý

Abstract Hydrocephalus (HCP) encompasses a large spectrum of clinical entities, with multiple distinguishing features. Consequently, several classification systems were proposed based on multiple criteria. Even though none of them thoroughly comprehend the conditions associated with HCP, many have been proved useful in current clinical practice. A multi-categorical classification could mitigate these difficulties, as proposed by some researchers. However, increasing complexity may lead to low applicability on a daily basis. The challenge of creating a practical and comprehensive system of classification for HCP remains one of the greatest missions for current neurosurgery research.

Keywords Classification of hydrocephalus · Normal pressure hydrocephalus · Genetics · Age of onset · Cerebrospinal fluid · Intracranial pressure

Abbreviations

CSF	Cerebrospinal fluid
ETV	Endoscopic third ventriculostomy
HC	Hydrocephalus
ICP	Intracranial pressure
iNPH	Idiopathic normal pressure hydrocephalus

L. C. M. Barros · V. Lomachinsky · P. Libý (✉)
Department of Neurosurgery, 2nd Faculty of Medicine, Charles University and Motol University Hospital, Prague, Czech Republic
e-mail: petr.liby@fnmotol.cz

L. C. M. Barros
e-mail: levicmaiabarros@gmail.com

V. Lomachinsky
e-mail: victor.lomachinsky@icloud.com

© The Author(s), under exclusive license to Springer Nature Switzerland AG 2023
O. Bradac (ed.), *Normal Pressure Hydrocephalus*,
https://doi.org/10.1007/978-3-031-36522-5_3

1 Introduction

Stratifying HCP is a major challenge for neurosurgery research. This heterogeneous group is composed of multiple conditions with varying pathophysiology, clinical symptoms, severity, and prognosis. Several classification systems have been proposed: obstructive vs absorptive; acquired vs congenital; genetic or CNS malformation-associated vs isolated; intraventricular obstructive vs extraventricular; simple vs complicated [1]. Although none is sufficient on its own, all systems listed have been proved useful in clinical practice. The present chapter's main goal is to present the most relevant hydrocephalus classification strategies in the current literature.

2 Hydrocephalus Definition

The complex variety of conditions related to hydrocephalus makes it difficult to define it. There is no internationally recognized definition of hydrocephalus, and multiple attempts were made based on the classification system adopted. One of the most accepted is Rekate's definition: "Hydrocephalus is an active distension of the ventricular system of the brain resulting from inadequate passage of cerebrospinal fluid from its point of production within the cerebral ventricles to its point of absorption into the systemic circulation" [2].

3 Treatment Strategies Based on HCP Type

Predicting clinical and radiological response to medical therapies such as shunt therapy or neuroendoscopic third ventriculostomy is vital in clinical practice. Individualizing patients with hydrocephalus in accord with its response to the offered therapy avoids unnecessary treatments and helps determine the best therapeutic approach for the patient [3].

Such an approach to HCP characterization can, for instance, be found within Kulkarni et al. proposed score for predicting endoscopic third ventriculostomy (ETV) success in the pediatric population. Based on age, etiology, and presence of a previous shunt, patients were subsequently stratified in score groups. Higher scores were associated with lower risk of ETV failure when compared to shunt therapy, even in early postoperative phase [4].

Interesting interplay can be found with other classification systems. Beni-Adani et al. has, for example, demonstrated a significant correlation between the HCP absorptive component and risk of ETV failure [1].

4 Categories of HCP

There are many ways of categorizing hydrocephalus. Criteria usually comprise age of onset, symptomatology, and response to the available treatments. Pathophysiological features such as disturbances in cerebrospinal fluid (CSF) and intracranial pressure dynamics are also often considered for stratification (Table 1).

4.1 Classification Based on Age of Onset

According to age of onset, hydrocephalus may be of fetal, neonatal, child, infantile, adult, and elderly onset. It is further possible to divide hydrocephalus in the newborn as congenital or acquired. The difference resides in whether it develops prenatal or

Table 1 An overview of relevant classification schemes

Author	Year	Concept	Notes
Dandy and Blackfan	1914	Communicating versus non-communicating	Choroid plexus as a site of CSF production, communicating between the lateral ventricles and the lumbar subarachnoid space
Rusell	1949	Obstructive versus non-obstructive	Obstruction in any location within major CSF pathways; non-obstructive including CSF overproduction (choroid plexus papilloma) or CSF hypoabsorption (sinus thrombosis)
Ransohoff et al	1960	Intraventricular and extraventricular obstructive HCP	Obstruction within the CSF circulation
Raimondi	1994	Excessive intracranial liquid other than blood	A pathological increase in "brain fluid" volume, both intraparenchymal and extraparenchymal
Mori et al	1995	HCP seen early in life/in adults	Further classified into eight types
Johnston and Teo	2000	Review of CSF dynamics	Limited understanding of CSF circulation
Beni-Adani et al	2006	Focus on newborns and infants, diverse classification	Four categories of obstructive–absorptive HCP spectrum with relevance to the treatment options
Oi and Di Rocco	2006	CSF circulation in the minor pathway HCP and the evolution theory in CSF dynamics	Dandy's and Russell's concepts correspond to "major pathways HCP," minor pathways considered for the first time as the direct cause of HCP (glymphatic system)
Rekate	2009	One of the most accepted definitions of HCP	All obstructive, focus on the site of obstruction

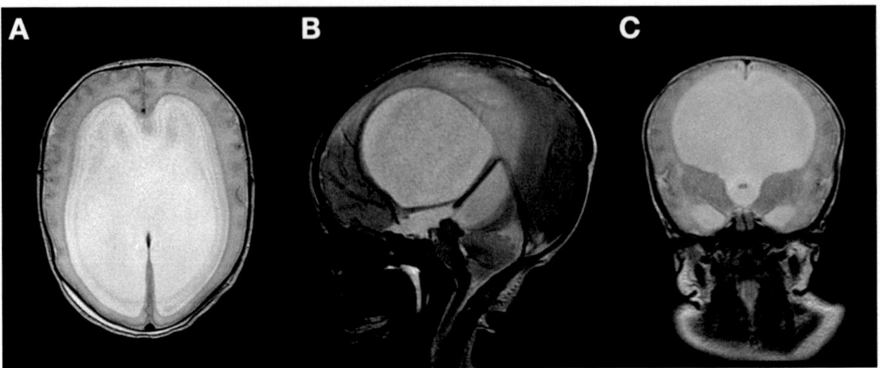

Fig. 1 Early postnatal T2W MRI demonstrating giant congenital triventricular HCP in three-day-old boy. (A, B, C) Axial, sagittal, and coronal T2W MRI depicted severe triventricular HCP. (B) Sagittal T2W MR image showed concave third floor and aqueductal stenosis

postnatal and carries a heavy impact on both management and prognosis [1]. Prenatal causes of hydrocephalus are, however, usually slowly progressive in nature, making an unambiguous differentiation between these categories not always feasible (Fig. 1) [1].

Based on the relationship between age of onset, neuronal developmental stages, and possible outcomes, Oi et al. [5] proposed in 1994 The Perspective Classification of Congenital Hydrocephalus (PCCH), stratifying hydrocephalus in the following clinico-embryological stages: stage I, hydrocephalus that develops between 8 and 21 weeks of gestation, during the neuronal cell proliferation process; stage II corresponding to development at 22 to 31 weeks of gestation, concurrently with the cell differentiation and migration period; stage III from 32 to 40 weeks of gestation, a period marked axonal maturation; stage V extending from 5 to 50 weeks of postnatal age, and is consistent with the myelination period of neuronal maturation.

The PCCH classification also includes linic-pathological types (primary, dysgenetic, and secondary hydrocephalus) and clinical categories (fetal, neonatal, and infantile) for better patient stratification. It is worth stressing that distinct linic-embryological stages have power of predicting neurological outcomes in patients within the same linic-pathological types. To this day, the correlation between PCCH stages and prognosis turns it into a very useful tool for assessing hydrocephalus patients [5].

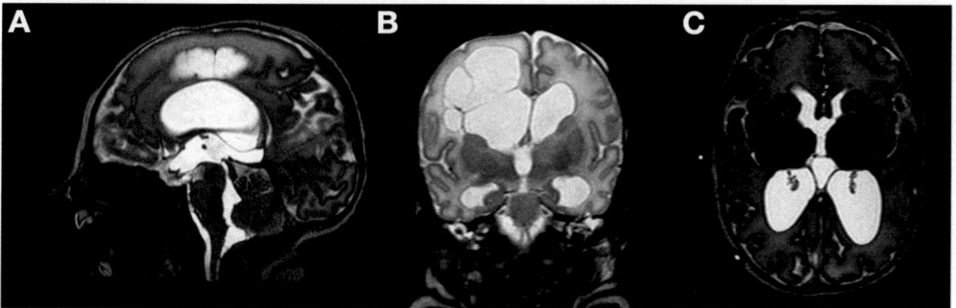

Fig. 2 Nearly two-month-old boy with posthemorrhagic hydrocephalus. (A) Sagittal T2W MRI showing posthemorrhagic pseudocyst formation above bowing corpus callosum, patent aqueduct, and signs of basilar arachnoiditis in basilar cisterns. (B) Coronal T2W MRI showing enlarged ventricular system with pseudocystic changes in right frontal lobe. (C) Axial T2W MRI showing dilated lateral ventricles

4.2 Classification Based on Underlying Cause

One of the simplest pathophysiological based classifications divides lesions in primary or secondary to an additional medical condition (e.g., dysgenetic, posthemorrhagic, postmeningitic, and posttraumatic) (Fig. 2). It is further possible to classify it as idiopathic if the cause is unknown [6].

4.3 Classification Based on Symptomatology and Chronology

The presence or lack of symptoms in hydrocephalus patients is also taken into account into many systems. Considering the head size, patients can be described as macrocephalic, microcephalic, or normocephalic. Distinct levels of consciousness correlate with distinct prognosis and the need for urgent therapy institution.

In addition, it is also often crucial to stratify HCP in both clinical course (progressive versus auto-limited) and chronology (acute versus chronic onset) [6].

Regarding course, while hydrocephalus progression is often devastating, the natural history is not always linear, and an invasive approach is not always warranted. For instance, in the case of arrested hydrocephalus, after an initial, progressive, phase, a new equilibrium is reached and spontaneous normalization of intracranial pressure follows. The patient is then left with macrocephaly and little to non-neurological deficits [7].

Chronology often dictates management. Acute settings are frequently more severe and, depending on pathophysiology, may require CSF diversion. Chronic conditions on the other hand sport more limited management options, and while they may be primary such as idiopathic normal pressure hydrocephalus, they are often second to another disease. A notable example is hydrocephalus ex-vacuo, a condition in which ventriculomegaly slowly develops due to reductions in encephalic volume [8].

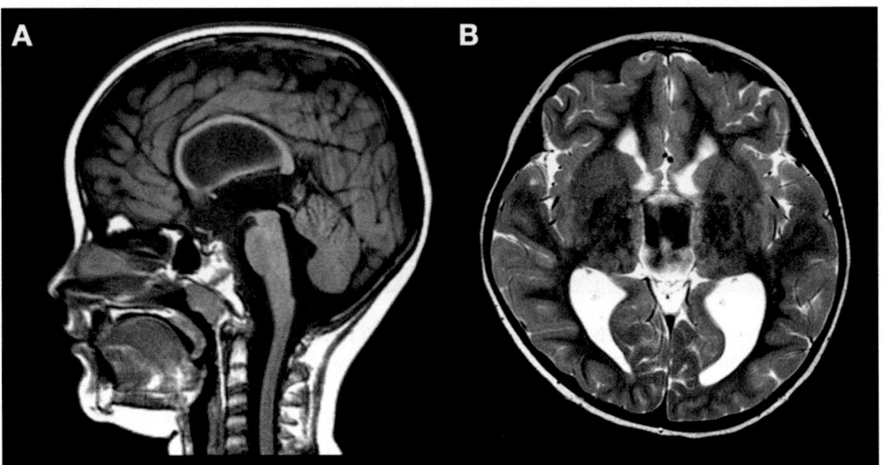

Fig. 3 Communicating HCP. Six-year-old girl with a picture of communicating HCP. (A) Sagittal T1W MRI showing corpus callosum bowing along with the bowing of lamina terminalis and floor of the third ventricle. Patent aqueduct is visible. (B) Dilated ventricles, especially third ventricle with CSF flow voids

4.4 Classification Based on CSF Dynamics

Considering CSF dynamics, two classifications are mostly used worldwide. They are Dandy's classification into communicating vs non-communicating and Russel's into obstructive vs non-obstructive [9, 10]. The first considers the CSF's ability to circulate from the lateral ventricle to the lumbar subarachnoid space and can be confirmed by dye injection. The second focuses on whether there is a presence of any sort of blockade in the major CSF pathway. These two classification systems are often used improperly as synonyms, which could contribute to negative outcomes whether the treatment chosen for hydrocephalus is based solely on them [6]. Dandy's classification, "communicating vs non-communicating" may still be the most practical due to direct impact on treatment strategy and thus indication to endoscopic solution or shunt (Figs. 3 and 4) [3].

4.5 Classification Based on Pressure Dynamics

As to pressure dynamics, it is possible to distinguish three main groups: normal, low-pressure and high-pressure hydrocephalus. Although intracranial pressure (ICP) is variable, and highly dependent on age, body posture, and comorbidities (Fig. 5), a clear pressure point cutoff is yet debatable [11].

An important example of HCP with inexpressive increases in intracranial pressures is idiopathic normal pressure hydrocephalus (iNPH). This was first described

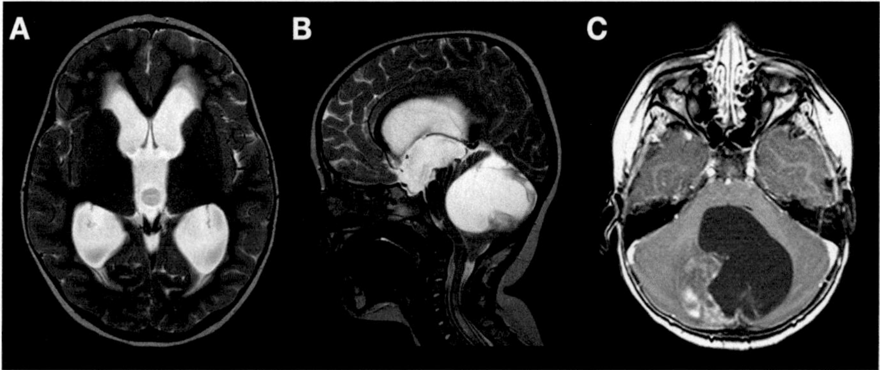

Fig. 4 Obstructive HCP due to posterior fossa tumor. Four-year-old girl with posterior fossa pilocytic astrocytoma (PA) and picture of obstructive triventricular HCP. (A) T2W MRI depicting ventricular system dilation with periventricular caps. (B) Coronal T2W MRI showing dilated third ventricle, bowing corpus callosum, and solid-cystic posterior fossa tumor with expansive behavior toward brain stem. (C) Enhanced axial T1W MRI depicting solid-cystic posterior fossa tumor, typical picture of PA

Fig. 5 Six-month-old boy with a picture of hydrocephalus on axial T2W MRI due to centrally located plexus papilloma. Lateral ventricles are asymmetric with transependymal edema predominantly in the right frontal lobe

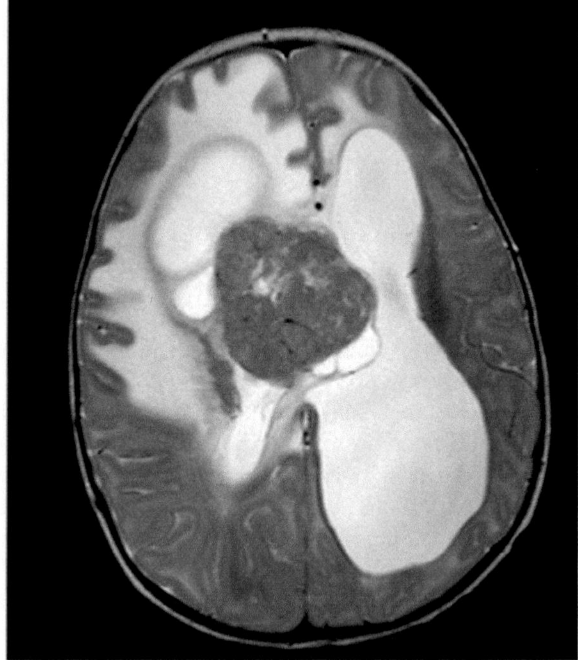

by Dr. Salomón Hakim in 1964 and is classically defined by a triad of a frontal gait ataxia, urinary incontinence, and subcortical dementia with short-term memory failure. It is a condition of an insidious nature, and its symptoms are thought to arise from progressive cortex compression over many years. Despite defining clinical and radiological traits of iNPH, the normal pressure HCP group also affords a large list of possible differential diagnosis and secondary causes are not always easy to dismiss. iNPH can mimic or occur concomitantly to a series of prevalent disorders in the elderly, such as arrested hydrocephalus, long-standing overt ventriculomegaly syndrome, and many more vascular, infectious, and neurodegenerative disorders. This severely diminishes both sensitivity and specificity of clinical diagnosis [12].

More infrequently, patients with symptoms of increased ICP could be classified as low-pressure or negative-pressure HCP [13]. This rare and heterogeneous condition is not yet fully understood. Some authors advocate that the differential pressure between the ventricular space and the subarachnoid space over cerebral convexity could lead to ventriculomegaly despite low or negative intracranial pressure (trans-mantle pressure theory) [14]. Patients usually have a poor prognosis and do not respond satisfactorily to routine shunt surgery [13]. Sub-atmospheric external ventricular drainage, endoscopic third ventriculostomy, and the use of a cervical tourniquet are reported to provide good outcomes in some case series [15, 16].

Forms of high-pressure hydrocephalus instead encompasses a far larger group that usually warrant more invasive measures such as ventriculoperitoneal shunting or endoscopic third ventriculostomy. This group can be further subdivided according to the mechanisms responsible for the pressure increase (such as obstruction or deficits in CSF absorption). More details are provided elsewhere in this chapter.

4.6 Classification Based on Genetics

Although genetic causes are often linked to poor prognosis, stratification based on genetics currently does not yield clinically relevant information on CSF circulation [1]. A notable exception represents X-linked HCP which usually demonstrates aqueduct stenosis. Remaining genetic aberrations with associated HCP should be analyzed on a case-by-case basis as points of mechanical obstruction, posterior fossa compression, venous drainage impairments, cardiovascular repercussions, and many other unique features carry, in each case, specific treatment directives.

Vein of Galen aneurysmal malformations (VGAMs), a rare group of malformations that account for approximately 30% of all pediatric vascular anomalies, are an interesting example of how a genetic-based condition has varying prognosis according to the mechanism responsible for the hydrodynamics disruption [17]. These units lead to HCP by both an underlying venous congestion and a mechanical, obstructive component. Management should be directed toward both mechanisms, and prognosis is intrinsically linked to the dominant element [18].

4.7 Current Multi-categorical Classification System

Numerous grouping systems were proposed in the last century. Unfortunately, they were usually limited to strict criteria, which led often to divergent and incomplete classification systems. The lack of standardized definition still poses a substantial challenge for neurosurgery communication worldwide, limiting the external validity of several hydrocephalus papers.

To mitigate these difficulties, Oi S published in 2010 a new comprehensive classification system: the multi-categorical hydrocephalus classification (Mc HC). The system classifies hydrocephalus within 10 categories (I: onset, II: cause, III: underlying lesion, IV: symptomatology, V: pathophysiology 1—CSF circulation, VI: pathophysiology 2—ICP dynamics, VII: chronology, VIII: post-shunt, IX: post-endoscopic ventriculostomy, and X: others) and 54 subcategories [6].

The advantages of a multi-categorical classification for such a complex condition as hydroccphalus include a thorough assessment of its many causes and their respective natural progression. In addition, it helps make hydrocephalus management more concise and individualized.

4.8 ASPECT Hydrocephalus System

An alternative way to visualize this multitude of conditions proposed recently by Birch Milan et al. is the ASPECT Hydrocephalus System [19]. The authors opted to abandon classification systems altogether, and rather invested in a parallel, non-hierarchical descriptive system. This model is aimed at expert and non-expert clinicians serving both as a checklist to ensure documentation of critical data and as a standardized coding to facilitate communication.

ASPECT stands for Anatomy, Symptoms, Previous interventions, Etiology, Complications, and Time. The driving principles behind the choice of these six traits are based on a goal to eliminate overlapping in diagnosis and classification, as currently noted within the ICD-10 and ICD-11 systems. The author's conception of hydrocephalus as a "pathological state in which abnormal CSF dynamics cause enlargement of one or more CSF compartments" is sufficiently broad not to be limited by the many controversies in pathophysiology but also sufficiently accurate to allow for the description of most clinically relevant scenarios (Fig. 6).

The anatomical focus of this model is an interesting way to systematize imaging analysis and provides a short, objective description that by itself has important patient management implications. As for the other components, the authors opted for a simple symptom analysis, focused on whether urgent treatment was warranted. Stepping from a view of HCP as a chronic condition, they further scanned the patient's history for previous interventions and related complications which tend to accumulate in the life of the affected individuals. Simplicity is also a defining trait of etiology description that took ICD-10 diagnostic list in consideration. Interestingly, only 10%

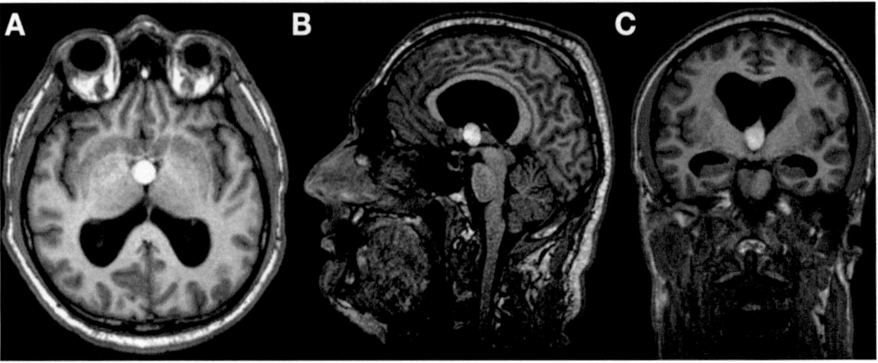

Fig. 6 Thirty-eight-year-old man with an obstructive hydrocephalus due to colloid cyst of third ventricle documented here on non-enhanced T1W MRI. Lateral ventricles are enlarged with normal-sized third and fourth ventricles

of the author's cohort had etiology labeled as unknown. Finally, the time component attempts to bridge the gap between age of onset and age at current evaluation also going from the premise of HCP as a condition that usually turns chronic.

The major limitations of the model revolve around the non-incorporation of advanced diagnostic tools (CSF analysis, biomarkers, genetic testing, etc.). It is a recent, promising model; however, further validation is still required to ensure clinical reliability.

5 Conclusion

In conclusion, classifying hydrocephalus remains challenging nowadays. Its complex nature does not allow a single criterion to comprehensively assess patients nor direct a therapeutic approach and predict neurological outcomes. A multi-categorical classification could mitigate these difficulties. However, it increases complexity, making it hard to replicate its use in daily practice. Stratifying these patients into distinct subgroups concerning management and prognosis could improve the quality of care among them. A promising new way to tackle the issue is the ASPECT system, unfortunately it still requires proper clinical validation. For now, a practical and thorough classification system is yet to be agreed upon.

6 Key Points

- Hydrocephalus (HCP) encompasses a broad spectrum of clinical entities, with multiple distinguishing features concerning pathophysiology, symptomatology, and age of onset.
- Several classification systems have been proposed according to age of onset, etiology, symptoms, chronology, CSF dynamics, and intracranial pressure dynamics.
- Although no classification system available is sufficient on its own, many have been proved useful in clinical practice.
- A multi-categorical classification could mitigate these difficulties. However, it increases complexity, making it hard to replicate its use in daily practice.

References

1. Beni-Adani L, Biani N, Ben-Sirah L, Constantini S. The occurrence of obstructive vs absorptive hydrocephalus in newborns and infants: relevance to treatment choices. Childs Nerv Syst. 2006;22(12):1543–63. https://doi.org/10.1007/s00381-006-0193-5.
2. Rekate H. A contemporary definition and classification of hydrocephalus. Semin Pediatr Neurol. 2009;16(1):9–15. https://doi.org/10.1016/j.spen.2009.01.002.
3. Alvi M, Brown D, Yolcu Y, Zreik J, Bydon M, Cutsforth-Gregory J, et al. Predictors of adverse outcomes and cost after surgical management for idiopathic normal pressure hydrocephalus: Analyses from a national database. Clini Neurol Neurosurg. 2020;197: 106178. https://doi.org/10.1016/j.clineuro.2020.106178.
4. Kulkarni AV, Drake JM, Kestle JR, et al. Predicting who will benefit from endoscopic third ventriculostomy compared with shunt insertion in childhood hydrocephalus using the ETV Success Score [published correction appears in J Neurosurg Pediatr. 2011 Feb;7(2):221] [published correction appears in J Neurosurg Pediatr. 2011 Feb;7(2):221]. J Neurosurg Pediatr. 2010;6(4):310–15. https://doi.org/10.3171/2010.8.PEDS103.
5. Oi S, Sato O, Matsumoto S. No to hattatsu = Brain and development. 1994;26(3):232–38.
6. Oi S. Classification of hydrocephalus: critical analysis of classification categories and advantages of "Multi-categorical Hydrocephalus Classification" (Mc HC). Childs Nerv Syst. 2011;27(10):1523–33. https://doi.org/10.1007/s00381-011-1542-6.
7. Vandertop W. Arrested hydrocephalus. Neuropediatrics. 2018;49(05):301–301. https://doi.org/10.1055/s-0038-1661350.
8. Kim M, Park S, Lee J, Kim H, Rhim J, Park S, et al. Differences in brain morphology between hydrocephalus ex vacuo and idiopathic normal pressure hydrocephalus. Psychiatry Invest. 2021;18(7);628–635. https://doi.org/10.30773/pi.2020.0352.
9. Russell DS. Observation on the pathology of hydrocephalus. Medical Research Council Special Report. 1949:112–13. https://doi.org/10.1001/archpedi.1950.04040020539018.
10. Dandy, W. Experimental hydrocephalus. Ann Surg. 1919;70(2):129–42. https://doi.org/10.1097/00000658-191908000-00001
11. Czosnyka M. Monitoring and interpretation of intracranial pressure. J Neurol Neurosurg Psychiatry. 2004;75(6):813–21. https://doi.org/10.1136/jnnp.2003.033126.
12. Relkin N, Marmarou A, Klinge P, Bergsneider M, Black P. Diagnosing idiopathic normal-pressure hydrocephalus. Neurosurgery. 2005;57(suppl_3):S2-4–S2-16. https://doi.org/10.1227/01.neu.0000168185.29659.c.

13. Wu X, Zang D, Wu X, Sun Y, Yu J, Hu J. Diagnosis and management for secondary low- or negative-pressure hydrocephalus and a new hydrocephalus classification based on ventricular pressure. World Neurosurg. 2019;124:e510–6. https://doi.org/10.1016/j.wneu.2018.12.123.
14. Diaz-Romero Paz R, Avendaño Altimira P, Coloma Valverde G, Balhen Martin C. A rare case of negative-pressure hydrocephalus: a plausible explanation and the role of transmantle theory. World Neurosurg. 2019;125:6–9. https://doi.org/10.1016/j.wneu.2019.01.117.
15. Casado Pellejero J, Moles Herbera J, Vázquez Sufuentes S, Orduna Martínez J, Rivero Celada D, Fustero de Miguel D. Hidrocefalia aguda a presión negativa: propuesta de manejo y valor de la ventriculostomía temprana. Neurocirugía. 2022;33(1):1–8. https://doi.org/10.1016/j.neu cir.2020.11.002.
16. Rekate H. Low or negative pressure hydrocephalus demystified. World Neurosurg. 2019;128:287–8. https://doi.org/10.1016/j.wneu.2019.05.032.
17. d'Avella D, Causin F. Hydrocephalus in vein of Galen malformation. Another paradigm shift in neurosurgery. Acta Neurochir. 2016;158:1285–8. https://doi.org/10.1007/s00701-016-2837-x.
18. Lomachinsky V, Taborsky J, Felici G, Charvat F, Benes V III, Liby P. Endoscopic third ventriculostomy in an infant with vein of Galen aneurysmal malformation treated by endovascular occlusion: case report and a review of literature. Neurochirurgie. 2022. https://doi.org/10.1016/j.neuchi.2021.12.001.
19. Milan JB, Jensen TS, Nørager N, Pedersen SS, Riedel CS, Toft NM, Ammar A, Foroughi M, Grotenhuis A, Perera A, Rekate H, Juhler M. The aspect hydrocephalus system: a non-hierarchical descriptive system for clinical use. Acta Neurochir. 2022. https://doi.org/10.1007/s00701-022-05412-6.

The Epidemiology of Normal Pressure Hydrocephalus

Jakub Táborský, Jana Blažková Jr., and Vladimír Beneš 3rd

Abstract Summarising accurate epidemiological data regarding normal pressure hydrocephalus (NPH) is a complex task: for example, defining NPH varies across guidelines, various methodological approaches are utilised, different populations are studied, clinical signs are sometimes difficult to distinguish from those of the normal ageing process, and radiological signs are not necessarily specific to NPH. It would thus be unwise to simplify the complex question of NPH epidemiology to a mean number as this would not reflect the diverse patient population, methods of patient selection, and data processing used by different authors. Taking into consideration the frequency of shunt surgery, NPH remains an underdiagnosed condition of potentially treatable dementia. Both the incidence and prevalence of NPH increase with age. NPH is probably more common among the male gender and shows interesting traits among specific patient populations. For future studies, a unified approach with standardised data recording and strict adherence to international guidelines is necessary.

Keywords Epidemiology of hydrocephalus · Normal pressure hydrocephalus · Incidence · Prevalence · Underdiagnosis

Abbreviations

AD	Alzheimer's disease
A-E guidelines	American-European guidelines for NPH diagnostics
ICP	Intracranial pressure
MRI	Magnetic resonance imaging
NIS	National inpatient sample
NPH	Normal pressure hydrocephalus
iNPH	Idiopathic normal pressure hydrocephalus

J. Táborský · J. Blažková Jr. · V. Beneš 3rd (✉)
Department of Neurosurgery, 2nd Faculty of Medicine, Charles University and Motol University Hospital, Prague, Czech Republic
e-mail: vladimir.benes@fnmotol.cz

O. Bradac (ed.), *Normal Pressure Hydrocephalus*,
https://doi.org/10.1007/978-3-031-36522-5_4

NIS   Nationwide inpatient sample
PD   Parkinson's disease

1 Introduction

Theoretically, an accurate assessment of normal pressure hydrocephalus (NPH) epidemiology should be a relatively easy task of counting the occurrence of patients at a given time in a defined population (prevalence), or newly diagnosed cases over a defined period of time (incidence). However, NPH is a complex diagnosis, and several factors complicate exact estimates. First, the definition of NPH and level of diagnosis are inconsistent across studies and guidelines. For example, the American-European (A-E) guidelines presented by Relkin et al. [1] usually provide higher prevalence numbers than the Japanese guidelines as demonstrated by Andersson [2], and furthermore, there have been three editions of Japanese guidelines (Figs. 1 and 2) [3–5]. Second, different population cohorts are evaluated—the general population in a given area [2], over a period of years [6] or with a specific medical condition such as schizophrenia [7, 8] or memory impairment [9]. Additionally, large registries [10, 11] or hospital records [12, 13] are queried. Third, inconspicuous clinical courses can be difficult to distinguish from other effects of ageing. Gait abnormality occurs in 35% of individuals older than 75 years of age [14], urinary incontinence affects up to 40% of women and 16% of men at this age [15]. Additionally, 15.1% of persons older than 70 years suffer from dementia and approximately 10, 8% from Alzheimer's disease (AD) [16]. Fourth, isolated radiological signs of NPH are not necessarily specific to this condition—in the general population older than 70 years of age, 20.7% have ventriculomegaly (defined as Evans index of >0.3) [17]. Fifth, all the mentioned findings, as well as NPH prevalence, increase with age and age thresholds majorly impact epidemiological results [2, 6, 11, 14–16]. Sixth, the incidence of NPH appears to be slightly increasing as recent studies [10] report higher incidence than the older ones [2, 18]. This may be due to the ageing population of economically strong countries, better patient referral, and higher focus on NPH diagnostics. Interestingly, a similar trend is observed in the incidence of dementia worldwide [16].

Gathering accurate epidemiological data under these circumstances is challenging and various methodological approaches have been employed. The most important findings for each methodology will be summarised; however, each methodology offers a different point of view on NPH epidemiology and has its strengths and weaknesses. Understanding these weaknesses is necessary to correctly interpret study results, and as will be shown, no firm conclusions regarding NPH epidemiology can be drawn.

	American-European guidelines by Relkin et al.	Japanese guidelines III. Edition by Nakajima et al.
Unlikely iNPH	• No evidence of ventriculomegaly • Signs of increased intracranial pressure such as papilledema • No component of the clinical triad of iNPH is present • Symptoms explained by other causes (e.g., spinal stenosis)	
Possible iNPH	History • subacute mode of onset • less than 3 months duration Brain imaging • evidence of cerebral atrophy Clinical symptoms of either • incontinence and / or cognitive impairment in the absence of an observable gait or balance disturbance • Gait disturbance or dementia alone Physiological • Opening pressure measurement not available or pressure outside the range required for probable INPH	• No causative neurological or non-neurological disorders • No apparent preceding disorders causing hydrocephalus Possible iNPH is diagnosed if the following criteria are met: • 1. More than one symptom in the clinical triad: gait disturbance, cognitive impairment, and urinary incontinence • 2. Above-mentioned clinical symptoms cannot be completely explained by other neurological or non-neurological disease. • 3. Preceding diseases possibly causing ventricular dilation (including subarachnoid hemorrhage, meningitis, head injury, congenital/developmental hydrocephalus, and aqueductal stenosis) are not obvious.

Probable iNPH	**I. History**
	• insidious onset
	• at least 3 to 6 month duration
	• above 40 years
	• no antecedent head trauma, hemorrhage, meningitis
	• progression over time
	• No other neurological, psychiatric or general medical conditions
	II. Brain imaging
	• Ventricular enlargement not entirely attributable to cerebral atrophy or congenital enlargement (Evan's index > 0.3)
	• No macroscopic obstruction to CSF flow
	• At least one of the following supportive features
	  1. Enlargement of the temporal horns of the lateral ventricles not entirely attributable to hippocampus atrophy
	  2. Callosal angle of 40 degrees or more
	  3. Evidence of altered brain water content, including periventricular signal changes on CT and MRI not attributable to microvascular ischemic changes or demyelination
	  4. An aqueductal or fourth ventricular flow void on MRI
	
	III. Clinical (more in table 2.)
	• Gait impairment must be present
	• plus at least one or both (cognitive impairment, urinary symptoms)
	IV. Physiological
	• CSF opening pressure between 5-18 mmHg
		Probable iNPH is diagnosed if a patient has all of the following three features.
		• 1. Meets the requirements for possible iNPH
		• 2. CSF pressure of 200 mmH2O or less and normal CSF content
		• 3. One of the following two investigational features:
		  • (a) Neuroimaging features of narrowing of the sulci and subarachnoid space over the high-convexity/ midline surface (DESH) with gait disturbance: small stride, shuffle, instability during walking, and increase in instability on turning
		  • (b) Improvement of symptoms after CSF tap test and/or drainage test

Definite iNPH		The diagnosis of definite iNPH is made when objective improvement of symptoms is shown after CSF shunt surgery. This category is synonymous with "shunt responder."

Fig. 1 Comparison of American-European and Japanese guidelines regarding the subtypisation of unlikely, possible, probable, and definite iNPH patients

American-European guidelines by Relkin et al.
Clinical symptoms expansion

By classic definitions, findings of gait/balance disturbance must be present, plus at least one other area of impairment in cognition, urinary symptoms, or both.

With respect to gait/balance, at least two of the following should be present and not be entirely attributable to other conditions

a. Decreased step height

b. Decreased step length

c. Decreased cadence (speed of walking)

d. Increased trunk sway during walking

e. Widened standing base

f. Toes turned outward on walking

f. Retropulsion (spontaneous or provoked)

g. En bloc turning (turning requiring three or more steps for 180 degrees)

h. Impaired walking balance, as evidenced by two or more corrections out of eight steps on tandem gait testing

With respect to cognition, there must be documented impairment (adjusted for age and educational attainment) and/or decrease in performance on a cognitive screening instrument (such as the Monumental State examination), or evidence of at least two of the following on examination that is not fully attributable to other conditions

a. Psychomotor slowing (increased response latency)

b. Decreased fine motor speed

c. Decreased fine motor accuracy

d. Difficulty dividing or maintaining attention

e. Impaired recall, especially for recent events

f. Executive dysfunction, such as impairment in multistep procedures, working memory, formulation of abstractions/similarities, insight

g. Behavioral or personality changes

To document symptoms in the domain of urinary continence, either one of the following should be present

a. Episodic or persistent urinary incontinence not attributable to primary urological disorders

b. Persistent urinary incontinence

c. Urinary and fecal incontinence

Or any two of the following should be present

a. Urinary urgency as defined by frequent perception of a pressing need to void

b. Urinary frequency as defined by more than six voiding episodes in an average 12-hour period despite normal fluid intake

c. Nocturia as defined by the need to urinate more than two times in an average night

Fig. 2 Expansion of the previous table in terms of clinical examination when assessing probable iNPH patients

2 Population-Based Studies

In these types of studies, the epidemiology of NPH is estimated in a defined population over a certain period of time, ideally yielding both incidence and prevalence. There are two ways to approach the population: (1) through a massive media information campaign aimed at the public, general practitioners, geriatric centres, nursing homes for the elderly and similar facilities. Patients are then referred for further testing; (2) randomly selected residents over a certain age (commonly over 65 years) are either contacted with a survey questionnaire focused on NPH symptoms or provided with an MRI screening offer. Afterwards selection criteria are applied and those patients who satisfy NPH criteria undergo additional testing. The response rates vary around 60%, and selection bias is unavoidable. Not responding due to NPH symptoms (dementia) would artificially lower the prevalence; on the contrary, healthy subjects may not feel the need to undergo testing, thus increasing the prevalence. Furthermore, unknown geographical factors could be influencing reported numbers. Despite these shortcomings, population-based studies represent the best attempts to clarify the true NPH epidemiology in the general population. The most important studies are briefly summarised.

2.1 Population-Based Studies Following the American-European Guidelines

A well-designed prospective study was conducted in Vestfold County, Norway in 2004–2005. The authors carried out a large patient recruitment campaign in a population of 220,000 inhabitants and eventually tested 63 patients (including CSF testing). Eventually, prevalence was calculated at 21.9/100,000 and incidence at 5.5/100,000/year for "probable" iNPH. Prevalence showed obvious age dependency ranging from 3.3/100,000 (50–59 years age group) to 93.3/100.000 ($\geq$ 80 years age group). No difference between genders was reported [19].

A representative sample of the elderly population ($\geq$ 70 years) in Swedish Gothenburg underwent neuropsychiatric evaluations and CT of the brain between 1986 and 2000. Following the A-E guidelines, the prevalence of probable iNPH was assessed at 0.2% among patients aged 70–79 years and 5.9% for those older than 80 years. Additionally, an Evans index of >0.3 was reported in 20.7% of investigated patients. Although men had higher prevalence in both age groups as well as in the Evans index, neither difference reached statistical significance [17].

Martin-Laez et al. presented a 10-year longitudinal prospective study on the incidence of iNPH in one Spanish region. Crude incidence over the study period was calculated at 3.25/100,000/year. The incidence rose exponentially with age and was higher in men than women. Considering favourable shunt response as the ultimate iNPH diagnosis, the incidence was estimated at 2.07/100,000/year [6].

Pyykko et al. collected data from four Finland hospitals with a defined catchment area from 1993 to 2010. In addition to standard testing, 24-hour ICP monitoring and frontal lobe brain biopsy were performed. Mean incidence over the study period was 4.84/100,000/year with a higher incidence of 14.6/100,000/year in patients over 70 years. Furthermore, the incidence increased during the study period, probably reflecting increased awareness among the referring practitioners and institutions [20].

Andersson et al. asked 1000 randomly selected patients over 65 years of age from Sweden to participate in a survey followed by a clinical and radiological investigation. The authors applied both diagnostic guidelines to the same study group and reported via modified (no CSF testing) A-E guidelines probable prevalence of 3.7%. An even higher prevalence of 8.9% was among patients over 80 years old. According to the Japanese guidelines, the prevalence of the same population was 1.5% and 3.8% among those older than 80 years. No significant difference between male and female patients was ascertained according to either guideline [2].

2.2 Population-Based Studies Following the Japanese Guidelines

Hiaroka et al. managed one of the first population-based studies focused on iNPH. In a group of 170 randomly selected patients older than 65 years in a rural Japan community, 2.9% showed clinical and MRI signs suggestive of iNPH [21]. A similar methodological approach and target age group in another geographically defined area showed slightly lower prevalence of "possible" iNPH (1.4%) [22].

Focusing on iNPH MRI features (ventricular enlargement and disproportional narrowing of cortical sulci) 12 patients were identified from a group of 790 subjects. However, only 4 of these had neurological symptoms of iNPH (0.51% prevalence). Interestingly, those who fulfilled only the brain imaging criteria without clinical features were followed for 4–8 years, and 2 out of 8 developed iNPH during this period [23]. A follow-up study after 5 additional years showed the prevalence of possible iNPH to be 0.3% (age 70) and 1.42% (age 80). Incidence was estimated at 120/100,000/year for patients older than 70 years [24].

Nakashita assessed the epidemiology of Parkinson's disease in a well-designed study in a rural Japanese town. Since the focus was on the elderly population, iNPH MRI and clinical features were examined as well. Of the 607 patients who underwent MRI, 20 showed positive findings, 17 with associated clinical symptoms: the prevalence of possible iNPH of 2.8% [18]. Neither of the abovementioned Japanese studies reported gender-specific prevalence or incidence.

In conclusion, population-based studies report prevalence and incidence rates of NPH rising exponentially with age, with the male gender being more commonly affected.

3 Hospital-Based Studies

Hospital-based studies derive data from medical or surgical records from single or multiple hospitals. Studies rely on inpatient data, outpatient data, or both. Overall limitations of hospital-based studies are diagnostic variability among hospitals, incomplete and unstandardized information, coding and administrative issues with data collection, case selection bias, retrospective data collection, and also duplicate admissions, which can raise final incidence and prevalence rates. Benefit appears when medical records are used to monitor the natural history of the disease [25, 26]. Bearing these shortcomings in mind, important studies are briefly summarised.

A large survey of 53 German hospitals focused on overall NPH management. The authors extrapolated treated NPH cases to the estimated German population to reach an iNPH incidence of 1.8/100.000/year. However, a wide variation between centres was observed with regard to preoperative testing, diagnostic criteria, the decision for shunt implantation, and other management issues, and the authors conclude that incidence may be even higher [27].

Tissel investigated retrospectively incidence rates via analysing surgical records of patients over 18 years in 6 neurosurgical departments in Sweden. Rather than focusing strictly on NPH, the overall epidemiology of hydrocephalus was studied. Nevertheless, an estimated overall incidence was 3.4/100.000/year for hydrocephalus, 1.6/100.000/year for NPH, and 0.9/100.000/year for iNPH. This study also nicely reflects regional differences in diagnostic criteria, surgical indications, and local awareness of hydrocephalus; the frequency of surgery for iNHP was 4 times higher in the most active centre compared to the least active one [13].

Search for patients with clinically suspected NPH at the Mayo Clinic database treated between 1995 and 2003 identified 41 cases giving a possible incidence of 3,74/100.000/year. Of these patients, 13 eventually received a shunt (incidence 1.19/100.000/year). Considering definite improvement at 3 years after shunting as NPH diagnosis confirmation, the incidence reached 0.36/100.000/year. All reported incidences were higher for those older than 50 years [12].

Bir retrospectively analysed the incidence of hydrocephalus during a 25-year span from hospital charts. All patients with hydrocephalus, regardless of aetiology, were included from a non-specified "population served by the hospital". They estimated overall hydrocephalus incidence at 17/100.000/year. NPH cases comprised 10.6% of all hydrocephalus patients, however no distinction between iNPH and secondary NPH was provided. In conclusion, this study provides a nice overview of hydrocephalus aetiology and demographics, although due to the mentioned reasons, no inference with regard to iNPH can be drawn besides peak age in the 9th decade of life [28].

Kuriyama et al. sent two surveys to 4220 Japanese centres in order to gather epidemiological data during the year 2012. The response rate was 42.7%. Diagnostic criteria of the Japanese iNPH guidelines (second edition) were applied. The estimated overall incidence was 10.2/100.000/year and rising with age (over 60 years 31.4/100 000/year). The reported age of onset was in the 70s in more than 50% of patients [29].

In conclusion, estimating epidemiological data from hospital-based studies is tedious; however, they provide useful insight into variations in NPH management, hydrocephalus demographics, and frequency of shunt surgeries.

4   Register Data Studies

As the title implies, these types of studies identify patient cohorts from national registers, insurance files or hospital registers. Studies work with large patient populations, hospital or surgical records, and diagnostic codes. Therefore, they allow stratification of patients by age, ethnicity, gender, comorbidities, socioeconomic status, and other followed data. Also, annual trends of incidence, surgical management, complication and local risk factors can be evaluated. Working with large numbers of patients, statistical significance can often be reached for the aforementioned demographic parameters. Similarly to hospital-based studies, problems with accurate coding, diagnostic variability and other administrative issues may limit drawn conclusions. The exact diagnostic workup for NPH is difficult to ascertain and probably varies across participating institutions. Furthermore, outcomes can usually be assessed only by discharge destination. Since NPH patients frequently reside in extended-care facilities, return discharge need not reflect eventual favourable outcomes. On the other hand, when compared to hospital-based studies, the register data are taken prospectively by independent researchers and at the time of analysis already exist, so there is limited to absent selection bias [25, 26].

Lemcke et al. [30] used anonymised data from a nationwide health-insurance provider representing approximately 10% of the German population. The period covered 10 years from 2003 to 2012 and used diagnostic codes to identify patients with NPH and iNPH. The incidence of shunt-treated iNPH was estimated at 1.08/100,000. The authors acknowledge a cohort that may have included a "large number of false positives and excluded false negatives". Due to a lack of widely employed and unified diagnostic criteria, a misclassification bias may have been introduced.

Rafi et al. used Nationwide Inpatient Sample (NIS) from the USA for collecting iNPH data on the incidence, gender, age group, income, and race/ethnicity during 2008–2016. NIS provides a 20% stratified sample of all community hospital discharges (more than 7 million discharge records from 4500 + hospitals). From this sample, the overall incidence of inpatient admission for iNPH was estimated to be 2.86/100,000/year with stable rates during the period covered. Subgroup analysis showed significantly higher incidence for males, the elderly population (e.g. 17.89/100,000/year for patients 65–84 years old), higher income status, rural residence, and white or black race. The differences may be due to better access to health care among affluent patients or genetic predisposition. Apart from the already mentioned limitations, this dataset represents inpatient discharges, thus patients not requiring hospitalisation or with incidental iNPH diagnosis would not be included [11].

Analysis of patients older than 60 years from the NIS (2007–2017) found the prevalence of iNPH to be 0.18%; again discharge codes for iNPH were used for identifying patients. Interestingly, only 21.6% of these patients underwent surgical management. This includes patients undergoing invasive testing procedures and endoscopic third ventriculostomy. In accordance with the previous study, a higher proportion of male and white patients was found. Interestingly, a greater use of laparoscopic shunt implantation in recent years was reported [10].

Analysis of large registers confirms results reported in other studies and allows for estimating management trends over long periods of time. In addition, important shortcomings in health care can be identified.

5 Meta-analyses and Systematic Reviews

Many of the above presented studies were included in systematic reviews and meta-analyses. These have to consider different iNPH definitions, methodological quality, different populations, time periods, and other potentially confounding factors. Important studies in other languages may also be missed in the search. Thus, the final review can only be as good as the studies that form its basis. Nevertheless, pooling together large numbers of patients may identify statistically significant traits, for which the individual study is underpowered.

Martín-Laéz summarised the results of 21 articles meeting the inclusion criteria. The authors pooled data from studies ($n = 7$) with random population sampling to reveal iNPH prevalence of 1.3% in subjects older than 60 years [6].

Of limited value regarding iNPH epidemiology is a systematic review published in 2018, since it does not distinguish between particular forms of hydrocephalus, secondary notwithstanding. This meta-analysis confirms an increasing prevalence in the elderly population: 175/100.000 for patients $\geq$65 years [31].

Zaccaria recently published a systematic review focused solely on the epidemiology of NPH. Crude prevalence reported in 10 analysed studies ranged from 10/100,000 to 29/100,000, while age-specific prevalence rose with age for both genders, notably for male patients. Crude incidence rates reported in 6 analysed studies ranged from 1.8/100,000/year to 7.3/100,000/year. Likewise, the incidence rose with age [32].

Unfortunately, systematic reviews and meta-analyses fail to bring additional information into NPH epidemiology, likely due to data heterogeneity, methodological differences of the included studies, lack of standardised reporting and other confounding factors. The need for unified and standardised data collection in the future cannot be emphasised more.

6　Other Epidemiological Studies

Several articles aimed to identify NPH patients in specific populations. Bech-Azeddine in a prospective study from a memory clinic found improvement after shunting in 8 patients from 400 (2%) who were referred for detailed evaluation. An elaborate protocol consisted of clinical and radiological evaluation (71 patients), invasive testing (35 patients), and eventual shunt implantation (13 patients). Interestingly, iNPH patients comprised 20% of those referred for clinical and radiological testing [33].

A prospective study in a similar setting of memory clinic was conducted in Tasmania. From a total of 408 consecutive patients with memory impairment, 62 (15.2%) were found to have iNPH, 29 received shunt and all but one improved at follow-up. Additionally, a minimum incidence of 11.9/100,000/year was reported based on population census. This increased with age; the highest being 120/100,000/year for patients older than 75 years [9].

Marmarou et al. investigated the prevalence of NPH among residents of assisted-living and extended-care facilities. They reported prevalence between 9 and 14% depending on the diagnostic criteria used. This would suggest a higher prevalence in healthcare centres in contrast with non-hospitalised patients [34]. Similarly, a remarkably high prevalence of iNPH of 14% was found in elderly patients with schizophrenia [7].

Screening the elderly population after falls led to diagnosis of possible iNPH in 18.7%, probable iNPH in 12.3% and definite iNPH in 10.6% (clinical improvement after shunting) [35].

Pyykko et al. investigated the causes of death of patients with NPH. Although dementia is one of the main NPH symptoms, these patients do not have a higher chance of death due to of dementia in comparison with the average population. The most frequent causes of death remain cardiovascular and cerebrovascular disease [20].

7　Clinical Relevance

Articles reporting incidence of shunt surgery for NPH found rates ranging from 0.91/100,000/year to 1.91/100,000/year [12, 13, 19]. These rates are far below the incidence of iNPH found in population-based studies, particularly in the elderly population. There may be several reasons: (1) limited awareness of NPH signs among the public and healthcare workers. A well-executed information campaign may help with improved patient referral [19]. (2) NPH symptoms are rather common in the elderly population: abnormal gait, cognitive decline or incontinence may be viewed as normal signs of ageing. (3) International guidelines require a relatively tedious protocol before shunting surgery is carried out and patients/relatives may refuse further testing/surgery. All of these and other factors mean that NPH is underdiagnosed and consequently undertreated.

8 Conclusion

Summarising accurate epidemiological data regarding NPH at this time is inadvisable due to the many shortcomings discussed above. It would be unwise to simplify the complex question of NPH epidemiology to a mean number as it would not reflect the diverse patient population, methods of patient selection and data processing used by different authors. Let us conclude that NPH remains an underdiagnosed condition of potentially treatable dementia whose incidence and prevalence increase with age is probably more common among the male gender and shows interesting traits among specific patient populations. For future studies, a unified approach with standardised data recording and strict adherence to international guidelines is necessary.

9 Key Points

- Incidence and prevalence of NPH increase with age.
- NPH is more common in men than in women.
- Incidence and prevalence of NPH are higher in recent studies.
- Study methodology greatly influences the results.
- American-European and Japanese guidelines give different epidemiological results.
- Future studies on large populations are needed.

References

1. Relkin N, et al. Diagnosing idiopathic normal-pressure hydrocephalus. Neurosurgery. 2005;57(3 Suppl):S4–16; discussion ii-v.
2. Andersson J, et al. Prevalence of idiopathic normal pressure hydrocephalus: a prospective, population-based study. PLoS ONE. 2019;14(5): e0217705.
3. Ishikawa M. Guideline committe for idiopathic normal pressure hydrocephalus, JSoNPH Clinical guidelines for idiopathic normal pressure hydrocephalus. Neurol Med Chir (Tokyo). 2004;44(4):222–3.
4. Mori E, et al. Guidelines for management of idiopathic normal pressure hydrocephalus: second edition. Neurol Med Chir (Tokyo). 2012 ;52(11):775–809.
5. Nakajima M, et al. Guidelines for management of idiopathic normal pressure hydrocephalus (third edition): endorsed by the Japanese society of normal pressure hydrocephalus. Neurol Med Chir (Tokyo). 2021;61(2):63–97.
6. Martin-Laez R, et al. Incidence of idiopathic normal-pressure hydrocephalus in northern Spain. World Neurosurg. 2016;87:298–310.

7. Yoshino Y, et al. Risk of idiopathic normal pressure hydrocephalus in older inpatients with schizophrenia. Int Psychogeriatr. 2016;28(5):863–8.

8. Yoshino Y, et al. Prevalence of possible idiopathic normal pressure hydrocephalus in older inpatients with schizophrenia: a replication study. BMC Psychiatry. 2020;20(1):273.

9. Razay G, Wimmer M, Robertson I. Incidence, diagnostic criteria and outcome following ventriculoperitoneal shunting of idiopathic normal pressure hydrocephalus in a memory clinic population: a prospective observational cross-sectional and cohort study. BMJ Open. 2019;9(12): e028103.

10. Alvi MA, et al. Prevalence and trends in management of idiopathic normal pressure hydrocephalus in the United States: insights from the national inpatient sample. World Neurosurg. 2021;145:e38–52.

11. Ghaffari-Rafi A, et al. Inpatient diagnoses of idiopathic normal pressure hydrocephalus in the United States: demographic and socioeconomic disparities. J Neurol Sci. 2020;418: 117152.

12. Klassen BT, Ahlskog JE. Normal pressure hydrocephalus: how often does the diagnosis hold water? Neurology. 2011;77(12):1119–25.

13. Tisell M, Hoglund M, Wikkelso C. National and regional incidence of surgery for adult hydrocephalus in Sweden. Acta Neurol Scand. 2005;112(2):72–5.

14. Verghese J, et al. Epidemiology of gait disorders in community-residing older adults. J Am Geriatr Soc. 2006;54(2):255–61.

15. Milsom I, Gyhagen M. The prevalence of urinary incontinence. Climacteric. 2019;22(3):217–22.

16. Cao Q, et al. The prevalence of dementia: a systematic review and meta-analysis. J Alzheimers Dis. 2020;73(3):1157–66.

17. Jaraj D, et al. Prevalence of idiopathic normal-pressure hydrocephalus. Neurology. 2014;82(16):1449–54.

18. Nakashita S, et al. Clinical assessment and prevalence of parkinsonism in Japanese elderly people. Acta Neurol Scand. 2016;133(5):373–9.

19. Brean A, Eide PK. Prevalence of probable idiopathic normal pressure hydrocephalus in a Norwegian population. Acta Neurol Scand. 2008;118(1):48–53.

20. Pyykko OT, et al. Incidence, comorbidities, and mortality in idiopathic normal pressure hydrocephalus. World Neurosurg. 2018;112:e624–31.

21. Hiraoka K, Meguro K, Mori E. Prevalence of idiopathic normal-pressure hydrocephalus in the elderly population of a Japanese rural community. Neurol Med Chir (Tokyo). 2008;48(5):197–99;discussion 199–200.

22. Tanaka N, et al. Prevalence of possible idiopathic normal-pressure hydrocephalus in Japan: the Osaki-Tajiri project. Neuroepidemiology. 2009;32(3):171–5.

23. Iseki C, et al. Asymptomatic ventriculomegaly with features of idiopathic normal pressure hydrocephalus on MRI (AVIM) in the elderly: a prospective study in a Japanese population. J Neurol Sci. 2009;277(1–2):54–7.

24. Iseki C, et al. Incidence of idiopathic normal pressure hydrocephalus (iNPH): a 10-year follow-up study of a rural community in Japan. J Neurol Sci. 2014;339(1–2):108–12.

25. Masi AT. Potential uses and limitations of hospital data in epidemiologic research. Am J Public Health Nations Health. 1965;55:658–67.

26. Thygesen LC, Ersboll AK. When the entire population is the sample: strengths and limitations in register-based epidemiology. Eur J Epidemiol. 2014;29(8):551–8.

27. Krauss JK, Halve B. Normal pressure hydrocephalus: survey on contemporary diagnostic algorithms and therapeutic decision-making in clinical practice. Acta Neurochir (Wien). 2004;146(4):379–88; discussion 388.

28. Bir SC, et al. Epidemiology of adult-onset hydrocephalus: institutional experience with 2001 patients. Neurosurg Focus. 2016;41(3):E5.

29. Kuriyama N, et al. Nationwide hospital-based survey of idiopathic normal pressure hydrocephalus in Japan: epidemiological and clinical characteristics. Brain Behav. 2017;7(3): e00635.

30. Lemcke J, et al. Nationwide incidence of normal pressure hydrocephalus (NPH) assessed by insurance claim data in Germany. Open Neurol J. 2016;10:15–24.
31. Isaacs AM, et al. Age-specific global epidemiology of hydrocephalus: systematic review, metanalysis and global birth surveillance. PLoS ONE. 2018;13(10): e0204926.
32. Zaccaria V, et al. A systematic review on the epidemiology of normal pressure hydrocephalus. Acta Neurol Scand. 2020;141(2):101–14.
33. Bech-Azeddine R, et al. Idiopathic normal-pressure hydrocephalus: evaluation and findings in a multidisciplinary memory clinic. Eur J Neurol. 2001;8(6):601–11.
34. Marmarou A, Young HF, Aygok GA. Estimated incidence of normal pressure hydrocephalus and shunt outcome in patients residing in assisted-living and extended-care facilities. Neurosurg Focus. 2007;22(4):E1.
35. Oike R, et al. Screening for idiopathic normal pressure hydrocephalus in the elderly after falls. Clin Neurol Neurosurg. 2021;205: 106635.

CSF Physiology

Adéla Bubeníková, Petr Skalický, Helen Whitley, and Ondřej Bradáč

Abstract The entire cerebral cavity surrounding the central nervous system has a volume of approximately 1700 ml. From this capacity, 150 ml stands for Cerebrospinal Fluid (CSF), watery fluid with a low concentration of protein and cellular components. CSF is mainly produced via plasma filtration and membrane secretion through choroid plexuses, a minority is secreted through secretion of ependymal surfaces of the cerebral ventricles and by the arachnoid layer. In the past few years, it has been observed that a fraction of CSF production is derived from perivascular spaces of cerebral capillaries, which is of further importance for the functioning of newly identified pseudolymphatic pathways called the glymphatic system. The classical model of CSF circulation was built upon the idea of unidirectional flow from the ventricles via cisterns and foramina into the subarachnoid spaces, and finally into the venous outflow from the brain. However, it seems that CSF circulation is much more complex, involving various kinetic mechanisms which are important for adequate osmotic and metabolic pathways in the central nervous system, and unmistakably vital for cerebral functioning. CSF pressure directly determines intracranial pressure, with physiological values from 3 to 4 mmHg in children younger than one year, and from 10 to 15 mmHg in healthy adults. Due to advances in the understanding of CSF physiology, and much more detailed imaging methods, we are able to introduce new concepts about the role of CSF in the brain, compare them to initial historical reports, and discuss possible implications for future research.

Keywords Cerebrospinal fluid · Physiology · Hydrocephalus · Anatomy · Cerebrospinal fluid circulation · Physiological mechanisms of hydrocephalus · Glymphatic system

A. Bubeníková · P. Skalický · O. Bradáč (✉)
Department of Neurosurgery, 2nd Medical Faculty, Charles University and Motol University Hospital, Prague, Czech Republic
e-mail: ondrej.bradac2@fnmotol.cz

A. Bubeníková · H. Whitley · O. Bradáč
Department of Neurosurgery and Neuro-Oncology, 1st Medical Faculty, Charles University and Military University Hospital, Prague, Czech Republic

© The Author(s), under exclusive license to Springer Nature Switzerland AG 2023
O. Bradac (ed.), *Normal Pressure Hydrocephalus*,
https://doi.org/10.1007/978-3-031-36522-5_5

Abbreviations

AQP   Aquaporin
BBB   Blood-brain barrier
BCB   Blood-cerebrospinal fluid barrier
CBB   Cerebrospinal fluid-brain barrier
CNS   Central nervous system
CSF   Cerebrospinal fluid
CVO   Circumventricular organ
ICP   Intracranial pressure
ISF   Interstitial fluid
MRI   Magnetic resonance imaging

1 Introduction

The first-ever attempts to describe the basic concepts of neuroscience, particularly those of neurophysiology and neuroanatomy, date back to the era of ancient Egyptians [1]. In recent years, a lot of effort has been invested into research in order to elucidate the role of cerebrospinal fluid (CSF), one of the essential compartments of the Central Nervous System (CNS). This has revealed that the mechanisms and functioning of CSF are more complex than previously believed.

The CSF space is formed by the intracerebral ventricles, the central spinal cord canal, and the subarachnoid spaces consisting of cisterns and sulci [2–4]. This is separated by the Blood-CSF Barrier (BCB) from the vascular system [5]. CSF is renewed approximately four times per 24 hours, the rate of CSF formation is roughly 0.4 ml per minute, and its volume is estimated to be 150 ml in healthy adults [2, 6]. Recent Magnetic Resonance Imaging (MRI) findings have proposed that the CSF volume is underestimated, proposing its range as high as 254–331 ml [7–10]. The choroid plexuses are considered to be the primary CSF production organs, nevertheless, approximately 20% of CSF is secreted via other pathways [11–13] and this number might be even higher. CSF is drained across perineural spaces into the lymphatics, whilst a minor part is absorbed into the venous circulatory system through arachnoid villi [11]. The CSF circulation is a complex combination of both uni- and bidirectional flow together with additional fluid exchange mechanisms [11, 14]. In addition to maintaining CNS homeostasis, CSF plays a vital role in overall physiological and pathophysiological pathways in the human body [15, 16]. Abnormal volume, impaired clearance functions, or metabolic changes of CSF may have a detrimental impact on cerebral performance and Intracranial Pressure (ICP) [17, 18] which is further described according to the well-known Monro-Kellie doctrine [19].

Several new findings challenge what is known about CSF physiology, and although results should be interpreted cautiously, there is a growing body of evidence that established beliefs should be revised. Such topics include the origins of CSF production, the concept of unidirectional (also known as bulk) flow, and CSF absorption via arachnoid villi [14, 20–23]. In this chapter, we describe historical hypotheses of CSF physiology, introduce up-to-date findings, and describe the current research trends in this topic.

2   A Brief Historical Insight

The oldest written report most likely mentioning CSF dates from 1500 BC in ancient Egypt (the era of the 16th and 17th dynasty). The so-called "Edwin Smith's Papyrus" is named after its purchaser [1, 24] and includes reports of 48 patients with cranial and spinal traumatic injuries, enriched by descriptions of symptoms, diagnosis, and conducted treatment. One of the patients experienced a skull fracture and "the rupture of meningeal membrane" accompanied by fluid leakage presumably referred to CSF [25, 26]. Centuries later, scholars in ancient Greece contributed to the essential improvement of the general knowledge about the human body (particularly Hippocrates, Aristotle, and Herophilus), but there are no preserved records of any CSF investigations [1, 27].

The "pneuma" theory of Ancient Greek medicine was built upon by Claudius Galen (129–216 AD) who differentiated between vital pneuma, which travelled in blood, and psychic pneuma, which went to the brain [28]. Pneuma generally referred to breath, air, or spirit, and it was described together with basic pulmonary and vascular physiology. Galen's theory also mentions the presence of pneuma along peripheral nerves [29]. At this time, there was already some knowledge of the ventricular system, but it was considered to be the origin of imagination (in lateral ventricles), cognition (the third ventricle), and finally memory (the fourth ventricle) [1, 30]. Following the mediaeval times, from which we have no significant scientific reports on CSF, the renaissance brought us an enormous number of discoveries across the natural sciences. Leonardo Da Vinci made critical contributions with his anatomical drawings and wax casts of the ventricular system which most likely belonged to an ox's brain [1, 31]. Galen's opposer, Andreas Vesalius, rewrote the description of human anatomy, and with his co-workers contributed to more accurate illustrations of the nervous system in the work *De humani corporis fabrica libri septem* [32, 33]. His university colleague, Costanzo Varolius, rejected the pneuma theory and proposed instead that it was "fluid", rather than spirits, which filled the ventricular system [34]. Italian anatomist Niccolo Massa mentioned a "watery excess", making the first reference to CSF circulation in 1532 [35]. The subarachnoid layer was not described until Gerardus Blasius coined the term "arachnoid" in 1666 and Raymond Viessens with Frederik Ruysch clarified its anatomy more in detail thereafter [36, 37]. In 1705, Antonio Pacchioni outlined the architecture of the arachnoid granulations, structures which bear his name to this day [38].

The generation of Alexander Monro, Jacobus Sylvius, Hubert von Luschka, and Francois Magendie further described anatomical landmarks within the ventricular system that bear these eponymous names. The CSF was for a long time referred to "liquor contugnii" after Italian physician Domenico Cotugno who was the first to describe the basics of CSF physiology [39], including CSF volume in 1764 [40]. Another milestone can be attributed to the neuroanatomist Magendie who extended Cotugno's publications and coined the term "liquid cerebrospinal", which is still used today [41]. After disclosing reports on CSF function, Heinrich Quincke performed a lumbar puncture to reduce ICP in patients experiencing subarachnoid haemorrhage, cerebral tumours, or hydrocephalus, and for diagnostic purposes [42, 43]. In 1893, Ludwig Lichtheim performed the first-ever CSF analysis in patients suffering from tubercular meningitis [44]. Investigations on CSF laboratory findings were improved due to new methods of bacterial cultivation and microbiological staining introduced by Hans Christian Gram in 1884 [1, 45]. Since then, the number of studies dedicated to CSF has been continually increasing and the progress in the field continuously helps to elucidate complex concepts of CSF (patho)physiology.

3 Anatomical Concept

3.1 *Ventricular System and Central Canal*

Familiarity with the anatomy of the ventricular system is a crucial step to a better understanding of CSF physiology and neurosurgical procedures. Two equivalent lateral ventricles localised in the cerebral hemispheres are the biggest landmarks of the ventricular system. Both morphologically resemble a C-shape further subdivided into five regions: three horns (anterior, posterior, and inferior), a single ventricular body, and finally the collateral trigone, also known as the atrium [46]. Via the foramen of Monro, the lateral ventricles are connected to the third ventricle. This communicates with the fourth ventricle through the so-called Sylvian aqueduct, a region of approximately 15 mm which is currently differentiated into three parts: pars anterior, antrum, and finally pars posterior. The pars anterior is a triangular structure beneath the posterior commissure which is morphologically continuous with the third ventricle. The aqueduct subsequently runs ventrally to the midbrain's tectum (antrum), between the inferior and superior colliculi and finally reaches the rhomboid fossa (pars posterior) [47]. CSF enters the subarachnoid space via three openings, the paired foramina of Luschka at the level of cerebellopontine angles and a single foramen of Magendie, caudal to the cerebellar nodule (Figs. 1, 2, 3A, B).

The cavity of the fourth ventricle extends into the central canal of the spinal cord up to its terminal point, the conus medullaris [48]. A layer of columnar ependymal cells lines the canal, and its exact location depends on specific spinal regions. In the cervical and thoracic region, the central canal runs ventrally. It runs centrally in the lumbar region and slightly dorsally in the conus medullaris region [49].

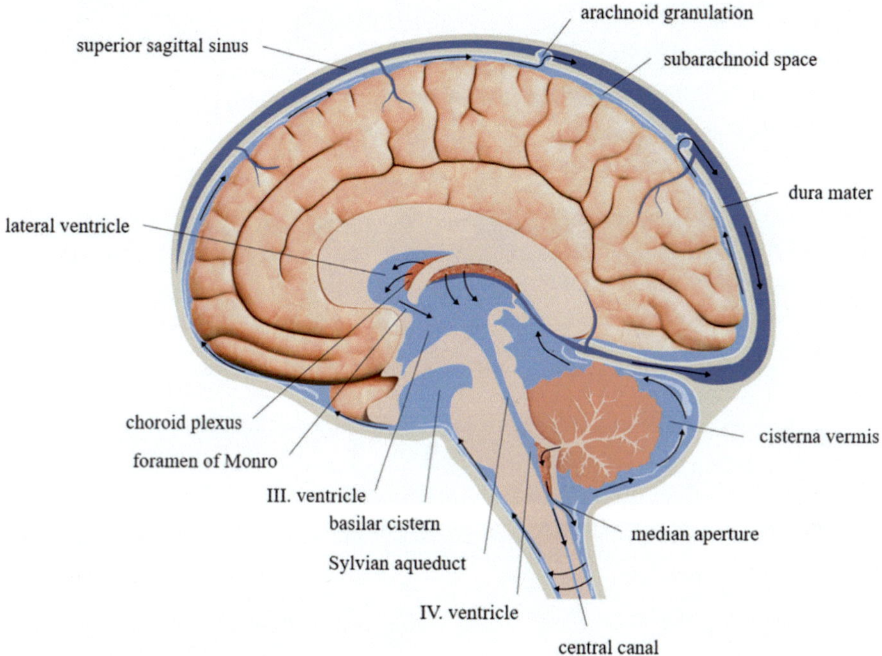

Fig. 1 Important anatomical landmarks of CSF circulation

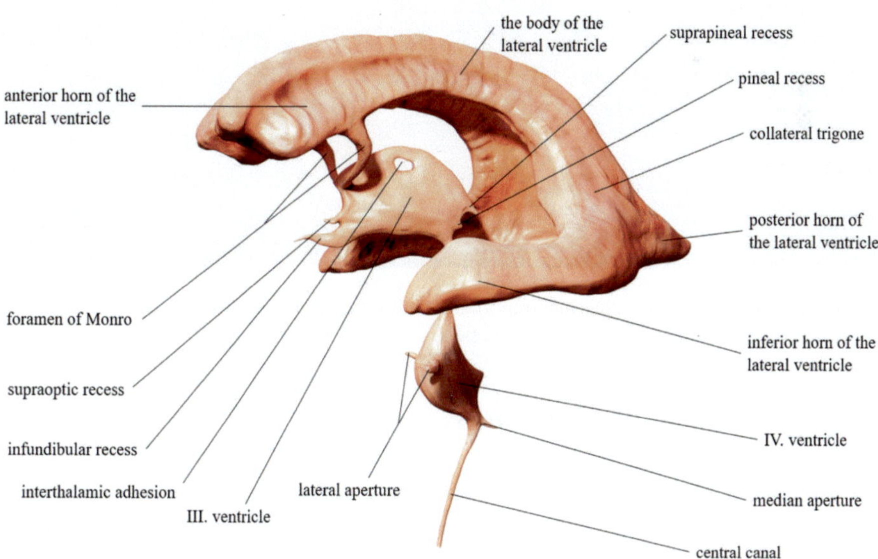

Fig. 2 Detailed anatomy of the ventricular system

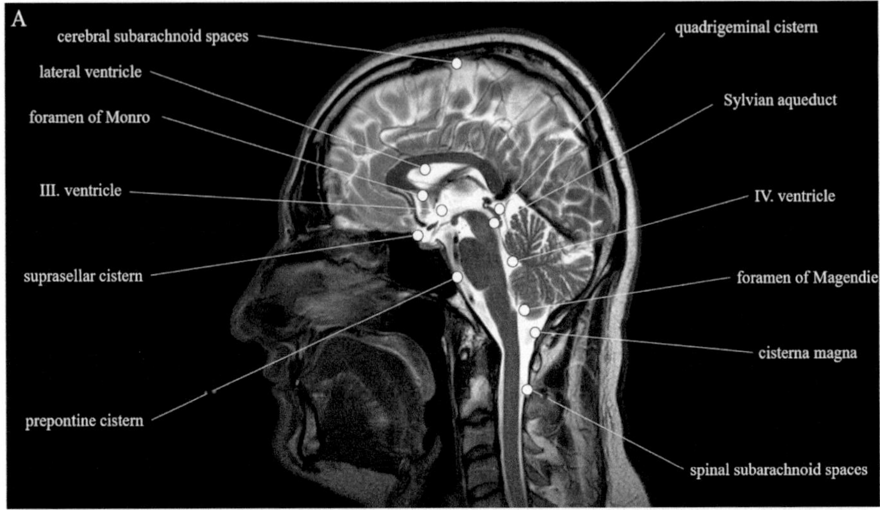

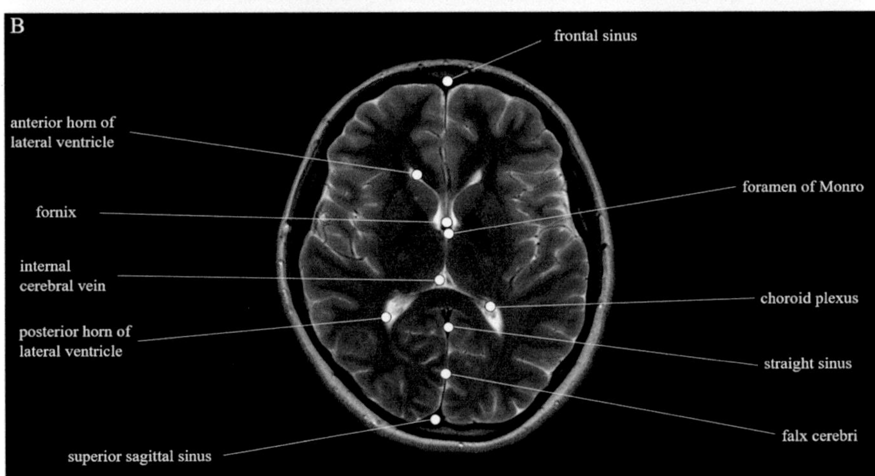

Fig. 3 MRI T2-WI scans depicting important landmarks of the ventricular system and CSF pathways on (A) sagittal and (B) axial projections

3.2 The Complexity of Barriers

The meticulous isolation of brain parenchyma, and the spinal cord from the rest of the body, is vital in order to ensure adequate regulation of metabolic interchange. This regulation is accomplished by three major landmarks: (1) Blood-Brain Barrier (BBB), (2) CSF-Brain Barrier (CBB, formed by the arachnoid layer), and (3) blood-CSF barrier (BCB) [50]. These barriers consist of epithelial and arachnoid cell compartments altogether with the cellular junctions allowing metabolic interchange between the body and the CNS.

Indisputably the most discussed of the aforementioned barriers is the BBB, a highly selective membrane-like structure formed by endothelial tight junctions from surrounding capillaries without the presence of fenestration [51]. Astrocytic endfeet in the Interstitial Fluid (ISF) ensheath the capillary walls and surrounding pericytes are ingrained into the capillary basal membrane which consists of two basal laminas [51, 52]. The BBB allows metabolites and smaller molecules to enter in accordance not only with passive or facilitated diffusion pathways but also through transmembrane active transport mechanisms. Interestingly, the overall surface of BBB accounts for 12–18 m^2 in the average adult [53] since it is present along the whole CNS. However, there are several regions in which it is significantly reduced. Such areas, known as Circumventricular Organs (CVOs), are unique structures characterised by higher permeability of metabolic interchange between the CNS and the rest of the body. This happens due to the construction of endothelial cells into gap junctions between endothelial cells, fenestrated capillaries, and their small size [54–56]. Instead of highly selective BBB, CVOs are primarily bordered by a layer of endothelium-like tanycytic cells [57]. CVOs can be classified into sensory and secretory, according to their physiological role [55]. The vast majority of hormones and complex metabolites are incapable (or only in reduced concentrations) of direct transportation across the BBB [58] and therefore require CVOs to enable such pathways. Sensory CVOs, namely the subfornical organ, organum vasculosum of the lamina terminalis, and the area postrema (nucleus tractus solitarii), are critical complex entities involved in hormonal regulation pathways as well as cardiovascular and immunological functioning [59, 60]. All sensory CVOs share a synaptic communication with paraventricular and supraoptic nuclei [61] which, according to up-to-date evidence, enable the hypothalamus to supervise the neuroendocrine and metabolic regulation [54]. Of note are afferent pathways directed to the organum vasculosum of the lamina terminalis from the subfornical organ, brainstem, hypothalamus, and the median preoptic nucleus. The efferent outputs from this region are focused to basal ganglia, and to stria medullaris [62]. The secretory CVOs consist of neurohypophysis, epiphysis, subcommissural organ, and eminentia medialis (hypothalamic arcuate nucleus) [63], all of which are responsible for neuroendocrine secretion [64]. The subcommissural organ is a more specific CVO due to the presence of increased concentrations of fenestrated capillaries when compared to the rest of CVOs, thus making the BBB less permeable [65]. Detailed anatomy of CVOS is depicted in Figs. 4, 5, and 6.

According to the highly selective nature of BBB in terms of allowing the substances and metabolites to enter the barrier, it has been a challenge to develop effective drug delivery pathways to the CNS. Approximately 98% of drugs with smaller molecular sizes, and basically all of those with larger (for example some of the viral vectors, peptides, antibodies etc.), are excluded by BBB [57, 66, 67]. Fortunately, the characteristic features of CVOs help to improve drug targeting and pharmacological treatment of various pathologies within the CNS [68, 69]. The overview of both CVOs' anatomical and physiological features is described in Table 1.

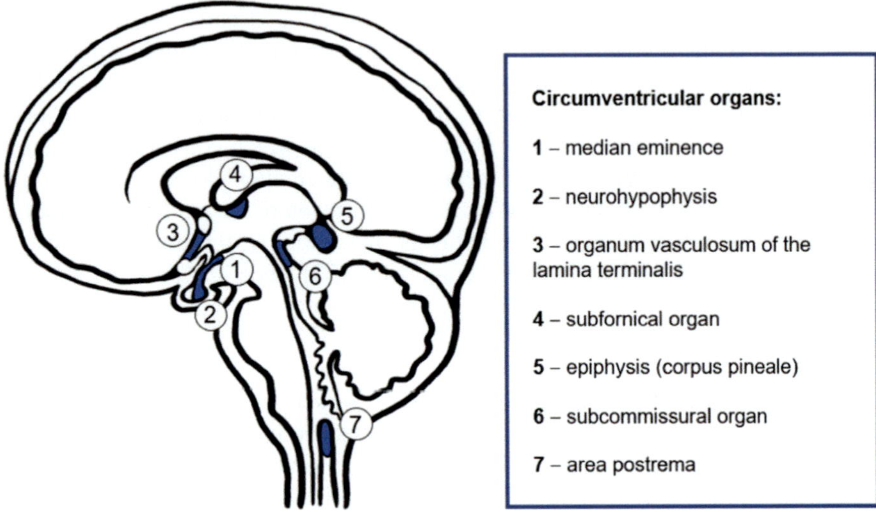

Fig. 4 Anatomy of circumventricular organs (CVOs)

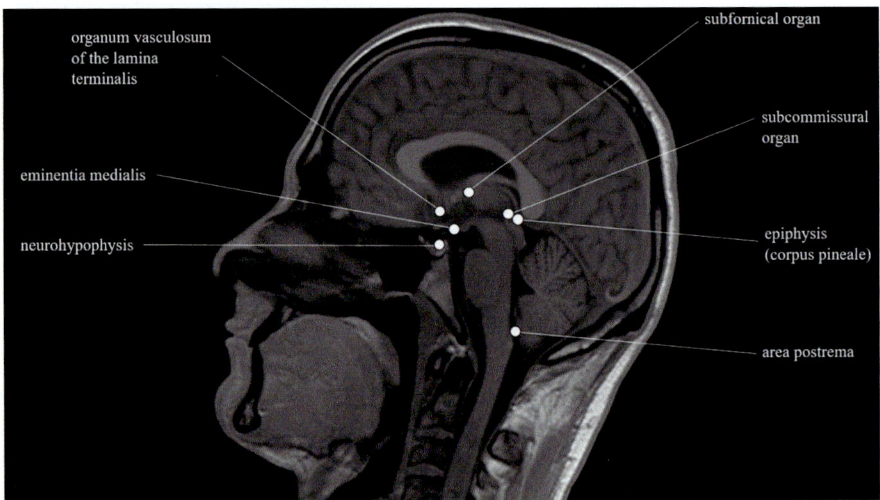

Fig. 5 Anatomy of circumventricular organs (CVOs) on MRI T1-WI

On the other hand, the BCB arises at the border between the capillaries of the choroid plexus inside the cerebral ventricles, which are characterised by fenestrations and the presence of gap, instead of tight junctions [52]. Unlike the BBB, the BCB comprises the endothelium of the pia mater with a single basal membrane (Fig. 6). This allows the motion of substances via ion channels and transmembrane enzymes, such as the Na^+/K^+-ATPase [5]. Furthermore, the BCB contains pinocytosis vesicles,

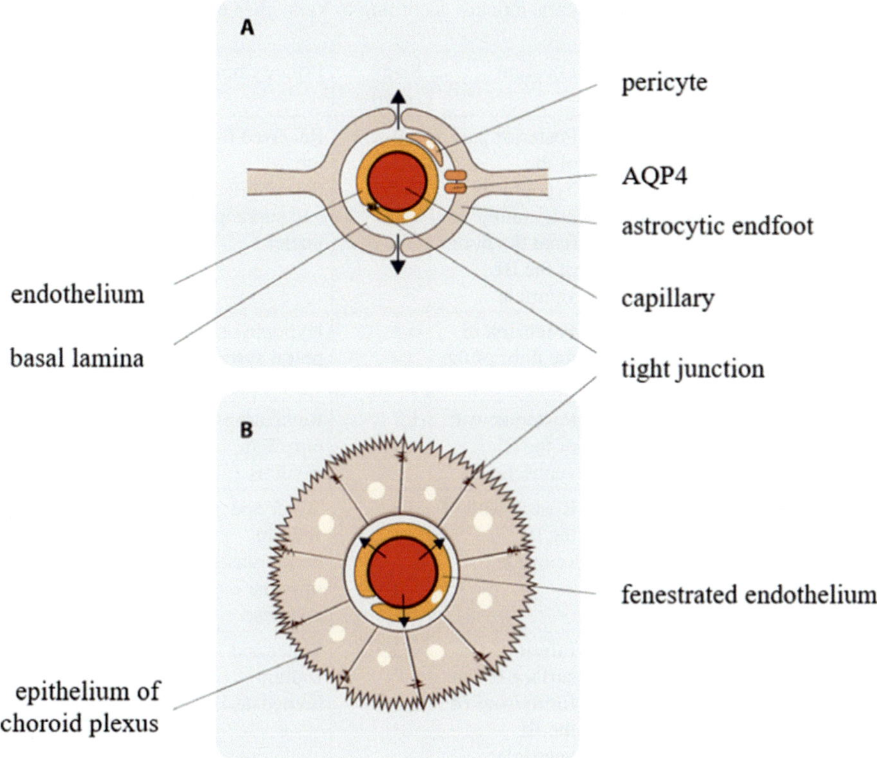

Fig. 6 The main anatomical differences between BBB and BCB that subsequently importantly involve their physiological functions

which are involved in the metabolism of protein filtration and their segregation [63, 64, 70]. In accordance with this description, Reiber in 1994 [71] defined a formula explaining that the reduction of CSF flow (for example in the case of impaired BCB function) is associated with the obstruction of vascular proteins inside the circulatory system, thus resulting in higher rates of transported proteins via the BCB into CSF [5, 64]. Conversely, the rates of CNS-derived proteins are not primarily influenced by BCB dysfunction [72].

4   CSF Composition

CSF is a clear, watery fluid with a low concentration of protein and cellular components. As we describe more in detail below, CSF is produced via plasma filtration and membrane secretion [50] and therefore, it differs in terms of its molecular content when compared to the blood plasma alone. Under normal circumstances, erythrocytes

Table 1 The overview of CVOs characteristics according to Verheggen et al. [69], licensed under CC-BY-4.0

	Type	Location	Size (mm)	Primary function	Hormones
Neurohypophysis	Secretory	Posterior part of the hypophysis originating from the floor of the III ventricle	1.0–2.9	Received from the paraventricular and supraoptic nuclei	Vasopressin, oxytocin
Median eminence	Secretory	Extension of the floor of the III ventricle	0.3	Hypophyseal portal system	Vasopressin, oxytocin
Pineal gland	Secretory	Posterior wall of the III ventricle	1.7	Regulating circadian rhythms	Melatonin
Subfornical organ	Sensory	Rostral wall of the III ventricle	0.2	Water and sodium homeostasis and immune response	Angiotensin II, cytokines
Ogranum vasculosum of the lamina terminalis	Sensory	Inferior surface of the fornix/roof of the III ventricle	0.3–0.6	Water and sodium homeostasis	Angiotensin II
Area postrema	Sensory	Floor of the IV ventricle	0.5	Opening the central canal, cardiovascular, and respiratory regulation and controlling the vomiting centre	Substance P

Besides the mentioned functions, CVOs are essential for allowing the inflammatory mediators to enter the CNS if any infections or pathological states are present. The paper is an Open Access article distributed under the terms of the Creative Commons Attribution License, which permits unrestricted use, distribution, and reproduction in any medium, provided the original work is properly credited

are not found in CSF, whilst some of the nucleated cells, predominantly lymphocytes and monocytes, are present. The most common CSF protein is albumin (50–70%), followed by immunoglobulins [15]. At this point, it should be noted that the CSF protein concentration and its flow rate vary since these measures are influenced by many factors, including the CSF sampling site, circadian variations, clearance, or physical effort [73, 74].

Unlike in other organ systems, the immunological mechanisms of the CSF do not involve any lymphatics in the traditional sense. Additionally, the presence of

Table 2 The comparison of CSF and blood plasma composition according to Hladky et al. [75], licensed under CC-BY-4.0

Component	Blood plasma	CSF
	Concentration/mg (100 ml)$^{-1}$	
Protein	6300 to 8500	16 to 38
Sugar	80 to 120	45 to 80
Amino acids	4.5 to 9	1.5 to 3
Creatinine	0.7 to 2	0.5 to 2.2
Uric acid	2.9 to 6.9	0.4 to 2.8
Urea	22 to 42	5 to 39
Cholesterol	100 to 150	trace
Lactic acid	10 to 32	8 to 25
Phosphate *	4.7	3.4
	Concentration/mmol kg^{-1}	
Na^+	150	147
K^+	4.63	2.86
Ca^{2+}	2.35	1.14
Mg^{2+}	0.8	1.1
Cl^-	99	113
$HCO3^-$	26.8	23.3
pH	7.4	7.3

* Inorganic. The paper is an Open Access article distributed under the terms of the Creative Commons Attribution License, which permits unrestricted use, distribution, and reproduction in any medium, provided the original work is properly credited

immunoglobulins in CSF is very low. Instead, immunological protection is accomplished by the system of CSF exchange across the extracellular space and microglial tissue [76]. In the elderly, however, the immunological activity of the microglial system is suppressed, which subsequently manifests by impaired function of specific proteins and other substances, therefore increasing the risk of neurodegenerative disease onset [77, 78].

5   CSF Functions

Primarily, CSF is responsible for the protection, waste clearance, and metabolic pathways in the CNS that we describe more in detail below. In most textbooks, CSF is described as a fluid providing mechanical protection of neuroaxis since it softens the external forces pushing against the skull in cases of traumatic injuries and reduces the effective weight of the brain itself. Normally, the brain weighs approximately 1500 g, and the fluid reduces this number by 30 times to an effective net weight of 50 g in total

[13, 15, 79, 80]. Moreover, CSF is responsible for maintaining CNS homeostasis as it regulates electrolyte and catabolite concentrations [81]. The majority of macromolecules that are not found in CSF in higher concentrations (for example amino acids, glucose etc.) are directed to the brain parenchyma primarily across the BBB [15, 82]. There are several substances, including methyltetrahydrofolate or vitamin C, which are transported into brain tissue directly from the CSF where they occur due to the previous process of blood plasma filtration [15, 82, 83].

6 CSF Mechanisms

6.1 Production and Secretion

In the majority of reports, the production of CSF is limited to approximately 500 ml per day which stands for roughly 0.3–0.4 ml per minute [84, 85], and a decreased CSF production rate has been observed in healthy elderly [86]. There is a well-established idea that the majority (60 85%) of CSF is secreted by the choroid plexuses and the tela choroidea (the lateral ventricles being the primary source) [20, 80, 87], whilst the rest is formed via extrachoroidal sources. Choroid plexuses are highly vascularised structures composed of a single layer of epithelium (cuboidal or cylindrical), their surface is ensheathed by microvilli [12, 88, 89]. The CSF secretion via the choroid plexus may be divided into two major stages. In the first stage, as a result of hydrostatic pressure, the blood plasma is passively filtered through the fenestrated capillaries of the choroidal endothelium. The second stage involves active CSF secretion across the apical side of the choroidal epithelium and into the ventricular system. Other studies additionally define the ependymal lining of the ventricular cavities as a secondary source of CSF secretion [90, 91]. It is important to note that CSF production is a selective mechanism, especially due to the tight junctions that are responsible for preventing paracellular motion of metabolites inside the ventricular cavity [92].

The filtration of blood plasma itself is a complex mechanism dependent on the activity of apical membrane Na^+/K^+-ATPase which maintains the ion concentration gradient across the cell membrane (Fig. 7) [92–94]. Released Na^+ is in accordance with Na^+/K^+-ATPase activity carried via one of three transporters (Na^+/H^+, Na^+-dependent $Cl^-/HCO3^-$, or $Na^+/HCO3^-$ transporter) [12, 75, 93–96]. These transporters are needed to control the motion of particles such as Cl^- and HCO_3^-, (specifically one Cl^- in exchange for one Na^+ and two $HCO3^-$) that cross the basolateral side of choroid epithelium to move according to the osmotic gradient to its apical side and finally reach CSF [93, 94]. Cl^- itself enters the ventricular system via K^+/CL^- or electroneutral apical $Na^+/K^+/2Cl^-$ co-transporter. The transport of abovementioned ions involves the osmotic balance, fundamental for H_2O secretion. One of the most important water co-transporters fundamental for CSF secretion, NKCC1, is found on the apical side of the choroid epithelium. It has been recently

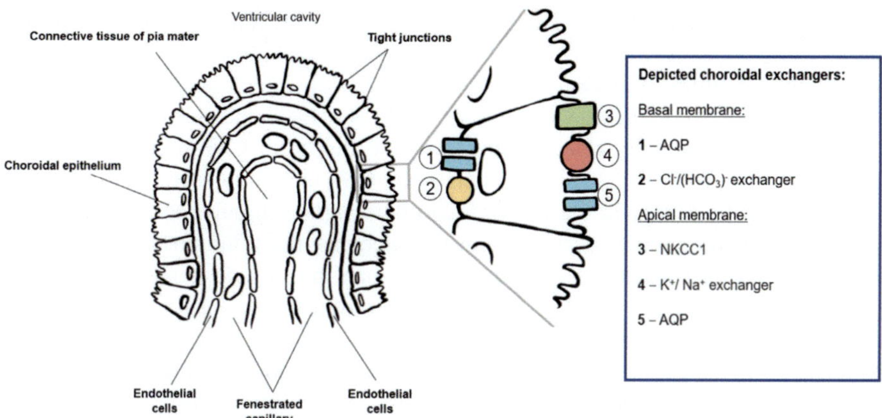

Fig. 7 Choroid plexus and its role in CSF production

shown that this bidirectional transporter is fundamental for water exchange within choroid plexuses in adults [97].

Interestingly, it has been observed in animal models (dog and rabbit) that the inhibition of Na^+/K^+-ATPase with ouabain, also known as g-strophanthin [98], causes a significant reduction of CSF production, by up to 80% [99, 100]. The motion of H_2O across the cellular membrane is accomplished and influenced by the expression of aquaporins (AQPs) in the choroid plexus, especially AQP1 [101]. AQPs, which to date consist of eleven members named AQP0 to AQP10 [102], are membrane channel proteins including a total of six transmembrane alpha helices with both terminal domains responsible for water transportation amongst cells [23, 103–105].

6.2 Classical Hypothesis and Its Criticism

Considered to be one of the fathers of neurosurgery, American physician and scientist Walter E. Dandy set the cornerstones for the classical model of CSF production in the first half of the twentieth century [20, 106]. The hypothesis is based on Dandy's surgical experiments involving unilateral choroid plexectomy and the bilateral obstruction of the foramen of Monro in a dog, both conducted in 1919 [107]. Dandy observed that ventricular dilation was not present if the choroid plexus was utterly removed, and therefore, he thought of choroid plexus as the origin of CSF production. Unfortunately, his experiments were performed on a single dog and never have been reproduced [20, 108]. In the 1970s, Milhorat with his colleagues [109–112], performed choroid plexectomy in a similar manner in a human and monkey, but could not confirm abnormal changes in the CSF production rate or its composition. Although Tamburrini et al. [113] endoscopically bilaterally removed choroid plexuses, they postoperatively did not find any significant changes in CSF secretion rate.

Almost a century after Dandy's findings, and with the classical model of CSF production preserved, Oreskovic and Klarica [114] revised and clarified the findings in the field, subsequently rejecting the classical model of CSF production. Other recent findings [108, 114, 115] have stated that CSF is mainly secreted in response to hydrostatic pressure via the cerebral capillaries. The impulse to investigate the origin of CSF production derives from the fact that the total surface of cerebral capillaries is approximately 5000 times larger than the surface of choroid plexuses of intracerebral ventricles [20], and therefore, cerebral capillaries may have a higher impact on CSF production than choroid plexuses alone. The mechanism of CSF production via the capillary system is believed to be dependent on the physiological involvement of intracranial hydrostatic pressure and metabolic pathways through the pia mater, ependymal tissue, and the interchange of intercellular elements inside the brain parenchyma [114, 116, 117].

Recently, the so-called "third model" [95] of CSF production was introduced by combining both the abovementioned theories about CSF secretion into a single mathematical model [118]. The authors investigated the role of Starling forces on water transport in the brain and propose that the model enables prediction of the effects of extracellular osmolarity, CSF, and blood on the intracranial motion of water, and thus may clarify a relationship between osmolarity itself and pathological states related to its impairment, including hydrocephalus or brain oedema.

6.3   Circulation and Dynamics

There are two major concepts explaining CSF circulation: (1) bulk flow and (2) pulsatile flow [5]. In the bulk flow model, hydrostatic forces cause a pressure gradient between the choroid plexuses inside the ventricular system (as the production site with higher pressure) and arachnoid granulations (as the absorption site with lower pressure), considering that the CSF flow is unidirectional (Fig. 8). This concept implies that the CSF flows from the lateral ventricles to the third ventricle via the foramen of Monro and subsequently to the fourth ventricle through the Sylvian aqueduct, where it enters the ventricular system to the central canal of the spinal cord or subarachnoid space via foramina of Luschka and Magendie. However, further investigations of CSF circulation, primarily by phase-contrast MRI, have doubted the bulk flow model, since CSF dynamics seems to be more complex and dependent on additional factors, including arterial pulsatile flow, jugular venous pressure, and respiratory waves. Therefore, the values of CSF pressure may also vary. Under normal circumstances, CSF pressure is around 10–15 mmHg in healthy adults and 3–4 mmHg in infants [2]. According to many recent suggestions [11, 117, 119], CSF circulation should be considered to be a combination of the bulk as well as the pulsatile flow, to-and-fro movement, and fluid exchange between the BBB and ISF.

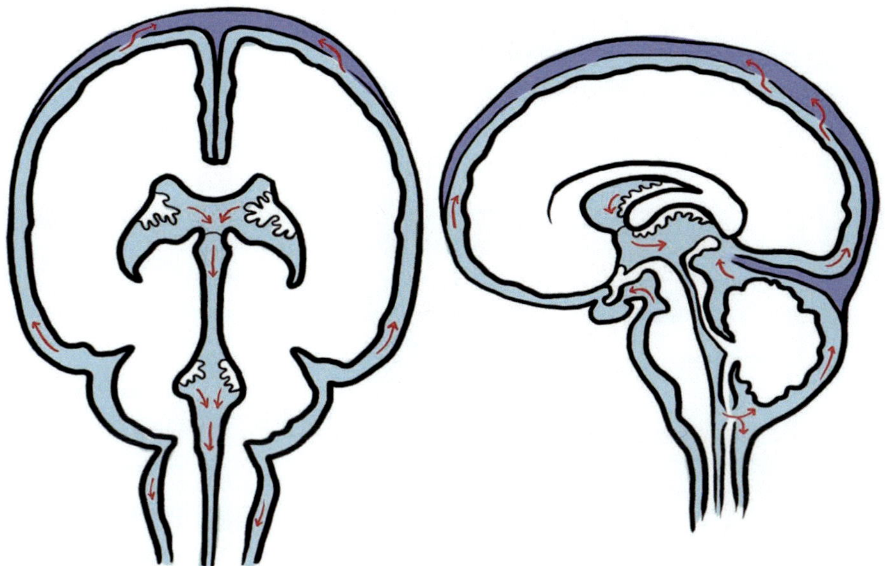

Fig. 8 Illustration of the CSF bulk flow model. Red arrows show the direction of CSF flow, according to the bulk model only unidirectional

6.4 The Glymphatic System

It has been recently hypothesised [120] that the perivascular spaces, also known as Virchow-Robin spaces, comprise a complex system of fluid interchange and waste clearance inside the brain comparable to the lymphatic pathways in other organ systems. Virchow-Robin spaces, formed from penetrating arterioles and ensheathed by a leptomeningeal cellular membrane and externally with glia limitans, are filled with CSF [95, 121]. The term "glymphatic system", referring to the combination of glial and lymphatic compartments involved in its functioning, was coined in 2012 by Iliff et al. [122] when they used *in vivo* two-photon microscopy in mice. They compared the functions of the perivascular space to a "conduit" of CSF drainage along the meninges, cranial nerves and vessels directed to the lymphatic system, and further subdivided the glymphatic pathway into four stages. In the first stage, CSF is transported from the basal cisterns into the cortical subarachnoid spaces, and from here it is directed into periarterial spaces in accordance with the bulk flow concept. In the second stage, CSF runs into the ISF via AQP4 channels found on astrocytic endfeet regions [5, 102, 103, 123, 124]. This process is critical since the mixture of CSF and ISF further enables waste solute removal [125]. The third and fourth stages include the fluid dispersion and subsequent transport of CSF and ISF directly into the perivenous spaces of the larger cerebral veins, eventually reaching the circulatory system (Fig. 9) [122, 125, 126].

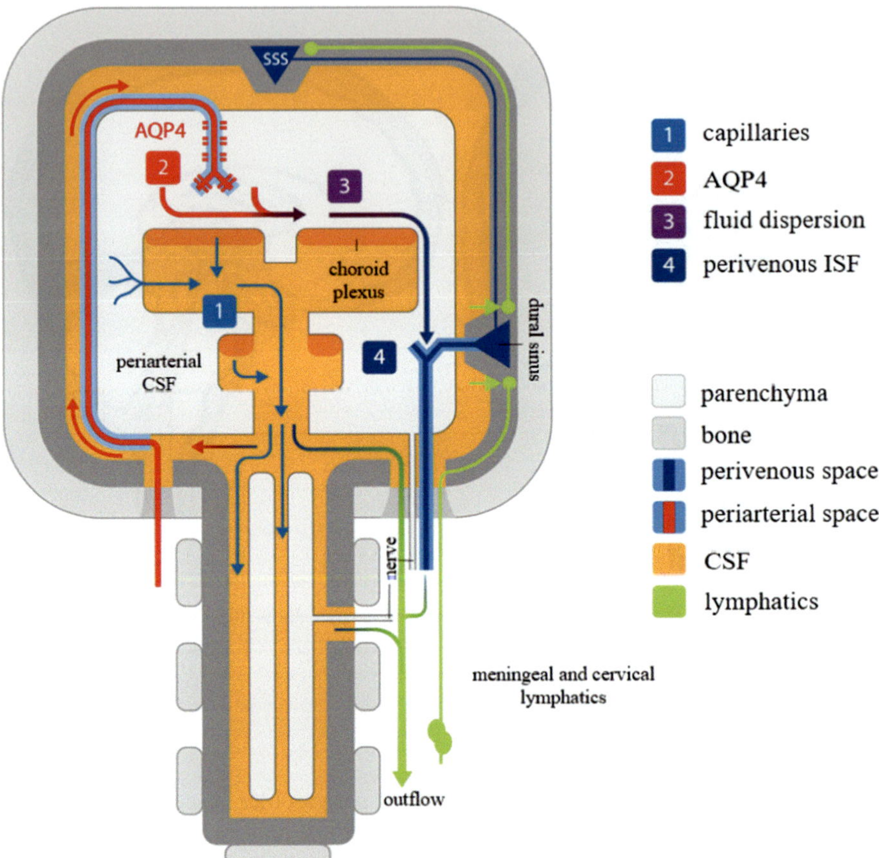

Fig. 9 Schematic diagram of glymphatic system functioning

In the CNS, the majority of the water volume is spread within intracellular space, whilst only approximately 32–40% falls into extracellular areas [95]. The latter comprises ISF, which surrounds the parenchymal cells, CSF, and blood vasculature (Fig. 10). Recent research dedicated to intracranial fluid movement has been proposed that the perivascular drainage of ISF occurs throughout the brain (Fig. 11) [119–121] rather than being limited to specific cerebral structures. Additionally, many studies have investigated the role of the glymphatic system in neurodegenerative disorders, particularly Alzheimer's disease, when considering the abnormal and altered accumulation of metabolites with subsequently increased toxicity, such as amyloid-beta or tau proteins [115, 127, 128]. It has been proposed that the glymphatic system plays a crucial role as an important clearance mechanism in removing neurodegeneration-related proteins. Its impairment may, therefore, enhance the progression of protein accumulation within the brain [129–132]. Dysfunction of or alterations in glymphatic

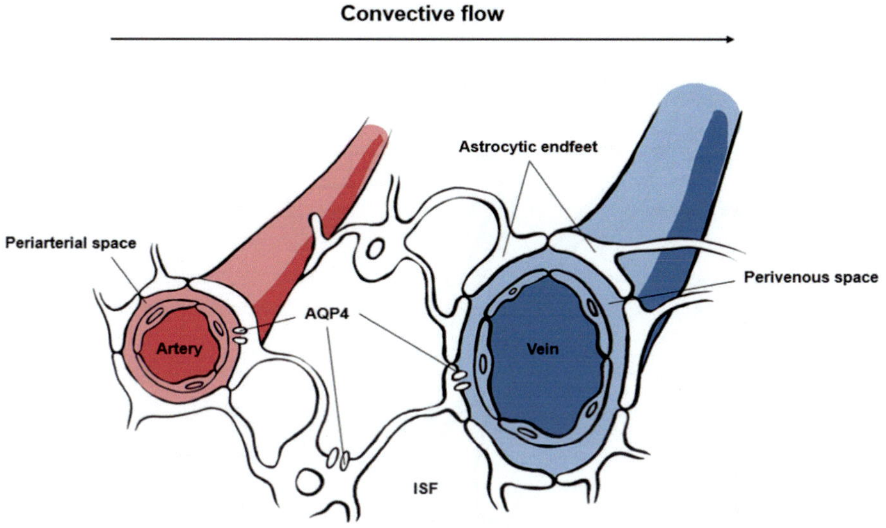

Fig. 10 The glymphatic pathway

pathways are mainly caused by abnormal AQP4 functioning or its reduced expression. Some studies suggest that deficiency of AQP4 may affect the regeneration of neurons after CNS traumatic injuries or, as mentioned above, the neurodegeneration itself [130, 133–135].

Interestingly, although the energy metabolism within the brain decreases approximately by 25% during sleep [136], recent findings [137] suggest that the glymphatic function is dramatically enhanced during sleep. Such results would imply that clearance of metabolic waste is primarily accomplished during sleep [95, 138, 139]. Although there is still a lack of studies dedicated to the topic, sufficient sleep duration seems to be of greater importance than previously believed and may be associated with long-term positive effects of glymphatic pathway functioning.

Despite an enormous amount of research dedicated to the concept of the glymphatic system, there is an existing controversy surrounding our understanding of it. The initial hypothesis of the glymphatic system is built on the idea of bulk flow being the main driving force of the fluid movement within the brain, i.e. the transfer of the CSF to ISF in the parenchyma. However, as we described earlier, bulk flow does not completely explain CSF movement since the CSF flow is much more complex and the explanation of its causes by unidirectional flow is inadequate [140]. Diffusion, rather than the bulk flow, is the decisive factor involved in the transportation of substances within the ISF. Interestingly, a recent study [141] questioned the extent of AQP4 involvement in the glymphatic pathway, based on mathematical modelling applying Navier-Stokes and convection-diffusion equations. The authors showed that the resistance against permeation of H_2O molecules via astrocytic endfeet is higher in comparison to the surrounding spaces between the individual endfeet and therefore, the movement of the extracellular fluid is not very likely supported by AQP4 water

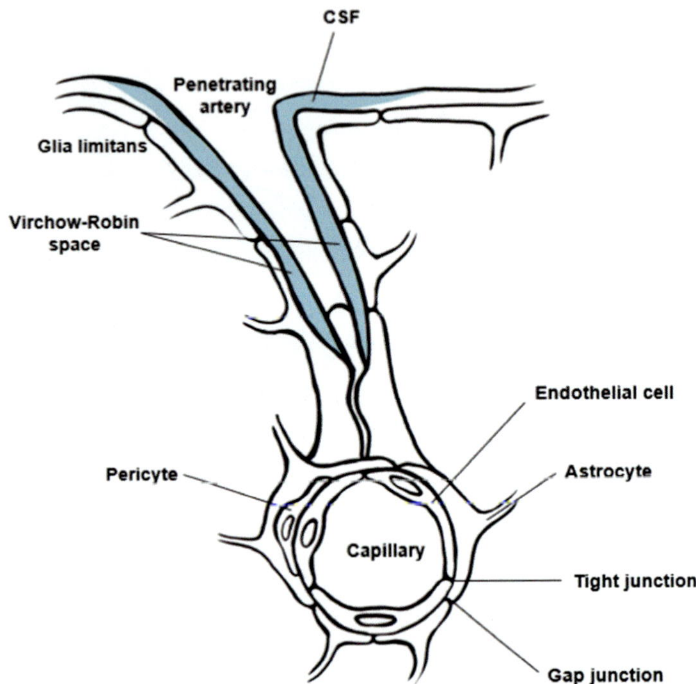

Fig. 11 The depiction of Virchow-Robin spaces in the neurovascular unit

permeability. Above all, although these studies have encouraging findings, there is still a need for larger and prospective studies in order to elucidate our concept of glymphatic functioning in more detail.

6.5   *Absorption*

Since Pacchioni in the eighteenth century described the "extrusions of the cranial membrane", now named arachnoid granulations, a lot of research has revealed contradictory findings about their role in CSF absorption processes. For a long time it was believed, in accordance with the aforementioned Dandy's surgical experiments [106, 107, 142] and Cushing's examinations [143], that CSF absorption is not primarily performed in the brain. It also should be noted that arachnoid granulations should not be interchangeably called arachnoid villi—villi are described as microscopic tissues, whereas granulations are recognisable by a naked eye [92, 144]. During the twentieth century, many researchers [145, 146] defined arachnoid villi and granulations as the primary CSF absorption sites. Further research, however, contradicts this. In

1974, Tripathi et al. [147, 148] described the existence of tight junctions inside the epithelial layers of arachnoid villi, and simultaneously proposed that there are no other openings that may serve as CSF absorption pathways. Later on, the structure of the villi was described more in detail—they are composed of four layers: a central core, cap cell, cell layer of arachnoid membrane, and a fibrous capsule [149, 150]. Instead of epithelium, which may or may not be present, arachnoid cells ensheath the villi, both in their internal and external membranes (Fig. 12).

According to the newest research in this field, the arachnoid villi themselves have only a minor role in CSF clearance, primarily in the case of increased ICP [151, 152]. Therefore, there must be different mechanisms involved in CSF absorption. CSF may be partiality absorbed via cranial and spinal nerve sheaths (primarily the optical, trigeminal, facial, auditory nerves, or lumbar spinal nerves [20]) ependymal tissue, extracellular fluid according to the pressure gradients, and directly to the ISF via perivascular spaces, which we already described above [14, 20, 117, 152, 153]. Based on historical and current research on additional CSF absorption sites, it is well established that the CSF drainage is impaired if the CSF pathways leading to the lymphatic system are obstructed [152]. Interestingly, the absorption of CSF may be additionally accomplished within the ventricular cavities through the transependymal exchange, finally resulting in full CSF absorption in the periventricular capillaries [8, 116].

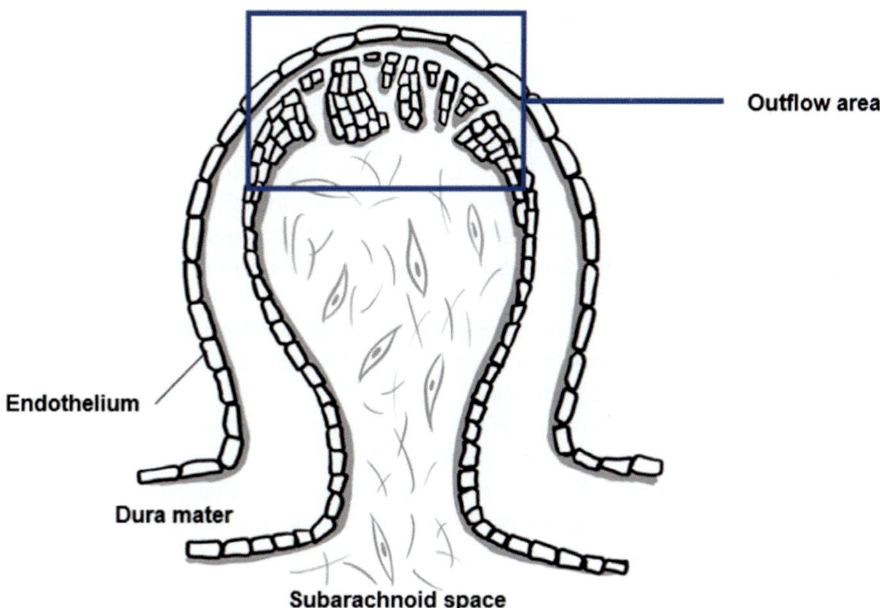

Fig. 12 The arachnoid villi and their function in CSF absorption mechanism

7 Conclusion

The classical model of CSF dynamics seems to be based on misinterpretations over time, without explicitly relevant evidence to support its statements. Recently introduced "new" models are becoming more widely accepted, with reproducible results. It is currently unclear how much and where the CSF is produced, but it is certain that the choroid plexuses are not a single CSF secretion origin. Nevertheless, they undeniably play a role in CSF formation together with the glymphatic system and the formation of CSF from cerebral capillaries. Rather than being unidirectional, CSF circulation seems to be a combination of many mechanisms dependent not only on the balance and regulation of CSF production and absorption, but also on overall physiological and pathophysiological changes in the human body. Recent findings devoted to the functional role of aquaporins, and other water transport channels imply an underestimated importance of water exchange in the understanding of CSF physiology since a lot of research so far has only considered only classical CSF flow concepts.

8 Key Points

- CSF secretion is not limited exclusively to choroid plexuses, and the arachnoid villi are not the only sites of CSF absorption.
- The production of CSF is most likely accomplished at various cerebral regions via several pathways. Attention should be paid to hypotheses of CSF production that correspond to hydrostatic and osmotic gradients along the cerebral capillaries and recent findings should be implemented for future research.
- CSF circulation should be considered to be a combination of both uni- and bidirectional flow concepts, to-and-fro movement, and fluid exchange mechanisms rather than taken unequivocally according to the classical, unfortunately misleading, bulk flow model.
- The glymphatic system plays a vital role in CSF metabolism and its detailed mechanism pathways should be elucidated more clearly in both physiological and pathophysiological conditions.
- The ISF and CSF are closely linked to maintaining homeostasis and providing the waste clearance mechanisms within the CNS.
- The role of arachnoid villi in CSF absorption has been overestimated. CSF is primarily absorbed via unique pathways into the lymphatic circulation, ependyma, and extracellular fluid.

Funding This chapter was supported by the Ministry of Health of the Czech Republic institutional grant no. NU23-04-00551.

References

1. Deisenhammer F. The history of cerebrospinal fluid. In: Deisenhammer F, Sellebjerg F, Teunissen CE, Tumani H, editors. Cerebrospinal fluid in clinical neurology. Cham: Springer International Publishing; 2015. p. 3–16. https://doi.org/10.1007/978-3-319-01225-4_1.
2. Sakka L, Coll G, Chazal J. Anatomy and physiology of cerebrospinal fluid. Eur Ann Otorhinolaryngol Head Neck Dis. 2011;128:309–16. https://doi.org/10.1016/j.anorl.2011.03.002.
3. Killer HE, Subramanian PS. Compartmentalized cerebrospinal fluid. Int Ophthalmol Clin. 2014;54:95–102. https://doi.org/10.1097/iio.0000000000000010.
4. Toro EF, Thornber B, Zhang Q, Scoz A, Contarino C. A computational model for the dynamics of cerebrospinal fluid in the spinal subarachnoid space. J Biomech Eng. 2019;141. https://doi.org/10.1115/1.4041551.
5. Tumani H, Huss A, Bachhuber F. The cerebrospinal fluid and barriers—anatomic and physiologic considerations. Handb Clin Neurol. 2017;146:21–32. https://doi.org/10.1016/B978-0-12-804279-3.00002-2.
6. Ghersi-Egea J-F, Strazielle N, Catala M, Silva-Vargas V, Doetsch F, Engelhardt B. Molecular anatomy and functions of the choroidal blood-cerebrospinal fluid barrier in health and disease. Acta Neuropathol. 2018;135:337–61. https://doi.org/10.1007/s00401-018-1807-1.
7. Hodel J, Lebret A, Petit E, Leclerc X, Zins M, Vignaud A, Decq P, Rahmouni A. Imaging of the entire cerebrospinal fluid volume with a multistation 3D SPACE MR sequence: feasibility study in patients with hydrocephalus. Eur Radiol. 2013;23:1450–8. https://doi.org/10.1007/s00330-012-2732-7.
8. Proulx ST. Cerebrospinal fluid outflow: a review of the historical and contemporary evidence for arachnoid villi, perineural routes, and dural lymphatics. Cell Mol Life Sci: CMLS. 2021;78:2429–57. https://doi.org/10.1007/s00018-020-03706-5.
9. Chazen JL, Dyke JP, Holt RW, Horky L, Pauplis RA, Hesterman JY, Mozley DP, Verma A. Automated segmentation of MR imaging to determine normative central nervous system cerebrospinal fluid volumes in healthy volunteers. Clin Imaging. 2017;43:132–5. https://doi.org/10.1016/j.clinimag.2017.02.007.
10. Alperin N, Bagci AM, Lee SH, Lam BL. Automated quantitation of spinal CSF volume and measurement of craniospinal CSF redistribution following lumbar withdrawal in idiopathic intracranial hypertension. Am J Neuroradiol. 2016;37:1957–63. https://doi.org/10.3174/ajnr.a4837.
11. Brinker T, Stopa E, Morrison J, Klinge P. A new look at cerebrospinal fluid circulation. Fluids Barriers CNS. 2014;11:10. https://doi.org/10.1186/2045-8118-11-10.
12. Damkier HH, Brown PD, Praetorius J. Cerebrospinal fluid secretion by the choroid plexus. Physiol Rev. 2013;93:1847–92. https://doi.org/10.1152/physrev.00004.2013.
13. Evolving concepts of cerebrospinal fluid physiology. Neurosurg Clin North Am;12:631–38. https://doi.org/10.1016/S1042-3680(18)30021-4.
14. Greitz D. Cerebrospinal fluid circulation and associated intracranial dynamics. A radiologic investigation using MR imaging and radionuclide cisternography. Acta Radiol Suppl. 1993;386:1–23.
15. Spector R, Robert Snodgrass S, Johanson CE. A balanced view of the cerebrospinal fluid composition and functions: focus on adult humans. Exp Neurol. 2015;273:57–68. https://doi.org/10.1016/j.expneurol.2015.07.027.
16. Wright BL, Lai JT, Sinclair AJ. Cerebrospinal fluid and lumbar puncture: a practical review. J Neurol. 2012;259:1530–45. https://doi.org/10.1007/s00415-012-6413-x.
17. Bothwell SW, Janigro D, Patabendige A. Cerebrospinal fluid dynamics and intracranial pressure elevation in neurological diseases. Fluids Barriers CNS. 2019;16. https://doi.org/10.1186/s12987-019-0129-6.
18. Vinje V, Eklund A, Mardal K-A, Rognes ME, Støverud K-H. Intracranial pressure elevation alters CSF clearance pathways. Fluids Barriers CNS. 2020;17. https://doi.org/10.1186/s12987-020-00189-1.

19. Wilson MH. Monro-Kellie 2.0: the dynamic vascular and venous pathophysiological components of intracranial pressure. J Cereb Blood Flow Metab. 2016;36:1338–50. https://doi.org/10.1177/0271678x16648711.

20. Chikly B, Quaghebeur J. Reassessing cerebrospinal fluid (CSF) hydrodynamics: a literature review presenting a novel hypothesis for CSF physiology. J Bodyw Mov Ther. 2013;17:344–54. https://doi.org/10.1016/j.jbmt.2013.02.002.

21. Greitz D, Greitz T, Hindmarsh T. We need a new understanding of the reabsorption of cerebrospinal fluid–II. Acta Paediatr. 1997;86:1148. https://doi.org/10.1111/j.1651-2227.1997.tb14828.x.

22. Igarashi H, Suzuki Y, Kwee IL, Nakada T. Water influx into cerebrospinal fluid is significantly reduced in senile plaque bearing transgenic mice, supporting beta-amyloid clearance hypothesis of Alzheimer's disease. Neurol Res. 2014;36:1094–8. https://doi.org/10.1179/1743132814y.0000000434.

23. Tait MJ, Saadoun S, Bell BA, Papadopoulos MC. Water movements in the brain: role of aquaporins. Trends Neurosci. 2008;31:37–43. https://doi.org/10.1016/j.tins.2007.11.003.

24. Van Middendorp JJ, Sanchez GM, Burridge AL. The Edwin Smith papyrus: a clinical reappraisal of the oldest known document on spinal injuries. Eur Spine J. 2010;19:1815–23. https://doi.org/10.1007/s00586-010-1523-6.

25. Clarke E, O'Malley CD. The human brain and spinal cord: a historical study illustrated by writings from antiquity to the twentieth century. In: Medical history, vol. 2. 2nd ed. Norman Neurosciences Series; 1996. https://doi.org/10.1017/S0025727300063948.

26. Wilkins RH. neurosurgical classic. XVII. J Neurosurg. 1964;21:240–4. https://doi.org/10.3171/jns.1964.21.3.0240.

27. Matsumae M, Sato O, Hirayama A, Hayashi N, Takizawa K, Atsumi H, Sorimachi T. Research into the physiology of cerebrospinal fluid reaches a new horizon: intimate exchange between cerebrospinal fluid and interstitial fluid may contribute to maintenance of homeostasis in the central nervous system. Neurol Med Chir. 2016;56:416–41. https://doi.org/10.2176/nmc.ra.2016-0020.

28. Quin CE. The soul and the pneuma in the function of the nervous system after Galen. J R Soc Med. 1994;87:393–5.

29. Woollam DH. The historical significance of the cerebrospinal fluid. Med Hist. 1957;1:91–114. https://doi.org/10.1017/s0025727300021025.

30. Sudhoff W. Die Lehre von den Hirnventrikeln in textlicher und graphischer Tradition des Altertums und Mittelalters. Arch Gesch Med. 1914;7:149–205.

31. Clark E. A catalogue of the drawings of Leonardo da Vinci in the collection of His Majesty the King at Windsor Castle; 1935.

32. Joutsivuo T. Vesalius and De humani corporis fabrica: Galen's errors and the change of anatomy in the sixteenth century. Hippokrates (Helsinki); 1997. p. 98–112.

33. Steele L. Andreas Vesalius and his De humani corporis Fabrica libri septem. Vesalius. 2014;20:5–10.

34. Varolius C. De Nervis Opticis nonnulisque aliis praeter communem opinionem in Humano capite observatis. Meietti Fratres, Padova 1573.

35. Delaidelli A, Moiraghi A. Respiration: a new mechanism for CSF circulation? J Neurosci. 2017;37:7076–8. https://doi.org/10.1523/JNEUROSCI.1155-17.2017.

36. Vieussens R. Neurographia universalis. Joannem Certe, Lyon 1685.

37. Ruysch F. Opera omnia anatomico-medico-chirurgica. Apud Janssonio-Waesbergios, Amsterdam 1737.

38. Pacchionus A. De Glandulis Conglobatis Durae Meningis Humanae indeque Ortis Lymphaticis ad Piam Meningem productis. Cesarius Leopodinus University, Rome 1705.

39. Di Ieva A, Yaşargil MG. Liquor cotunnii: the history of cerebrospinal fluid in Domenico Cotugno's work. Neurosurgery. 2008;63:352–58; discussion 358. https://doi.org/10.1227/01.Neu.0000320438.99843.9f.

40. Cotugno D. De Ischiade Nervosa Commentarius. Fratrem Simonios, Neapolis 1764.

41. Magendie F. Recherches physiologiques et cliniques sur le liquide céphalo-rachidien ou cérébro-spinal. Paris: Méquignon-Marvis fils; 1842.

42. Quincke H. Die Lumbalpunction des Hydrocephalus. Berl Klin Wochenschr 1891, 28.

43. Quincke H. Über Hydrocephalus. Verh Congress Innere Med 1891.

44. Lichtheim L. Re: the proposal of Quincke to withdraw cerebrospinal fl uid by lumbar puncture in cases of brain disease. Dtsch Med Wochenschr 1893, 19.

45. Coico R. Gram staining. Curr Protoc Microbiol. 2005;Appendix 3:Appendix 3C https://doi. org/10.1002/9780471729259.mca03cs00.

46. Stratchko L, Filatova I, Agarwal A, Kanekar S. The Ventricular system of the brain: anatomy and normal variations. Semin Ultrasound CT MR. 2016;37:72–83. https://doi.org/10.1053/j. sult.2016.01.004.

47. Rubino JM, Hogg JP. Neuroanatomy, Cerebral Aqueduct (Sylvian). In: StatPearls. Treasure Island (FL): StatPearls Publishing, Copyright © 2021, StatPearls Publishing LLC.; 2021.

48. Storer KP, Toh J, Stoodley MA, Jones NR. The central canal of the human spinal cord: a computerised 3-D study. J Anat. 1998;192:565–72. https://doi.org/10.1046/j.1469-7580. 1998.19240565.x.

49. Saker E, Henry BM, Tomaszewski KA, Loukas M, Iwanaga J, Oskouian RJ, Tubbs RS. The human central canal of the spinal cord: a comprehensive review of its anatomy, embryology, molecular development, variants, and pathology. Cureus. 2016. https://doi.org/10.7759/cur eus.927.

50. Di Terlizzi R, Platt S. The function, composition and analysis of cerebrospinal fluid in companion animals: part I—function and composition. Vet J. 2006;172:422–31. https://doi. org/10.1016/j.tvjl.2005.07.021.

51. Daneman R, Prat A. The Blood-Brain Barrier. Cold Spring Harb Perspect Biol. 2015;7: a020412. https://doi.org/10.1101/cshperspect.a020412.

52. D'Agata F, Ruffinatti F, Boschi S, Stura I, Rainero I, Abollino O, Cavalli R, Guiot C. Magnetic nanoparticles in the central nervous system: targeting principles, applications and safety issues. Molecules. 2017;23:9. https://doi.org/10.3390/molecules23010009.

53. Abbott NJ, Patabendige AA, Dolman DE, Yusof SR, Begley DJ. Structure and function of the blood-brain barrier. Neurobiol Dis. 2010;37:13–25. https://doi.org/10.1016/j.nbd.2009. 07.030.

54. Ganong WF. Circumventricular organs: definition and role in the regulation of endocrine and autonomic function. Clin Exp Pharmacol Physiol. 2000;27:422–7. https://doi.org/10.1046/j. 1440-1681.2000.03259.x.

55. Kaur C, Ling EA. The circumventricular organs. Histol Histopathol. 2017;32:879–92. https:/ /doi.org/10.14670/hh-11-881.

56. Kiecker C. The origins of the circumventricular organs. J Anat. 2018;232:540–53. https://doi. org/10.1111/joa.12771.

57. Pandit R, Chen L, Götz J. The blood-brain barrier: physiology and strategies for drug delivery. Adv Drug Deliv Rev. 2020;165–166:1–14. https://doi.org/10.1016/j.addr.2019.11.009.

58. Jeong JK, Dow SA, Young CN. Sensory circumventricular organs, neuroendocrine control, and metabolic regulation. Metabolites. 2021;11:494. https://doi.org/10.3390/metabo110 80494.

59. McKinley MJ, McAllen RM, Davern P, Giles ME, Penschow J, Sunn N, Uschakov A, Oldfield BJ. The sensory circumventricular organs of the mammalian brain. Adv Anat Embryol Cell Biol. 2003;172:III–XII,1–122, back cover. https://doi.org/10.1007/978-3-642-55532-9.

60. Fry M, Ferguson AV. The sensory circumventricular organs: brain targets for circulating signals controlling ingestive behavior. Physiol Behav. 2007;91:413–23. https://doi.org/10. 1016/j.physbeh.2007.04.003.

61. Fry M, Hoyda TD, Ferguson AV. Making sense of it: roles of the sensory circumventricular organs in feeding and regulation of energy homeostasis. Exp Biol Med (Maywood). 2007;232:14–26.

62. Ferguson AV, Bains JS. Electrophysiology of the circumventricular organs. Front Neuroendocrinol. 1996;17:440–75. https://doi.org/10.1006/frne.1996.0012.

63. Saunders NR, Daneman R, Dziegielewska KM, Liddelow SA. Transporters of the blood-brain and blood-CSF interfaces in development and in the adult. Mol Aspects Med. 2013;34:742–52. https://doi.org/10.1016/j.mam.2012.11.006.

64. Solár P, Zamani A, Kubíčková L, Dubový P, Joukal M. Choroid plexus and the blood–cerebrospinal fluid barrier in disease. Fluids Barriers CNS. 2020;17. https://doi.org/10.1186/s12987-020-00196-2.

65. Cottrell GT, Ferguson AV. Sensory circumventricular organs: central roles in integrated autonomic regulation. Regul Pept. 2004;117:11–23. https://doi.org/10.1016/j.regpep.2003.09.004.

66. Pardridge WM. The blood-brain barrier: bottleneck in brain drug development. NeuroRx. 2005;2:3–14. https://doi.org/10.1602/neurorx.2.1.3.

67. Neuwelt E, Abbott NJ, Abrey L, Banks WA, Blakley B, Davis T, Engelhardt B, Grammas P, Nedergaard M, Nutt J, et al. Strategies to advance translational research into brain barriers. Lancet Neurol. 2008;7:84–96. https://doi.org/10.1016/s1474-4422(07)70326-5.

68. Johanson CE, Duncan JA, Stopa EG, Baird A. Enhanced prospects for drug delivery and brain targeting by the choroid plexus–CSF route. Pharm Res. 2005;22:1011–37. https://doi.org/10.1007/s11095-005-6039-0.

69. Verheggen ICM, De Jong JJA, Van Boxtel MPJ, Postma AA, Verhey FRJ, Jansen JFA, Backes WH. Permeability of the windows of the brain: feasibility of dynamic contrast-enhanced MRI of the circumventricular organs. Fluids Barriers CNS. 2020;17. https://doi.org/10.1186/s12987-020-00228-x.

70. Livrea P, Trojano M, Simone IL, Zimatore GB, Pisicchio L, Logroscino G, Cibelli G. Heterogeneous models for blood-cerebrospinal fluid barrier permeability to serum proteins in normal and abnormal cerebrospinal fluid/serum protein concentration gradients. J Neurol Sci. 1984;64:245–58. https://doi.org/10.1016/0022-510x(84)90173-4.

71. Reiber H. Flow rate of cerebrospinal fluid (CSF)—a concept common to normal blood-CSF barrier function and to dysfunction in neurological diseases. J Neurol Sci. 1994;122:189–203. https://doi.org/10.1016/0022-510X(94)90298-4.

72. Süssmuth SD, Reiber H, Tumani H. Tau protein in cerebrospinal fluid (CSF): a blood–CSF barrier related evaluation in patients with various neurological diseases. Neurosci Lett. 2001;300:95–8. https://doi.org/10.1016/S0304-3940(01)01556-7.

73. Nilsson C, Ståhlberg F, Thomsen C, Henriksen O, Herning M, Owman C. Circadian variation in human cerebrospinal fluid production measured by magnetic resonance imaging. Am J Physiol. 1992;262:R20-24. https://doi.org/10.1152/ajpregu.1992.262.1.R20.

74. Xu Q, Yu S-B, Zheng N, Yuan X-Y, Chi Y-Y, Liu C, Wang X-M, Lin X-T, Sui H-J. Head movement, an important contributor to human cerebrospinal fluid circulation. Sci Rep. 2016;6:31787. https://doi.org/10.1038/srep31787.

75. Hladky SB, Barrand MA. Mechanisms of fluid movement into, through and out of the brain: evaluation of the evidence. Fluids Barriers CNS. 2014;11:26. https://doi.org/10.1186/2045-8118-11-26.

76. Wake H, Moorhouse AJ, Jinno S, Kohsaka S, Nabekura J. Resting microglia directly monitor the functional state of synapses in vivo and determine the fate of ischemic terminals. J Neurosci. 2009;29:3974–80. https://doi.org/10.1523/jneurosci.4363-08.2009.

77. Kan MJ, Lee JE, Wilson JG, Everhart AL, Brown CM, Hoofnagle AN, Jansen M, Vitek MP, Gunn MD, Colton CA. Arginine deprivation and immune suppression in a mouse model of Alzheimer's disease. J Neurosci. 2015;35:5969–82. https://doi.org/10.1523/jneurosci.4668-14.2015.

78. Streit WJ, Xue QS. The brain's aging immune system. Aging Dis. 2010;1:254–61.

79. Puntis M, Reddy U, Hirsch N. Cerebrospinal fluid and its physiology. Anaesth Intensive Care Med. 2016;17:611–2. https://doi.org/10.1016/j.mpaic.2016.09.012.

80. Davson H, Welch K, Segal MB. Physiology and pathophysiology of the cerebrospinal fluid. Edinburgh: Churchill Livingstone; 1987.

81. Han CY, Backous DD. Basic principles of cerebrospinal fluid metabolism and intracranial pressure homeostasis. Otolaryngol Clin North Am. 2005;38:569–76. https://doi.org/10.1016/j.otc.2005.01.005.

82. Spector R, Johanson CE. The nexus of vitamin homeostasis and DNA synthesis and modification in mammalian brain. Mol Brain. 2014;7:3. https://doi.org/10.1186/1756-660 6-7-3.

83. Spector R, Johanson CE. Vitamin transport and homeostasis in mammalian brain: focus on Vitamins B and E. J Neurochem. 2007;103:425–38. https://doi.org/10.1111/j.1471-4159. 2007.04773.x.

84. Silverberg GD, Mayo M, Saul T, Rubenstein E, McGuire D. Alzheimer's disease, normal-pressure hydrocephalus, and senescent changes in CSF circulatory physiology: a hypothesis. Lancet Neurol. 2003;2:506–11. https://doi.org/10.1016/s1474-4422(03)00487-3.

85. Ekstedt J. CSF hydrodynamic studies in man. 2. Normal hydrodynamic variables related to CSF pressure and flow. J Neurol, Neurosurg Psychiatry. 1978;41:345–53. https://doi.org/10. 1136/jnnp.41.4.345.

86. May C, Kaye JA, Atack JR, Schapiro MB, Friedland RP, Rapoport SI. Cerebrospinal fluid production is reduced in healthy aging. Neurology. 1990;40:500–3. https://doi.org/10.1212/ wnl.40.3_part_1.500.

87. McComb JG. Recent research into the nature of cerebrospinal fluid formation and absorption. J Neurosurg. 1983;59:369–83. https://doi.org/10.3171/jns.1983.59.3.0369.

88. Banizs B, Pike MM, Millican CL, Ferguson WB, Komlosi P, Sheetz J, Bell PD, Schwiebert EM, Yoder BK. Dysfunctional cilia lead to altered ependyma and choroid plexus function, and result in the formation of hydrocephalus. Development. 2005;132:5329–39. https://doi. org/10.1242/dev.02153.

89. Lun MP, Monuki ES, Lehtinen MK. Development and functions of the choroid plexus–cerebrospinal fluid system. Nat Rev Neurosci. 2015;16:445–57. https://doi.org/10.1038/nrn 3921.

90. Brown PD, Davies SL, Speake T, Millar ID. Molecular mechanisms of cerebrospinal fluid production. Neuroscience. 2004;129:955–68. https://doi.org/10.1016/j.neuroscience.2004. 07.003.

91. Johanson CE, Duncan JA, Klinge PM, Brinker T, Stopa EG, Silverberg GD. Multiplicity of cerebrospinal fluid functions: New challenges in health and disease. Cerebrospinal Fluid Res. 2008;5:10. https://doi.org/10.1186/1743-8454-5-10.

92. Plog BA, Nedergaard M. The glymphatic system in central nervous system health and disease: past, present, and future. Annu Rev Pathol. 2018;13:379–94. https://doi.org/10.1146/annurev-pathol-051217-111018.

93. Praetorius J, Nielsen S. Distribution of sodium transporters and aquaporin-1 in the human choroid plexus. Am J Physiol Cell Physiol. 2006;291:C59-67. https://doi.org/10.1152/ajpcell. 00433.2005.

94. Praetorius J. Water and solute secretion by the choroid plexus. Pflügers Arch Eur J Physiol. 2007;454:1–18. https://doi.org/10.1007/s00424-006-0170-6.

95. Jessen NA, Munk ASF, Lundgaard I, Nedergaard M. The glymphatic system: a beginner's guide. Neurochem Res. 2015;40:2583–99. https://doi.org/10.1007/s11064-015-1581-6.

96. Hladky SB, Barrand MA. Fluid and ion transfer across the blood–brain and blood–cerebrospinal fluid barriers; a comparative account of mechanisms and roles. Fluids Barriers CNS. 2016;13. https://doi.org/10.1186/s12987-016-0040-3.

97. Xu H, Fame RM, Sadegh C, Sutin J, Naranjo C, Della S, Cui J, Shipley FB, Vernon A, Gao F, et al. Choroid plexus NKCC1 mediates cerebrospinal fluid clearance during mouse early postnatal development. Nat Commun. 2021;12. https://doi.org/10.1038/s41467-020-20666-3.

98. Dobler S, Dalla S, Wagschal V, Agrawal AA. Community-wide convergent evolution in insect adaptation to toxic cardenolides by substitutions in the Na, K-ATPase. Proc Natl Acad Sci. 2012;109:13040–5. https://doi.org/10.1073/pnas.1202111109.

99. Vates TS Jr, Bonting SL, Oppelt WW. NA-K activated adenosine triphosphatase formation of cerebrospinal fluid in the cat. Am J Physiol. 1964;206:1165–72. https://doi.org/10.1152/ajp legacy.1964.206.5.1165.

100. Pollay M, Hisey B, Reynolds E, Tomkins P, Stevens FA, Smith R. Choroid plexus Na+/ K+-activated adenosine triphosphatase and cerebrospinal fluid formation. Neurosurgery. 1985;17:768–72. https://doi.org/10.1227/00006123-198511000-00007.

101. Oshio K, Song Y, Verkman AS, Manley GT. Aquaporin-1 deletion reduces osmotic water permeability and cerebrospinal fluid production. In: Springer Vienna; 2003. p. 525–28. https://doi.org/10.1007/978-3-7091-0651-8_107.

102. King LS, Kozono D, Agre P. From structure to disease: the evolving tale of aquaporin biology. Nat Rev Mol Cell Biol. 2004;5:687–98. https://doi.org/10.1038/nrm1469.

103. Nagelhus EA, Ottersen OP. Physiological roles of aquaporin-4 in brain. Physiol Rev. 2013;93:1543–62. https://doi.org/10.1152/physrev.00011.2013.

104. Fu D, Lu M. The structural basis of water permeation and proton exclusion in aquaporins (Review). Mol Membr Biol. 2007;24:366–74. https://doi.org/10.1080/09687680701446965.

105. Nakada T. Virchow-Robin space and aquaporin-4: new insights on an old friend. Croat Med J. 2014;55:328–36. https://doi.org/10.3325/cmj.2014.55.328.

106. Dandy WE. Where is cerebrospinal fluid absorbed? JAMA. 1929;92:2012–14.

107. Dandy WE. Experimental hydrocephalus. Ann Surg. 1919;70:129–42.

108. Miyajima M, Arai H. Evaluation of the production and absorption of cerebrospinal fluid. Neurol Med Chir. 2015;55:647–56. https://doi.org/10.2176/nmc.ra.2015-0003.

109. Milhorat TH. Choroid plexus and cerebrospinal fluid production. Science. 1969;166:1514–6. https://doi.org/10.1126/science.166.3912.1514.

110. Milhorat TH, Hammock MK, Chien T, Davis DA. Normal rate of cerebrospinal fluid formation five years after bilateral choroid plexectomy Case report. J Neurosurg. 1976;44:735–9. https://doi.org/10.3171/jns.1976.44.6.0735.

111. Milhorat TH. Structure and function of the choroid plexus and other sites of cerebrospinal fluid formation. Int Rev Cytol. 1976;47:225–88. https://doi.org/10.1016/s0074-7696(08)600 90-x.

112. Milhorat TH, Hammock MK, Fenstermacher JD, Levin VA. Cerebrospinal fluid production by the choroid plexus and brain. Science. 1971;173:330–2. https://doi.org/10.1126/science. 173.3994.330.

113. Tamburrini G, Caldarelli M, Di Rocco F, Massimi L, D'Angelo L, Fasano T, Di Rocco C. The role of endoscopic choroid plexus coagulation in the surgical management of bilateral choroid plexuses hyperplasia. Childs Nerv Syst. 2006;22:605–8. https://doi.org/10.1007/s00 381-006-0070-2.

114. Oresković D, Klarica M. The formation of cerebrospinal fluid: nearly a hundred years of interpretations and misinterpretations. Brain Res Rev. 2010;64:241–62. https://doi.org/10. 1016/j.brainresrev.2010.04.006.

115. Carare RO, Hawkes CA, Weller RO. Afferent and efferent immunological pathways of the brain. Anatomy, function and failure. Brain Behav Immun. 2014;36:9–14. https://doi.org/10. 1016/j.bbi.2013.10.012.

116. Bulat M, Klarica M. Fluid filtration and reabsorption across microvascular walls: control by oncotic or osmotic pressure? (secondary publication). Croat Med J. 2014;55:291–8.

117. Bulat M, Klarica M. Recent insights into a new hydrodynamics of the cerebrospinal fluid. Brain Res Rev. 2011;65:99–112. https://doi.org/10.1016/j.brainresrev.2010.08.002.

118. Buishas J, Gould IG, Linninger AA. A computational model of cerebrospinal fluid production and reabsorption driven by Starling forces. Croat Med J. 2014;55:481–97. https://doi.org/10. 3325/cmj.2014.55.481.

119. Greitz D, Hannerz J. A proposed model of cerebrospinal fluid circulation: observations with radionuclide cisternography. Am J Neuroradiol. 1996;17:431.

120. Nedergaard M, Goldman SA. Brain drain. Sci Am. 2016;314:44–9. https://doi.org/10.1038/ scientificamerican0316-44.

121. Kulik T, Kusano Y, Aronhime S, Sandler AL, Winn HR. Regulation of cerebral vasculature in normal and ischemic brain. Neuropharmacology. 2008;55:281–8. https://doi.org/10.1016/ j.neuropharm.2008.04.017.

122. Iliff JJ, Wang M, Liao Y, Plogg Benjamin A, Peng W, Gundersen Georg A, Benveniste H, Vates GE, Deane R, Goldman Steven A, et al. A paravascular pathway facilitates CSF flow through the brain parenchyma and the clearance of interstitial solutes, including Amyloid β. Sci Transl Med. 2012;4:147ra111–147ra111. https://doi.org/10.1126/scitranslmed.3003748.

123. Yang C, Huang X, Huang X, Mai H, Li J, Jiang T, Wang X, Lü T. Aquaporin-4 and Alzheimer's disease. J Alzheimers Dis. 2016;52:391–402. https://doi.org/10.3233/JAD-150949.

124. Verkman AS, Smith AJ, Phuan P-W, Tradtrantip L, Anderson MO. The aquaporin-4 water channel as a potential drug target in neurological disorders. Expert Opin Ther Targets. 2017;21:1161–70. https://doi.org/10.1080/14728222.2017.1398236.

125. Benveniste H, Liu X, Koundal S, Sanggaard S, Lee H, Wardlaw J. The glymphatic system and waste clearance with brain aging: a review. Gerontology. 2019;65:106–19. https://doi.org/10.1159/000490349.

126. Louveau A, Plog BA, Antila S, Alitalo K, Nedergaard M, Kipnis J. Understanding the functions and relationships of the glymphatic system and meningeal lymphatics. J Clin Investig. 2017;127:3210–9. https://doi.org/10.1172/jci90603.

127. Weller RO, Subash M, Preston SD, Mazanti I, Carare RO. Clearance of Aβ from the brain in Alzheimer's disease: perivascular drainage of amyloid-β peptides from the brain and its failure in cerebral amyloid angiopathy and Alzheimer's disease. Brain Pathol. 2007;18:253–66. https://doi.org/10.1111/j.1750-3639.2008.00133.x.

128. Hawkes CA, Härtig W, Kacza J, Schliebs R, Weller RO, Nicoll JA, Carare RO. Perivascular drainage of solutes is impaired in the ageing mouse brain and in the presence of cerebral amyloid angiopathy. Acta Neuropathol. 2011;121:431–43. https://doi.org/10.1007/s00401-011-0801-7.

129. Da Mesquita S, Louveau A, Vaccari A, Smirnov I, Cornelison RC, Kingsmore KM, Contarino C, Onengut-Gumuscu S, Farber E, Raper D, et al. Functional aspects of meningeal lymphatics in ageing and Alzheimer's disease. Nature. 2018;560:185–91. https://doi.org/10.1038/s41586-018-0368-8.

130. Xu Z, Xiao N, Chen Y, Huang H, Marshall C, Gao J, Cai Z, Wu T, Hu G, Xiao M. Deletion of aquaporin-4 in APP/PS1 mice exacerbates brain Aβ accumulation and memory deficits. Mol Neurodegeneration. 2015;10. https://doi.org/10.1186/s13024-015-0056-1.

131. Iliff JJ, Chen MJ, Plog BA, Zeppenfeld DM, Soltero M, Yang L, Singh I, Deane R, Nedergaard M. Impairment of glymphatic pathway function promotes tau pathology after traumatic brain injury. J Neurosci. 2014;34:16180–93. https://doi.org/10.1523/jneurosci.3020-14.2014.

132. Zou W, Pu T, Feng W, Lu M, Zheng Y, Du R, Xiao M, Hu G. Blocking meningeal lymphatic drainage aggravates Parkinson's disease-like pathology in mice overexpressing mutated α-synuclein. Transl Neurodegeneration. 2019;8. https://doi.org/10.1186/s40035-019-0147-y.

133. Auguste KI, Jin S, Uchida K, Yan D, Manley GT, Papadopoulos MC, Verkman AS. Greatly impaired migration of implanted aquaporin-4-deficient astroglial cells in mouse brain toward a site of injury. FASEB J. 2007;21:108–16. https://doi.org/10.1096/fj.06-6848com.

134. Liu L, Lu Y, Kong H, Li L, Marshall C, Xiao M, Ding J, Gao J, Hu G. Aquaporin-4 deficiency exacerbates brain oxidative damage and memory deficits induced by long-term ovarian hormone deprivation and D-galactose injection. Int J Neuropsychopharmacol. 2012;15:55–68. https://doi.org/10.1017/s1461145711000022.

135. Wu Q, Zhang Y-J, Gao J-Y, Li X-M, Kong H, Zhang Y-P, Xiao M, Shields CB, Hu G. Aquaporin-4 mitigates retrograde degeneration of rubrospinal neurons by facilitating edema clearance and glial scar formation after spinal cord injury in mice. Mol Neurobiol. 2014;49:1327–37. https://doi.org/10.1007/s12035-013-8607-3.

136. Madsen PL, Schmidt JF, Wildschiødtz G, Friberg L, Holm S, Vorstrup S, Lassen NA. Cerebral O_2 metabolism and cerebral blood flow in humans during deep and rapid-eye-movement sleep. J Appl Physiol. 1985;1991(70):2597–601. https://doi.org/10.1152/jappl.1991.70.6.2597.

137. Xie L, Kang H, Xu Q, Chen MJ, Liao Y, Thiyagarajan M, O'Donnell J, Christensen DJ, Nicholson C, Iliff JJ, et al. Sleep drives metabolite clearance from the adult brain. Science. 2013;342:373–7. https://doi.org/10.1126/science.1241224.

138. Benveniste H, Heerdt PM, Fontes M, Rothman DL, Volkow ND. Glymphatic system function in relation to anesthesia and sleep states. Anesth Analg. 2019;128:747–58. https://doi.org/10.1213/ane.0000000000004069.

139. Gordleeva S, Kanakov O, Ivanchenko M, Zaikin A, Franceschi C. Brain aging and garbage cleaning. Semin Immunopathol. 2020;42:647–65. https://doi.org/10.1007/s00281-020-00816-x.

140. Symss NP, Oi S. Theories of cerebrospinal fluid dynamics and hydrocephalus: historical trend. J Neurosurg Pediatr. 2013;11:170–7. https://doi.org/10.3171/2012.3.Peds0934.
141. Cushing H. Studies on the cerebro-spinal fluid: I Introduction. J Med Res. 1914;31:1–19.
142. Pollay M. The function and structure of the cerebrospinal fluid outflow system. Cerebrospinal Fluid Res. 2010;7:9. https://doi.org/10.1186/1743-8454-7-9.
143. Weed LH. Studies on cerebro-spinal fluid. No. III: the pathways of escape from the subarachnoid spaces with particular reference to the arachnoid villi. J Med Res. 1914;31:51–91.
144. Shulman K, Yarnell P, Ransohoff J. Dural sinus pressure: in normal and hydrocephalic dogs. Arch Neurol. 1964;10:575–80. https://doi.org/10.1001/archneur.1964.00460180041003.
145. Tripathi R. Tracing the bulk outflow route of cerebrospinal fluid by transmission and scanning electron microscopy. Brain Res. 1974;80:503–6. https://doi.org/10.1016/0006-8993(74)910 33-6.
146. Tripathi BJ, Tripathi RC. Vacuolar transcellular channels as a drainage pathway for cerebrospinal fluid. J Physiol. 1974;239:195–206. https://doi.org/10.1113/jphysiol.1974.sp0 10563.
147. Kida S, Yamashima T, Kubota T, Ito H, Yamamoto S. A light and electron microscopic and immunohistochemical study of human arachnoid villi. J Neurosurg. 1988;69:429–35. https://doi.org/10.3171/jns.1988.69.3.0429.
148. Yamashima T. Ultrastructural study of the final cerebrospinal fluid pathway in human arachnoid villi. Brain Res. 1986;384:68–76. https://doi.org/10.1016/0006-8993(86)91220 5.
149. Cserr HF, Knopf PM. Cervical lymphatics, the blood-brain barrier and the immunoreactivity of the brain: a new view. Immunol Today. 1992;13:507–12. https://doi.org/10.1016/0167-569 9(92)90027-5.
150. Mollanji R, Bozanovic-Sosic R, Silver I, Li B, Kim C, Midha R, Johnston M. Intracranial pressure accommodation is impaired by blocking pathways leading to extracranial lymphatics. Am J Physiol Regul Integr Comp Physiol. 2001;280:R1573-1581. https://doi.org/10.1152/ajp regu.2001.280.5.R1573.
151. Leinonen V, Vanninen R, Rauramaa T. Cerebrospinal fluid circulation and hydrocephalus. Handb Clin Neurol. 2017;145:39–50. https://doi.org/10.1016/b978-0-12-802395-2.00005-5.
152. Mollanji R, Bozanovic-Sosic R, Zakharov A, Makarian L, Johnston MG. Blocking cerebrospinal fluid absorption through the cribriform plate increases resting intracranial pressure. Am J Physiol Regul Integr Comp Physiol. 2002;282:R1593–1599. https://doi.org/10.1152/ajpregu.00695.2001.
153. Oresković D, Whitton PS, Lupret V. Effect of intracranial pressure on cerebrospinal fluid formation in isolated brain ventricles. Neuroscience. 1991;41:773–7. https://doi.org/10.1016/0306-4522(91)90367-w.

Pathophysiology of NPH

Adéla Bubeníková, Petr Skalický, and Ondřej Bradáč

Abstract Over the past decades, there have been various hypotheses and theories discussing the aetiology of Normal Pressure Hydrocephalus (NPH). This reversible form of dementia, as an entity characterised by the famous clinical triad of symptoms: gait impairment, urinary incontinence, and cognitive deficit, represents a complex vicious cycle of pathophysiological mechanisms simultaneously involving each other, rather than being a consequence of one well-defined cause. Despite a lot of effort to fully understand the pathogenesis of the disease, a clear cause and exact pathophysiological pathways remain unclear. Pathophysiological factors including the impairment of glymphatic system, reduced arterial pulsatility, associated metabolic and osmotic disbalances, astrogliosis, or neuroinflammation are known to contribute to the disease's pathogenesis, and lead to NPH manifestation. In this chapter, we summarise both historical and current conceptions of NPH pathophysiology, in relation to typical clinical and radiological findings.

Keywords Normal pressure hydrocephalus · Pathophysiology · Glymphatic system · Hydrocephalus · Abnormal cerebrospinal fluid dynamics

Abbreviations

AQP	Aquaporin
BBB	Blood-brain barrier
CFAP	Cilia- and flagella-associated protein
CI	Confidence interval
CiNPHT	Comprehensive idiopathic normal-pressure hydrocephalus theory

A. Bubeníková · P. Skalický · O. Bradáč (✉)
Department of Neurosurgery, 2nd Medical Faculty, Charles University and Motol University Hospital, Prague, Czech Republic
e-mail: ondrej.bradac2@fnmotol.cz

A. Bubeníková · O. Bradáč
Department of Neurosurgery and Neuro-Oncology, 1st Medical Faculty, Charles University and Military University Hospital, Prague, Czech Republic

O. Bradac (ed.), *Normal Pressure Hydrocephalus*,
https://doi.org/10.1007/978-3-031-36522-5_6

CNS	Central nervous system
CSAS	Cortical subarachnoid spaces
CSF	Cerebrospinal fluid
DTI-ALPS	Diffusion tensor image analysis along the perivascular space
ICP	Intracranial pressure
iNPH	Idiopathic normal pressure hydrocephalus
LIAS	Late-onset idiopathic aqueductal stenosis
MRI	Magnetic resonance imaging
NPH	Normal pressure hydrocephalus
OR	Odds ratio
OSA	Obstructive sleep apnoea
PCD	Primary cilia dyskinesia
sNPH	Secondary normal pressure hydrocephalus

1 Introduction

One of the potentially reversible neuropsychiatric conditions, normal pressure hydrocephalus (NPH), is a specific entity of adult-onset hydrocephalus [1, 2]. Below, the attention is paid to two major subgroups of NPH. In the case of the first, known as idiopathic NPH (iNPH), the exact causes of the disease onset are previously not known, but occur primarily in the elderly [3–5]. On the contrary, secondary NPH (sNPH) may be experienced at any age since it is a result of initial pathological factors, such as subarachnoid or intracerebral haemorrhage, stroke, tumour, or infection [6, 7]. These groups need to be differentiated in order to deliver the best treatment outcome and future prognosis for each patient.

In the last few decades, the widely discussed issue about NPH has been the absence of disease-specific diagnostic measures, mainly due to the range of concurrent neurodegeneration-related comorbidities, leading to a serious problem of under-diagnoses [3, 8–10]. NPH is characterised by a clinical triad of cognitive deficit, gait impairment, urinary incontinence [11], and features of ventriculomegaly without the increase of Intracranial Pressure (ICP). The complete triad, however, may not be seen in all patients with NPH. The cornerstones of NPH pathogenesis are primarily set upon the alterations of Cerebrospinal Fluid (CSF) dynamics, and additionally on possible vascular, neuropathological changes, and neuroinflammatory factors [12–14]. In recent years, the impairment of the glymphatic system has been observed as another potential link between the abnormal CSF hydrodynamics and neurodegeneration, further reflecting typical NPH manifestation [15–17]. A few investigated genetic predispositions are believed to be involved in disease development as well [18].

The pathophysiology of NPH, rather than taken as a single and simple mechanism of the disease development, is a complex entity of many pathological states contemporary dependent and involving each other. In this chapter, we aim to summarise the historical and modern understandings of NPH pathophysiology that are fundamental for adequate treatment and prospective research.

2 Historical Understanding of NPH Pathophysiology

The cornerstones of NPH pathophysiology are based on famous research by Hakim and Adams from 1965 [11]. Later on, their findings were expanded and replenished by new concepts of CSF physiology and the pathogenesis of hydrocephalus [19, 20]. Although the exact determinants and mechanisms of NPH pathogenesis have been continuously investigated in several studies [14, 21, 22] (Table 1), up-to-date knowledge in the field remains incomplete. Hoff and Barber [23] studied features of posttraumatic NPH in elderly patients in 1974, proposing that the pressure gradient across the cerebral mantle may influence the ventricular expansion in NPH. Twenty years later, Raimondi [24] fundamentally contributed to understanding the association between ICP and CSF pulsatility which we introduce more in detail below. The previous theories introduced by Hoff and his colleagues had to be questioned, particularly because of their contradictory results in relation to Pascal's hydrodynamic law. The vascular factors and disturbed hemodynamics in patients with idiopathic intracranial hypertension were investigated by Bateman in 2004 [25]. Due to advances in utilising concepts of CSF hydrodynamics, several reports [14, 21, 22, 26, 27] subsequently improved the pathophysiological descriptions of the disease since alterations of CSF behaviour present one of the most discussed factors involving the NPH manifestation. In a recent hemodynamic theory, increased intracerebral blood volume is believed to be associated with increased ICP in obstructive hydrocephalus, particularly due to hemodynamic factors involving venous stenoses or elevated intracranial venous pressure. These findings were similarly investigated in iNPH since the compression of cortical veins and reduced cerebral blood flow are typically observed in iNPH patients. Before utilising the knowledge about the glymphatic system, a renewed concept [28] of iNPH pathophysiological mechanisms was disclosed. This theory summarised and reviewed up-to-date information together with the individual clinical data from iNPH patients. The authors compared iNPH to a vicious cycle of pathophysiological mechanisms simultaneously involving each other. Despite all effort that has been made to stop the pathophysiological cycle, so far it has been only possible to regulate or slow down the disease progression. In recent years, the concept of glymphatic system involvement in NPH development has been studied in more detail, although these investigations are primarily limited to animal models. With the advances in available technical equipment, it has been possible to analyse waste clearance mechanisms in NPH patients non-invasively, therefore enabling the study of metabolic alterations and osmotic disbalances which result in the typical pathophysiological features of NPH and its clinical manifestation. The summary of several pathophysiological determinants of disease progression is presented in Fig. 1, where we present a new diagram and pathophysiological theory through expansion of the Comprehensive theory from 2017 [28] with up-to-date findings.

Table 1 Review of historical theories about iNPH pathophysiology and renewed concepts of CSF hydrodynamics related to the disease manifestation

Year	Authors	Title
1965	Hakim and Adams	Hakim–Adams Theory [11]
1974	Hoff and Barber	Transcerebral mantle pressure gradient [23]
1993	Greitz	Restricted arterial pulsation hydrocephalus [19]
1994	Raimondi	A unifying theory for definition and classification of hydrocephalus [24]
2004	Bateman	Hemodynamic theory of venous congestion [25]
2006	Oi and Di Rocco	Evolution theory in cerebrospinal fluid dynamics and minor pathway hydrocephalus [26]
2008	Rekate	Importance of cortical subarachnoid space in understanding hydrocephalus [21]
2012	Iliff et al.	A paravascular pathway facilitates CSF flow through the brain parenchyma and the clearance of interstitial solutes, including amyloid β [29]
2013	Preuss	Pulsatile vector theory [14]
2013	Chikly and Quaghebeur	Reassessing CSF hydrodynamics and novel hypothesis [30]
2013	Xie et al.	Sleep drives metabolite clearance from the adult brain [31]
2014	Krishnamurthy and Li	Osmotic gradient theory [22]
2016	Matsumae et al.	Intimate exchange between cerebrospinal fluid and interstitial fluid [27]
2017	Ammar et al.	The comprehensive idiopathic normal-pressure hydrocephalus theory (CiNPHT) [28]
2018	Eide and Hansson	Astrogliosis and impaired aquaporin-4 and dystrophin systems in idiopathic normal pressure hydrocephalus [32]
2018	Ringstad et al.	Brain-wide glymphatic enhancement and clearance in humans assessed with MRI [33]
2019	Román et al.	Sleep-disordered breathing and idiopathic normal-pressure hydrocephalus: recent pathophysiological advances [34]
2019	Eide and Ringstad	Delayed clearance of cerebrospinal fluid tracer from entorhinal cortex in idiopathic normal pressure hydrocephalus: a glymphatic magnetic resonance imaging study [35]
2020	Eide and Hansson	Blood-brain barrier leakage of blood proteins in idiopathic normal pressure hydrocephalus [36]

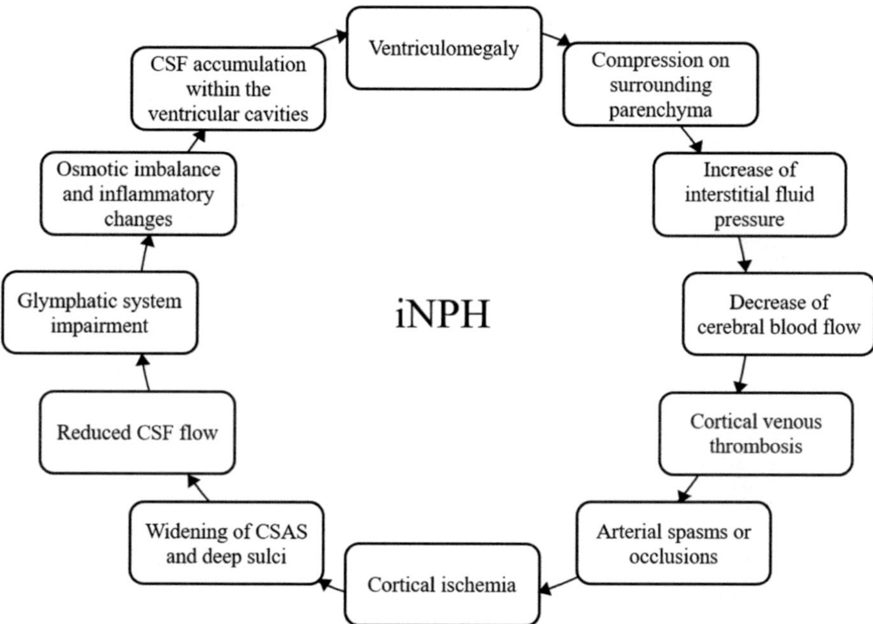

Fig. 1 Brief summary of NPH pathophysiology according to the Comprehensive Idiopathic Normal Pressure Hydrocephalus Theory introduced (CiNPHT) by Ammar et al. in 2017 [23] expanded by up-to-date findings of the glymphatic system, metabolic changes, and neuroinflammatory involvement

3 Alteration of CSF Dynamics and Vascular Factors

According to Adam and Hakim's model of NPH pathophysiology [11], the expansion of intracerebral ventricles is initially caused by the pressure on the surrounding brain parenchyma. The subsequent ventriculomegaly is considered to be a compensation mechanism responsible for the return of ICP to its normal values. The abnormal CSF dynamics are a factor that primarily contribute to such a state [13, 14]. Hakim explained the mechanism of normal pressure maintenance within the ventricular cavities according to the well-known Pascal's law of fluid mechanics. Pascal's equation says that the pressure is equal to the force divided by the area on which it acts and is the same in all directions at a specific point in a fluid at rest. In the case of NPH, we measure the pressure inside the ventricles filled with CSF. At first, both pressure and forces pushing on the ventricular walls are increasing. When the pressure inside the ventricles reaches its maximal value, it decreases to a balanced, stabilised level, but the forces continue to rise with the growing expansion of ventricular cavities [37]. The universal concept of hydrocephalus pathophysiology was studied by Bering and Pappenheimer [38–40], who investigated the impaired CSF motion within the brain in animal models. At this time, i.e., during the sixties of the twentieth century, the classical hypothesis of unidirectional flow was doubted together with the concept of CSF secretion through the filtration of blood plasma via choroid plexuses. Nowadays,

CSF flow is considered to be a combination of bulk and pulsatile flow, accompanied by to-and-fro movement and additional fluid exchange mechanisms [19, 41] which have been described in the previous chapter in more detail. These factors play a vital role in understanding the concepts of NPH pathophysiology.

In the case of sNPH, the abnormal CSF dynamics results from the adhesions of the subarachnoid space or arachnoid granulations, as the accumulation of proteins and cellular compartments from intracranial tumours, haemorrhagic processes or infections may cause an abnormally increased viscosity of CSF [6, 42]. Such a state is typically associated with impaired absorption mechanisms of CSF, and therefore leads to ventricular dilatation. It has been observed in cases of some tumours, e.g., acoustic neuromas [42], that the CSF protein concentrations are, in the vast majority of patients, increased [43]. The hydrocephalus itself may be managed surgically in both sNPH and iNPH. However, the outcomes of surgical treatment are generally better in the case of sNPH. This may be partly attributed to the duration of preclinical development of the disease, as the manifestation of sNPH tends to be much shorter compared to iNPH [44].

However, the CSF dynamics in iNPH differ from those in sNPH, since sNPH has different primary causes of hydrocephalus onset. Due to the ageing process, associated neurodegeneration and initially increased CSF pressure, the compliance of the intracranial parenchyma decreases. This subsequently causes the restriction of CSF flow into the convexity and subarachnoid spaces, resulting in ventricular dilatation [45] (Fig. 1). Since the production of CSF is not disturbed, the secretion exceeds the capacity for absorption, which is reduced due to alterations in brain compliance and CSF dynamics [5, 46, 47]. In a recent meta-analysis [48], the resistance to CSF outflow, Rout, was shown to be a useful parameter for predicting shunt responsiveness. A value of 12 mmHg/ml/min was defined as a suitable predictor of shunt responsiveness in iNPH patients. It has been proposed in a randomised study [49] that this value was found in 83% of iNPH cases. Interestingly, the impaired CSF drainage in iNPH might be associated with the elevation of venous pressure caused by the stenosis of cerebral venous sinuses [50], and reduced flow velocity of the superior sagittal sinus [51]. Benabid et al. [52] reported that an increase in sagittal sinus pressure by 3–4 mmHg might correlate with the termination of the CSF outflow through arachnoid granulations (Fig. 2).

Due to the dilatation of intracerebral ventricles, which is typically associated with ischemic processes and the increase of interstitial fluid, the compliance of periventricular parenchyma is reduced (Fig. 3). This is a state known as "stiff ventricles" [28]. The ventricular tension leads to compression and occlusion of small arteries, subsequently causing ischemia. The surrounding tissue loses its integrity, the compliance of the brain parenchyma is reduced, and the pulse wave transmission decreases. These processes result in what is called transependymal transition (also known as transependymal oedema or periventricular lucency) which is a state that typifies the accumulation of interstitial fluid along the periventricular tissue (Fig. 4) [56]. This might result in the disease progression, considering the osmotic imbalance in the periventricular white matter and analogous intracellular alterations [47, 57, 58]. The periventricular CSF is very likely to be absorbed, via two possible mechanisms:

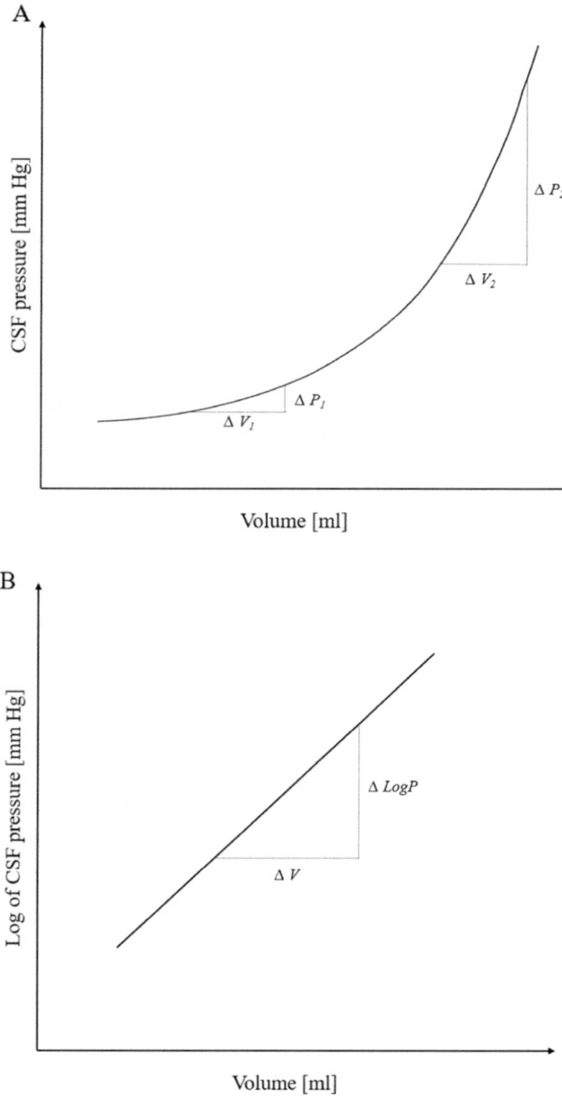

Fig. 2 The compliance (C) is the ability of cerebral parenchyma to adapt to external processes influencing the intracranial environment. It is defined through the formula: $C = \frac{\Delta V}{\Delta P}$ or $C = \frac{dV}{dP}$, where V stands for the volume and P for pressure. The first graph (A) shows an exponential increase of CSF pressure when the three intracranial compartments (i.e., CSF, brain parenchyma, and blood according to the Monro-Kellie doctrine [53]) reach their maximal levels. In the second graph (B), the same measures are depicted on a semilog scale which is a linear function of constant values derived from the slope of the line. Such distribution may be considered as the extra fluid compartment needed for the increase of CSF pressure ten-fold [54, 55]

(1) through the perivascular spaces along with the upstream blood flow of cerebral arteries or (2) directly into the capillaries [59]. The hyperdynamic behaviour of CSF in iNPH influences the elevation of CSF pulsatility, whilst the arterial pulsatility is decreased. This might be, above all, explained according to the Windkessel mechanism [13, 60] which proposes that the central arteries, primarily the aorta, serve as a reservoir of ejected blood from the heart during the systole. Subsequently, diastole is responsible for the motion of the ejected blood to the peripheries (Fig. 5). Due to the physiological changes during ageing, arteries become less compliant and as a consequence, the arterial pulsatility is reduced. This further causes the elevation of the pulsatile flow within the Sylvian aqueduct since it compensates for decreased arterial pulsatility [47, 61, 62]. These findings further indicate the involvement of changes in blood vessel elasticity and subsequent alteration in the transmission of pulse waves, associated with changes in arterial pressure during the cardiac cycle [62, 63]. Of note are recent findings dedicated to investigations of CSF circulation and hydrodynamics in phase-contrast MRI and their 3D reconstructions [64, 65]. Since NPH is technically limited to the ventricular system, spinal subarachnoid spaces, primarily at the site of the foramen magnum, form a compensatory mechanism for stabilisation of CSF hyperdynamic behaviour.

The alterations of ICP pulse waves were investigated by Eide and Stanisic in 2010 [66]. According to their findings derived from the monitoring of 40 definite iNPH patients, the amplitude of ICP pulse wave was a determinant of shunt-responsive or shunt-non-responsive samples. Their study outlines the association between the ICP, CSF pressure, and the compliance of intracerebral parenchyma since any alterations

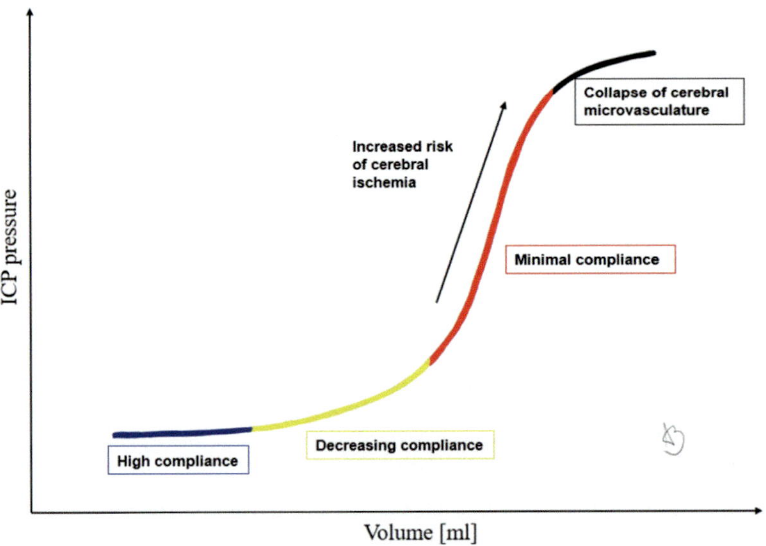

Fig. 3 The well-known pressure-volume curve for the ICP, divided into four stages that relate to the extent of compensatory reserves and analogous behaviour of brain compliance

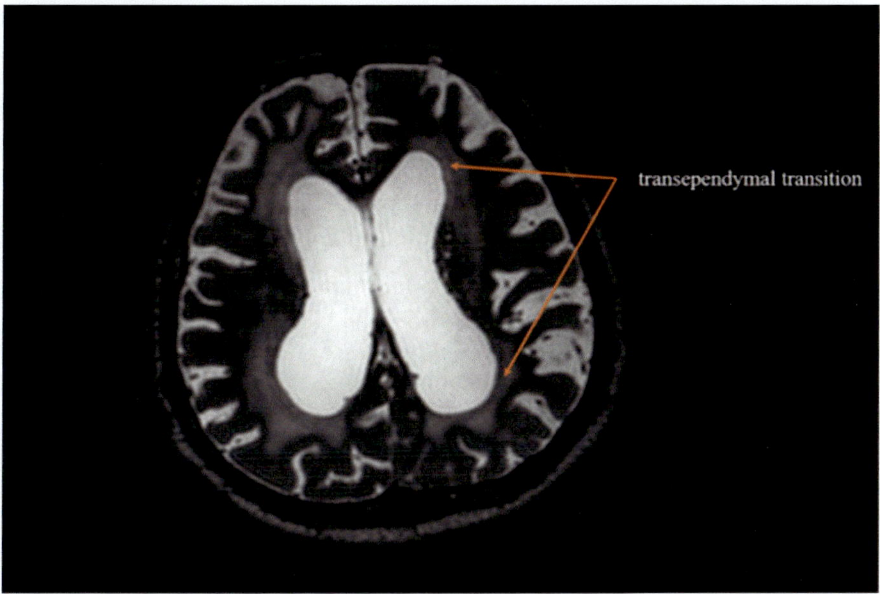

Fig. 4 Ventriculomegaly and transependymal transition shown on MRI T2-WI

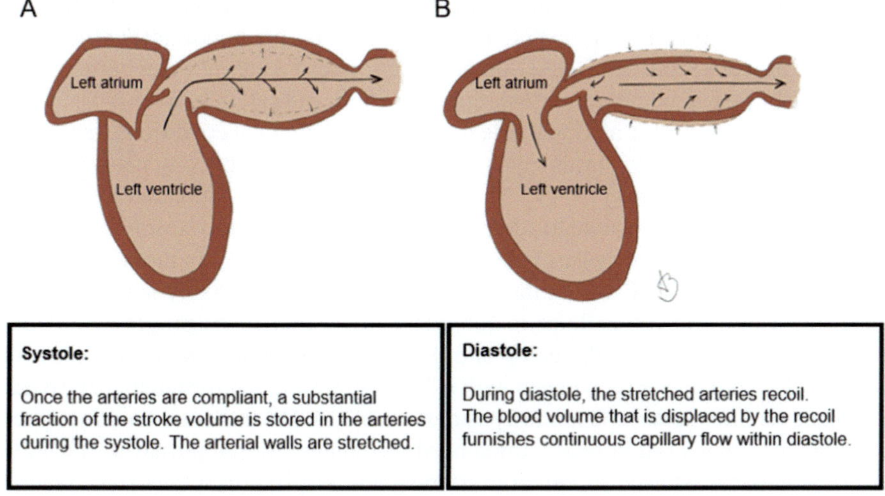

Systole:	**Diastole:**
Once the arteries are compliant, a substantial fraction of the stroke volume is stored in the arteries during the systole. The arterial walls are stretched.	During diastole, the stretched arteries recoil. The blood volume that is displaced by the recoil furnishes continuous capillary flow within diastole.

Fig. 5 Windkessel mechanism explained more in detail. This mechanism is generally important for damping the fluctuation in blood pressure over the cardiac cycle and it enables to maintain organ perfusion during ventricular diastole. However, this mechanism continually diminishes with age. In the elderly, the previously elastic arteries are less compliant due to elastin loss and fragmentation. A reduced Windkessel effect results in elevated pulse pressure that may subsequently involve the onset of hypertension or other diseases of the cardiovascular system. In the case of iNPH, the reduced arterial pulsatility causes elevation of the CSF pulsatile flow and thus has an impact on the progression of hydrocephalus and ventriculomegaly

of the mentioned variables reflect neurophysiological changes and development of cognitive deficits [44, 54, 55]. The ICP pulse waves in iNPH and Late-onset Idiopathic Aqueductal Stenosis (LIAS) were investigated in a recent study [67]. Higher ICP values were measured in LIAS when compared to iNPH subjects, whilst the ratio of the heartbeat related pulse wave amplitude (calculated in the frequency domain and the time domain) was higher in iNPH patients. These findings verify the hypothesis that high ICP pulse waves amplitudes have a role in the pathophysiology of the disease.

4   Glymphatic System Impairment

Water exchange mechanisms within the CNS have been widely discussed in accordance with a recently described concept of the so-called glymphatic system [17, 68]. This system serves as a complex of waste clearance formed by astrocytes, perivascular spaces, and lymphatic compartments. The CSF drainage is directed along the meninges, cranial nerves, and vessels through the perivascular (also known as Virchow-Robin) spaces, into the lymphatics to be absorbed [29, 69]. CSF enters the CNS at the level of subarachnoid spaces in the convexity, moving into the interstitial fluid via aquaporin 4 (AQP4) channels. AQP4s are transmembrane proteins primarily found at the astrocytic perivascular endfeet [70]. They are also on the glia limitans interna and glia limitans externa [71, 72]. These proteins are important for the water exchange processes and facilitate a number of processes including water homeostasis within the brain parenchyma [73, 74], fluid secretion, and cell migration [71]. Moreover, AQP4 proteins play a critical role in various pathological conditions, including cerebral oedema, traumatic brain injury, mesial temporal lobe epilepsy, neuromyelitis optica, and hydrocephalus [75–79]. The way in which AQP4 is impaired depends on the specific type of hydrocephalus. In certain types it might be the reason for reduced drainage and in others the cause of elevated CSF production [71]. In the case of NPH, the accumulation of CSF within the ventricular cavities most likely leads to AQP4 impairment in astrocytic cellular membranes. AQP4 undergoes progressive depolarisation in accordance with ageing and therefore exacerbates the unusual flow of perivascular fluid in elderly patients with iNPH [29, 80–82]. Unfortunately, the exact mechanism of this process is not fully understood [71]. The impaired function of the glymphatic system is additionally influenced by reduced arterial pulsatility, changes in the vascular resistance in cerebral arteries, and respiration waves [83]. Due to ageing, the cerebral microvasculature mechanically remodels in accordance with atherosclerosis, calcifications, and arterial stiffening [84, 85]. Many recent studies have confirmed the link between restricted arterial pulsations and reduced glymphatic functioning and have considered its consequences in terms of impaired CSF pulsatility and disturbed cerebral perfusion [70, 83, 86, 87].

The pioneers of investigating the glymphatic system in iNPH were Ringstad et al. in 2018 [33] and Eide et al. in 2019 [35]. Their findings suggested reduced efficiency of glymphatic functioning when compared to controls. Eide et al. [35] observed delayed removal of CSF tracer gadobutrol along the glymphatic drainage pathways into the lymphatics, using contrast-enhanced MRI. In recent years, the functioning of waste clearance via glymphatic system was studied by non-invasive imaging, namely diffusion tensor image analysis along with the perivascular space (DTI-ALPS) analyses [88–90], where the motion of H_2O molecules within the cerebral white matter is depicted under DTI. It has been verified that DTI-ALPS analyses serve as an effective diagnostic approach to demonstrate impaired glymphatic functioning instead of using invasive tests [91]. Furthermore, the loss of AQP4 has been confirmed in iNPH patients when compared to a control group of subjects experiencing epilepsy, subarachnoid haemorrhage, or brain carcinogenesis [80]. The reduced AQP4 expression in NPH is most likely additionally associated with dysfunction of blood–brain barrier permeability and neuroinflammatory changes [80]. Accordingly, the disturbance of CSF clearance is associated with the accumulation of amyloid beta and analogous neurotoxic substances which may be involved in neuroinflammatory pathways and the processes of astrogliosis, and thus influences CSF perfusion within the brain [92, 93] (Fig. 6).

Recent findings suggest that glymphatic functioning is in physiological conditions dramatically enhanced during sleep [31]. Therefore, metabolic waste clearance via the glymphatic system might be disturbed in NPH, and moreover might be associated with sleep abnormalities to some extent [15, 94, 95]. This might be also an age-related process since the glymphatic decline is probably associated with deep sleep deficiency and non-rapid eye movement in the elderly [87, 96, 97]. It should be noted that iNPH may be closely linked to obstructive sleep apnoea, being present in over 90.3% of iNPH patients [34]. The inspiratory motions against tongue-blocked air influx typically contribute to intracranial venous hypertension in iNPH, considering increased intrathoracic negative pressure and decreased return of venous blood to the brain [34]. However, the vast majority of research investigating the physiological role of the glymphatic system in terms of CSF clearance mechanisms have been devoted to animal models [98–100] and further research in humans is needed in order to elucidate the role of the glymphatic system in NPH and its involvement in disease progression. Of note is that AQP channels may serve as potential drug therapy targets to control the fluid exchange in hydrocephalus, but as of yet there has been no practical research to verify such statements [71].

5 Neuropathological Changes

The compression of the brain parenchyma due to ventricle dilation subsequently leads to pathophysiological changes in the periventricular space and subcortical damage. The mechanical stress on the periventricular white matter causes damage of white matter axons, resulting in altered intraneuronal biochemical processes, hypoxia, and ischemia [28]. Moreover, due to the reduced CSF drainage, ventriculomegaly, and reduced cerebral compliance, the cerebral blood flow decreases (Fig. 7) which might result in the progression of disease symptomatology considering the reduced

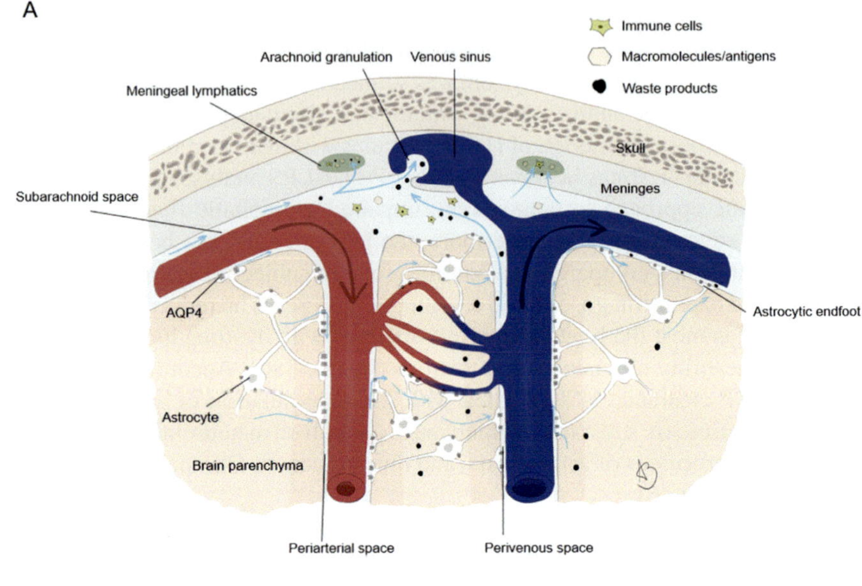

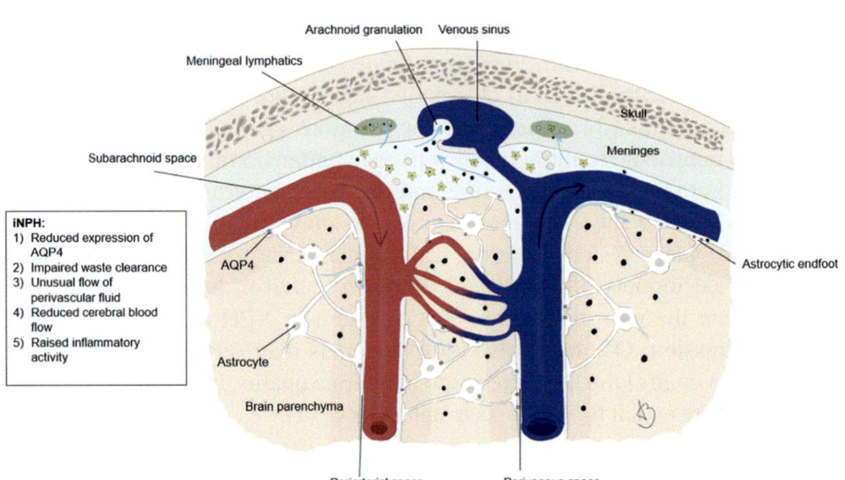

Fig. 6 The comparison of the glymphatic system functioning in healthy individuals (A) and in iNPH (B)

metabolic intercellular communication. For example, decreased cerebral blood flow through the frontal lobe correlates with the severity of urinary incontinence and the reduced flow via basal ganglia was found to influence the gait disturbance. Impaired glymphatic function in accordance with the abovementioned pathophysiological mechanisms contributes to disease progression. The pressure and compression on the periventricular corticospinal tract leads to stretching of sacral nerve fibres and loss of supraspinal control. This results in loss of voluntary bladder contractions and urinary incontinence. Similarly, when the motor fibres are compressed, the metabolic changes in the intra-axonal environment contribute to the progression of neurological deficits, characteristically gait apraxia [101–103]. It has been recently proposed [104] that the motor dysfunction may not be only due to the corticospinal tract compression, but also due to the disturbance of locomotion. Due to the subcortical damage and associated axonal loss, research has been trying to identify biomarkers typical for such a state. However, recent findings reveal contradictory results and there are no disease-specific markers of subcortical damage used for identification of NPH or for any diagnostic purposes [105]. This happens due to the high concurrence of neurodegenerative comorbidities, which are also characterised by increased concentrations of these biomarkers [5, 106–109].

In 2018, Yin et al. [110] investigated alterations in the grey matter using reconstructions of structural networks between regional grey matter volumes under the screening of 3D T1-WI MRI. 29 possible iNPH patients were compared to 30 healthy controls. The authors found that the global network modularity was larger in the iNPH ($p < 0.05$) and the hubs of the iNPH network were primarily localised within the limbic lobe and temporal regions, whilst the hubs of healthy controls were primarily limited to the frontal lobe. It is possible that the connections of the structural networks are reduced due to disease progression and its typical manifestation [111].

5.1 Metabolic Changes and Neuroinflammation

In accordance with hypoxia, ischemia, and hypoperfusion, the energy metabolism of neurons is disturbed, leading to abnormal metabolic pathways and triggering inflammatory involvement [112–114]. For example, one study found high rates of accumulated lactate within ventricular cavities in iNPH due to the reduced cerebral blood flow [114], but further MRI investigations did not verify such findings [115]. Interestingly, older individuals commonly experience vitamin D deficiency, which might correlate with clinical manifestation and radiological features similar to iNPH [116]. Considering the abnormal CSF hydrodynamics and associated vascular and inflammatory factors, dysfunction of the Blood-Brain Barrier (BBB) has been found in many disorders after CNS injury [13]. When compared to healthy controls, iNPH patients typically manifest with increased BBB leakage, associated with fibrinogen extravasation or astrogliosis [36, 117]. It has been verified in several studies [118–120] that the concentrations of pro- and anti-inflammatory biomarkers are increased in patients with iNPH but distinguishing from other neurodegenerative comorbidities is a challenge since the neuroinflammation is often present in neurodegenerative diseases, typically contributing to disease progression. Particularly interleukin 1 (IL-1), tumour necrosis factor-alpha (TNF-α), IL-β1, IL-6, IL-10, TGF-β1 are the most discussed inflammatory biomarkers in the literature. Their CSF concentrations might

Healthy control

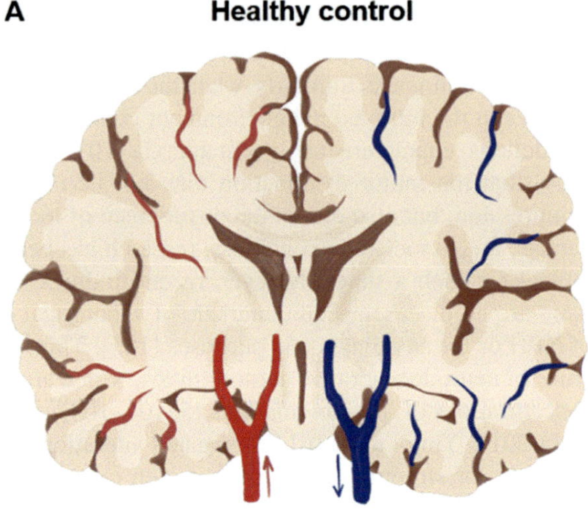

iNPH

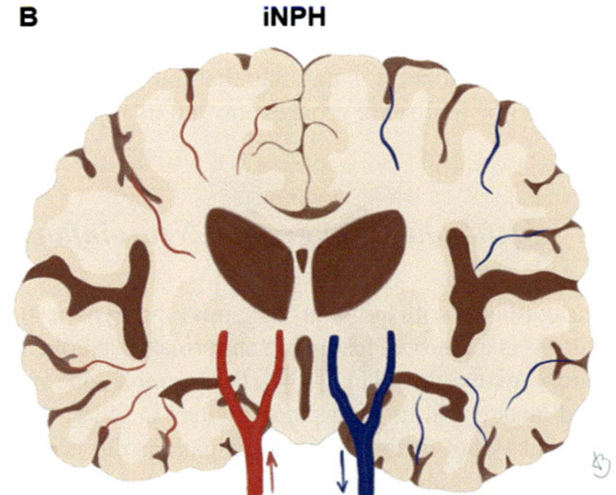

Fig. 7 Hemodynamics and reduced cerebral blood flow (A) in healthy controls, compared to (B) iNPH

be increased, but so far results are heterogeneous and their role in iNPH pathogenesis is unclear [121–123].

Recent studies are paying attention to astrogliosis processes in iNPH. Astrogliosis is defined as a defence mechanism of reactive astrocytes which are involved in epairmen pathways responding to CNS damage [124]. Primarily, Glial Fibrillary Acidic Protein (GFAP) is a typical biomarker of reactive astrocytes found in iNPH affected brains [32]. Statistical results depicting the differences between iNPH and healthy controls in GFAP concentrations correlated with worse CSF dynamic changes in terms of decreased compliance of brain parenchyma or parenchymal stiffness [32, 125].

6 Genetic Aspects

In the vast majority of cases, NPH occurs sporadically, however, recent studies [126–128] have described the existence of familial patterns related to the disease onset. The first description of inheritable NPH is dated to 1984 when Portenoy et al. [129] found two siblings diagnosed with NPH—a 74-year-old female and her 67-year-old brother, both manifesting with the complete triad of NPH. Further on, another report published in 2011 [130] showed a potential genetic aspect to NPH in two sisters, a 72- and 73-year-old. These findings were subsequently expanded by a study from Takahashi et al. [131] where the familial pattern of the disease was inherited in an autosomal-dominant fashion. This was described in four patients from three family generations (another four patients were diagnosed only with suspected NPH). In 2016 [132], genetic risk for shunt-responsive and definite iNPH was examined by investigating a copy number loss in intron 2 of the SFMBT1 gene. This study proposed that 26% of shunt-responsive and definite iNPH patients had intronic copy number loss in the SFMBT1 gene, whilst the same genetic abnormality was found in 4.2% of healthy elderly individuals (odds ratio (OR) $= 7.94$, 95% confidence interval (CI) $= 2.82-23.79$, p $= 1.8 \times 10^{-5}$) and in 6.3% of patients with Parkinson's disease (OR $= 5.18$, 95% CI $= 1.1-50.8$, $p = 0.038$). A study genotyping Norwegian and Finnish patients experiencing iNPH had similar results [18]. The copy number loss in intron 2 of SFMBT1 gene was found in 21% of Norwegian (OR $= 4.7$, $p < 0.0001$) and 10% of Finnish (OR $= 1.9$, $p = 0.0078$) iNPH patients, compared to 5.4% controls who also presented with his genetic change.

More recently, Morimoto et al. [128] performed whole-exome sequencing on a Japanese family with several members diagnosed with iNPH in 2019. The authors identified a missense mutation in the gene encoding the cilia- and flagella-associated protein 43 (CFAP43) which is responsible for male infertility and several abnormal morphological variations of sperm flagella, resulting in unusual functions [133, 134]. It has been suggested that the ciliary dysfunction may affect various tissues besides the testes, including the ependymal cells within choroid plexuses [128]. In a study by Yang et al. published in 2021 [135], 53 unrelated iNPH patients underwent whole-exome sequencing. In 15% of the participants, two types of heterozygous deletions in the CWH43 gene were identified with 6.6-fold and 2.7-fold enrichment when compared to the average population sample. Despite all the research which has been disclosed, more evidence and investigations are needed for clearer elucidation of genetic patterns in NPH pathogenesis. Further information about the genetic factors of the disease will be described in a separate chapter in this book.

7 Conclusion

The pathophysiology of NPH is a complex system of interacting mechanisms dependent on many factors which contribute to the disease progression. Due to the enormous amount of research on NPH pathophysiology and a new concept of the glymphatic system, we are becoming more familiar with the cerebrovascular and neuroinflammatory determinants that contribute to disease progression. However, besides a lot of promising research and reports in the field, the understanding of NPH pathogenesis and pathophysiology remains incomplete. Many findings need to be reproduced or clarified in correlation with clinical examinations, autopsy findings, and diagnostic measures which are essential for clearer differentiation between NPH and other neurodegenerative disorders. The treatment itself, now limited only to surgical implantation of the shunt system, might progressively evolve in terms of pharmacological and surgical approaches in disease management. Unfortunately, despite a lot of effort invested into iNPH research, findings so far cannot unequivocally define the initial cause of the disease. It is not certain why the manifestation of the disease is diverse and why patients with similar radiological and clinical features often respond to current treatment strategies differently. Further research needs to be made in order to elucidate pathophysiological concepts of iNPH more clearly (Fig. 8).

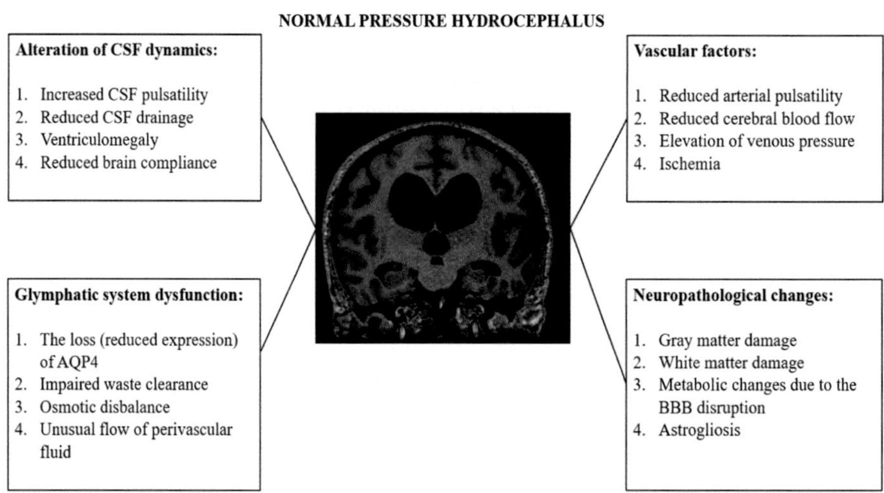

Fig. 8 Summary of pathophysiological mechanisms influencing the pathogenesis of iNPH

8   Key Points

- Ventricular expansion is initially caused by the pressure on the brain parenchyma and consequent ventriculomegaly is considered a compensation mechanism responsible for the return of ICP to its normal values.
- The dilatation of intracerebral ventricles is accompanied by increased CSF pulsatility, but reduced absorption of CSF. The physical stress on the periventricular white matter is responsible for axonal damage and their loss, resulting in alterations of intraneuronal biochemical processes, hypoxia, and ischemia.
- "Stiff ventricles" are one of the typical pathophysiological features of NPH. The compliance of periventricular parenchyma is reduced due to the increase of interstitial fluid, reduced plasticity of surrounding ependyma, and potentially the presence of ischemic processes.
- The exact pathophysiological mechanisms of the glymphatic system impairment in NPH have not been yet elucidated. It is most likely caused by abnormal CSF hydrodynamics which results in a disbalance of intracellular osmotic and metabolic pathways due to loss or disfigurement of AQP4 transmembrane channels. These channels remain vital for maintaining adequate water homeostasis in the brain.
- iNPH may be associated with obstructive sleep apnoea, but the exact mechanism of such a state needs to be investigated more in detail.
- The genetic factors involved in NPH onset are currently being investigated but it is certain that some NPH patients share a genetic predisposition to the disease onset.

Funding   This chapter was supported by the Ministry of Health of the Czech Republic institutional grant no. NU23-04-00551.

References

1. Filis AK, Aghayev K, Vrionis FD. Cerebrospinal fluid and hydrocephalus: physiology, diagnosis, and treatment. Cancer Control. 2017;24:6–8. https://doi.org/10.1177/107327481702 400102.
2. Gavrilov GV, Gaydar BV, Svistov DV, Korovin AE, Samarcev IN, Churilov LP, Tovpeko DV. Idiopathic normal pressure hydrocephalus (Hakim-Adams syndrome): clinical symptoms, diagnosis and treatment. Psychiatr Danub. 2019;31:737–44.
3. Martín-Láez R, Caballero-Arzapalo H, López-Menéndez L, Arango-Lasprilla JC, Vázquez-Barquero A. Epidemiology of idiopathic normal pressure hydrocephalus: a systematic review of the literature. World Neurosurg. 2015;84:2002–9. https://doi.org/10.1016/j.wneu.2015. 07.005.

4. Nakajima M, Yamada S, Miyajima M, Ishii K, Kuriyama N, Kazui H, Kanemoto H, Suehiro T, Yoshiyama K, Kameda M, et al. Guidelines for management of idiopathic normal pressure hydrocephalus (third edition): endorsed by the Japanese society of normal pressure hydrocephalus. Neurol Med Chir (Tokyo). 2021;61:63–97. https://doi.org/10.2176/nmc.st.2020-0292.

5. Jeppsson A, Zetterberg H, Blennow K, Wikkelsø C. Idiopathic normal-pressure hydrocephalus: pathophysiology and diagnosis by CSF biomarkers. Neurology. 2013;80:1385–92. https://doi.org/10.1212/WNL.0b013e31828c2fda.

6. Daou B, Klinge P, Tjoumakaris S, Rosenwasser RH, Jabbour P. Revisiting secondary normal pressure hydrocephalus: does it exist? A review. Neurosurg Focus. 2016;41:E6. https://doi.org/10.3171/2016.6.focus16189.

7. Wang C, Du HG, Yin LC, He M, Zhang GJ, Tian Y, Hao BL. Analysis of related factors affecting prognosis of shunt surgery in patients with secondary normal pressure hydrocephalus. Chin J Traumatol. 2013;16:221–4.

8. Brean A, Fredø HL, Sollid S, Müller T, Sundstrøm T, Eide PK. Five-year incidence of surgery for idiopathic normal pressure hydrocephalus in Norway. Acta Neurol Scand. 2009;120:314–6. https://doi.org/10.1111/j.1600-0404.2009.01250.x.

9. Brean A, Eide PK. Prevalence of probable idiopathic normal pressure hydrocephalus in a Norwegian population. Acta Neurol Scand. 2008;118:48–53. https://doi.org/10.1111/j.1600-0404.2007.00982.x.

10. Jaraj D, Rabiei K, Marlow T, Jensen C, Skoog I, Wikkelso C. Prevalence of idiopathic normal-pressure hydrocephalus. Neurology. 2014;82:1449–54. https://doi.org/10.1212/wnl.0000000000000342.

11. Hakim S, Adams RD. The special clinical problem of symptomatic hydrocephalus with normal cerebrospinal fluid pressure. Observations on cerebrospinal fluid hydrodynamics. J Neurol Sci. 1965;2:307–27. https://doi.org/10.1016/0022-510x(65)90016-x.

12. Reiber H. Flow rate of cerebrospinal fluid (CSF)—a concept common to normal blood-CSF barrier function and to dysfunction in neurological diseases. J Neurol Sci. 1994;122:189–203. https://doi.org/10.1016/0022-510X(94)90298-4.

13. Wang Z, Zhang Y, Hu F, Ding J, Wang X. Pathogenesis and pathophysiology of idiopathic normal pressure hydrocephalus. CNS Neurosci Ther. 2020;26:1230–40. https://doi.org/10.1111/cns.13526.

14. Preuss M, Hoffmann KT, Reiss-Zimmermann M, Hirsch W, Merkenschlager A, Meixensberger J, Dengl M. Updated physiology and pathophysiology of CSF circulation–the pulsatile vector theory. Childs Nerv Syst. 2013;29:1811–25. https://doi.org/10.1007/s00381-013-2219-0.

15. Benveniste H, Liu X, Koundal S, Sanggaard S, Lee H, Wardlaw J. The glymphatic system and waste clearance with brain aging: a review. Gerontology. 2019;65:106–19. https://doi.org/10.1159/000490349.

16. Reeves BC, Karimy JK, Kundishora AJ, Mestre H, Cerci HM, Matouk C, Alper SL, Lundgaard I, Nedergaard M, Kahle KT. Glymphatic system impairment in Alzheimer's disease and idiopathic normal pressure hydrocephalus. Trends Mol Med. 2020;26:285–95. https://doi.org/10.1016/j.molmed.2019.11.008.

17. Plog BA, Nedergaard M. The glymphatic system in central nervous system health and disease: past, present, and future. Annu Rev Pathol. 2018;13:379–94. https://doi.org/10.1146/annurev-pathol-051217-111018.

18. Korhonen VE, Helisalmi S, Jokinen A, Jokinen I, Lehtola J-M, Oinas M, Lönnrot K, Avellan C, Kotkansalo A, Frantzen J, et al. Copy number loss in SFMBT1 is common among Finnish and Norwegian patients with iNPH. Neurology Genet. 2018;4: e291. https://doi.org/10.1212/nxg.0000000000000291.

19. Greitz D. Cerebrospinal fluid circulation and associated intracranial dynamics. A radiologic investigation using MR imaging and radionuclide cisternography. Acta Radiol Suppl. 1993;386:1–23.

20. Floyd Domer R. Basic physiology of cerebrospinal fluid outflow. Exp Eye Res. 1977;25:323–32. https://doi.org/10.1016/S0014-4835(77)80029-8.

21. Rekate HL, Nadkarni TD, Wallace D. The importance of the cortical subarachnoid space in understanding hydrocephalus. J Neurosurg: Pediatr PED. 2008;2:1–11. https://doi.org/10.3171/PED/2008/2/7/001.

22. Krishnamurthy S, Li J. New concepts in the pathogenesis of hydrocephalus. Transl Pediatr. 2014;3:185–94. https://doi.org/10.3978/j.issn.2224-4336.2014.07.02.

23. Hoff J, Barber R. Transcerebral mantle pressure in normal pressure hydrocephalus. Arch Neurol. 1974;31:101–5. https://doi.org/10.1001/archneur.1974.00490380049005.

24. Raimondi AJ. A unifying theory for the definition and classification of hydrocephalus. Childs Nerv Syst. 1994;10:2–12. https://doi.org/10.1007/bf00313578.

25. Bateman GA. Idiopathic intracranial hypertension: priapism of the brain? Med Hypotheses. 2004;63:549–52. https://doi.org/10.1016/j.mehy.2004.03.014.

26. Oi S, Di Rocco C. Proposal of "evolution theory in cerebrospinal fluid dynamics" and minor pathway hydrocephalus in developing immature brain. Childs Nerv Syst. 2006;22:662–9. https://doi.org/10.1007/s00381-005-0020-4.

27. Matsumae M, Sato O, Hirayama A, Hayashi N, Takizawa K, Atsumi H, Sorimachi T. Research into the physiology of cerebrospinal fluid reaches a new horizon: intimate exchange between cerebrospinal fluid and interstitial fluid may contribute to maintenance of homeostasis in the central nervous system. Neurol Med Chir. 2016;56:416–41. https://doi.org/10.2176/nmc.ra.2016-0020.

28. Ammar A, Abbas F, Issawi W, Fakhro F, Batarfi L, Hendam A, Hasen M, Shawarby M, Al-Jehani H. Idiopathic normal-pressure hydrocephalus syndrome: Is it understood? The comprehensive idiopathic normal-pressure hydrocephalus theory (CiNPHT). In; 2017. p. 67–82. https://doi.org/10.1007/978-3-319-61304-8_5.

29. Iliff JJ, Wang M, Liao Y, Plogg Benjamin A, Peng W, Gundersen Georg A, Benveniste H, Vates GE, Deane R, Goldman Steven A, et al. A paravascular pathway facilitates CSF flow through the brain parenchyma and the clearance of interstitial solutes, including amyloid β. Sci Transl Med. 2012;4:147ra111–147ra111. https://doi.org/10.1126/scitranslmed.3003748.

30. Chikly B, Quaghebeur J. Reassessing cerebrospinal fluid (CSF) hydrodynamics: a literature review presenting a novel hypothesis for CSF physiology. J Bodyw Mov Ther. 2013;17:344–54. https://doi.org/10.1016/j.jbmt.2013.02.002.

31. Xie L, Kang H, Xu Q, Chen MJ, Liao Y, Thiyagarajan M, O'Donnell J, Christensen DJ, Nicholson C, Iliff JJ, et al. Sleep drives metabolite clearance from the adult brain. Science. 2013;342:373–7. https://doi.org/10.1126/science.1241224.

32. Eide PK, Hansson HA. Astrogliosis and impaired aquaporin-4 and dystrophin systems in idiopathic normal pressure hydrocephalus. Neuropathol Appl Neurobiol. 2018;44:474–90. https://doi.org/10.1111/nan.12420.

33. Ringstad G, Valnes LM, Dale AM, Pripp AH, Vatnehol S-AS, Emblem KE, Mardal K-A, Eide PK. Brain-wide glymphatic enhancement and clearance in humans assessed with MRI. JCI Insight. 2018;3. https://doi.org/10.1172/jci.insight.121537.

34. Román GC, Jackson RE, Fung SH, Zhang YJ, Verma AK. Sleep-disordered breathing and idiopathic normal-pressure hydrocephalus: recent pathophysiological advances. Curr Neurol Neurosci Rep. 2019;19. https://doi.org/10.1007/s11910-019-0952-9.

35. Eide PK, Ringstad G. Delayed clearance of cerebrospinal fluid tracer from entorhinal cortex in idiopathic normal pressure hydrocephalus: a glymphatic magnetic resonance imaging study. J Cereb Blood Flow Metab. 2019;39:1355–68. https://doi.org/10.1177/0271678x18760974.

36. Eide PK, Hansson HA. Blood-brain barrier leakage of blood proteins in idiopathic normal pressure hydrocephalus. Brain Res. 2020;1727: 146547. https://doi.org/10.1016/j.brainres.2019.146547.

37. Keong NCH, Pena A, Price SJ, Czosnyka M, Czosnyka Z, Pickard JD. Imaging normal pressure hydrocephalus: theories, techniques, and challenges. Neurosurg Focus. 2016;41:E11. https://doi.org/10.3171/2016.7.focus16194.

38. Bering EA Jr, Sato O. Hydrocephalus: changes in formation and absorption of cerebrospinal fluid within the cerebral ventricles. J Neurosurg. 1963;20:1050–63. https://doi.org/10.3171/jns.1963.20.12.1050.

39. Pappenheimer JR, Heisey SR, Jordan EF, Downer Jd. Perfusion of the cerebral ventricular system in unanesthetized goats. Am J Physiol-Legacy Content. 1962;203:763–74. https://doi.org/10.1152/ajplegacy.1962.203.5.763.

40. Pappenheimer JR, Miller TB, Goodrich CA. Sleep-promoting effects of cerebrospinal fluid from sleep-deprived goats. Proc Natl Acad Sci. 1967;58:513–7. https://doi.org/10.1073/pnas.58.2.513.

41. Brinker T, Stopa E, Morrison J, Klinge P. A new look at cerebrospinal fluid circulation. Fluids Barriers CNS. 2014;11:10. https://doi.org/10.1186/2045-8118-11-10.

42. Pirouzmand F, Tator CH, Rutka J. Management of hydrocephalus associated with vestibular schwannoma and other cerebellopontine angle tumors. Neurosurgery. 2001;48:1246–53; discussion 1253–1244. https://doi.org/10.1097/00006123-200106000-00010.

43. Xiao F, Lv S, Zong Z, Wu L, Tang X, Kuang W, Zhang P, Li X, Fu J, Xiao M, et al. Cerebrospinal fluid biomarkers for brain tumor detection: clinical roles and current progress. Am J Transl Res. 2020;12:1379–96.

44. Marmarou A, Foda MA, Bandoh K, Yoshihara M, Yamamoto T, Tsuji O, Zasler N, Ward JD, Young HF. Posttraumatic ventriculomegaly: hydrocephalus or atrophy? A new approach for diagnosis using CSF dynamics. J Neurosurg. 1996;85:1026–35. https://doi.org/10.3171/jns.1996.85.6.1026.

45. Miyati T, Mase M, Kasai H, Hara M, Yamada K, Shibamoto Y, Soellinger M, Baltes C, Luechinger R. Noninvasive MRI assessment of intracranial compliance in idiopathic normal pressure hydrocephalus. J Magn Reson Imaging. 2007;26:274–8. https://doi.org/10.1002/jmri.20999.

46. Tisell M, Tullberg M, Månsson JE, Fredman P, Blennow K, Wikkelsø C. Differences in cerebrospinal fluid dynamics do not affect the levels of biochemical markers in ventricular CSF from patients with aqueductal stenosis and idiopathic normal pressure hydrocephalus. Eur J Neurol. 2004;11:17–23. https://doi.org/10.1046/j.1351-5101.2003.00698.x.

47. Chrysikopoulos H. Idiopathic normal pressure hydrocephalus: thoughts on etiology and pathophysiology. Med Hypotheses. 2009;73:718–24. https://doi.org/10.1016/j.mehy.2009.04.044.

48. Kim DJ, Kim H, Kim YT, Yoon BC, Czosnyka Z, Park KW, Czosnyka M. Thresholds of resistance to CSF outflow in predicting shunt responsiveness. Neurol Res. 2015;37:332–40. https://doi.org/10.1179/1743132814y.0000000454.

49. Boon AJ, Tans JT, Delwel EJ, Egeler-Peerdeman SM, Hanlo PW, Wurzer HA, Avezaat CJ, de Jong DA, Gooskens RH, Hermans J. Dutch normal-pressure hydrocephalus study: randomized comparison of low- and medium-pressure shunts. J Neurosurg. 1998;88:490–5. https://doi.org/10.3171/jns.1998.88.3.0490.

50. Bateman GA. The pathophysiology of idiopathic normal pressure hydrocephalus: cerebral ischemia or altered venous hemodynamics? Am J Neuroradiol. 2008;29:198–203. https://doi.org/10.3174/ajnr.a0739.

51. Kuriyama N, Tokuda T, Yamada K, Akazawa K, Hosoda M, Sakai K, Watanabe Y, Nakagawa M. Flow velocity of the superior sagittal sinus is reduced in patients with idiopathic normal pressure hydrocephalus. J Neuroimaging. 2011;21:365–9. https://doi.org/10.1111/j.1552-6569.2011.00592.x.

52. Benabid AL, De Rougemont J, Barge M. Cerebral venous pressure, sinus pressure and intracranial pressure. Neurochirurgie. 1974;20:623–32.

53. Wilson MH. Monro-Kellie 2.0: the dynamic vascular and venous pathophysiological components of intracranial pressure. J Cereb Blood Flow Metab. 2016;36:1338–50. https://doi.org/10.1177/0271678x16648711.

54. Kayis C, Aygok GA. Cerebrospinal fluid dynamics and infusion techniques. In: Rigamonti D, editors. Adult hydrocephalus. Cambridge: Cambridge University Press; 2014. p. 139–49. https://doi.org/10.1017/CBO9781139382816.014.

55. Marmarou A, Shulman K, Rosende RM. A nonlinear analysis of the cerebrospinal fluid system and intracranial pressure dynamics. J Neurosurg. 1978;48:332–44. https://doi.org/10.3171/jns.1978.48.3.0332.

56. Kim H, Jeong E-J, Park D-H, Czosnyka Z, Yoon BC, Kim K, Czosnyka M, Kim D-J. Finite element analysis of periventricular lucency in hydrocephalus: extravasation or transependymal CSF absorption? J Neurosurg. 2016;124:334–41. https://doi.org/10.3171/2014.11.jns141382.

57. Bulat M, Klarica M. Recent insights into a new hydrodynamics of the cerebrospinal fluid. Brain Res Rev. 2011;65:99–112. https://doi.org/10.1016/j.brainresrev.2010.08.002.

58. Mascalchi M, Arnetoli G, Inzitari D, Dal Pozzo G, Lolli F, Caramella D, Bartolozzi C. Cine-MR imaging of aqueductal CSF flow in normal pressure hydrocephalus syndrome before and after CSF shunt. Acta Radiol. 1993;34:586–92.

59. Czosnyka M, Czosnyka Z, Momjian S, Pickard JD. Cerebrospinal fluid dynamics. Physiol Meas. 2004;25:R51-76. https://doi.org/10.1088/0967-3334/25/5/r01.

60. Egnor M, Wagshul M, Madsen J, Zou R, McCormack E, Hazel R, McAllister P. The cerebral Windkessel and its relevance to hydrocephalus: the notch filter model of cerebral blood flow. Cerebrospinal Fluid Res. 2006;3. https://doi.org/10.1186/1743-8454-3-s1-s48.

61. Israelsson H, Carlberg B, Wikkelsö C, Laurell K, Kahlon B, Leijon G, Eklund A, Malm J. Vascular risk factors in INPH. Neurology. 2017;88:577–85. https://doi.org/10.1212/wnl.0000000000003583.

62. Hamilton RB, Scalzo F, Baldwin K, Dorn A, Vespa P, Hu X, Bergsneider M. Opposing CSF hydrodynamic trends found in the cerebral aqueduct and prepontine cistern following shunt treatment in patients with normal pressure hydrocephalus. Fluids Barriers CNS. 2019;16. https://doi.org/10.1186/s12987-019-0122-0.

63. Yatsushiro S, Sunohara S, Hayashi N, Hirayama A, Matsumae M, Atsumi H, Kuroda K. Cardiac-driven pulsatile motion of intracranial cerebrospinal fluid visualized based on a correlation mapping technique. Magn Reson Med Sci. 2018;17:151–60. https://doi.org/10.2463/mrms.mp.2017-0014.

64. Hentschel S, Mardal KA, Løvgren AE, Linge S, Haughton V. Characterization of cyclic CSF flow in the foramen magnum and upper cervical spinal canal with MR flow imaging and computational fluid dynamics. Am J Neuroradiol. 2010;31:997–1002. https://doi.org/10.3174/ajnr.a1995.

65. Sass LR, Khani M, Natividad GC, Tubbs RS, Baledent O, Martin BA. A 3D subject-specific model of the spinal subarachnoid space with anatomically realistic ventral and dorsal spinal cord nerve rootlets. Fluids Barriers CNS. 2017;14. https://doi.org/10.1186/s12987-017-0085-y.

66. Eide PK, Stanisic M. Cerebral microdialysis and intracranial pressure monitoring in patients with idiopathic normal-pressure hydrocephalus: association with clinical response to extended lumbar drainage and shunt surgery. J Neurosurg. 2010;112:414–24. https://doi.org/10.3171/2009.5.Jns09122.

67. Green LM, Wallis T, Schuhmann MU, Jaeger M. Intracranial pressure waveform characteristics in idiopathic normal pressure hydrocephalus and late-onset idiopathic aqueductal stenosis. Fluids Barriers CNS. 2021;18. https://doi.org/10.1186/s12987-021-00259-y.

68. Jessen NA, Munk ASF, Lundgaard I, Nedergaard M. The glymphatic system: a beginner's guide. Neurochem Res. 2015;40:2583–99. https://doi.org/10.1007/s11064-015-1581-6.

69. Nakada T. Virchow-Robin space and aquaporin-4: new insights on an old friend. Croat Med J. 2014;55:328–36. https://doi.org/10.3325/cmj.2014.55.328.

70. Rasmussen MK, Mestre H, Nedergaard M. The glymphatic pathway in neurological disorders. The Lancet Neurology. 2018;17:1016–24. https://doi.org/10.1016/s1474-4422(18)30318-1.

71. Desai B, Hsu Y, Schneller B, Hobbs JG, Mehta AI, Linninger A. Hydrocephalus: the role of cerebral aquaporin-4 channels and computational modeling considerations of cerebrospinal fluid. Neurosurg Focus. 2016;41:E8. https://doi.org/10.3171/2016.7.focus16191.

72. Badaut J, Lasbennes F, Magistretti PJ, Regli L. Aquaporins in brain: distribution, physiology, and pathophysiology. J Cereb Blood Flow Metab. 2002;22:367–78. https://doi.org/10.1097/00004647-200204000-00001.

73. Nagelhus EA, Ottersen OP. Physiological roles of aquaporin-4 in brain. Physiol Rev. 2013;93:1543–62. https://doi.org/10.1152/physrev.00011.2013.
74. Verkman AS, Smith AJ, Phuan P-W, Tradtrantip L, Anderson MO. The aquaporin-4 water channel as a potential drug target in neurological disorders. Expert Opin Ther Targets. 2017;21:1161–70. https://doi.org/10.1080/14728222.2017.1398236.
75. Ke C, Poon WS, Ng HK, Pang JC, Chan Y. Heterogeneous responses of aquaporin-4 in oedema formation in a replicated severe traumatic brain injury model in rats. Neurosci Lett. 2001;301:21–4. https://doi.org/10.1016/s0304-3940(01)01589-0.
76. Qi LL, Fang SH, Shi WZ, Huang XQ, Zhang XY, Lu YB, Zhang WP, Wei EQ. CysLT2 receptor-mediated AQP4 up-regulation is involved in ischemic-like injury through activation of ERK and p38 MAPK in rat astrocytes. Life Sci. 2011;88:50–6. https://doi.org/10.1016/j.lfs.2010.10.025.
77. Ribeiro Mde C, Hirt L, Bogousslavsky J, Regli L, Badaut J. Time course of aquaporin expression after transient focal cerebral ischemia in mice. J Neurosci Res. 2006;83:1231–40. https://doi.org/10.1002/jnr.20819.
78. Misu T, Fujihara K, Kakita A, Konno H, Nakamura M, Watanabe S, Takahashi T, Nakashima I, Takahashi H, Itoyama Y. Loss of aquaporin 4 in lesions of neuromyelitis optica: distinction from multiple sclerosis. Brain. 2007;130:1224–34. https://doi.org/10.1093/brain/awm047.
79. Eid T, Lee TSW, Thomas MJ, Amiry-Moghaddam M, Bjornsen LP, Spencer DD, Agre P, Ottersen OP, De Lanerolle NC. Loss of perivascular aquaporin 4 may underlie deficient water and K+ homeostasis in the human epileptogenic hippocampus. Proc Natl Acad Sci. 2005;102:1193–8. https://doi.org/10.1073/pnas.0409308102.
80. Hasan-Olive MM, Enger R, Hansson HA, Nagelhus EA, Eide PK. Loss of perivascular aquaporin-4 in idiopathic normal pressure hydrocephalus. Glia. 2019;67:91–100. https://doi.org/10.1002/glia.23528.
81. Haj-Yasein NN, Vindedal GF, Eilert-Olsen M, Gundersen GA, Skare O, Laake P, Klungland A, Thoren AE, Burkhardt JM, Ottersen OP, et al. Glial-conditional deletion of aquaporin-4 (Aqp4) reduces blood-brain water uptake and confers barrier function on perivascular astrocyte endfeet. Proc Natl Acad Sci. 2011;108:17815–20. https://doi.org/10.1073/pnas.1110655108.
82. Vindedal GF, Thoren AE, Jensen V, Klungland A, Zhang Y, Holtzman MJ, Ottersen OP, Nagelhus EA. Removal of aquaporin-4 from glial and ependymal membranes causes brain water accumulation. Mol Cell Neurosci. 2016;77:47–52. https://doi.org/10.1016/j.mcn.2016.10.004.
83. Ringstad G, Vatnehol SAS, Eide PK. Glymphatic MRI in idiopathic normal pressure hydrocephalus. Brain. 2017;140:2691–705. https://doi.org/10.1093/brain/awx191.
84. Kass DA, Shapiro EP, Kawaguchi M, Capriotti AR, Scuteri A, Degroof RC, Lakatta EG. Improved arterial compliance by a novel advanced glycation end-product crosslink breaker. Circulation. 2001;104:1464–70. https://doi.org/10.1161/hc3801.097806.
85. Semba RD, Nicklett EJ, Ferrucci L. Does accumulation of advanced glycation end products contribute to the aging phenotype? J Gerontol A Biol Sci Med Sci. 2010;65A:963–75. https://doi.org/10.1093/gerona/glq074.
86. Tan C, Wang X, Wang Y, Wang C, Tang Z, Zhang Z, Liu J, Xiao G. The pathogenesis based on the glymphatic system, diagnosis, and treatment of idiopathic normal pressure hydrocephalus. Clin Interv Aging. 2021;16:139–53. https://doi.org/10.2147/cia.s290709.
87. Yamada S, Ishikawa M, Nozaki K. Exploring mechanisms of ventricular enlargement in idiopathic normal pressure hydrocephalus: a role of cerebrospinal fluid dynamics and motile cilia. Fluids Barriers CNS. 2021;18. https://doi.org/10.1186/s12987-021-00243-6.
88. Taoka T, Masutani Y, Kawai H, Nakane T, Matsuoka K, Yasuno F, Kishimoto T, Naganawa S. Evaluation of glymphatic system activity with the diffusion MR technique: diffusion tensor image analysis along the perivascular space (DTI-ALPS) in Alzheimer's disease cases. Jpn J Radiol. 2017;35:172–8. https://doi.org/10.1007/s11604-017-0617-z.
89. Taoka T, Naganawa S. Neurofluid dynamics and the glymphatic system: a neuroimaging perspective. Korean J Radiol. 2020;21:1199. https://doi.org/10.3348/kjr.2020.0042.

90. Rammo R, Nagel S. The importance of non-invasive imaging in understanding the glymphatic system in normal pressure hydrocephalus. Parkinsonism Relat Disord. 2021;82:158. https://doi.org/10.1016/j.parkreldis.2021.01.007.

91. Bae YJ, Choi BS, Kim J-M, Choi J-H, Cho SJ, Kim JH. Altered glymphatic system in idiopathic normal pressure hydrocephalus. Parkinsonism Relat Disord. 2021;82:56–60. https://doi.org/10.1016/j.parkreldis.2020.11.009.

92. Chen Z, Liu C, Zhang J, Relkin N, Xing Y, Li Y. Cerebrospinal fluid Aβ42, t-tau, and p-tau levels in the differential diagnosis of idiopathic normal-pressure hydrocephalus: a systematic review and meta-analysis. Fluids Barriers CNS. 2017;14. https://doi.org/10.1186/s12987-017-0062-5.

93. Bech-Azeddine R, Hogh P, Juhler M, Gjerris F, Waldemar G. Idiopathic normal-pressure hydrocephalus: clinical comorbidity correlated with cerebral biopsy findings and outcome of cerebrospinal fluid shunting. J Neurol Neurosurg Psychiatry. 2007;78:157–61. https://doi.org/10.1136/jnnp.2006.095117.

94. Benveniste H, Heerdt PM, Fontes M, Rothman DL, Volkow ND. Glymphatic system function in relation to anesthesia and sleep states. Anesth Analg. 2019;128:747–58. https://doi.org/10.1213/ane.0000000000004069.

95. Gordleeva S, Kanakov O, Ivanchenko M, Zaikin A, Franceschi C. Brain aging and garbage cleaning. Semin Immunopathol. 2020;42:647–65. https://doi.org/10.1007/s00281-020-00816-x.

96. Kang J-E, Lim Miranda M, Bateman Randall J, Lee James J, Smyth Liam P, Cirrito John R, Fujiki N, Nishino S, Holtzman DM. Amyloid-β dynamics are regulated by orexin and the sleep-wake cycle. Science. 2009;326:1005–7. https://doi.org/10.1126/science.1180962.

97. Ohayon MM, Carskadon MA, Guilleminault C, Vitiello MV. Meta-analysis of quantitative sleep parameters from childhood to old age in healthy individuals: developing normative sleep values across the human lifespan. Sleep. 2004;27:1255–73. https://doi.org/10.1093/sleep/27.7.1255.

98. Kalani MYS, Filippidis AS, Rekate HL. Hydrocephalus and aquaporin's: the role of aquaporin-1. In: Springer Vienna; 2012. p. 51–54. https://doi.org/10.1007/978-3-7091-0923-6_11.

99. Hua Y, Ying X, Qian Y, Liu H, Lan Y, Xie A, Zhu X. Physiological and pathological impact of AQP1 knockout in mice. Biosci Rep. 2019;39:BSR20182303. https://doi.org/10.1042/bsr20182303.

100. Castañeyra-Ruiz L, González-Marrero I, Carmona-Calero EM, Abreu-Gonzalez P, Lecuona M, Brage L, Rodríguez EM, Castañeyra-Perdomo A. Cerebrospinal fluid levels of tumor necrosis factor alpha and aquaporin 1 in patients with mild cognitive impairment and idiopathic normal pressure hydrocephalus. Clin Neurol Neurosurg. 2016;146:76–81. https://doi.org/10.1016/j.clineuro.2016.04.025.

101. Gleason PL, Black PM, Matsumae M. The neurobiology of normal pressure hydrocephalus. Neurosurg Clin N Am. 1993;4:667–75.

102. Md J, Biagioni M. Normal pressure hydrocephalus. In: StatPearls. Treasure Island: StatPearls Publishing. Copyright ©; 2020.

103. Tang YM, Yao Y, Xu S, Li X, Hu F, Wang H, Ding J, Wang X. White matter microstructural damage associated with gait abnormalities in idiopathic normal pressure hydrocephalus. Front Aging Neurosci. 2021;13: 660621. https://doi.org/10.3389/fnagi.2021.660621.

104. Thompson PD. Frontal lobe ataxia. Handb Clin Neurol. 2012;103:619–22. https://doi.org/10.1016/b978-0-444-51892-7.00044-9.

105. Agren-Wilsson A, Lekman A, Sjöberg W, Rosengren L, Blennow K, Bergenheim AT, Malm J. CSF biomarkers in the evaluation of idiopathic normal pressure hydrocephalus. Acta Neurol Scand. 2007;116:333–9. https://doi.org/10.1111/j.1600-0404.2007.00890.x.

106. Lin Y-S, Lee W-J, Wang S-J, Fuh J-L. Levels of plasma neurofilament light chain and cognitive function in patients with Alzheimer or Parkinson disease. Sci. Rep. 2018;8. https://doi.org/10.1038/s41598-018-35766-w.

107. Olsson B, Portelius E, Cullen NC, Sandelius Å, Zetterberg H, Andreasson U, Höglund K, Irwin DJ, Grossman M, Weintraub D, et al. Association of cerebrospinal fluid neurofilament light protein levels with cognition in patients with dementia, motor neuron disease, and movement disorders. JAMA Neurol. 2019;76:318. https://doi.org/10.1001/jamaneurol.2018.3746.

108. Mattsson N, Andreasson U, Zetterberg H, Blennow K. Association of plasma neurofilament light with neurodegeneration in patients with Alzheimer disease. JAMA Neurol. 2017;74:557. https://doi.org/10.1001/jamaneurol.2016.6117.

109. Tullberg M, Rosengren L, Blomsterwall E, Karlsson JE, Wikkelsö C. CSF neurofilament and glial fibrillary acidic protein in normal pressure hydrocephalus. Neurology. 1998;50:1122. https://doi.org/10.1212/WNL.50.4.1122.

110. Yin L-K, Zheng J-J, Tian J-Q, Hao X-Z, Li C-C, Ye J-D, Zhang Y-X, Yu H, Yang Y-M. Abnormal gray matter structural networks in idiopathic normal pressure hydrocephalus. Front Aging Neurosci. 2018;10:356–356. https://doi.org/10.3389/fnagi.2018.00356.

111. Khoo HM, Kishima H, Tani N, Oshino S, Maruo T, Hosomi K, Yanagisawa T, Kazui H, Watanabe Y, Shimokawa T, et al. Default mode network connectivity in patients with idiopathic normal pressure hydrocephalus. J Neurosurg. 2016;124:350–8. https://doi.org/10.3171/2015.1.jns141633.

112. Glenn TC, Kelly DF, Boscardin WJ, McArthur DL, Vespa P, Oertel M, Hovda DA, Bergsneider M, Hillered L, Martin NA. Energy dysfunction as a predictor of outcome after moderate or severe head injury: indices of oxygen, glucose, and lactate metabolism. J Cereb Blood Flow Metab. 2003;23:1239–50. https://doi.org/10.1097/01.wcb.0000089833.23606.7f.

113. Kondziella D, Sonnewald U, Tullberg M, Wikkelso C. Brain metabolism in adult chronic hydrocephalus. J Neurochem. 2008;106:1515–24. https://doi.org/10.1111/j.1471-4159.2008.05422.x.

114. Tarnaris A, Toma AK, Pullen E, Chapman MD, Petzold A, Cipolotti L, Kitchen ND, Keir G, Lemieux L, Watkins LD. Cognitive, biochemical, and imaging profile of patients suffering from idiopathic normal pressure hydrocephalus. Alzheimers Dement. 2011;7:501–8. https://doi.org/10.1016/j.jalz.2011.01.003.

115. Lundin F, Tisell A, Dahlqvist Leinhard O, Tullberg M, Wikkelso C, Lundberg P, Leijon G. Reduced thalamic N-acetylaspartate in idiopathic normal pressure hydrocephalus: a controlled 1H-magnetic resonance spectroscopy study of frontal deep white matter and the thalamus using absolute quantification. J Neurol Neurosurg Psychiatry. 2011;82:772–8. https://doi.org/10.1136/jnnp.2010.223529.

116. Lee C, Seo H, Yoon S-Y, Chang SH, Park S-H, Hwang J-H, Kang K, Kim C-H, Hahm MH, Park E, et al. Clinical significance of vitamin D in idiopathic normal pressure hydrocephalus. Acta Neurochir. 2021;163:1969–77. https://doi.org/10.1007/s00701-021-04849-5.

117. Eidsvaag VA, Hansson H-A, Heuser K, Nagelhus EA, Eide PK. Brain capillary ultrastructure in idiopathic normal pressure hydrocephalus: relationship with static and pulsatile intracranial pressure. J Neuropathol Exp Neurol. 2017;76:1034–45. https://doi.org/10.1093/jnen/nlx091.

118. Lee J-H, Park D-H, Back D-B, Lee J-Y, Lee C-I, Park K-J, Kang S-H, Cho T-H, Chung Y-G. Comparison of cerebrospinal fluid biomarkers between idiopathic normal pressure hydrocephalus and subarachnoid hemorrhage-induced chronic hydrocephalus: a pilot study. Med Sci Monit. 2012;18:PR19–PR25. https://doi.org/10.12659/msm.883586.

119. Sosvorova L, Kanceva R, Vcelak J, Kancheva L, Mohapl M, Starka L, Havrdova E. The comparison of selected cerebrospinal fluid and serum cytokine levels in patients with multiple sclerosis and normal pressure hydrocephalus. Neuro Endocrinol Lett. 2015;36:564–71.

120. Sosvorova L, Vcelak J, Mohapl M, Vitku J, Bicikova M, Hampl R. Selected pro- and anti-inflammatory cytokines in cerebrospinal fluid in normal pressure hydrocephalus. Neuro Endocrinol Lett. 2014;35:586–93.

121. Schirinzi T, Sancesario GM, Di Lazzaro G, D'Elia A, Imbriani P, Scalise S, Pisani A. Cerebrospinal fluid biomarkers profile of idiopathic normal pressure hydrocephalus. J Neural Transm. 2018;125:673–9. https://doi.org/10.1007/s00702-018-1842-z.

122. Boyd FT, Cheifetz S, Andres J, Laiho M, Massagué J. Transforming growth factor-β receptors and binding proteoglycans. J Cell Sci. 1990;1990:131–8. https://doi.org/10.1242/jcs.1990.supplement_13.12.

123. Hinck AP, Archer SJ, Qian SW, Roberts AB, Sporn MB, Weatherbee JA, Tsang MLS, Lucas R, Zhang B-L, Wenker J, et al. Transforming growth factor β1: three-dimensional structure in solution and comparison with the X-ray structure of transforming growth factor β2. Biochemistry. 1996;35:8517–34. https://doi.org/10.1021/bi9604946.

124. Sofroniew MV. Astrogliosis. Cold Spring Harb Perspect Biol. 2015;7: a020420. https://doi.org/10.1101/cshperspect.a020420.

125. Zhou B, Zuo YX, Jiang RT. Astrocyte morphology: diversity, plasticity, and role in neurological diseases. CNS Neurosci Ther. 2019;25:665–73. https://doi.org/10.1111/cns.13123.

126. Huovinen J, Kastinen S, Komulainen S, Oinas M, Avellan C, Frantzen J, Rinne J, Ronkainen A, Kauppinen M, Lönnrot K, et al. Familial idiopathic normal pressure hydrocephalus. J Neurol Sci. 2016;368:11–8. https://doi.org/10.1016/j.jns.2016.06.052.

127. McGirr A, Cusimano MD. Familial aggregation of idiopathic normal pressure hydrocephalus: novel familial case and a family study of the NPH triad in an iNPH patient cohort. J Neurol Sci. 2012;321:82–8. https://doi.org/10.1016/j.jns.2012.07.062.

128. Morimoto Y, Yoshida S, Kinoshita A, Satoh C, Mishima H, Yamaguchi N, Matsuda K, Sakaguchi M, Tanaka T, Komohara Y, et al. Nonsense mutation in CFAP43 causes normal-pressure hydrocephalus with ciliary abnormalities. Neurology. 2019;92:e2364–74. https://doi.org/10.1212/wnl.0000000000007505.

129. Portenoy RK, Berger A, Gross E. Familial occurrence of idiopathic normal-pressure hydrocephalus. Arch Neurol. 1984;41:335–7. https://doi.org/10.1001/archneur.1984.04050150117029.

130. Cusimano MD, Rewilak D, Stuss DT, Barrera-Martinez JC, Salehi F, Freedman M. Normal-Pressure Hydrocephalus: Is There a Genetic Predisposition? Can J Neurol Sci/Journal Canadien des Sciences Neurologiques. 2011;38:274–81. https://doi.org/10.1017/s031716710001146x.

131. Takahashi Y, Kawanami T, Nagasawa H, Iseki C, Hanyu H, Kato T. Familial normal pressure hydrocephalus (NPH) with an autosomal-dominant inheritance: a novel subgroup of NPH. J Neurol Sci. 2011;308:149–51. https://doi.org/10.1016/j.jns.2011.06.018.

132. Sato H, Takahashi Y, Kimihira L, Iseki C, Kato H, Suzuki Y, Igari R, Sato H, Koyama S, Arawaka S, et al. A segmental copy number loss of the SFMBT1 gene is a genetic risk for shunt-responsive, idiopathic normal pressure hydrocephalus (iNPH): a case-control study. PLoS ONE. 2016;11: e0166615. https://doi.org/10.1371/journal.pone.0166615.

133. Tang S, Wang X, Li W, Yang X, Li Z, Liu W, Li C, Zhu Z, Wang L, Wang J, et al. Biallelic mutations in CFAP43 and CFAP44 cause male infertility with multiple morphological abnormalities of the sperm flagella. Am J Hum Genet. 2017;100:854–64. https://doi.org/10.1016/j.ajhg.2017.04.012.

134. Coutton C, Vargas AS, Amiri-Yekta A, Kherraf Z-E, Ben Mustapha SF, Le Tanno P, Wambergue-Legrand C, Karaouzène T, Martinez G, Crouzy S, et al. Mutations in CFAP43 and CFAP44 cause male infertility and flagellum defects in Trypanosoma and human. Nat Commun. 2018;9. https://doi.org/10.1038/s41467-017-02792-7.

135. Yang HW, Lee S, Yang D, Dai H, Zhang Y, Han L, Zhao S, Zhang S, Ma Y, Johnson MF, et al. Deletions in CWH43 cause idiopathic normal pressure hydrocephalus. EMBO Mol Med. 2021;13. https://doi.org/10.15252/emmm.202013249.

Genetic Aspects of iNPH

Tomáš Moravec, Helen Whitley, Zdeněk Musil, and Ondřej Bradáč

Abstract Idiopathic Normal Pressure Hydrocephalus (iNPH) is a complex and multifactorial condition. Although the disease appears to occur sporadically, the presence of familial subtypes and new investigations of candidate genes suggest a genetic component to the pathogenesis. Whilst pedigree studies of iNPH provide the starting point for evidence of genetic risk factors, functional analysis of candidate genes and their mutations offers insight into possible molecular mechanisms underlying the disorder. We have reviewed the current literature and identified 7 genes or gene groups likely to be involved in iNPH pathogenesis. Currently, the genes with the most evidence for a crucial role are *CFAP43*, *SFMBT1*, and *CWH43*. Animal models are indispensable for understanding genetic disease. As iNPH is multifactorial and complex, animal models are an appropriate tool for untangling genetic, epigenetic, and environmental risks in a disease involving interconnected pathological processes. We also describe results from animal studies of candidate genes, as reverse genetic approaches can uncover the function and underlying pathogenic mechanisms of iNPH genes.

Keywords Genetics · Hydrocephalus · Normal pressure hydrocephalus · CFAP43 · SFMBT1 · CWH43 · Epigenetic factors

Moravec and Whitley contributed equally to this work and share first authorship.

T. Moravec · H. Whitley · O. Bradáč (✉)
Department of Neurosurgery and Neurooncology, 1st Faculty of Medicine, Charles University and Military University Hospital, Prague, Czech Republic
e-mail: ondrej.bradac2@fnmotol.cz

Z. Musil
Institute of Biology and Medical Genetics, 1st Faculty of Medicine, Charles University and General University Hospital, Prague, Czech Republic

Department of Anatomy, 3rd Faculty of Medicine, Charles University, Prague, Czech Republic

O. Bradáč
Department of Neurosurgery, 2nd Faculty of Medicine, Charles University and Motol University Hospital, Prague, Czech Republic

© The Author(s), under exclusive license to Springer Nature Switzerland AG 2023
O. Bradac (ed.), *Normal Pressure Hydrocephalus*,
https://doi.org/10.1007/978-3-031-36522-5_7

Abbreviations

A1R	A1 receptor
A2AR	A2A receptor
Aβ	Amyloid beta
AβPP	Amyloid beta precursor protein
AD	Alzheimer disease
ALS	Amyotrophic lateral sclerosis
APOE	Apolipoprotein E
AQP	Aquaporin
C9ORF72	Chromosome 9 open reading frame 72
CFAP43	Cilia- and flagella-associated protein 43
CNV	Copy number variations
CSF	Cerebrospinal fluid
DNA	Deoxyribonucleic acid
ELISA	Enzyme-linked immunosorbent assay
ET	Essential tremor
ETINPH	Essential tremor normal pressure hydrocephalus
FAB	Frontal assessment battery
FTL	Frontotemporal lobe dementia
GPI	Glycosylphosphatidylinositol
GWAS	Genome-wide association study
iNPH	Idiopathic normal pressure hydrocephalus
MBT	Malignant brain tumour
MMSE	Mini mental state exam
OR	Odds ratio
PCD	Primary ciliary dyskinesia
qPCR	Quantitative polymerase chain reaction
SNP	Single nucleotide polymorphism
WES	Whole exome sequencing

1 Introduction

Idiopathic normal pressure hydrocephalus (iNPH) is a neurodegenerative disorder of the elderly, characterised by ventriculomegaly and the classic Hakim's triad of incontinence, gait disturbance, and dementia. This multi-factors disorder involves a complex interplay of neuroinflammation, vascular changes, and CSF hyper-dynamism. The advances in understanding of pathogenesis are complemented by an increasing number of genetic studies, which suggest possible molecular mechanisms and help to elucidate the underlying disease process.

Other forms of hydrocephalus, such as congenital or infantile types, have a known genetic component. They are often associated with genetic syndromes, several causative genes are already known, and the disease manifests in infancy. However, since iNPH is a disease of the elderly, a simple cause-and-effect relationship is unlikely. Any predisposing genetic factors do not affect the phenotype unless additional triggers are present. These may be environmental factors, epigenetic mechanisms, or other processes associated with ageing. iNPH represents a number of complex traits, and variations in gene expression and penetrance is to be expected. This also means that identifying one genetic marker for analysis is problematic.

Identifying genetic risk factors has many potential advantages. Genetic markers could aid the problematic differentiation of iNPH from closely related diseases such as AD or other types of dementia. This would firmly establish iNPH as a known disease entity and standardise diagnosis, which is currently based on response to treatment. Patients with iNPH-associated mutations could benefit from earlier interventions or prophylaxis treatment, lessening disease burden. Still, the majority of current genetic studies are relatively small or incomplete, and larger more comprehensive projects are needed to comprehensively identify iNPH-associated variants. Additionally, candidate genes identified in the studies require full functional analysis before any clinical relevance can be established. Such analysis requires multidisciplinary approaches, as supported by genetically modifiable animal models of disease.

2 Familial Studies of iNPH

Long considered sporadic, an increasing number of cohort studies and pedigree analyses are revealing that iNPH aggregates in families. These observations form the earliest suggestions that iNPH has a heritable component. The first account of familial occurrence of iNPH was a 1984 case report describing shunt-responsive iNPH in siblings [1]. Subsequently, McGirr et al. [2] investigated the prevalence of Hakim's triad amongst family members of patients with iNPH, finding six of the 20 probands had first degree relatives with more than two symptoms of the triad. The incidence amongst iNPH relatives was 7.1%, whilst in the control group the incidence was 0.7% (OR = 11.53). A larger study investigated a cohort of 375 shunted iNPH patients, describing the pedigrees of all families with more than one case of iNPH [3]. 4.8% of patients from 12 different pedigrees had at least one relative with iNPH, and 11% had relatives with two or more of the classical triad of iNPH symptoms. This study also characterised the difference between familial iNPH and sporadic iNPH. The familial type was associated with a threefold increased risk of clinical dementia, according to multivariate logistic regression analysis. A familial subtype of iNPH was proposed by Takahashi et al. in a case report of a family with iNPH in three generations [4]. Four patients had clinical and MRI features consistent with iNPH, and a family interview revealed that an additional four members have suspected iNPH, although the diagnosis was not confirmed. According to the pedigree analysis, the condition appeared to be inherited in an autosomal dominant pattern. A 2011 case report of two siblings with iNPH also suggested a genetic component to the disease [5], although in this case two elderly siblings shared environmental exposures and comorbidities. Another report of two siblings with iNPH suggests a genetic predisposition amongst the children of the patients. [6] Both patients had daughters who complained of urinary continence, but without gait or cognitive defects. These observations imply variations in gene expressivity, due to factors such as age and other environmental influences. Pedigree analyses may also lead to the identification of subclinical iNPH in a target population, allowing earlier intervention and lowering the disease burden.

A subtype of iNPH with a genetic cause was described in 2008. This condition was characterised by the development of Essential Tremor (ET) in young adulthood followed by iNPH when elderly [7]. The condition was named Essential Tremor Idiopathic Normal Pressure Hydrocephalus (ETINPH), and a follow up study uncovered the genetic aetiology. Using genome-wide linkage, a locus was mapped to chromosome 19q12-13.31 [8]. Several genes in this region are expressed in the nervous system, and functional analysis on these genes could offer insights into the pathogenic processes involved in both ETINPH and iNPH. Notable genes include ATP*1A3* and *PSEN2*. *ATP1A3* encodes the Na(+)/K(+)-ATPase pump. A mutation in this gene causes rapid-onset dystonia-parkinsonism [9]. *PSEN2* encodes Presenilin 2, which processes amyloid beta precursor protein (AβPP). Changes in amyloid metabolism have a known involvement in Alzheimer's disease (AD) pathogenesis and are hypothesised to have a role in the disease process of iNPH.

3   Candidate Genes Associated with iNPH

Several studies on the genetic basis of iNPH have yielded positive results. Genome-Wide Association Studies (GWAS) and Whole Exome Sequencing (WES) have identified genes and loci that are compelling candidates for disease. The important genes associated with iNPH are described in the following paragraphs. A summary of each gene described and can be found in Table 1: Summary of candidate genes.

3.1   *Cilia- and Flagella-Associated Protein 43*, CFAP43

Current evidence indicates that CSF flow is generated and restrained by the synchronised beats of motile cilia, such as those found on the surface of the ependymal cells that line the brain ventricles. Mutations in *CFAP43* on chromosome 10, are associated with ciliary dysfunction. This gene is preferentially expressed in the testes, epithelial linings of the airways and trachea, the ependymal cells lining the brain ventricles, and the choroid plexus. Functions include cilium movement in epithelia, sperm axoneme assembly, and brain development. Subcellular localisation is the cytoskeleton and cilium axoneme [10]. A Japanese family with multiple members who had iNPH was analysed using WES. This identified a loss of function variant of *CFAP4* associated with the disease. The proband was a 55-year-old woman presenting with the

Table 1 Summary of candidate genes

Gene name	Gene product	Mutation/ variant/ expression change	Function	Localisation	Loci	References
CFAP43	Cilia- and flagella-associated protein 43	Nonsense, loss of function C > T	Cilium movement, sperm axoneme assembly, and brain development	Cytoskeleton and cilium axoneme	Ch10 q 25.1	Morimoto et al. [10]
SFMBT1	Scm like with four Mbt domains 1	Copy number loss of intron 2	Chromatin modification	Smooth muscle and endothelium of vasculature, ependymal cells lining the ventricles, and cells of the choroid plexus	Ch 3p 21.1	Kato et al. [11], Sato et al. [12], Korhonen et al. [13]
CWH43	"Cell wall biogenesis protein 43"	Loss of function deletion	Incorporates ceramide into the glycosylphosphatidylinositol (GPI) anchor in yeast	Apical surface of ependymal cells and choroid plexus	Ch 4 p11	Yang et al. [14]
C9ORF72	Chromosome 9 open reading frame 72	Full or intermediate repeat expansion (20–30 repeats)	Endosomal trafficking, actin regulation	Neuronal cytoplasm, presynaptic terminals	Ch 9p21.2	Korhonen et al. [15]
APOE3	Apolipoprotein E3	Allelic variant	Transports lipids and cholesterol to lymphatics	Vesicles	Ch 19q13. 32	Gudmundsson et al. [16], Huovinen et al. [3], Laiterä et al. [17]
TTR	Transthyretin	Decreased expression in iNPH (17 × decrease)	Transports thyroxine and retinol	choroid plexus, retina, liver	Ch 18 q 12.1	Laiterä et al. [18]

(continued)

Table 1 (continued)

Gene name	Gene product	Mutation/ variant/ expression change	Function	Localisation	Loci	References
AβPP	Amyloid beta precursor protein	Increased expression in iNPH (3 ×)	Binds cell surface proteins, cleaved into defined fragments	Throughout CNS, concentrated in neuronal synapses	Ch 21q21.3	Laiterä et al. [18]
ADAM10	Disintegrin and metalloproteinase domain-containing protein 10	Increased expression iNPH	Adhesion and proteolysis, dendritic spine formation	Ubiquitous throughout CNS	Ch 15q21.3	Laiterä et al. [18]
NME8	Thioredoxin domain-containing protein 3 (TXNDC3)	Allelic variant	DNA damage repair, ciliary maturation	Ciliated cells, cilium axoneme	Ch 7 p14.1	Huovinen et al. [19]
A1R and A2AR	Adenosine 1 receptor and adenosine 2A receptor	Decreased expression in iNPH	Adenosine signalling	A1R—cortex, hippocampus, cerebellum, A2AR—striatum, olfactory bulb	A1R—Ch 1q32.1 A2AR—Ch 22 q11.23	Casati et al. [20]

Hakim triad of symptoms. She presented with gait disturbance, cognitive impairment as indicated by MMSE 24/30 and FAB 3/18, and urinary incontinence. Five family members were recruited for sequencing. After filtering our simple missense variants, 72 gene variants were found. One nonsense mutation that segregated with the disease was identified. This was found at chr10:105893468 with the change C > T, in the gene *CFAP43*. To confirm pathogenic ciliary ultrastructure, nasal mucosa was analysed by TEM, revealing many abnormal cilia. The study also included results from mouse experiments which were subsequently performed, knocking out an ortholog of *CFAP43* with CRISPR-Cas9 technology. The mice exhibited a hydrocephalus phenotype with morphologic abnormality of motile cilia. These results strongly suggest that CFAP43 could be responsible for normal pressure hydrocephalus, challenging the concept that iNPH is "idiopathic" [21].

3.2 Histone-Associated Genes Products: SFMBT1

SFMBT1 is a product of a histone-associated gene called *SFMBT1*, which has recently gained attention for its possible role in CSF flow and absorption. SFMBT1 is localised in the smooth muscle, vascular endothelium, ependymal cells lining the ventricles, and cells of the choroid plexus. The gene is located on chromosome 3p 21.1 which encodes a protein consisting of 866 amino acid residues. The protein contains 4 Malignant Brain Tumour (MBT) repeat domains. This MBT domain is a "chromatin reader", a protein that binds to post-translational modifications on histone tails. MBT domains bind to mono- and di-methylated histone lysines *in vitro* and down-regulate gene transcription via interaction with various repressors [11]. Several studies have shown that copy number loss of SFMBT1 seems to be a risk factor for iNPH [12, 13, 22].

A GWAS for CNVs using DNA from blood samples of eight possible iNPH patients and 110 controls showed that 50% of the iNPH group had heterozygous copy number loss in SFMBT1. The loss was within the intron 2 of the gene. One of the 110 controls also had this mutation (0.9%). This study also analysed shunt-responsive patients with definite iNPH, finding that five (65%) of the eight patients had the same mutation at the same locus [12]. A further study on SFMBT1 showed by PCR analyses that 26% of iNPH patients ($n = 50$) had a copy number loss in intron 2 of the SFMBT1 gene, compared to 4.2% of healthy elderly controls ($n = 191$); (OR $= 7.94$, 95%CI: 2.82–23.79, $p = 1.8 \times 10^{-5}$). The authors suggest that this specific mutation in SFMBT1 may be a genetic risk factor for definitive, shunt-responsive iNPH [13]. Korhoen et al. analysed *SFMBT1* variation by quantitative PCR (qPCR) in 567 NPH Finnish and 377 Norwegian patients with iNPH. Copy number loss in intron 2 of *SFMBT1* was found in 10% of Finnish and 21% of Norwegian patients. (OR $= 1.9, p = 0.0078$ and OR $= 4.7, p < 0.0001$ respectively). The variant did not correlate with the outcome of shunt surgery. This large cohort provides further evidence for a genetic aspect to iNPH pathogenesis [22]. Although it is still unknown whether copy number loss of SFMBT1 causes definitive, shunt-responsive iNPH, there is strong evidence that this specific mutation is a risk factor for the disease. Given the known molecular functions of SFMBT1 in localisation to ependymal cell and choir plexus, and involvement in chromatin modification, it seems likely that iNPH pathogenesis involves disturbed epigenetic mechanisms.

3.3   Genes Encoding Cell Membrane-Associated Proteins: CWH43 and AQP

A hallmark feature of iNPH pathology is hyper-dynamic CSF flow. Cell membrane proteins with possible roles in CSF homeostasis may have a role in the development of disease. *CWH43 is a gene* involved in membrane structure, encoding a protein that fixates certain proteins to the cell membrane. Brain aquaporins are encoded by genes *AQP1* and *AQP4* and have also been hypothesised to play a role in CSF homeostasis.

CWH43 encodes a membrane protein called "Cell wall biogenesis protein 43", which incorporates ceramide into the glycosylphosphatidylinositol (GPI) anchor, fixing proteins to the membrane [14]. This functional analysis was performed in yeast, and the exact function in multicellular organisms is still unknown. A WES study by Yang et al. on 53 unrelated iNPH patients identified two heterozygous loss of function deletions in *CWH43* [23]. 15% of the iNPH patients were significantly enriched compared to the general population (6.6-fold and 2.7-fold). Using CRISPR9/Cas9 technology, the authors also generated a modified mouse line heterozygous for *CWH43* deletion. The animals presented communicating hydrocephalus with ventriculomegaly, gait and balance disturbances. Electron microscopy revealed decreased number of ependymal cilia, and expression studies revealed decreased localisation of GPI-anchored proteins on apical surfaces of the choroid plexus and ependymal cells. Interestingly, there is some evidence that *CWH43* deletion leads to decreased L1CAM signalling [24]. L1CAM is a known cause of congenital hydrocephalus. The evidence for *CWH43* as a risk factor underlying iNPH symptomatology is compelling.

Brain aquaporins (AQP1 and AQP4, encoded by genes *AQP1 and AQP4* respectively) were included in our review due to their involvement in maintaining CSF homeostasis [25]. Hiraldo-González et al. examined AQP1 and AQP4 protein levels in CSF with ELISA in 179 subjects, 81 with possible NPH. No aquaporin elevation in CSF was found. AQP1 and AQP4 analysis showed no promising results as a biomarker of iNPH [26]. The search for a genetic marker in *AQP* genes, therefore, seems unwarranted.

3.4   Chromosome 9 Open Reading Frame 72, C9ORF72

Chromosome 9 open reading frame 72 is a protein found in neuronal cytoplasm and presynaptic terminals, encoded by the gene *C9ORF72*. Known functions include endosomal trafficking and regulation of actin dynamics. Mutations in the gene consist of hexanucleotide repeat expansions. These mutations are known to be associated with Frontotemporal Dementia (FTD) and Amylotrophic Lateral Sclerosis (ALS). [15] The expansion was investigated in a large cohort of possible iNPH patients ($n = 487$) and age matched controls ($n = 432$). Results showed the mutation in 1.6% of the iNPH cohort, and was not found in the control population. This study also found that carriers of the mutation exhibited symptoms earlier than non-carriers [27]. Although the authors suggest that analysis of *C9ORF72* expansion should be considered for patients with symptoms of iNPH, the study is limited by the lack of standardised diagnostic criteria in the iNPH population. This means that the population under investigation could have included patients with atypical parkinsonism, FTD, or other neurodegenerative dementias.

3.5   Genes Involved in Amyloid Metabolism

Altered amyloid processing is hypothesised to play a critical role in iNPH pathogenesis. It has been shown that iNPH patients have lower CSF levels of amyloid beta (Aβ) and lower levels of soluble precursor proteins [28]. Additionally, the concomitance of Alzheimer's disease (AD) and iNPH as confirmed on brain tissue biopsy has led to speculation that NPH and AD share a pathophysiological background. Aβ accumulation is well established as a cause of AD. Products of the *APOE* gene group are involved in the regulation of Aβ. Notably, the allele *APOE4* is known to cause amyloid build-up in the brain in AD [16]. Studies searching for an association between *APOE4* or *APOE3* genotypes and the iNPH phenotype have not shown any clear correlation. Gudmindson et al. clinically evaluated 15 patients meeting the criteria for ventriculoperitoneal shunt insertion. The patients were genotyped, and all were found to be homozygous for *APOE3* genotype [29]. However this study was too small to draw general conclusions. A previously mentioned large cohort study ($n = 375$ of shunt-operated patients) ruled out an association between iNPH and the *APOE4* genotype [3]. Yang el. Al. analysed the distribution of six different *APOE* alleles in 77 iNPH patients, finding similar genotype distributions in iNPH and controls. [17] Although the *APOE4* allele was found more frequently in the iNPH group, this was not significantly different to the control population. The *APOE4* allele Odds Ratio (OR) for the iNPH population was 0.90, and the 95% confidence intervals (CI) were 0.50–1.60. For AD, this was considerably smaller (OR = 5.34, CI = 4.10–7.00). This reconfirms the status of *APOE4* in AD pathogenesis, but does not shed any light on the involvement of amyloid metabolism in iNPH. Similarly, a study of AD-associated loci and their possible roles in iNPH found that these loci did not have a statistically significant effect on Aβ accumulation in iNPH [30]. The association of APOE4 and iNPH was also ruled out again by Pyykko et al. who genotyped 202 patients with iNPH and 687 controls. They found that *APOE4* is not a risk factor for NPH [31]. In a single case study, Cusimano et al. reported two sisters with iNPH, hypothesising a genetic involvement. Genotyping for APOE was carried out, revealing that both were homozygous for the APOE3 allele [5]. However, the generalisability of a case report is limited. Overall, whilst it seems that the *APOE3* allele could be associated with iNPH in a way that is unclear, a role for *APOE4* seems unlikely.

Another gene product known to be involved in amyloid disease is transthyretin, encoded by *TTR*. A genome-wide association study (GWAS) with 35,000 probes was performed in 22 iNPH patients and 8 healthy controls [32]. Results showed a 17-fold decrease in *TTR* expression in iNPH. Transthyretin is a known biomarker for neuronal stress, showing increased expression in the rat choroid plexus in response to increased glucocorticoid hormones [18].

Other genes with differential expression profiles included *AβPP*, encoding amyloid beta protein precursor (AβPP), which increased threefold in iNPH and *ADAM10*, encoding a protein involved in AβPP proteolysis, also showed increased expression [32]. Both gene products are expressed in the CNS, and their differential expression in iNPH provides some evidence that alterations in amyloid metabolism have a part to play in iNPH pathogenesis. However, there is no clear relationship between genotype and phenotype.

3.6 NME8

NME family member 8 encodes thioredoxin domain-containing protein 3 (TXNDC3), which is also known as spermatid-specific thioredoxin-2 (Sptrx-2). The protein products serve as intranuclear transcriptional regulators, have a role in DNA damage repair, and are involved in ciliary function. TXNDC3 possesses exonuclease activity with a preference for single stranded DNA [33]. The NME8 transcript is thought to be implicated in ciliary function, by an unknown mechanism. The transcript is probably required in the final stages of cilia maturation, yet the specific function and effect on the maturation period is still unknown [34]. The clinical manifestation of NME8 mutation is known as primary ciliary dyskinesia (PCD) [19].

Huovinen et al. analysed SNPs in a large cohort of shunted iNPH patients ($n = 188$) and controls ($n = 688$). SNPs in *NME8* revealed allelic variation between iNPH patients and controls ($p = 0.014$) [35]. Variants were not linked to neuropathological changes in biopsy samples, however, periventricular changes were more frequent in the iNPH group ($p = 0.017$). This large study provides more evidence for an underlying genetic mechanism, and *NME8* is a compelling candidate given its role in ciliary maturation.

3.7   Adenosine Receptors A1R and A2AR

Adenosine and its receptors have known roles in vasodilation and protecting tissue from inflammation [20]. It has been hypothesised that cerebrovascular disease has a role in iNPH aetiology. Casati et al. performed gene and protein expression studies on peripheral blood mononuclear cells from iNPH patients and healthy controls [36]. The results suggested down-regulation of adenosine receptors A1 and A2A in iNPH, suggesting changes to the adenosine system in disease pathogenesis. The adenosine system has known roles in the vascular system and immune processes in states of disease. The high prevalence of cardiovascular disease amongst iNPH patients and the possibility of altered immune functions may explain these observations.

4   Future Studies: Animal Models and Functional Analysis

Reverse genetic studies that attempt to establish a link between a candidate gene and its role in iNPH are currently lacking in the literature. Techniques such as targeted mutations, gene silencing, or modifying gene expression aim to elucidate biological functions of a gene product and its role in pathogenesis. With the use of animal models, the effect of gene alterations can be seen in a whole organism. Animal models of iNPH include knockout mouse lines for candidate iNPH genes *CWH43* and *CFAP43*. Mice lacking the gene *CCNO* express a phenotype strikingly similar to iNPH. Additionally, *Drosophila melanogaster* offers a battery of sophisticated genetic tools for functional analysis, which has led to a deeper understanding of the functions of domains iNPH candidate gene SFMBT1.

4.1   Cyclin O, CCNO

The *CCNO* gene encodes an atypical cyclin, cyclin O, necessary for the generation of motile cilia [37]. It has been proposed that mutations constitute part of the molecular basis of iNPH. Complete or partial loss of CCNO lead to defective cilia in the pendymal, and consequently disrupted CSF flow. In the human population, this manifests as PCD. However, *CCNO -/-* mice have striking similarities to human iNPH patients. The animals survive severe communicating hydrocephalus by compensating for increased ICP with a thinner brain parenchyma [38]. Interestingly, *CCNO +/-* heterozygous mice develop hydrocephalus with lower penetrance than their homozygous counterparts [39]. Although many aspects of CCNO are promising, many genes involved in cilia development are linked to higher comorbidity in younger age, and thus have limited potential in iNPH diagnostics.

4.2 Drosophila Studies of SFMBT1

Drosophila offers a powerful and sophisticated toolbox to analyse the various functions of genes involved in disease. Functional analysis of the Malignant Brain Tumour (MBT) domain in candidate gene *SFMBT1* was first reported in *Drosophila* gene *dL3mbt* [40, 41]. Mutations in the MBT domain of *dL3mbt* caused malignant overgrowth in the larval brain, implicating a tumour-suppressing function of *dL3mbt* and the importance of the MBT domain [40, 41]. Different MBT proteins have been identified in various protein complexes, suggesting that MBT proteins have distinct functional activities and modes of action in regulating chromatin. Mammalian SFMBT1 contains four MBT repeat domains that are essential for mediating histone H3 N-terminal tail binding and transcriptional repression [41]. In *Drosophila*, *dSfmbt* contains four MBT repeats and is a polycomb protein because *dSfmbt* knockout displays a classic polycomb phenotype with strong and widespread derepression of HOX genes [42]. *dSfmbt* is part of the Pho repressive complex, which contains the DNA-binding protein Pho and recruits other polycomb proteins, mediating transcriptional silencing at target loci [43]. The MBT repeat domain of *dSfmbt* preferentially binds to mono- or di-methylated lysine containing histone peptides [21].

5 Conclusion

The genetic analysis of iNPH patients offers promising results. Pedigree analysis has revealed that iNPH is a complex trait, without a Mendelian inheritance pattern. This suggests a high level of genetic heterogeneity, variable expression, and penetrance, with multiple genes involved. Approaches such as GWAS and WES have made some way towards identifying these genes. *CFAP43* is a promising candidate, being identified in a family with heritable iNPH, and *CFAP43-/-* mice appear to have a hydrocephalus phenotype. *SFMBT1* is interesting because it is involved in histone modification, implying expression changes in other genes via epigenetic control. This is in keeping with the theory that iNPH involves multiple genes. Large cohort studies provide strong evidence that *SFMBT1* is a risk factor for iNPH. A heterozygous loss of function *CWH43* mutations was identified by WES in 53 unrelated patents, and a *CWH43+/-* mice exhibited hydrocephalus, ventriculomegaly, and gait disturbances. *C9ORF72* mutations may also be associated with iNPH, with carriers of the mutation exhibiting symptoms earlier than non-carriers. Other possible candidates include genes involved in amyloid metabolism, *NME8* involved in ciliary function, and adenosine receptors. As several of the discovery cohorts in the studies reviewed were rather small, genetic studies of iNPH need larger cohorts and multi-centre approaches. Genotyping iNPH patients has revealed some promising biomarkers, which could be used to differentiate iNPH from other neurodegenerative disorders. Larger cohorts would uncover rare variants as of yet unknown, and establish the common variants with small effect-size. Larger and more comprehensive studies are needed before the clinical utility of this preliminary data can be fully realised.

6 Key Points

- Current genetic studies suggest that idiopathic NPH might not be idiopathic after all.
- iNPH is a complex trait with genetic risk factors.
- Underlying mechanisms involve a complex interplay of genetic, epigenetic, and environmental factors.
- *CFAP43* is a strong candidate gene confirmed in human iNPH with family aggregation. 15% of iNPH patients have *CFAP45* polymorphism when compared to the general population. *CFAP43-/-* mice have a hydrocephalus phenotype.
- Several studies on *SFMBT1* have shown an association with iNPH.
- A heterozygous loss of function mutations in *CWH43* is associated with iNPH, and mouse models of *CWH43 +/-* have a hydrocephalus phenotype.
- The allelic variant of *NME8* has been confirmed in patients with NPH.
- Aquaporin has shown little potential in diagnosing NPH.
- Genes involved in amyloid metabolism and adenosine signalling are likely to have a role.
- Larger cohorts are needed to discover rare variants, and to establish common variants with small effect-size.
- Animal studies are needed for functional analysis of candidate genes.

References

1. Portenoy RK, Berger A, Gross E. Familial occurrence of idiopathic normal-pressure hydrocephalus. Arch Neurol. 1984;41(3):335–37.
2. McGirr A, Cusimano MD. Familial aggregation of idiopathic normal pressure hydrocephalus: novel familial case and a family study of the NPH triad in an iNPH patient cohort. J Neurol Sci. 2012;321(1–2):82–8.
3. Huovinen J, Kastinen S, Komulainen S, et al. Familial idiopathic normal pressure hydrocephalus. J Neurol Sci. 2016;368:11–8.
4. Cusimano MD, et al. Normal-pressure hydrocephalus: is there a genetic predisposition? Can J Neurol Sci. 2011;38(2):274–81.
5. Liouta E, Liakos F, Koutsarnakis C, Katsaros V, Stranjalis G. Novel case of familial normal pressure hydrocephalus. Psychiatry Clin Neurosci. 2014;68(7):583–4.
6. Zhang J, Williams MA, Rigamonti D. Heritable essential tremor-idiopathic normal pressure hydrocephalus (ETINPH). Am J Med Genet A. 2008;146A(4):433–9.
7. Zhang J, Carr CW, Rigamonti D, Badr A. Genome-wide linkage scan maps ETINPH gene to chromosome 19q12-13.31. Hum Hered. 2010;69(4):262–67.
8. Geyer HL, Bressman SB. Rapid-onset dystonia-parkinsonism. Handb Clin Neurol. 2011;100:559–62.

9. Rachev E, et al. CFAP43 modulates ciliary beating in mouse and Xenopus. Dev Biol. 2020;459(2):109–25.

10. Morimoto Y, Yoshida S, Kinoshita A, Satoh C, Mishima H, Yamaguchi N, et al. Nonsense mutation in CFAP43 causes normal-pressure hydrocephalus with ciliary abnormalities. Neurology. 2019;92(20):e2364–74.

11. Kato T, Sato H, Takahashi Y, A genetic risk factor for idiopathic normal pressure hydrocephalus (iNPH). Fluids Barriers CNS. 2015;12(Suppl 1):O51.

12. Sato H, Takahashi Y, Kimihira L, Iseki C, Kato H, Suzuki Y, et al. A segmental copy number loss of the SFMBT1 gene is a genetic risk for shunt-responsive, idiopathic normal pressure hydrocephalus (iNPH): a case-control study. PLoS One. 2016;11(11):e0166615.

13. Korhonen VE, et al. Copy number loss in SFMBT1 is common among Finnish and Norwegian patients with iNPH. Neurol Genet. 2018;4(6): e291.

14. Yang HW, et al. Deletions in CWH43 cause idiopathic normal pressure hydrocephalus. EMBO Mol Med. 2021;13(3): e13249.

15. Korhonen VE, Remes AM, Helisalmi S, et al. Prevalence of C9ORF72 expansion in a large series of patients with idiopathic normal-pressure hydrocephalus. Dement Geriatr Cogn Disord. 2019;47(1–2):91–103.

16. Gudmundsson G, Kristjansdottir G, Cook E, Olafsson I. Association of ApoE genotype with clinical features and outcome in idiopathic normal pressure hydrocephalus (iNPH): a preliminary report. Acta Neurochir (Wien). 2009;151(11):1511–2.

17. Laiterä T, Paananen J, Helisalmi S, et al. Effects of Alzheimer's disease-associated risk loci on amyloid-β accumulation in the brain of idiopathic normal pressure hydrocephalus patients. J Alzheimers Dis. 2017;55(3):995–1003.

18. Laiterä T, Kurki MI, Pursiheimo JP, et al. The expression of transthyretin and amyloid-β protein precursor is altered in the brain of idiopathic normal pressure hydrocephalus patients. J Alzheimers Dis. 2015;48(4):959–968.

19. Huovinen J, et al. Alzheimer's disease-related polymorphisms in shunt-responsive idiopathic normal pressure hydrocephalus. J Alzheimers Dis. 2017;60(3):1077–85.

20. Casati M, Arosio B, Gussago C, et al. Down-regulation of adenosine A1 and A2A receptors in peripheral cells from idiopathic normal-pressure hydrocephalus patients. J Neurol Sci. 2016;361:196–9.

21. Bonasio R, Lecona E, Reinberg D. MBT domain proteins in development and disease. Semin Cell Dev Biol. 2010;21(2):221–30.

22. Ghugtyal V, et al. CWH43 is required for the introduction of ceramides into GPI anchors in Saccharomyces cerevisiae. Mol Microbiol. 2007;65(6):1493–502.

23. Yang D, Yang H, Luiselli G, et al. Increased plasmin-mediated proteolysis of L1CAM in a mouse model of idiopathic normal pressure hydrocephalus. Proc Natl Acad Sci U S A. 2021;118(33): e2010528118.

24. Trillo-Contreras JL, et al. Combined effects of aquaporin-4 and hypoxia produce age-related hydrocephalus. Biochim Biophys Acta Mol Basis Dis. 2018;1864(10):3515–26.

25. Hiraldo-González L, et al. Evaluation of aquaporins in the cerebrospinal fluid in patients with idiopathic normal pressure hydrocephalus. PLoS ONE. 2021;16(10): e0258165.

26. Cavallieri F, Mandrioli J, Rosafio F, et al. C9ORF72 and parkinsonism: Weak link, innocent bystander, or central player in neurodegeneration? J Neurol Sci. 2017;378:49–51.

27. Jeppsson H, Höltta M, Zetterberg H, Blennow K, Wikkelsø C, Tullberg M. Amyloid mis-metabolism in idiopathic normal pressure hydrocephalus. Fluids Barriers CNS. 2016;13(1):13.

28. Kawamura K, et al. Cerebrospinal fluid amyloid-β oligomer levels in patients with idiopathic normal pressure hydrocephalus. J Alzheimers Dis. 2021;83(1):179–90.

29. Yang Y, et al. The APOE genotype in idiopathic normal pressure hydrocephalus. PLoS ONE. 2016;11(7): e0158985.

30. Pyykkö OT, Helisalmi S, Koivisto AM, et al. APOE4 predicts amyloid-β in cortical brain biopsy but not idiopathic normal pressure hydrocephalus. J Neurol Neurosurg Psychiatry. 2012;83(11):1119–24.

31. Martinho A, Gonçalves I, Costa M, Santos CR. Stress and glucocorticoids increase transthyretin expression in rat choroid plexus via mineralocorticoid and glucocorticoid receptors. J Mol Neurosci. 2012;48(1):1–13.
32. Puts GS, et al. Nuclear functions of NME proteins. Lab Invest. 2018;98(2):211–8.
33. Boissan M, Dabernat S, Peuchant E, et al. The mammalian Nm23/NDPK family: from metastasis control to cilia movement. Mol Cell Biochem. 2009;329:51–62.
34. Duriez B, et al. A common variant in combination with a nonsense mutation in a member of the thioredoxin family causes primary ciliary dyskinesia. Proc Natl Acad Sci U S A. 2007;104(9):3336–41.
35. Ohta A, Sitkovsky M. Role of G-coupled adenosine receptors in down regulation of inflammation and protection from tissue damage. Nature. 2001;414(6866):916–20.
36. Wallmeier J, et al. Motile ciliopathies. Nat Rev Dis Primers. 2020;**6**(1):77
37. Núñez-Ollé M, Stracker TH, Gil-Gómez G. CCNO mutations in NPH? Aging (Albany NY). 2018;10(2):158–9.
38. Núñez-Ollé M, et al. Constitutive Cyclin O deficiency results in penetrant hydrocephalus, impaired growth and infertility. Oncotarget. 2017;8(59):99261–73.
39. Gateff E, Löffler T, Wismar J. A temperature-sensitive brain tumor suppressor mutation of Drosophila melanogaster: developmental studies and molecular localization of the gene. Mech Dev. 1993;41(1):15–31.
40. Wismar J, et al. The Drosophila melanogaster tumor suppressor gene lethal(3)malignant brain tumor encodes a proline-rich protein with a novel zinc finger. Mech Dev. 1995;53(1):141–54.
41. Klymenko T, et al. A Polycomb group protein complex with sequence-specific DNA-binding and selective methyl-lysine-binding activities. Genes Dev. 2006;20(9):1110–22.
42. Simon JA, Kingston RE. Mechanisms of polycomb gene silencing: knowns and unknowns. Nat Rev Mol Cell Biol. 2009;10(10):697–708.
43. Grimm C, et al. Molecular recognition of histone lysine methylation by the polycomb group repressor dSfmbt. Embo J. 2009;28(13):1965–77.

Diagnosis of NPH

Clinical Symptoms and Examination

Jan Laczó and Martina Laczó

Abstract Idiopathic Normal Pressure Hydrocephalus (iNPH) is one of the treatable clinical entities and, therefore, it is very important to identify and examine the clinical symptoms that lead to the accurate diagnosis. The chapter provides an overview and description of the major clinical symptoms, including gait disturbance, urinary incontinence, and cognitive impairment, as well as the most frequent minor clinical symptoms of iNPH. The emphasis is also placed on the description of the "red flags", the symptoms and signs that make the diagnosis of iNPH less likely or may even question the diagnosis and indicate a different underlying aetiology. Next, the chapter discusses, in detail, differential diagnosis of iNPH and describes how to distinguish iNPH from the most common diseases that present with all three or some of the major clinical symptoms and thus may mimic iNPH. Finally, the most important clinical information about iNPH is summarised.

Keywords Atypical parkinsonian syndromes · Cervical myelopathy · Chronic obstructive hydrocephalus · Lumbosacral spinal stenosis · Neurosyphilis · Parkinson's disease · Peripheral neuropathy · Secondary normal pressure hydrocephalus · Subcortical ischemic vascular disease · Vitamin B_{12} deficiency

Abbreviations

CSF	Cerebrospinal fluid
CT	Computed tomography
iNPH	Idiopathic normal pressure hydrocephalus
LOVA	Longstanding overt ventriculomegaly in adults
LIAS	Late-onset idiopathic aqueductal stenosis
MRI	Magnetic resonance imaging
PaVM	Panventriculomegaly

J. Laczó (✉) · M. Laczó
Memory Clinic, Department of Neurology, Second Faculty of Medicine and Motol University Hospital, Charles University, Prague, Czech Republic
e-mail: jan.laczo@fnmotol.cz

REM   Rapid eye movement
SPECT   Single-photon emission computed tomography

1   Introduction

Idiopathic normal pressure hydrocephalus (iNPH) is a syndrome of older adults that is characterised by the triad of major clinical symptoms including gait disturbance, urinary incontinence, and cognitive impairment in the presence of ventriculomegaly and normal Cerebrospinal Fluid (CSF) pressure [1]. However, the complete clinical triad is not required to suspect iNPH. The major clinical symptoms vary greatly in the onset, presentation, severity, progression, and response to shunting. Minor clinical symptoms are present irregularly and include dizziness, sleep disorders, sexual dysfunction, and headache. The symptoms of iNPH also occur in patients with other neurological diagnoses such as cerebrovascular and neurodegenerative diseases, and their manifestations may be affected by chronic comorbidities (e.g., hip and knee osteoarthritis, prostate adenoma, and pelvic floor insufficiency) [2]. The diagnosis of iNPH is thus challenging and requires the exclusion of other diagnoses that would completely explain the patient's symptoms. It is of great importance to purposefully look for clinical symptoms and findings that are not commonly present in iNPH (i.e., red flags) and can aid the differential diagnosis. The complete diagnostic process of iNPH includes a detailed medical history documenting insidious onset and slow progression of the symptoms, clinical/neurological examination showing one or more of the major clinical symptoms, brain imaging (i.e., CT or more preferably MRI) with enlarged lateral and third ventricles in the absence of CSF flow obstruction and atrophy, and finally specific tests of CSF drainage (i.e., tap test and external lumbar drainage) or CSF hydrodynamics (i.e., infusion testing) [3].

2   Overview of Clinical Symptoms

2.1   *Major Symptoms*

Gait disturbance, urinary incontinence, and cognitive impairment are the major symptoms of iNPH and their combination creates the classic clinical triad first described by Hakim and Adams in 1965 [1]. However, the complete clinical triad occurs in about only 50% of patients [9]. Patients with iNPH should present with one or more of the major symptoms (typically gait disturbance) starting insidiously and progressing slowly over at least three to six months with the usual age of onset after the age of 60 and at least after the age of 40 [3, 4]. Importantly, the diagnosis of iNPH requires that the major clinical symptoms are not completely explained by other neurological or non-neurological diseases. Extensive and detailed medical history and examination of each symptom together with radiological examination are, therefore, required to determine if a given symptom is due to iNPH or other diseases.

Gait Disturbance

Nearly all patients with iNPH have gait disturbance, which is typically either the first or the worst symptom [5]. It is also the first symptom to improve after treatment [6]. Gait disturbance progresses without treatment, and in the advanced stages, patients are unable to walk without assistance and may end up bedridden. Gait disturbance is characterised as an apraxia of gait. The gait is broad-based, short-stepped with decreased cadence leading to decreased gait velocity, and ataxic with irregular step length and feet rotated outwards [34]. A typical shuffling, also described as a magnetic gait, is caused by reduced step height and insufficient dorsiflexion of the forefoot [7]. Patients have difficulties standing up and initiating gait, they turn en bloc using multiple steps and may experience sudden, transient blocks of movement (i.e., freezing episodes), particularly when turning, navigating through narrow spaces or approaching obstacles. Balance and postural stability are impaired and retropulsion that may lead to backward falls occurs in some patients. Importantly, compared to patients with Parkinson's disease, gait-associated movements of the trunk and upper limbs, in particular arm swing, are not impaired in patients with iNPH [8].

Urinary Incontinence

About 50 to 75% of patients with iNPH have urinary symptoms that usually accompany gait disturbance and cognitive impairment, and very rarely occur as an isolated symptom [4, 9]. They are twofold less likely to improve after treatment compared to gait disturbance [6]. Urinary symptoms are the result of a neurogenic bladder dysfunction due to reduced central inhibition with detrusor overactivity, which was observed in 95% of patients with iNPH [10]. The most common urinary symptoms are urinary urgency with difficulty inhibiting bladder emptying and increased daytime (i.e., pollakiuria) and nighttime (i.e., nocturia) urinary frequency [11]. Urge incontinence occurs in the later stages and can progress to complete incontinence in the advanced stages. Patients with iNPH are usually aware of the urinary urge and incontinence without awareness of urinary urge is not characteristic of iNPH. Of note, gait disturbance and cognitive impairment can also contribute to urinary incontinence, especially in the advanced stages [11]. Voiding symptoms including retardation in initiating urination, prolongation and poor flow, sensation of post-void residual, straining, and intermittency are less common in patients with iNPH [11]. In the advanced stages, even faecal incontinence may occur [4].

Cognitive Impairment

About 80% of patients with iNPH have cognitive impairment [4, 9], which is rarely the first or the predominant clinical symptom. It is also the least likely symptom of the clinical triad to improve after treatment, especially when the impairment is severe [12]. Cognitive impairment in patients with iNPH is characterised by slowing of processing and psychomotor speed, attentional and working memory deficits, executive dysfunction, and impaired delayed recall improved with cueing with relatively intact delayed recognition on episodic memory tests, all of which are referred to as a "frontal-subcortical" profile of cognitive impairment, and also by visuospatial impairment including visuoperceptual and visuoconstructional deficits [13]. In the early stages, cognitive impairment does not interfere with everyday activities and patients present with mild cognitive impairment. In the later stages, cognitive impairment gradually leads to loss of independence in activities of daily living and patients present with dementia. Patients with iNPH usually present with neuropsychiatric and behavioural symptoms, the most common being apathy [14]. Amongst other neuropsychiatric symptoms, depression, irritability, and agitation occur in about one-third of patients with iNPH, whilst hallucinations and delusions are much less common [14, 15].

2.2 Minor Symptoms

Minor clinical symptoms include dizziness, sleep disorders, sexual dysfunction, and headache. These symptoms are not typical of iNPH, but may occur in patients with iNPH. They are not given as much attention as the main clinical symptoms, but if present they can be distressing for the patients.

Dizziness

Patients with iNPH commonly complain of feeling dizzy and unstable when standing and walking, and are afraid of falling. For this reason, they may use their hands to get up and touch the surrounding furniture when walking. Dizziness is usually associated with gait disturbance and postural instability, improves after treatment [16], and can be evaluated using specific clinical grading scales [17].

Sleep Disorders

Sleep disorders have been reported in patients with iNPH and sleep-disordered breathing/obstructive sleep apnea in particular has been frequently associated with iNPH [18–20]. The pathophysiological mechanism of this association remains unclear. Sleep-disordered breathing, unlike increased daily need for sleep [21], does not seem to respond to therapy [18].

Sexual Dysfunction

Sexual dysfunction seems to be a frequent but underdiagnosed symptom in patients with iNPH, which may occur several years before the onset of the major clinical symptoms [22]. Sexual dysfunction also has the potential for restoration after treatment [22].

Headache

Unlike hydrocephalus with increased intracranial pressure, iNPH usually does not cause chronic headache and only occasionally patients with iNPH report mild dull headache or head fullness [23]. However, headache including unilateral and postural headache is a commonly occurring problem in shunt-treated patients with iNPH and should, therefore, be specifically asked about during postoperative follow-ups [24, 25].

3 Red Flags—Exclusion Criteria

The typical clinical symptoms of iNPH include a combination of symmetric gait disturbance characterised as gait apraxia, which is a primary symptom, increased urinary frequency and urgency with or without incontinence, and cognitive impairment of a frontal-subcortical profile with visuospatial deficit starting insidiously over months and progressing slowly over years. A clinical presentation that is different from this is suspected to be of a different aetiology. Acute onset and fluctuation of clinical symptoms is not typical for iNPH and may suggest secondary NPH, vascular aetiology or the presence of comorbidities. Medical history of moderate to severe headache, visual or hearing impairments, oculomotor disorder, speech disorder, swallowing difficulties, rotational vertigo, nausea, vomiting, facial and limb weakness, sensory impairment, paresthesia, and neck or back pain associated with the onset of one or more major clinical symptoms raises suspicion of other intracranial or intraspinal pathology. Neurological examination in patients is normal except for findings associated with the major clinical symptoms. There should be no abnormal findings on cranial nerves, which would indicate other intracranial pathology, no signs of hemiparesis suggestive of other brain pathology or paraparesis suggestive of spinal cord pathology or nerve root compression. Upper motor neuron findings including spasticity and hyperreflexia are not typical for iNPH and may indicate vascular ischemic changes. Lower motor neuron findings including muscle atrophy and hyporeflexia or areflexia should not be present in iNPH and may indicate polyneu-ropathy or nerve root compression. Patients with iNPH should also not have any cerebellar symptoms including ataxia and intention tremor, or extrapyramidal symp-toms including resting tremor, bradykinesia, rigidity, and hyperkinetic dyskinesias that would be suggestive of neurodegenerative diseases. Spinal ataxia, i.e., ataxia and instability markedly worsening in the dark, is characteristic for spinal cord pathology and polyneuropathy but should not be present in iNPH. Gait disturbance should be symmetric and, therefore, lateralising findings should increase suspicion of other diseases. Incontinence without urinary urgency or awareness of urinary symptoms should question the diagnosis of iNPH. Severe memory deficits with poor recall, which does not benefit from cueing, and impaired recognition, agnosia or aphasia are not typical for iNPH and should raise concerns for other causes of cognitive impairment such as Alzheimer's disease, multi-infarct dementia, or frontotemporal dementia. Visual hallucinations are very atypical in iNPH and are suggestive of dementia with Lewy bodies. Also, delirium is not typical of iNPH and implies the presence of another disease or comorbidity. A cause other than iNPH should be considered in patients with progressive cognitive impairment with or without urinary symptoms who do not have gait disturbance. In the case of gait disturbance and urinary symptoms without cognitive impairment, it is necessary to look for spinal cord pathology or nerve root compression.

4   Differential diagnosis

The major clinical symptoms are frequently found in many other diseases that can mimic iNPH. A detailed medical history, careful clinical/neurological examination, and radiological examination (i.e., preferably MRI) are, therefore, required to make a correct diagnosis and differentiate other diseases from iNPH. The most challenging differential diagnosis is for diseases that present with all three major clinical symp-toms including secondary NPH and chronic obstructive hydrocephalus, subcortical ischemic vascular disease, Parkinson's disease, atypical parkinsonian syndromes (i.e., progressive supranuclear palsy, corticobasal degeneration, multiple system atrophy, and dementia with Lewy bodies), vitamin B_{12} deficiency, neurosyphilis, medication side effects, and combinations of diseases. However, diseases that present with two major clinical symptoms may also be challenging for differential diag-nosis. These include cervical myelopathy, lumbosacral spinal stenosis, peripheral neuropathy, and combinations of diseases. Diseases that present with only one clin-ical symptom (i.e., gait disturbance in spinocerebellar degeneration, degenerative arthritis and peripheral vascular disease, urinary incontinence in prostatic hyper-trophy, pelvic-floor abnormalities and interstitial cystitis, and cognitive impairment in Alzheimer's disease, frontotemporal dementia and major depression) may be less challenging for differential diagnosis. However, it is still important to identify or rule out these diseases that should be treated before evaluating iNPH.

4.1   Diseases with Three Major Clinical Symptoms

Secondary Normal Pressure Hydrocephalus and Chronic Obstructive Hydrocephalus

Secondary NPH, similar to iNPH, is a communicating hydrocephalus with no visible obstruction of the CSF pathways. In secondary NPH, there should be evidence of the pre-existing condition in medical history that could interfere with CSF resorption (e.g., subarachnoid haemorrhage, meningitis, traumatic brain injury, or brain surgery). The onset of clinical symptoms in secondary NPH is usually more rapid than in iNPH. The differential diagnosis is based primarily on the patient´s medical history and brain imaging. In contrast, chronic obstructive hydrocephalus is a non-communicating type of hydrocephalus, which typically has aqueductal stenosis or fourth ventricle outlet occlusion. This type of hydrocephalus includes different pathological entities of congenital or developmental aetiology, such as Longstanding Overt Ventriculomegaly in Adults (LOVA) [26], Panventriculomegaly (PaVM) [27], persistent Blake's pouch cyst [28], and Late-onset Idiopathic Aqueductal Stenosis (LIAS) [29], the latter of which could also be of secondary aetiology. Chronic obstructive hydrocephalus has a similar clinical presentation to iNPH and secondary NPH, but it is more commonly associated with headaches. It should be noted that patients with iNPH and secondary NPH may also report milder headaches that are typically characterised as the pressure in the head. The diagnosis of chronic obstructive hydrocephalus requires brain imaging to evaluate the size of the ventricles and possible CSF pathway obstructions. CSF drainage tests should be performed in all subtypes of communicating hydrocephalus, however, they should be avoided in cases of obstructive hydrocephalus.

Subcortical Ischemic Vascular Disease

Subcortical ischemic vascular disease is caused by microvascular ischemic changes in the deep white matter and the periventricular region leading to disruption of subcortical neural circuits. The clinical symptoms are similar to those observed in iNPH and include cognitive impairment of a frontal-subcortical profile, gait apraxia, and urinary symptoms. Clinical symptoms usually present with an insidious onset and progressive decline. However, unlike iNPH, the stepwise progression and fluctuation of symptoms can also occur. Patients with subcortical ischemic vascular disease more frequently have vascular risk factors in their medical history (e.g., arterial hypertension, diabetes, and smoking) and upper motor neuron findings upon clinical examination including spasticity and hyperreflexia. Mild focal neurological deficits may also be present. However, differentiating between subcortical ischemic vascular disease and iNPH is very challenging due to the similar clinical presentation and frequent overlap between the two diagnoses. Brain MRI is used to evaluate the extent of white matter lesions and degree of ventricular enlargement and is essential for the diagnosis. CSF drainage tests and tests of CSF hydrodynamics are also important for the differential diagnosis.

Parkinson's Disease

Parkinson's disease is a neurodegenerative disease associated with degeneration of the dopaminergic neurons in the substantia nigra. The clinical symptoms include gradually progressing motor symptoms with asymmetric resting tremor, bradykinesia, and rigidity (i.e., extrapyramidal symptoms), as well as non-motor symptoms with hyposmia, depression and Rapid Eye Movement (REM) sleep behaviour disorders. Gait disturbance with freezing and postural instability, cognitive impairment of a frontal-subcortical profile, autonomic dysfunction including orthostatic hypotension, urogenital dysfunction and constipation, together with swallowing and speech difficulties are also present to some degree in a majority of patients. If patients with Parkinson's disease show predominantly asymmetric extrapyramidal symptoms in the upper and lower limbs and typical non-motor symptoms, its differentiation from iNPH is not very challenging. Clinical findings of swallowing and speech difficulties in patients with Parkinson's disease may also be useful for the differential diagnosis. However, if gait impairment is a prominent symptom, the differential diagnosis becomes more challenging. The finding of a broad-based and atactic gait with irregular step length and feet rotated outwards associated with preserved or increased reciprocal arm swing during gait increases the probability of an iNPH diagnosis. It may also be helpful in the differential diagnosis that cognitive impairment in Parkinson's disease typically does not develop until several years after the onset of motor symptoms, in contrast to iNPH. Enlarged ventricles on brain imaging and positive tests of CSF drainage and hydrodynamics are suggestive of iNPH, whilst a good response to levodopa treatment and decreased striatal dopamine transporter uptake on ^{123}I-ioflupane SPECT make a diagnosis of Parkinson's disease more likely.

Atypical Parkinsonian Syndromes

Atypical parkinsonian syndromes are a heterogeneous group of neurodegenerative disorders that share certain clinical symptoms with Parkinson's disease (e.g., extrapyramidal symptoms, gait disturbance, cognitive impairment, and autonomic dysfunction with bladder dysfunction) and generally progress more rapidly and respond poorly to levodopa treatment. They commonly include progressive supranuclear palsy, corticobasal syndrome, multiple system atrophy, and dementia with Lewy bodies. In the differential diagnosis between atypical parkinsonian syndromes and iNPH, clinicians should specifically look for symptoms that are typical for these syndromes and are not present in iNPH. Progressive supranuclear palsy can be distinguished from iNPH by the presence of early gait instability with unexplained falls, supranuclear gaze palsy, axial rigidity, dysphagia and dysarthric speech. However, if gait disturbance is a prominent symptom (i.e., in the variant "pure akinesia with gait freezing"), the differential diagnosis becomes more challenging. In corticobasal syndrome, the distinguishing symptoms are markedly asymmetric extrapyramidal symptoms, predominantly in the upper limbs, with or without dystonia and myoclonus, orobuccal or ideomotor limb apraxia, cortical sensory deficit, and alien limb phenomenon (i.e., involuntary movements of the limb along with a sense of estrangement). Multiple system atrophy can be distinguished from iNPH by the presence of extrapyramidal symptoms, early postural instability with falls, dysarthria, upper motor neuron signs, sleep disturbance (e.g., REM sleep behaviour disorder), and early marked autonomic failure including orthostatic hypotension. In the parkinsonian type of multiple system atrophy, other distinguishing symptoms are axial dystonia, anterocollis (i.e., dropped head), high-frequency limb tremor with or without myoclonic component, and respiratory or laryngeal stridor. In the cerebellar type of multiple system atrophy, other distinguishing symptoms are cerebellar limb and gait ataxia, and oculomotor disturbances including nystagmus. Dementia with Lewy bodies can be distinguished from iNPH by the presence of extrapyramidal symptoms, fluctuations in cognition and alertness, recurrent visual hallucinations, REM sleep behaviour disorder, and early cognitive impairment with prominent visuospatial deficit. Brain imaging in atypical parkinsonian syndromes can show atrophy of the midbrain and superior cerebellar peduncles in progressive supranuclear palsy, asymmetric frontoparietal atrophy in corticobasal syndrome, bilateral hypointensities in the posterolateral putamen, representing iron deposition, and slitlike hyperintensity in the lateral margin of the putamen on T2-weighted images in the parkinsonian type of multiple system atrophy, and olivopontocerebellar atrophy with or without pontine gliosis on T2-weighted images (i.e., the hot cross bun sign) in the cerebellar type of multiple system atrophy. Dopamine transporter SPECT with ^{123}I-ioflupane typically shows asymmetric reduction in striatal uptake in atypical parkinsonian syndromes.

Vitamin B$_{12}$ Deficiency

Vitamin B$_{12}$ deficiency is usually due to limited dietary intake or malabsoprtion. It leads to subacute combined degeneration of the spinal cord, affecting the posterior and lateral columns of the spinal cord, and peripheral neuropathy. Careful clinical/neurological examination may reveal clinical symptoms that differ from those typical of iNPH. Degeneration of posterior columns leads to loss of proprioception, sensory ataxia, and paresthesia, whilst degeneration of lateral columns leads to spasticity and hyperreflexia (i.e., upper motor neuron findings) as well as muscle weakness. Peripheral neuropathy is manifested by paresthesia, decreased or absent ankle reflexes, limb weakness, and sensory ataxia. Sensory ataxia is characterised by gait disturbance and difficulty in maintaining balance, especially in the absence of visual cues (e.g., in the dark or with closed eyes). This manifests as a positive Romberg's sign, which should not be present in iNPH. Vitamin B$_{12}$ deficiency is associated with cognitive impairment characterised by slowing of psychomotor speed and memory deficits [30]. Some patients may develop urinary incontinence, which makes differential diagnosis more challenging. The diagnosis of vitamin B_{12} deficiency is based on laboratory testing with characteristic findings of low serum vitamin B_{12} levels, elevated methylmalonic acid and homocysteine plasma levels and haematological abnormalities (i.e., macrocytosis and anaemia). MRI of the spinal cord shows typical hyperintensities in the dorsal columns of the cervical and upper thoracic spinal cord on T2-weighted images.

Neurosyphilis

Neurosyphilis is an infection of the central nervous system caused by Treponema pallidum that occurs 10 to 20 years after the initial infection if not treated with antibiotics. Neurosyphilis causes damage to the posterior columns of the spinal cord and the dorsal root ganglia, the so-called "tabes dorsalis". The most promi nent clinical finding is gait disturbance in the form of sensory ataxic gait due to loss of proprioceptive input. A characteristic feature of neurosyphilis is that gait disturbance worsens in the dark and balance is markedly impaired when standing with the eyes closed (i.e., positive Romberg's sign), which is not typical for iNPH. Other typical symptoms of neurosyphilis include paresthesia, lightning-like pain and areflexia in lower limbs, and Argyll Robertson pupils, which constrict to accommodation but not to light. These symptoms are not found in iNPH. Neurosyphilis, similar to iNPH, causes cognitive impairment with predominantly impaired memory, attention, and executive function. Neuropsychiatric and behavioural symptoms are frequently associated with neurosyphilis, the most common being personality changes with or without aggressive behaviour, psychosis with paranoid delusions, hallucinations and illusions, as well as mood disorders including mania and depression. Except for depression, these symptoms are not typical of hydrocephalus [31]. Patients with neurosyphilis may present with urinary incontinence due to neurogenic bladder. The diagnosis of syphilis is based on the cerebrospinal fluid analysis, where pleocytosis and increased protein concentration are usually present, and positivity of the Venereal Disease Research Laboratory test.

Medication Side Effects

Certain drugs can have side effects such as gait disturbance, motor symptoms, and cognitive impairment that resemble those in Parkinson's disease and atypical parkinsonian syndromes. The so-called drug-induced Parkinsonism is triggered by drugs that affect dopamine receptors. These drugs include antipsychotics, more frequently typical than atypical, gastrointestinal prokinetics and antiemetics, calcium channel blockers (e.g., flunarizine and cinnarizine), dopamine-depleting drugs (e.g., reserpine and tetrabenazine), antiepileptic drugs (e.g., valproic acid and phenytoin), mood stabilisers (e.g., lithium), and antidepressants (e.g., selective serotonin reuptake inhibitors) [32]. In addition, antipsychotic drugs can induce urinary incontinence [33]. The differential diagnosis between iNPH and drug-induced Parkinsonism is similar to that between iNPH and other parkinsonian syndromes. However, drug-induced Parkinsonism has a poor response to levodopa treatment, has normal striatal dopamine transporter uptake on ^{123}I-ioflupane SPECT, and is reversible after discontinuation of the drug, although the symptoms may persist for weeks to months after stopping the treatment [32].

4.2 Diseases with Two Major Clinical Symptoms

Cervical Myelopathy

Cervical myelopathy is frequently caused by degenerative cervical spondylosis with spinal canal stenosis and leads to gait disturbance and urinary problems. Patients usually have a medical history of neck pain. The most prominent clinical finding in cervical myelopathy is gait disturbance characterised by sensory ataxia (i.e., ataxia that is markedly impaired in the dark or with the eyes closed). Clinical/neurological examination also reveals upper motor neuron findings in lower limbs (i.e., hyper-reflexia, increased muscle tone, and a positive Babinski sign). None of these clinical findings are typical for iNPH. Urinary problems, including urgency and incontinence due to neurogenic bladder, may occur as the disease progresses. Imaging of the cervical spine reveals myelopathy and spondylosis with spinal canal stenosis. The ventricles should not be enlarged on brain imaging and tests of CSF drainage and hydrodynamics are negative. Increased protein concentration is usually present in CSF.

Lumbosacral Spinal Stenosis

Lumbosacral spinal stenosis can lead to nerve root compression, causing gait disturbance and urinary incontinence without urgency. Gait disturbance typically worsens with increasing walking distance. Patients usually have neurogenic claudication (i.e., pain in the lower back and lower limbs with or without numbness and weakness in the legs) when walking a longer distance. The symptoms in lumbosacral spinal stenosis are markedly reduced when patients bend over or change their position (e.g., sit or lie down). In contrast, gait disturbance in iNPH does not depend on walking distance or forward bending. In lumbosacral spinal stenosis, step length may be shortened, but shuffling that is typical for iNPH is usually not present. Clinical/neurological examination can reveal lower motor neuron findings (i.e., muscle atrophy and hyporeflexia or areflexia). In severe stenosis, bladder dysfunction with urinary incontinence without urgency may develop. In the advanced stages, walking may be impossible and urinary retention may be present due to compression of the cauda equina. Imaging of the lumbosacral spine reveals spinal canal stenosis and tests of CSF drainage and hydrodynamics, preferably performed at a higher level than the stenosis, are negative.

Peripheral Neuropathy

Peripheral neuropathy is caused by damage of the peripheral nerves, including motor, sensory, autonomic, or multiple nerve types simultaneously. The most common causes of peripheral neuropathy in older adults are diabetes, vitamin B deficiency, medication (e.g., chemotherapy), excessive alcohol consumption, tumours (e.g., paraneoplastic syndrome), autoimmune diseases, or idiopathic aetiology. Gait disturbance is caused by sensory ataxia due to loss of proprioception in the lower limbs and typically worsens in the dark. Muscle weakness due to motor nerve damage can also contribute to gait disturbance. Damage to sensory and autonomic nerves can cause bladder dysfunction with voiding difficulties. The typical clinical symptoms of peripheral neuropathy are paresthesia, numbness, sensory impairment, muscle weakness, and neuropathic pain in the lower limbs. None of these symptoms should be present in patients with iNPH. Clinical/neurological examination can reveal lower motor neuron findings (i.e., muscle atrophy and hyporeflexia or areflexia) with or without paresis and hypoesthesia for various qualities, including loss of vibration sense. The diagnosis of peripheral neuropathy can be verified by nerve conduction studies and needle electromyography.

Diseases with One Major Clinical Symptom

There are a number of diseases that can have one clinical symptom characteristic of iNPH. Gait disturbance can be present in degenerative arthritis of hips, knees, and ankles, peripheral vascular disease with typical claudications, and also in spinocerebellar ataxia with impaired limb coordination. Isolated urinary urgency and incontinence can be present in prostate hypertrophy, pelvic-floor abnormalities, and interstitial cystitis. Cognitive impairment is typically present in a number of neurodegenerative diseases and in major depression. Specifically, patients with Alzheimer's disease have severe memory deficits with poor recall that does not benefit from cueing and impaired recognition, as well as anomic aphasia and agnosia. Depending on the variant of the disease, patients with frontotemporal dementia have personality changes and socially inappropriate behaviour or various types of aphasia. Almost all patients with neurodegenerative diseases may also have urinary incontinence and gait disturbance in the very advanced stages, which makes their differentiation from iNPH more challenging. Patients with major depression usually have cognitive impairment of a frontal-subcortical profile similar to that found in iNPH. All of these diseases should be ruled out or identified and treated, if possible, before evaluating iNPH.

5 Conclusion

Gait disturbance, urinary incontinence and cognitive impairment are the major clinical symptoms of iNPH. Minor clinical symptoms, including dizziness, sleep disorders, sexual dysfunction, and headache, may also be present in patients with iNPH. It is of great importance to accurately identify the typical major clinical symptoms of iNPH and to specifically look for clinical symptoms and findings that are not usually present in iNPH and may point to the other diagnoses, the red flags. In the differential diagnosis, it is particularly important to keep in mind diseases that present with all three major clinical symptoms, including other types of hydrocephalus (i.e., secondary NPH and chronic obstructive hydrocephalus), subcortical ischemic vascular disease, Parkinson's disease, atypical parkinsonian syndromes, vitamin B_{12} deficiency, neurosyphilis and medication side effects. Careful examination of the major clinical symptoms along with evaluation of specific findings on brain imaging is essential to identify patients who should be referred for specific tests of CSF drainage or hydrodynamics to confirm the diagnosis of iNPH.

6 Key Points

- Gait disturbance, urinary incontinence, and cognitive impairment are the major clinical symptoms, which are together present in about 50% of patients with iNPH.
- Gait disturbance is characterised as an apraxia of gait (i.e., broad-based and short-stepped gait with irregular step length, reduced step height and turning en bloc using multiple steps) with preserved arm swing.
- The most common urinary symptoms are urinary urgency and increased urinary frequency together with urge incontinence in the later stages.
- Cognitive impairment is characterised by slowing of psychomotor speed, attentional and working memory deficits, executive dysfunction, episodic memory deficits with preserved recognition and visuospatial impairment, and is usually accompanied by neuropsychiatric and behavioural symptoms, the most common of which is apathy.
- The minor clinical symptoms are present irregularly and include dizziness, sleep disorders, sexual dysfunction, and headache.
- Acute onset and fluctuation of clinical symptoms is not typical for iNPH.
- Neurological examination in patients is normal except for findings associated with the major clinical symptoms.
- Upper motor neuron findings may indicate vascular ischemic changes, lower motor neuron findings may indicate polyneuropathy or nerve root compression, cerebellar or extrapyramidal symptoms are suggestive of neurodegenerative diseases and spinal ataxia is characteristic of spinal cord pathology and polyneuropathy.

- Severe memory deficits, agnosia, aphasia, and visual hallucinations should raise concerns about another diseases causing cognitive impairment.
- In the case of progressive cognitive impairment without gait disturbance regardless of urinary symptoms, other diseases should be considered.
- If gait disturbance and urinary symptoms without cognitive impairment are present, spinal cord pathology and nerve root compression have to be excluded.
- The differential diagnosis of iNPH is most challenging for diseases that present with three major clinical symptoms including secondary NPH, chronic obstructive hydrocephalus, subcortical ischemic vascular disease, Parkinson's disease, atypical parkinsonian syndromes, vitamin B_{12} deficiency, neurosyphilis, and medication side effects.
- Diseases that present with two major clinical symptoms and may mimic iNPH include cervical myelopathy, lumbosacral spinal stenosis, and peripheral neuropathy.
- Also diseases that present with one major clinical symptom should be ruled out or identified and treated, if possible, before evaluating iNPH.

References

1. Hakim S, Adams RD. The special clinical problem of symptomatic hydrocephalus with normal cerebrospinal fluid pressure. Observations on cerebrospinal fluid hydrodynamics. J Neurol Sci. 1965;2(4):307–27. https://doi.org/10.1016/0022-510x(65)90016-x.
2. Gallia GL, Rigamonti D, Williams MA. The diagnosis and treatment of idiopathic normal pressure hydrocephalus. Nat Clin Pract Neurol. 2006;2(7):375–81. https://doi.org/10.1038/ncpneuro0237.
3. Mori E, Ishikawa M, Kato T, Kazui H, Miyake H, Miyajima M, et al. Guidelines for management of idiopathic normal pressure hydrocephalus: second edition. Neurol Med Chir (Tokyo). 2012;52(11):775–8. https://doi.org/10.2176/NMC.52.775.
4. Relkin N, Marmarou A, Klinge P, Bergsneider M, McL Black P. Diagnosing idiopathic normal-pressure hydrocephalus. Neurosurgery. 2005;57(3 Suppl):S24–S216. https://doi.org/10.1227/01.NEU.0000168185.29659.C5.
5. Giannini G, Palandri G, Ferrari A, Oppi F, Milletti D, Albini-Riccioli L, et al. A prospective evaluation of clinical and instrumental features before and after ventriculo-peritoneal shunt in patients with idiopathic normal pressure hydrocephalus: the Bologna PRO-Hydro study. Parkinsonism Relat Disord. 2019;66:117–24. https://doi.org/10.1016/J.PARKRELDIS.2019.07.021.
6. McGirt MJ, Woodworth G, Coon AL, Thomas G, Williams MA, Rigamonti D. Diagnosis, treatment, and analysis of long-term outcomes in idiopathic normal-pressure hydrocephalus. Neurosurgery. 2005;57(4):699–705. https://doi.org/10.1093/NEUROSURGERY/57.4.699.
7. Stolze H, Kuhtz-Buschbeck JP, Drücke H, Jöhnk K, Diercks C, Palmié S, et al. Gait analysis in idiopathic normal pressure hydrocephalus–which parameters respond to the CSF tap test? Clin Neurophysiol. 2000;111(9):1678–86. https://doi.org/10.1016/S1388-2457(00)00362-X.
8. Kuba H, Inamura T, Ikezaki K, Inoha S, Nakamizo A, Shono T, et al. Gait disturbance in patients with low pressure hydrocephalus. J Clin Neurosci. 2002;9(1):33–6. https://doi.org/10.1054/jocn.2001.1010.

9. Hashimoto M, Ishikawa M, Mori E, Kuwana N. Diagnosis of idiopathic normal pressure hydrocephalus is supported by MRI-based scheme: a prospective cohort study. Cerebrospinal Fluid Res. 2010;7. https://doi.org/10.1186/1743-8454-7-18.

10. Sakakibara R, Uchiyama T, Kanda T, Uchida Y, Kishi M, Hattori T. Urinary dysfunction in idiopathic normal pressure hydrocephalus. Brain Nerve. 2008;60(3):233–9.

11. Sakakibara R, Kanda T, Sekido T, Uchiyama T, Awa Y, Ito T, et al. Mechanism of bladder dysfunction in idiopathic normal pressure hydrocephalus. Neurourol Urodyn. 2008;27(6):507–10. https://doi.org/10.1002/NAU.20547.

12. Poca MA, Mataró M, Matarín MDM, Arikan F, Junqué C, Sahuquillo J. Is the placement of shunts in patients with idiopathic normal-pressure hydrocephalus worth the risk? Results of a study based on continuous monitoring of intracranial pressure. J Neurosurg. 2004;100(5):855–66. https://doi.org/10.3171/JNS.2004.100.5.0855.

13. Picascia M, Zangaglia R, Bernini S, Minafra B, Sinforiani E, Pacchetti C. A review of cognitive impairment and differential diagnosis in idiopathic normal pressure hydrocephalus. Funct Neurol. 2015;30(4):217–28. https://doi.org/10.11138/FNEUR/2015.30.4.217.

14. Kito Y, Kazui H, Kubo Y, Yoshida T, Takaya M, Wada T, et al. Neuropsychiatric symptoms in patients with idiopathic normal pressure hydrocephalus. Behav Neurol. 2009;21(3):165–74. https://doi.org/10.3233/BEN-2009-0233.

15. Kanemoto H, Kazui H, Suzuki Y, Sato S, Kishima H, Yoshimine T, et al. Effect of lumboperitoneal shunt surgery on neuropsychiatric symptoms in patients with idiopathic normal pressure hydrocephalus. J Neurol Sci. 2016;361:206–12. https://doi.org/10.1016/J.JNS.2016.01.001.

16. Blomsterwall E, Svantesson U, Carlsson U, Tullberg M, Wikkelsö C. Postural disturbance in patients with normal pressure hydrocephalus. Acta Neurol Scand. 2000;102(5):284–91. https://doi.org/10.1034/J.1600-0404.2000.102005284.X.

17. Meier U. The grading of normal pressure hydrocephalus. Biomed Tech (Berl). 2002;47(3):54–8. https://doi.org/10.1515/BMTE.2002.47.3.54.

18. Kristensen B, Malm J, Rabben T. Effects of transient and persistent cerebrospinal fluid drainage on sleep disordered breathing in patients with idiopathic adult hydrocephalus syndrome. J Neurol Neurosurg Psychiatry. 1998;65(4):497–501. https://doi.org/10.1136/JNNP.65.4.497.

19. Román GC, Verma AK, Zhang YJ, Fung SH. Idiopathic normal-pressure hydrocephalus and obstructive sleep apnea are frequently associated: a prospective cohort study. J Neurol Sci. 2018;395:164–8. https://doi.org/10.1016/J.JNS.2018.10.005.

20. Riedel CS, Milan JB, Juhler M, Jennum P. Sleep-disordered breathing is frequently associated with idiopathic normal pressure hydrocephalus but not other types of hydrocephalus. Sleep 2022;45(3). https://doi.org/10.1093/SLEEP/ZSAB265.

21. Tisell M, Hellström P, Ahl-Börjesson G, Barrows G, Blomsterwall E, Tullberg M, et al. Long-term outcome in 109 adult patients operated on for hydrocephalus. Br J Neurosurg. 2006;20(4):214–21. https://doi.org/10.1080/02688690600852324.

22. Missori P, Scollato A, Formisano R, Currà A, Mina C, Marianetti M, et al. Restoration of sexual activity in patients with chronic hydrocephalus after shunt placement. Acta Neurochir (Wien). 2009;151(10):1241–4. https://doi.org/10.1007/S00701-009-0331-4.

23. Edwards RJ, Britz GW, Marsh H. Chronic headaches due to occult hydrocephalus. J R Soc Med. 2003;96(2):77–8. https://doi.org/10.1258/JRSM.96.2.77.

24. Larsson J, Israelsson H, Eklund A, Malm J. Epilepsy, headache, and abdominal pain after shunt surgery for idiopathic normal pressure hydrocephalus: the INPH-CRasH study. J Neurosurg. 2018;128(6):1674–83. https://doi.org/10.3171/2017.3.JNS162453.

25. Israelsson H, Larsson J, Eklund A, Malm J. Risk factors, comorbidities, quality of life, and complications after surgery in idiopathic normal pressure hydrocephalus: review of the INPH-CRasH study. Neurosurg Focus. 2020;49(4):E8–E8. https://doi.org/10.3171/2020.7.FOCUS20466.

26. Oi S, Shimoda M, Shibata M, Honda Y, Togo K, Shinoda M, et al. Pathophysiology of long-standing overt ventriculomegaly in adults. J Neurosurg. 2000;92(6):933–40. https://doi.org/10.3171/JNS.2000.92.6.0933.

27. Kageyama H, Miyajima M, Ogino I, Nakajima M, Shimoji K, Fukai R, et al. Panventriculomegaly with a wide foramen of Magendie and large cisterna magna. J Neurosurg. 2016;124(6):1858–66. https://doi.org/10.3171/2015.6.JNS15162.
28. Cornips EMJ, Overvliet GM, Weber JW, Postma AA, Hoeberigs CM, Baldewijns MMLL, et al. The clinical spectrum of Blake's pouch cyst: report of six illustrative cases. Childs Nerv Syst. 2010;26(8):1057–64. https://doi.org/10.1007/S00381-010-1085-2.
29. Fukuhara T, Luciano MG. Clinical features of late-onset idiopathic aqueductal stenosis. Surg Neurol. 2001;55(3):132–6. https://doi.org/10.1016/S0090-3019(01)00359-7.
30. Moore E, Mander A, Ames D, Carne R, Sanders K, Watters D. Cognitive impairment and vitamin B12: a review. Int Psychogeriatr. 2012;24(4):541–56. https://doi.org/10.1017/S10416 10211002511.
31. Friedrich F, Aigner M. Psychiatric manifestations of neurosyphilis. In: Sato NS, editor. Syphilis—recognition, description and diagnosis. London: IntechOpen; 2011. https://doi.org/10.5772/20662.
32. Shin HW, Chung SJ. Drug-induced parkinsonism. J Clin Neurol 2012;8(1):15–21. https://doi.org/10.3988/JCN.2012.8.1.15.
33. Arasteh A, Mostafavi S, Zununi Vahed S, Mostafavi Montazeri SS. An association between incontinence and antipsychotic drugs: a systematic review. Biomed Pharmacother. 2021;142(112027). https://doi.org/10.1016/J.BIOPHA.2021.112027.
34. Ishikawa M, Yamada S, Yamamoto K. Agreement study on gait assessment using a video-assisted rating method in patients with idiopathic normal-pressure hydrocephalus. PLoS One 2019;14(10). https://doi.org/10.1371/JOURNAL.PONE.0224202.

Differential Diagnosis of Gait and Balance Impairment in Idiopathic Normal Pressure Hydrocephalus

Ota Gál, Martina Hoskovcová, and Jiří Klempíř

Abstract Difficulties with gait and balance are a key component of normal pressure hydrocephalus (NPH) pathology. They contribute to the symptomatic triad of NPH together with cognitive and urinary impairment. However, not all of these symptoms are always present in each patient. Although the pathophysiology of NPH gait and balance impairment has not yet been fully elucidated, a multilevel cortical and subcortical dysfunction including midbrain compression and atrophy likely plays a role. Impairment of all modalities of postural stability corresponds to the typical manifestation of frontal gait pathology which involves short steps, widened base of support, and reduced foot-floor clearance as well as other signs described in this chapter. Sixty to eighty per cent of NPH patients are at risk of falls. Other gait phenotypes might be present in NPH patients due to various neurological and non-neurological comorbidities. Early diagnosis and treatment of NPH using ventriculoperitoneal shunting usually lead to significant improvement in gait and balance. Thus, this chapter elaborates on the neurological differential diagnostics of NPH with specific focus on gait impairment.

Keywords Normal pressure hydrocephalus · Gait · Gait apraxia · Balance · Postural instability · Differential diagnosis · Parkinsonian syndrome · Urinary dysfunction · Cognitive impairment · Response to shunting

Ota Gál, Martina Hoskovcová, Jiří Klempíř contributed equally.

O. Gál · M. Hoskovcová · J. Klempíř (✉)
Department of Neurology and Centre of Clinical Neuroscience, First Faculty of Medicine, Charles University and General University Hospital in Prague, Prague, Czech Republic
e-mail: jiri.klempir@vfn.cz

J. Klempíř
Department of Anatomy, First Faculty of Medicine, Charles University and General University Hospital in Prague, Prague, Czech Republic

Abbreviations

BOS   Base of support
CBD   Corticobasal degeneration
CBS   Corticobasal syndrome
CoP   Centre of pressure
DLB   Dementia with Lewy bodies
FGA   Functional gait assessment
FOG   Freezing of gait
Inph   Idiopathic normal pressure hydrocephalus
MSA   Multiple system atrophy
NPH   Normal pressure hydrocephalus
PD   Parkinson's disease
PSP   Progressive supranuclear palsy
PSP-RS   PSP-Richardson's syndrome
sNPH   Secondary normal pressure hydrocephalus
VP   Vascular Parkinsonism

1   Introduction

Idiopathic normal pressure hydrocephalus (iNPH) typically presents with the triad of gait difficulty, urinary incontinence, and cognitive decline. Bladder symptoms of NPH are high urinary frequency, complete urinary incontinence, and rarely faecal incontinence. Common signs of mental disorders are slow psychomotor speed, inattentiveness, memory impairment, affective indifference, and apathy. Other non-constant symptoms include headache, dizziness/vertigo, extended need of sleep, sexual dysfunction, and behavioural changes. However, the complete syndrome is present in only 50–75% of the patients [1]. iNPH occurs after the age of 60 in approximately one-third of all cases, and its prevalence continues to increase with age. In clinical practice, **secondary NPH** (sNPH) is often encountered. Therefore, it is sometimes difficult to distinguish iNPH from other neurological (Table 1) and non-neurological (Table 2) aetiologies, which can even be combined independently with the symptoms of iNPH. For the elderly, we often use the term "multifactorial gait disorder" in such cases. In any case, it is necessary to recognise the symptoms, including the dominant type of gait disorder (Table 3) and accordingly search for provoking aetiology (Tables 1, 2, and 3) [2, 3].

Table 1 Differential diagnosisof idiopathicnormal pressure hydrocephalus

Secondary normal pressure hydrocephalus
Chronic obstructive hydrocephalus
Parkinson's disease
Atypical Parkinsonian syndromes
Secondary Parkinsonian syndromes
Cerebrovascular disease
Brain atrophy
Cervical myelopathy
Lumbar spinal canal stenosis
Secondary normal pressure hydrocephalus

Table 2 Non-neurological causes of gait disorders

Pain
Visual impairment
Hearing impairment
Orthopaedic disorders
Rheumatologic disorders
Cardiorespiratory problems
Side effects of drugs
Visual impairment

2 NPH Gait Impairment

2.1 *Characteristics and Terminology of NPH Gait Impairment*

Gait disturbance is one of the cardinal clinical signs of normal pressure hydrocephalus (NPH). It is characterised by markedly **decreased step length** accompanied by **broadening base of support** (BOS) and **reduced foot-floor clearance** which **resembles** the **cautious walking of a person on ice**. Depending on which one of these main signs is emphasised, NPH gait has been described as **magnetic** (reduced foot-floor clearance), **marche à petits pas** and **lower half/body Parkinsonism** (small steps), or **broad-based** (wide BOS). Since the additional features characteristic of the NPH gait includes balance problems and pronounced fear of falls (see Sect. 2.3), it is sometimes termed **astasia-abasia-basophobia**. However, two additional names are more frequently used, namely **gait apraxia** and **frontal gait disorder.** These are both a type of high-level gait disorder. The former term highlights the fact that this gait disturbance cannot be explained simply on the basis of upper or lower motor neuron lesions or impaired coordination. In this sense, it can be called apraxia. The latter emphasises similarities with the gait phenotype seen in frontal lobe lesions (see Sect. 3.1).

Table 3 Basic types of gait disorders due to neurological causes

Gait pattern	Gait characteristics	Common aetiologies
Spastic gait	Hip and knee pathology depends mainly on whether anterior muscles (quadriceps femoris and especially rectus femoris) or posterior muscles (gluteus maximus and/or hamstrings) being more overactive. The former pathology causes premature termination of the stance phase, which decreases gait speed and step length on the non-paretic side. In the swing, an overactive quadriceps hinders knee flexion, thus "making the limb longer" and forces the patient to compensate (typically by circumducting the limb) to not trip. In the latter pathology, the overactive muscles hinder hip flexion in the initial swing phase which leads to a reduced step length on the paretic side. Hamstrings also contribute to this by preventing knee re-extension in the terminal swing Distal (ankle and foot) pathology is primarily caused by triceps surae and tibialis posterior. In the former case, soleus leads to tripping in the first half of the swing phase (when the knee is flexed) or when walking down the stairs and also to knee hyperextension in mid stance. Tiptoeing in the second half of the swing phase (when the knee is extended) or when walking up the stairs is a consequence of muscle overactivity of the gastrocnemii. In the latter case, tibialis posterior causes equinovarus where the lateral side of the toe touches the ground at initial contact	Lesions of the corticospinal tract vascular, traumatic, hereditary, autoimmune, infectious, neoplasia
Flaccid paresis	The foot drags, scuffs, or catches with walking. In some patients, a compensatory high-stepping gait develops, making use of hip flexor strength to allow foot clearance	Lumbar radiculopathy, lumbar stenosis, trauma, neuropathy, lower motor neuron lesions
Myopathic gait	Waddling gait and abnormal pelvic tilt with each step because of limb girdle weakness	Myopathy (drug-induced, critical conditions, hormonal, inclusion body myositis), sarcopenia, deconditioning, myasthenic syndrome
Parkinsonian gait	Narrow-based gait with reduced stride length; the feet barely clear the floor. Posture is stooped and arm swing reduced when walking. The forward centre of gravity causes increasingly faster, short steps (hurrying or "festinating"). Turning is by small steps rather than pivoting	Parkinson's disease, atypical Parkinsonian syndromes, secondary Parkinsonian syndromes

(continued)

Table 3 (continued)

Gaitpattern	Gaitcharacteristics	Common aetiologies
Apraxia of (frontal)gait	Gaitmay appear cautious or "magnetic". There is difficulty initiating or maintaining walking. There may be inappropriate or counterproductive postural responses, short shuffling steps, disequilibrium, and start and turn hesitation. Base of support is widened	iNPH, sNPH, vascular disorders of the brain, especially in the case of involvement of the white matter of the frontal lobes, neurodegenerative disease
Cerebellargait	Thegaitmay appear to be stumbling, lurching, staggering, reeling, drunken, or slow, with reduced step length and a wide base. Associated features can include other signs of cerebellar dysfunction, including scanning and slow speech, finger-nose and heel-shin dysmetria, and dyssynergia	Hereditary and sporadic cerebellar neurodegeneration, stroke, tumours, alcohol
Vestibulargait	Deviation on walking depending on the type of vestibular pathology. Thegaitvaries from an occasional stumble to frank veering. The legs are slightly spread, and stride length is slightly reduced. Stamping on the spot with eyes closed demonstrates veering (Unterberger test). Often associated with nystagmus	Lesion of brainstem or cerebellum—stroke or expansive processes, vestibular system disorders
Sensory ataxia	Gaitis high stepping and stamping and may be slightly wide based. Stride length is normal or a little reduced. Thegaitdeteriorates markedly without visual control	Sensory neuropathy, compressive myelopathy, paraneoplastic disorder, vitamin B12 deficiency
Functionalgaitdisorder	An inconsistent and incongruentgaitpattern that does not correspond to thegaitdisorders described above	Heterogeneous, multifactorial, bio-psycho-social factors

2.2 Mechanism of Gait Apraxia in NPH

Pathophysiology of gait impairment in NPH is far from understood. Several mechanisms have been proposed including **midbrain compression and atrophy**, in particular of the rostral part as well as mesencephalic locomotor region and its efferents to the medullary reticular formation [4–8]. However, these findings have been challenged [9]. Since several **descending cortical tracts** (fronto-ponto-cerebellar connections, corticospinal tracts controlling lower limbs, and the frontal cortico-subcortical basal ganglia loop) are localised near the ventricles, they **might be compressed**, and their function disturbed as well [4, 10, 11]. Also, **reduced short intracortical inhibition** (frontal and prefrontal) and **increased corticospinal excitability** probably contribute to gait disturbance in NPH [10, 12]. Alternatively, **decreased regional cerebral blood flow** in frontal and periventricular areas such

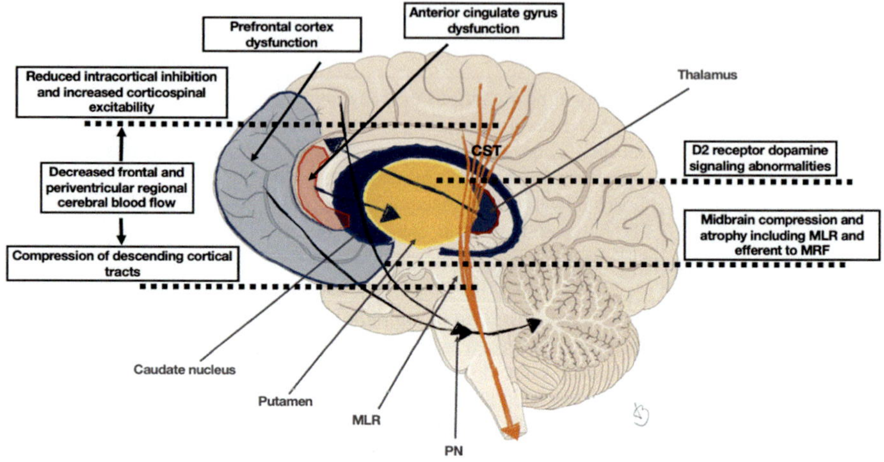

Fig. 1 Summary of NPH gait pathophysiology hypotheses

as the thalamus, basal ganglia, bilateral frontal middle gyri, and the left temporal parahippocampal cortex has been suggested to play a role [4, 13–17]. **Dysfunction of the dorsolateral prefrontal and anterior cingulate cortex** related to attention and executive function may also contribute to NPH gait pathology [10, 11, 18, 19]. Finally, **postsynaptic D2 receptor dopamine signalling abnormalities** in the dorsal putamen including the somatotopic representation of the foot have been reported in NPH patients [5, 20]. See Fig. 1 for summary and Fig. 2 for comparison with gait and balance control.

2.3   Clinical and Instrumental Gait Characteristics

As noted, the basic characteristics of gait in NPH are **decreased step length, broadened BOS,** and **reduced foot-floor clearance**. These characteristics typically manifest first [22]. Shortened step or stride length and not decreased cadence (reported only inconsistently in various studies) have been shown to be the main cause of **decreased gait velocity** seen in these patients [23]. Co-contractions of proximal muscles have been suggested as a possible mechanism for the decreased step length [12] which often does not even exceed the length of the patient's foot [24]. Reduced foot-floor clearance is necessarily accompanied by **reduced step height** and insufficient forefoot extension [22] and may be described as shuffling gait. The broadened BOS—typically exceeding the length of the patient's foot [24]—might be considered a compensatory mechanism along with **external foot rotation**, *en bloc* **gait**, and slightly **crouched posture** for disturbed balance (see below).

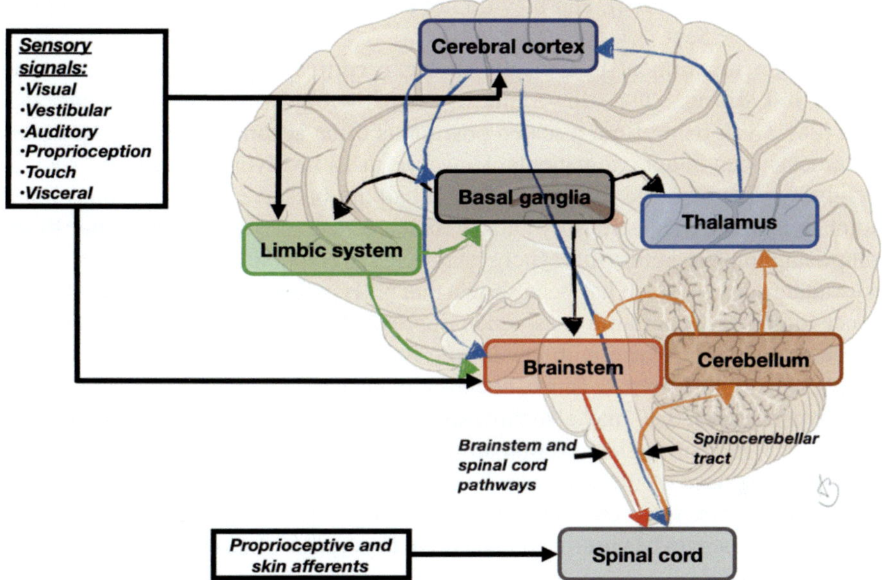

Fig. 2 Summary of gait and balance control. Adapted from Takakusaki [21]. Gait and balance control: "Multisensory signals from the visual, vestibular, auditory, somatosensory (proprioceptive), and visceral receptors act on various sites in the central nervous system. These signals may provide cognitive and emotional references to the cerebral cortex and limbic system, respectively, so that the subject may elicit either voluntary movements or emotional motor behaviour depending on the context. In each case, automatic process of postural control, such regulation of postural muscle tone and basic postural reflexes, by the brainstem and spinal cord is required. On the other hand, cognitive postural control is particularly important when the subject learns motor skills and behaves in unfamiliar circumstance" [21]. See Takakusaki [21] for further explanation

Frontal gait pathology characterised by the above-mentioned triad **may not be the most prevalent gait phenotype in real-life** NPH patients due to NPH severity and various neurological and non-neurological comorbidities [3]. In a relatively large sample size ($n = 80$), Morel [2] has shown that other clinical gait abnormalities were the most common (hemiparetic or ataxic gait; 30%) followed by normal (absence of any clinical gait abnormalities; 29%), frontal (26%), and Parkinsonian (short and/ or shuffling steps, flexed posture, reduced arm swing, and normal base; 15%) gait phenotypes. It must be noted however, that the **Parkinsonian gait phenotype shares many characteristics** with the NPH frontal one: slowness of movement, decreased step length, difficulties with gait initiation as well as fragmented and *en bloc* turning (>3 steps/180° turn; [24]), often associated with freezing of gait. **Freezing** can be seen in NPH patients with predominant supplementary motor area damage along with good response to external cues reported by some authors [12, 25] and denied by others [26, 27]. However, **as opposed to Parkinson's disease** (PD), patients with NPH gait pathology have **preserved arm swing**, **more upright posture**, and

symmetrical impairment, and they do not suffer from tremor and do not respond to levodopa (see Sect. 3.3).

NPH gait impairment is typically in **clear contrast to the performance in supine and sitting**, suggesting a link of the pathology with weight-bearing positions [28]. Even rising from a seated position is often accompanied by purposeless movements seen in apraxic patients. However, tasks involving lower limbs such as cycling, writing with the foot, or kicking a ball are preserved which implies intact motor strength as well as sensory and cerebellar functions. **Apraxia of upper limbs** comprising impaired grasp-lift synergy and force overshooting has recently received more attention [29–31]. It has been shown that NPH patients also have poorer performance in various upper limb tests which improve after shunting. Upper limb performance was also correlated with lower limb function and cognition in these studies. Reflexes are usually normal. Since, however, many NPH patients are older and suffer from hypertension, they may also have spasticity and Babinski sign due to previous strokes [32]. In neurological examination, **frontal lobe signs** including grasp reflex and grasp response of the toes may be present as well as **Parkinsonian features** [33]. Furthermore, some characteristics of NPH gait pathology (i.e. gait speed and stride length) seem to be specifically **sensitive to cognitive but not motor dual-task interference** [34].

With respect to balance (Table 4), the following pathology can be seen in NPH patients. **Steady-state** NPH balance impairment **in standing** is characterised by an **increased trunk sway**, a **larger displacement of the centre of pressure** (CoP) **in the frontal plane, faster velocity of the backward movement** in positions with the eyes open, neutral or **forward directed inclination,** and often **broad-based stance**. The stance of NPH subjects is often, but not universally broad-based and tandem stance is very difficult or practically impossible. In marked gait or postural ataxia, patients cannot stand with their feet together and their eyes opened, which, however, already goes beyond quiet stance since standing with feet together or in tandem loads proactive balance. Some authors have suggested that an NPH patient's **perception of their vertical axis may be distorted** with regard to their backward tilt. This might be due to bilateral central vestibular dysfunction of the thalamus [35] or pontine postural centre misinterpretation of the vertical axis [36]. As a consequence, these patients are positioned near the posterior limit of stability and thus show a compensatory forward-directed inclination. However, backward-tilted vertical axis resembles the situation of falling forwards, which accounts for faster backward mean CoP velocity [36]. This might be the reason why—paradoxically—these patients show spontaneous and provoked **retropulsion** despite the forward-leaning posture [37–39].

In an otherwise healthy subject, distortion of the vertical axis can be compensated for by other sensory inputs since the patients' sensory weighting and information is not disturbed. However, patients with NPH do not seem to be able to utilise visual inputs for such compensation, perhaps due to **impaired sensory integration**. Thus, impaired central integration of sensory stimuli (visual and/or vestibular) might be one of the factors of impaired balance seen in NPH [35, 36, 40–43].

With respect to **reactive balance in standing**, NPH patients performed worse than controls and even PD patients in the shoulder tug test (a variant of the Pull

Table 4 Description of balance modalities related to balance assessment

Balance modality	Description
Steady state	The ability to control the centre of mass in relationship to BOS in sitting, standing, or walking without any external or internal perturbations
Reactive	The ability to control the centre of mass in relationship to BOS during unexpected perturbations in sitting, standing, or walking
Proactive	The ability to control the centre of mass in relationship to BOS during expected perturbations in sitting, standing, or walking

See Shumway-Cook and Woollacott [51] for further details. Steady-state, reactive, and proactive balance modalities are assessed in sitting, standing, and walking with/without sensory (vestibular, somatosensory, visual) interference and/or dual-task

test) [44]. Moreover, their **proactive standing balance** is compromised not only in standing with feet together or in tandem stance as noted before, but also in the multidirectional leaning test with predominantly impaired balance in the frontal plane [45]. The authors speculate that this mediolateral balance impairment may be the cause of widened BOS which would thus again be a compensatory mechanism. Similarly, Nikaido [46] found impaired proactive balance instance in various tasks of the Berg Balance Scale (especially item 14, standing on one leg).

Balance during walking has also been studied by Nikaido [46] using functional gait assessment (FGA), which comprises several tasks loading proactive balance modality in walking as well as vestibular interference and walking with eyes closed. As compared to age-related controls provided in Walker [47], NPH non-fallers in Nikaido [46] scored worse by nearly 25% and fallers by 50%. FGA items with specifically good predictive value with respect to falls were change in gait speed, gait with horizontal head turns, gait and pivot turn, step over obstacle, gait with narrow BOS, and gait with eyes closed. In fact, **60–80% of NPH patients fall** according to various studies [34, 48, 49] and the **factors associated with the risk of falling** are— amongst others—instrumentally measured temporal **gait variability** and **dynamic balance dysfunction** as reflected in FGA [50]. Clinically, using tandem gait to assess proactive balance impairment in walking can be used (Tsakanikas and Relkin [38]: >2 foot corrections/8 steps with open eyes).

Given the phenomenology of gait impairment which—as noted—resembles the cautious walking of a person on ice, and given the fact that balance is consistently impaired both in stance and in walking, **it is tempting to speculate** that most of the NPH **gait pathology** or perhaps even its three basic characteristics (decreased step length, broad BOS, and magnetism) are **compensatory mechanisms for impaired balance**. When walking on ice, one spontaneously slightly crouches, broadens BOS, decreases step height and length, externally rotates the feet, increases trunk muscle tone decreasing pelvis and shoulder girdle movement, and flexes and slightly abducts the upper limbs, all of this to lower the centre of gravity and improve stability. However, this hypothesis remains to be tested.

3 Clinical Characteristics and Differential Diagnosis

3.1 Characteristics of Frontal Lobe Dysfunction

Apraxia of gait is a very common feature that occurs in various types of central nervous system disorders. When the **frontal lobes** are **affected bilaterally**, the key areas for programming the walking pattern are affected (see Fig. 2). The **prefrontal cortex** is important in the cognitive control of motor performance. Loss of white matter integrity in major anterior projection fibres (thalamic radiations, corticofugal motor tracts) and adjacent association fibres (corpus callosum, superior fronto-occipital fasciculus, short association fibres) show the **greatest covariance with poorer gait**. White matter lesions probably contribute to age-related gait decline by disconnecting motor networks served by these tracts [52].

Apraxia manifests as a cautious and slow gait [53] (see Sect. 2.3). The stride length is shortened on a normal or slightly wide base, and there may be **hesitation** (a few preliminary steps on the spot are taken before takeoff), freezing, and *en bloc* turns. The gait can also appear "magnetic", as if the feet are stuck to the floor (reduced step height) [54]. Definitions and **variants of freezing of gait are described in PD** and other Parkinsonian syndromes. Frontal disequilibrium is characterised by inappropriate or counterproductive postural and locomotion responses. The patient may be easily displaced backwards, precipitating falls (pull test). Fear of falling and anxiety associated with walking are common.

Since frontal regions are tightly connected with cerebellar structures via pontine nuclei, the phenomenology may comprise ataxia (wide-based and lurching gait). Thus, some authors use the term **frontal ataxia** interchangeably with frontal apraxia. However, during examination of the patient's cerebellar functions in bed, no cerebellar disorders are present. On the contrary, there are often signs of an upper motor neuron lesion on the lower limbs (hyperreflexia, positive Babinski reflex, spasticity, unilateral paresis). Neurological findings on the upper limbs are often normal or only slightly altered [55]. **Psychomotor tempo** tends to slow down, and signs of cortical or subcortical **cognitive deficits** appear. These include **other variants of apraxia, pseudobulbar affect**, and prefrontal syndrome. Computed tomography or magnetic resonance imaging of the brain shows **white matter lesions** of the frontal lobes (usually small vessel vascular disease) [56] and also various neurodegenerative disorders such as Alzheimer dementia, fronto-temporal dementia, Parkinsonian syndromes, and including NPH. Typical Parkinsonian symptoms such as asymmetric resting tremor, bradykinesia, and rigidity suggest comorbidity with PD.

3.2 Normal Pressure Hydrocephalus

Gait apraxia is considered to be the typical gait pattern in iNPH. However, small-step Parkinsonian gait is also described, as well as ataxic wide-based gait [2, 3, 57, 58].

Table 5 Gait characteristic in idiopathic normal pressure hydrocephalus

Gait characteristics	Abnormal findings
10-m walking test	>13 steps, taking >10 s
Step breadth	Distance between toes >1 feet length
Step length	<1—foot distance between the heel of the front foot and the toe of the rear foot
360° turn	>4 steps
Foot placement	Foot position correction >25% of steps

The triad of decreased stride length, decreased foot-floor clearance, and a broad-based gait have been described in NPH. In clinical practice, the **number of steps and seconds needed to walk 10 m** at a free pace is assessed in particular, followed by an ordinal gait assessment (Table 5) [59, 60]. Stance, postural reactions, and gait can be measured much more comprehensively (Table 6 and Fig. 3) [24].

The clinical distinction between **iNPH and sNPH** is often difficult clinically because the pathophysiology of iNPH is still unclear [61]. However, the patient's history can help us, especially if symptoms of NPH appear after subarachnoid haemorrhage, meningitis, intracerebral haemorrhage, brain tumour, or head trauma [2, 3, 62]. Secondary NPH can occur at any age and affects both sexes equally [63]. From a practical point of view, however, the **diagnostic and therapeutic procedure is the same** for both variants of NPH. Usually, improvement in walking (stride length) is achieved after performing a tap test, during which we take 30–50 ml of cerebrospinal fluid. Improvement of gait is usually noticeable after 2 h and within 24 h at the latest. Compared to gait, cognitive performance and urinary incontinence improve proportionally less. The tap test can be repeated up to three times on consecutive days. The negativity of the tap test does not necessarily mean a contraindication of surgery procedure, and therefore, if in doubt, a lumbar infusion test can be recommended [64]. After the introduction of a ventriculoperitoneal shunt, gait disturbances tend to improve the most compared to the other symptoms of the triad [65]. The improvement of gait lasts longer than that of the other symptoms. With sNPH, results may be less satisfactory.

3.3 *Parkinsonian Syndromes*

Distinguishing between PD and other Parkinsonian syndromes in the early stages of the disease can be problematic. In 90% of cases, it is PD. Atypical Parkinsonian syndromes, with the exception of dementia with Lewy bodies, are very rare. Atypical Parkinsonian syndromes include multiple system atrophy, progressive supranuclear palsy, and corticobasal degeneration. Important differentials of the secondary

Table 6 Classification gait and posture (Souza [24])

Parameters	Description		
En bloc turning	Requiring three or more steps for turning 180 degrees		
Dynamic balance or imbalance	Patient is asked to walk 8 steps putting one foot in front of the other (tandem gait). Imbalance was considered to be present when correction steps were needed on two or more attempts		
En bloc gait	Reduced rotation of the pelvic and scapular girdles and decreased mobility of the upper limbs		
Festination	Accelerated gait at least once in the total path		
*Postural reflex	Score		Shoulder tug test
	0		Patient stands without taking a step
	1		Patient takes a step and remains stable
	2		Patient takes more than one step and keeps his/her balance
	3		Patient takes several steps and needs to be held
	4		Patient falls backward without taking a step
Freezing	Characterised by at least one episode of sudden deceleration or a break (feet almost stuck to floor) in gait during free walking		
Hesitant gait	Hesitation at the beginning and end of the course		
"Magnetism" or shuffling gait	Step height decreased during free walking		
Broad-based gait	Distance between toes >1 own foot length (Fig. 2 B)		
Decreased step length (*petit pas*)	Distance from heel of front foot to toes of rear foot <1 own foot length (Fig. 2 C)		
Foot angle	Toes turned outward on walking (Fig. 2 D)		
Trunk flexion	A healthy person remains standing upright with his/her head up, chest out, and abdomen held in		
Lateral flexion of the trunk	Flexion of the trunk to one side whilst walking spontaneously		
Gait cadence (Reference value for normality)	Gender	Age: 60–69 years	Age: 70–79 years
	Female	148 steps per minute (SD ± 23.07)	129.5 steps per minute (SD ± 21.79)
	Male	**Not given	119.4 steps per minute (SD ± 11.07)

*Assessment of postural reflexes. The examiner must stand behind the patient, pull the patient's shoulders suddenly and briskly, and then analyse if there is retropulsion. The examiner should always be prepared to hold the patient when performing this test; otherwise, a person with a loss of postural reflexes may fall. The patient must be informed of the details of the test beforehand. A score of higher than 1 indicates impaired postural reflexes; SD: standard deviation;

**Value for females was used; gait cadence: number of steps per minute; reference normality values of the preceding decade were used for patients older than 80 years

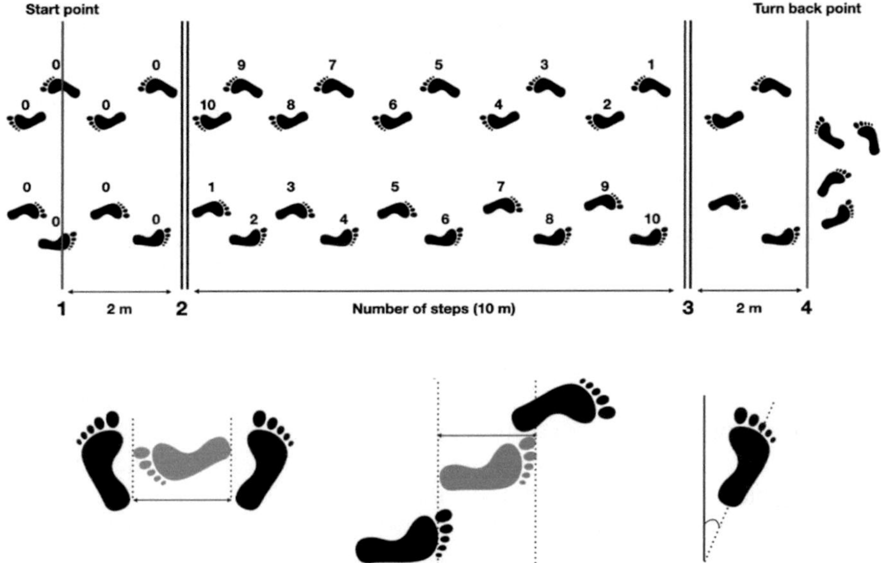

Fig. 3 Classification gait and posture (Souza [24])

Parkinsonian syndromes include vascular Parkinsonism, less so NPH and drug-induced Parkinsonism. In clinical practice, **concomitant occurrence** of cerebrovascular disease, Alzheimer's disease, and NPH **is not rare** [2, 3]. Gait impairment and balance impairment associated with a higher risk of falls are pivotal features of Parkinsonian syndromes (Table 6) [66].

Parkinson's Disease

PD typically manifests asymmetrically with **resting tremor, bradykinesia, rigidity,** and, in more advanced stages, **postural instability** (Table 6). After the administration of an adequate dose of **dopaminergic medication**, there is a **clear improvement** in the clinical condition. Insufficient or no effect of dopaminergic stimulation raises the suspicion of another aetiology. The occurrence of gait and balance disorders, manifestations of autonomic dysfunction, and a significant cognitive deficit in the first years of disease progression further casts doubt on this diagnosis. In such a case, an asymmetric presynaptic deficit of dopamine receptors in the striatum is evidence for PD (123-I Ioflupane).

In PD, an **asymmetric** reduction of **synkinesias** or a subtle narrowing of the base support appears already in the early stages [67]. Axial symptoms are more pronounced only in more advanced stages or in people in a hypodopaminergic state. When sitting, a forward flexion of posture appears across the entire body axis including the neck, trunk, and extremities [68]. **Camptocormia or lateral trunk**

flexion is common [69]. As the disease progresses, it is difficult to stand up from a sitting position on the first attempt, without the support of hands or another person. The base tends to narrow as the disease progresses and is associated with instability in the mediolateral plane, usually due to vascular involvement of the brain [70]. Performance in gait and postural instability tests (timed up and go, pull test, tandem gait) may be preserved until advanced stages [71]. Freezing of the gait is an inherent part of the advanced stages of the disease.

Freezing of gait (FOG) is a brief, episodic absence, or marked reduction of forward progression of the feet despite the intention to walk [72]. FOG usually lasts a few seconds. It most often appears in PD simultaneously with balance impairment, gait disorders, and cognitive dysfunction [18]. FOG can also occur in other Parkinsonian syndromes and neurodegenerative diseases. There are several classifications of FOG [73]. For the needs of differential diagnosis of FOG and NPH, the phenotypic classification of Fahn [74] (Table 7) and also Schaafsma [75] (Table 8) may be helpful. In PD, FOG can also involve speech, face, and arms and can be dependent on the current state of dopaminergic stimulation [73, 76, 77] (Table 9).

PD patients with cognitive impairment have slower gait speed, step length, and stride length than those without cognitive impairment. Amongst cognitive domains, registration, attention/calculation, and visuospatial function positively correlated with step length and stride length. Visuospatial function is significantly associated with speed. Severity of cognitive dysfunction is associated with worsening of dynamic balance, especially in dual-task conditions [78].

Multiple System Atrophy

In multiple system atrophy (MSA), symptoms of **autonomic dysfunction, Parkinsonian, cerebellar**, and **later pyramidal** syndrome appear. The non-motor manifestations of MSA mainly include pain, orthostatic hypotension, urogenital, gastrointestinal, respiratory disorders, sleep disorders, behaviour, and cognitive deficits. In clinical practice, the phenotype is divided into either dominant Parkinsonian or cerebellar types. However, in time these types combine with the progression of the disease.

Compared to PD, the disease **progresses rapidly**, and patients are usually immobile due to **balance and gait disorders** (Table 7) within five years of the onset of neurological symptoms. Parkinsonian syndrome can be resistant to levodopa from the onset of motor symptoms. Levodopa helps in high doses (1500–2000 mg/day) and only partially, and its effectiveness can disappear at any time. Although the morphological examination of the brain may be normal at the beginning of the clinical manifestation of MSA, magnetic resonance imaging in MSA shows 50% sensitivity and 90% specificity [79].

Impairments of voluntary movement and rigidity are typically more pronounced in the neck and trunk. Patients often have forward flexion of the neck (**antecollis**), which is out of proportion to the degree of anteflexion in the other parts of the body

Table 7 Slow unsteady gait and other axial features in Parkinsonian disorders (modified by Raccagni [66])

Disease	Axial features
Parkinson's disease	Narrow-based Mediolateral stability Capable to ride a bicycle Festination Freezing of gait Normal tandem gait
Multiple system atrophy	Broad-based Not capable of riding a bicycle Mediolateral instability Disproportionate antecollis Autonomic failure Non-neurogenic orthostatic Hypotension-related falls Abnormal tandem gait Freezing of gait
Progressive supranuclear palsy	Broad-based Not capable of riding a bicycle Mediolateral instability Careless gait Rocket sign Backwards falls Freezing of gait Abnormal tandem gait
Corticobasal syndrome	Broad-based Not capable of riding a bicycle Mediolateral instability Marked asymmetry Fixed foot dystonia Repeated falls Abnormal tandem gait Freezing of gait
Lewy body dementia	Broad-based Not capable of riding a bicycle Mediolateral instability Repeated falls Abnormal tandem gait Freezing of gait
Vascular Parkinsonism	Broad-based Not capable of riding a bicycle Mediolateral instability No or minimal upper limb Bradykinesia/rigidity Repeated falls Abnormal tandem gait Freezing of gait

(continued)

Table 7 (continued)

Disease	Axial features
Normal pressure hydrocephalus	Broad-based Frontal ataxia Not capable of riding a bicycle Mediolateral instability Preserved reciprocal arm swing Repeated falls Abnormal tandem gait Freezing of gait

Table 8 Phenotypical freezing of gait manifestation [74]

Phenotype	Situation
Start hesitation	When patient initiates walking
Turn hesitation	During turning
Apparent hesitation in tight quarters	Passing through doorways
Destination–hesitation	When the patient approaches a target
Open space hesitation	Appears spontaneously

Table 9 Phenotypical freezing of gait patterns [75]

Phenotype	Description
Trembling in place	The patient attempts to move the feet to overcome the block and produce short and incomplete steps—i.e. alternating trembling (3–8 Hz) of the legs—remaining in the same place
Shuffling	The patient moves forward with very short steps
Akinetic freezing	The patient experiences a total arrest of the movement of the legs and feet

[80]. The trunk often flexes tonically to the sides (**Pisa syndrome**) [81]. A broad-based stance is noticeable during verticalisation after rising from a chair and when standing. Additionally, this action can be aggravated by **orthostatic hypotension** and leads to frequent falls.

There are problems with the initiation of walking, the step is shortened, **sensory tricks typically do not help** with freezing, synkinesias disappear, turns are difficult, and in advanced stages, there is an apraxic gait. Some individuals show signs of cerebellar and brainstem damage (midline cerebellar ataxia) [82]. Gait variability parameters reflect the major axial impairment and postural instability displayed by MSA patients compared to PD patients and controls [83]. FOG is more common in MSA Parkinsonian variants [84]. Proactive and reactive postural instability is a **frequent** cause of **falls** without warning signs and without impairment of consciousness. The **pull test and tandem gait are often positive within 3 years** of the onset of the disease.

Clinical evidence implies that patients with MSA and progressive supranuclear palsy have larger postural instability and gait difficulty impairment than PD patients. When instrumentally measured, stride length, gait velocity, toe off angle, and parameters representing gait variability (stance time variability, swing time variability, stride time variability, stride length variability) significantly differ between PD and the above-mentioned atypical Parkinsonian syndromes [85].

Progressive Supranuclear Palsy

Progressive supranuclear palsy (PSP) is an atypical Parkinsonian syndrome and a tauopathy. The main clinical symptoms include **oculomotor dysfunctions**, **early postural instability** (Table 7), **symmetrical hypokinetic-rigid syndrome** with **axial predominance**, and **cognitive decline**. Loss of balance and **frequent falls** are the most common early signs of PSP. Affected individuals have problems with walking, including poor coordination and an unsteady, lurching gait. Other movement abnormalities develop as the disease progresses, including unusually slow movements (bradykinesia), clumsiness, and stiffness of the trunk muscles. The symptom variability and rate of progression depend on disease subtype. Diagnostics are based on clinical symptoms; magnetic resonance remains the most useful auxiliary method.

In **PSP-Richardson's syndrome** (PSP-RS), the rate of disease progression (including gait and posture disorders) and responsiveness to treatment is similar to that of MSA. PSP-RS patients show increased measures of dynamic instability compared to other variant syndromes of PSP and PD, mainly during a dual-task (walking whilst serial subtracting 7 starting from 100). The correlation analysis showed a significant relationship between gait parameters and visuospatial, praxic, and attention abilities in PSP-RS only. Other variants of PSP present with worse gait parameters than PD. PSP-RS presents with greater gait dynamic instability in the early stages compared to other phenotypes [86].

The main symptom of **PSP with progressive gait freezing** is the development of akinesia and freezing during the first year of the disease, hesitation when initiating, festination, pulses and eventually stuttering in speech, writing, and other motor activities [87]. Freezing and akinesia may be the only symptoms of this variant for a long time. Bradykinesia and limb rigidity may also develop without improvement after administration of levodopa. In later stages, instability with falls and oculomotor disorders appear. Given that patients often reach the classic picture of PSP-RS after more than 10 years, or never reach it, this option seems to be slightly more favourable than the others.

In **PSP with dominant postural instability**, postural instability may be the only dominant symptom for a long time. Instability can be recognised by the pull test: more than two steps back within 3 years of the first symptoms of the disease. A higher degree of certainty is then represented by references of unprovoked falls back [88]. Patients develop supranuclear visual paresis only at a very late stage of the disease, or never develop it, as well as other motor symptoms and cognitive or behavioural disorders.

The **corticobasal variant of PSP** is manifested by limb apraxia, dystonia, impairment of cortical sensory functions, and alien hand syndrome. These symptoms are very often asymmetric in correspondence with asymmetric contralateral hemispheric atrophy. There is also speech and facial apraxia, myoclonus, and manifestations of pyramidal system involvement.

In general, many PSP patients have a backward dropping of the head (**retrocollis**) when sitting [89] and may rise from a chair far too rapidly due to frontal disinhibition only to topple backwards into the chair ("**rocket sign**") [89]. Upright stance is impaired, base of support is broad, and patients have a tendency to backward drift [90]. During the posturographic examination, deviations of the centre of gravity are described in PSP, mainly in the anteroposterior plane typically in connection with axial rigidity. The stability pattern differs from MSA patients, where deviations of centre of gravity occur in both the anteroposterior and mediolateral planes, due to the ataxic component. Balance is significantly more impaired compared to patients with PD [91]. Sudden internal and external perturbation can lead to severe instability [92]. Postural instability and falls are early motor signs of PSP. The pull test, timed up and go test, and tandem gait test are highly sensitive, but not specific. Frontal disinhibition is attributed to ignorance of significant postural instability during walking when patients move disproportionately quickly with abrupt stops and turns [93]. In addition, downward gaze makes orientation in space and mobility difficult. FOG also contributes to falls. The temporal-spatial gait characteristics (cadence and stride length) of PSP and PD are largely similar, but progression in PSP is quicker [94].

Observations lead to the assumption of faulty motor planning and limitation of myotatic stretching reflexes in spinal impairment and possibly also impairment of vestibular processing [92]. Amongst other things, abnormal central integration of sensory inputs probably also plays a role [95, 96].

Dementia with Lewy Bodies

The clinical features of dementia with Lewy bodies (DLB) depend on the underlying form of the disease. In the common form, **dementia is the prominent feature**, whilst in the pure form, Parkinsonian features are more prominent initially. Approximately, 20% of patients do not have any Parkinsonian features (Table 7). Neuropsychological deficits that have been described include **aphasia, dyscalculia, and apraxia**. A psychotic state develops in approximately 20% of patients. **Depression, auditory and visual hallucinations, and paranoid ideation** may occur. These patients are more likely to have cognitive adverse effects with levodopa therapy in early stages than patients with PD.

Gait disorders are common in people with dementia (including vascular dementia and Alzheimer's disease), and a number of studies have documented various changes in the walking patterns of people with dementia compared to controls [97]. These changes include decreased velocity and stride length and increased variability. Falls in people with dementia have been associated with changes in walking patterns [98].

After Alzheimer's disease, DLB is now thought to be the **second most common form of neurodegenerative dementia** making up 15–25% of cases [99]. Patients with DLB walk with reduced velocity and stride length compared to people with Alzheimer´s disease [100–103]. The spatiotemporal gait characteristics of people with Alzheimer´s disease and DLB are similar, but significantly different from the normal population [102, 104]. A quantitative gait assessment identified key differences in domains of pace, step length, rhythm, and postural control that distinguish early DLB from early PD [105].

Corticobasal Syndrome

The most common presentation of corticobasal cegeneration CBD is the corticobasal cyndrome (CBS), which is a constellation of **cortical and asymmetric akinetic-rigid, poorly levodopa-responsive Parkinsonism, dystonia, myoclonus, limb clumsiness, and ideomotor apraxia** [106, 107]. In the early stages, the upper limbs are affected sooner and more severely. CBD can present with diverse clinical phenotypes, including a non-fluent, agrammatic primary progressive aphasia syndrome, dysexecutive and visuospatial syndrome, various behavioural disorders, prominent pseudobulbar syndrome with dysarthria, frontal-type gait disorder [108] as well as a progressive supranuclear palsy-like syndrome (see above) [106, 107].

Asymmetric neurological findings are evident even when sitting (dystonia, rigidity, myoclonus, or tremor). **Alien hand** ("useless arm") is a typical symptom of CBS. A broad BOS when standing up from a sitting position and postural instability are early symptoms (Table 7) [109]. FOG, apraxia of gait, bradykinesia, a widened base, leg stiffness interfering with walking, reduced stride length, and start or turn hesitations are common symptoms [53]. CBS is related to regional grey matter loss in the basal ganglia/thalamus, frontal, parietal, and temporal lobes.

Vascular Parkinsonism

The diagnosis of vascular varkinsonism (VP) is based on the co-occurrence of **Parkinsonism** with various **pyramidal** and **ataxic** and non-motor symptoms, such as **cognitive changes** or **urinary incontinence**, which are confirmed by **morphological findings of cerebrovascular disease** [110]. There are three subtypes of VP: (1) the acute/subacute **post-stroke VP** subtype presents with (sub)acute onset of Parkinsonism, which is usually asymmetric. (2) The more frequent **insidious onset VP** subtype presents with progressive Parkinsonism with lack/insufficiency of levodopa responsiveness, prominent gait and postural disorders, a mixed shuffling-ataxic gait pattern, upper motor neurons signs, or incontinence. (3) Vascular lesions gradually contribute to the Parkinsonian syndrome in mixed idiopathic PD or other neurodegenerative **Parkinsonism and cerebrovascular disease,** particularly the features of gait and postural instability (Table 7). VP accounts for around 10% of all cases of Parkinsonian syndromes [111].

In VP, voluntary motor skills of the upper limbs are unaffected or only mildly impaired. Such an impairment would manifest as akinesia, bradykinesia, rigidity, or resting tremor. Instead, typical features of VP are postural instability and a broad-based gait. Compared to PD, postural tremor appears more often in VP [112]. With verticalisation, a widened base and postural instability typically appear in the early stages of the disease [113]. A broad-based, unsteady stance is a sensitive but non-specific symptom during full standing [89]. Posture is characterised by relatively upright posture and straight legs with extension of knees and hips (Table 7) [114]. Typically, gait is unsteady, broad-based and start hesitations are common, and shuffling steps occur. In some individuals, there is also reduced bilateral arm synkinesias and loss of the normal synergy, fluency and dynamic interplay of arms, trunk, and legs. Also, a limited sideway turning of the head, neck, and shoulder is often present, as well as walking *en bloc* [111, 113, 114]. For frontal lobe impairments, a broad BOS together with variable step length can sometimes mimic cerebellar ataxia, but when examining the cerebellar functions of the lower limbs whilst sitting or lying down, findings are normal (frontal ataxia) [113]. Festination and FOG are common in VP. FOG episodes tend to be broad based in VP patients, unlike the more narrow-based FOG episodes in PD patients [115]. Movement disorders together with a progressive cognitive deficit often lead to immobilisation and loss of self-sufficiency.

3.4 Other Disorders

In this section, diagnoses which are often mentioned in the differential diagnosis of NPH are briefly described, because their confusion with NPH is less probable. However, they may occur in coincidence with NPH and thus complicate the diagnostic process (Tables 1, 2, 3, and 6) [2, 3].

Drug-induced Parkinsonism is triggered by drugs that affect dopamine receptors (antipsychotics, antiemetics, dopamine-depleting drugs, calcium channel blockers). In such cases, the patient's medical history is important.

Cervical myelopathy with gait ataxia and urinary disorders are complications of degenerative cervical spondylosis with spinal canal stenosis in the elderly. Magnetic resonance imaging and possibly cerebrospinal fluid tests will help establish the correct diagnosis.

Lumbar spinal canal stenosis can shorten walking distance and is usually associated with back and leg pain. Step length can be reduced, but shuffling is not usually present. Patients recover when bending over or changing position. In contrast to walking problems, cycling is usually not impaired. Urination difficulties only occur in more advanced stages and again more often in the elderly. Spinal imaging will show spinal canal stenosis.

Neurosyphilis can cause gait disorders (spinal ataxia, paresis), neurogenic bladder, cognitive impairment, and behavioural changes. Diagnosis is based on cerebrospinal fluid analysis.

Vitamin B$_{12}$ deficiency due to limited dietary intake or malabsorption can cause degeneration of posterior and lateral columns of the spinal cord and peripheral neuropathy resulting in loss of proprioception, sensory ataxia, paraesthesias, and upper motor neuron signs as well as muscle weakness. Slowing of psychomotor speed, memory deficits, and urinary incontinence may develop. To confirm the diagnosis, evidence of a critically low serum level of vitamin B$_{12}$, elevation of methylmalonic acid, and homocysteine plasma levels is crucial. Accompanying symptoms include anaemia and macrocytosis. Magnetic resonance of the spinal cord can show hyperintensities in the dorsal columns of cervical and upper thoracic spinal cord on T2-weighted images.

4 Conclusion

Gait and balance impairment is often the first and key symptom of NPH. Besides the frontal gait phenotype with a typical triad—decreased step length, broad BOS, and magnetism—other gait phenotypes may be present. Therefore, neurological differential diagnosis is crucial, especially distinguishing the NPH pathology from PD and other Parkinsonian and frontal lobe syndromes, as well as disorders with ataxic gait or general gait and balance disturbances of the elderly.

5 Key Points

- Gait impairment is often the first and the most dominant symptom in NPH.
- Typical NPH gait impairment is characterised by markedly decreased step length accompanied by broadening of base of support and reduced foot-floor clearance which resembles the cautious walking of a person on ice.
- Due to various neurological and non-neurological comorbidities, other gait phenotypes (including hemiparetic, ataxic, or Parkinsonian) may be present besides the frontal one which makes differential diagnosis challenging.
- The Parkinsonian gait phenotype shares many similarities with the frontal one: slowness of movement, decreased step length, difficulties with gait initiation as well as fragmented, and *en bloc* turning often associated with freezing of gait.
- NPH gait is often described as magnetic (reduced foot-floor clearance), *marche à petits pas* and lower half/body Parkinsonism (small steps), or broad-based (wide base of support). It is also sometimes termed astasia-abasia-basophobia, gait apraxia, or frontal gait disorder.
- Several mechanisms of gait apraxia have been proposed including midbrain compression and atrophy, descending cortical tracts compression, reduced short intracortical inhibition and increased corticospinal excitability, decreased regional cerebral blood flow in frontal and periventricular areas, dysfunction of dorsolateral prefrontal, and anterior cingulate cortex or postsynaptic D2 receptor dopamine

signalling abnormalities in the dorsal putamen including the somatotopic representation of the foot.

- NPH balance impairment is characterised by an increased trunk sway, a larger displacement of the centre of gravity in the frontal plane, faster velocity of the backward movement in positions with the eyes open, neutral or forward directed inclination, and often broad-based stance. Proactive (multidirectional leaning), reactive (pull test), and dynamic balance is impaired leading to frequent falls.
- Diagnosis of NPH and the selection of suitable candidates for ventriculoperitoneal shunting are based on balance and gait improvement (especially speed and number of steps) after lumbar infusion test or intracranial pressure monitoring.
- In properly selected patients, gait and balance are improved the most and the longest after ventriculoperitoneal shunting.

Funding Supported by the project National Institute for Neurological Research (Programme EXCELES, ID Project No. LX22NPO5107)—funded by the European Union—Next Generation EU; Charles University: Cooperation Program in Neuroscience; General University Hospital in Prague project MH CZ-DRO-VFN64165.

References

1. Mori K. Management of idiopathic normal-pressure hydrocephalus: a multi-institutional study conducted in Japan. J Neurosurg. 2001;95:970–3.
2. Morel E, Armand S, Assal F, Allali G. Is frontal gait a myth in normal pressure hydrocephalus? J Neurol Sci. 2019;15(402):175–9.
3. Morel E, Armand S, Assal F, Allali G. Normal pressure hydrocephalus and CSF tap test response: the gait phenotype matters. J Neural Transm (Vienna). 2021;128(1):121–5.
4. Lee PH, Yong SW, Ahn YH, Huh K. Correlation of midbrain diameter and gait disturbance in patients with idiopathic normal pressure hydrocephalus. J Neurol. 2005;252:958–63.
5. Ouchi Y, Nakayama T, Kanno T, et al. In vivo presynaptic and postsynaptic striatal dopamine functions in idiopathic normal pressure hydrocephalus. J Cereb Blood Flow Metab. 2007;27:803–10.
6. Mocco J, Tomey MI, Komotar R, et al. Ventriculoperitoneal shunting of idiopathic normal pressure hydrocephalus increases midbrain size: a potential mechanism for gait improvement. Neurosurgery. 2006;59(4):B47–9.
7. Akiguchi I, Ishii M, Watanabe Y, et al. Shunt-responsive parkinsonism and reversible white matter lesions in patients with idiopathic NPH. J Neurol. 2008;255:1392–9.
8. Tullberg M, Jensen C, Ekholm S, Wikkelsø C. Normal pressure hydrocephalus: vascular white matter changes on MR images must not exclude patients from shunt surgery. Am J Neuroradiol. 2001;22:1665–73.
9. Hiraoka K, Yamasaki H, Takagi M, et al. Is the midbrain involved in the manifestation of gait disturbance in idiopathic normal-pressure hydrocephalus? J Neurol. 2011;258:820–5.
10. Armand S, Allet L, Landis T, et al. Interest of dualtask-related gait changes in idiopathic normal pressure hydrocephalus. Eur J Neurol. 2011;18:1081–4.
11. Aoki Y, Kazui H, Pascual-Marqui RD, Ishii R, Yoshiyama K, Kanemoto H, Suzuki Y, Sato S, Azuma S, Suehiro T, Matsumoto T, Hata M, Canuet L, Iwase M, Ikeda M. EEG resting-state networks responsible for gait disturbance features in idiopathic normal pressure hydrocephalus. Clin EEG Neurosci. 2019;50(3):210–8.

12. Chistyakov AV, Hafner H, Sinai A, et al. Motor cortex disinhibition in normal-pressure-hydrocephalus. J Neurosurg. 2012;116:453–9.
13. Dumarey NE, Massager N, Laureys S, et al. Voxel-based assessment of spinal tap test-induced regional cerebral blood l ow changes in normal pressure hydrocephalus. Nucl Med Commun. 2005;26:757–63.
14. Sasaki H, Ishii K, Kono AK, et al. Cerebral perfusion pattern of idiopathic normal pressure hydrocephalus studied by SPECT and statistical brain mapping. Ann Nucl Med. 2007;21:39–45.
15. Momjian S, Owler BK, Czosnyka Z, et al. Pattern of white matter regional cerebral blood flow and autoregulation in normal pressure hydrocephalus. Brain. 2004;127:965–72.
16. Ishii K, Hashimoto M, Hayashida K, et al. A multicenter brain perfusion SPECT study evaluating idiopathic normal-pressure hydrocephalus on neurological improvement. Dement Geriatr Cogn Disord. 2011;32:1–10.
17. Kobayashi S, Tateno M, Utsumi K, Takahashi A, Morii H, Saito T. Two-layer appearance on brain perfusion SPECT in idiopathic normal pressure hydrocephalus: a qualitative analysis by using easy Z-score imaging system, eZIS. Dement Geriatr Cogn Disord. 2009;28:330–7.
18. Yogev-Seligmann G, Hausdorf JM, Giladi N. The role of executive function and attention in gait. Mov Disord. 2008;23(3):329–42.
19. Allali G, Assal F, Kressig R, et al. Impact of impaired executive function on gait stability. Dement Geriatr Cogn Disord. 2008;26:364–9.
20. Nakayama T, Ouchi Y, Yoshikawa E, et al. Striatal D2 receptor availability after shunting in idiopathic normal pressure hydrocephalus. J Nucl Med. 2007;48:1981–6.
21. Takakusaki K. Functional neuroanatomy for posture and gait control. J Mov Disord. 2017;10(1):1–17.
22. Kehler U. Clinical characteristics and differential diagnosis. In: Fritsch MJ, Kehler U, Meier U, editors. Normal pressure hydrocephalus. Stuttgart/New York/Delhi/Rio: Thieme; 2014.
23. Stolze H, Kuhtz-Buschbeck JP, Drücke H, Jöhnk K, Illert M, Deuschl G. Comparative analysis of the gait disorder of normal pressure hydrocephalus and Parkinson's disease. J Neurol Neurosurg Psychiatry. 2001;70(3):289–97.
24. De Souza RKM, Rocha SFBD, Martins RT, Kowacs PA, Ramina R. Gait in normal pressure hydrocephalus: characteristics and effects of the CSF tap test. Arq Neuropsiquiatr. 2018;76(5):324–31.
25. Liston R, Mickelborough J, Bene J, Tallis R. A new classification of higher level gait disorders in patients with cerebral multi-infarct states. Age Ageing. 2003;32(3):252–8.
26. Forssberg H, Johnels B, Steg G. Is parkinsonian gait caused by a regression to an immature walking pattern? Adv Neurol. 1984;40:375–9 PMID: 6695614.
27. Suteerawattananon M, Morris GS, Etnyre BR, Jankovic J, Protas EJ. Effects of visual and auditory cues on gait in individuals with Parkinson's disease. J Neurol Sci. 2004;219(1–2):63–9.
28. Rajput A, Rajupt AH. Old age and Parkinson's disease. In: Koller WC, Melamed E, editors. Handbook of clinical neurology, Vol. 84 (3rd series) Parkinson's disease and related disorders, Part II. p. 427–44.
29. Sirkka J, Parviainen M, Jyrkkänen HK, Koivisto AM, Säisänen L, Rauramaa T, Leinonen V, Danner N. Upper limb dysfunction and activities in daily living in idiopathic normal pressure hydrocephalus. Acta Neurochir (Wien). 2021;163(10):2675–83.
30. Gallagher RM, Marquez J, Osmotherly P. Cognitive and upper limb symptom changes from a tap test in Idiopathic normal pressure hydrocephalus. Clin Neurol Neurosurg. 2018;174:92–6.
31. Nowak DA, Topka HR. Broadening a classic clinical triad: the hypokinetic motor disorder of normal pressure hydrocephalus also affects the hand. Exp Neurol. 2006;198(1):81–7.
32. Rosenberg GA. BrainEdema and disorders of cerebrospinal fluid circulation. In: Jankovic J, Mazziotta JC, Pomeroy SL, Newman NJ, editors. Bradley and Daroff's neurology in clinical practice. Edinburgh/Lonfon/New York/Oxford/Philadelphia/St Louis/Sidney: Elsevier; 2022.
33. Molde K, Söderström L, Laurell K. Parkinsonian symptoms in normal pressure hydrocephalus: a population-based study. J Neurol. 2017;264(10):2141–8.

34. Selge C, Schoeberl F, Zwergal A, Nuebling G, Brandt T, Dieterich M, Schniepp R, Jahn K. Gait analysis in PSP and NPH: dual-task conditions make the difference. Neurology. 2018;90(12):e1021–8.

35. Selge C, Schoeberl F, Bergmann J, Kreuzpointner A, Bardins S, Schepermann A, Schniepp R, Koenig E, Mueller F, Brandt T, Dieterich M, Zwergal A, Jahn K. Subjective body vertical: a promising diagnostic tool in idiopathic normal pressure hydrocephalus? J Neurol. 2016;263(9):1819–27.

36. Blomsterwall E, Svantesson U, Carlsson U, Tullberg M, Wikkelsö C. Postural disturbance in patients with normal pressure hydrocephalus. Acta Neurol Scand. 2000;102(5):284–91.

37. Relkin N, Marmarou A, Klinge P, Bergsneider M, Black PM. Diagnosing idiopathic normal-pressure hydrocephalus. Neurosurgery. 2005;57(3 Suppl):S4–16; discussion ii-v.

38. Tsakanikas D, Relkin N. Normal pressure hydrocephalus. Semin Neurol. 2007;27(1):58–65.

39. Hunter-Smith D, Pappas C, Devarajan S. Clinical inquiries. How can you best diagnose idiopathic normal pressure hydrocephalus? J Fam Pract. 2007;56(11):947–9. PMID: 17976345.

40. Bäcklund T, Frankel J, Israelsson H, Malm J, Sundström N. Trunk sway in idiopathic normal pressure hydrocephalus-quantitative assessment in clinical practice. Gait Posture. 2017;54:62–70.

41. Lundin F, Ledin T, Wikkelsø C, Leijon G. Postural function in idiopathic normal pressure hydrocephalus before and after shunt surgery: a controlled study using computerized dynamic posturography (EquiTest). Clin Neurol Neurosurg. 2013;115(9):1626–31.

42. Abram K, Bohne S, Bublak P, Karvouniari P, Klingner CM, Witte OW, Guntinas-Lichius O, Axer H. The effect of spinal tap test on different sensory modalities of postural stability in idiopathic normal pressure hydrocephalus. Dement Geriatr Cogn Dis Extra. 2016;6(3):447–57.

43. Czerwosz L, Szczepek E, Blaszczyk JW, Sokolowska B, Dmitruk K, Dudzinski K, Jurkiewicz J, Czernicki Z. Analysis of postural sway in patients with normal pressure hydrocephalus: effects of shunt implantation. Eur J Med Res. 2009;14(Suppl 4):53–8.

44. Bugalho P, Alves L, Miguel R. Gait dysfunction in Parkinson's disease and normal pressure hydrocephalus: a comparative study. J Neural Transm (Vienna). 2013;120(8):1201–7.

45. Nikaido Y, Akisue T, Kajimoto Y, Tucker A, Kawami Y, Urakami H, Iwai Y, Sato H, Nishiguchi T, Hinoshita T, Kuroda K, Ohno H, Saura R. Postural instability differences between idiopathic normal pressure hydrocephalus and Parkinson\'s disease. Clin Neurol Neurosurg. 2018;165:103–7.

46. Nikaido Y, Kajimoto Y, Akisue T, Urakami H, Kawami Y, Kuroda K, Ohno H, Saura R. Dynamic balance measurements can differentiate patients who fall from patients who do not fall in patients with idiopathic normal pressure hydrocephalus. Arch Phys Med Rehabil. 2019;100(8):1458–66.

47. Walker ML. Reference group data for the functional gait assessment. Phys Ther. 2007;(87)11:1468–77.

48. Nikaido Y, Akisue T, Kajimoto Y, Ikeji T, Kawami Y, Urakami H, Sato H, Nishiguchi T, Hinoshita T, Iwai Y, Kuroda K, Ohno H, Saura R. The effect of CSF drainage on ambulatory center of mass movement in idiopathic normal pressure hydrocephalus. Gait Posture. 2018;63:5–9.

49. Nikaido Y, Akisue T, Urakami H, Kajimoto Y, Kuroda K, Kawami Y, Sato H, Ohta Y, Hinoshita T, Iwai Y, Nishiguchi T, Ohno H, Saura R. Postural control before and after cerebrospinal fluid shunt surgery in idiopathic normal pressure hydrocephalus. Clin Neurol Neurosurg. 2018;172:46–50.

50. Nikaido Y, Urakami H, Akisue T, Okada Y, Katsuta N, Kawami Y, Ikeji T, Kuroda K, Hinoshita T, Ohno H, Kajimoto Y, Saura R. Associations among falls, gait variability, and balance function in idiopathic normal pressure hydrocephalus. Clin Neurol Neurosurg. 2019;183: 105385.

51. Shumway-Cook A, Woollacott M. Motor control. Philadelphia: Wolters Kluwer; 2022.

52. de Laat KF, Tuladhar AM, van Norden AG, et al. Loss of white matter integrity is associated with gait disorders in cerebral small vessel disease. Brain. 2011;134:73.
53. Nutt JG, Marsden CD, Thompson PD. Human walking and higher-level gait disorders, particularly in the elderly. Neurology. 1993;43(2):268–79.
54. Verghese J, Lipton RB, Hall CB, Kuslansky G, Katz MJ, Buschke H. Abnormality of gait as a predictor of non-Alzheimer's dementia. N Engl J Med. 2002;347(22):1761–8.
55. Hou Y, Yang S, Li Y, Qin W, Yang L, Hu W. Association of enlarged perivascular spaces with upper extremities and gait impairment: an observational, prospective cohort study. Front Neurol. 2022;26(13): 993979.
56. van der Holst HM, Tuladhar AM, Zerbi V, van Uden IWM, de Laat KF, van Leijsen EMC, Ghafoorian M, Platel B, Bergkamp MI, van Norden AGW, Norris DG, van Dijk EJ, Kiliaan AJ, de Leeuw FE. White matter changes and gait decline in cerebral small vessel disease. Neuroimage Clin. 2017;7(17):731–8.
57. Stolze H, Kuhtz-Buschbeck JP, Drücke H, Jöhnk K, Diercks C, Palmié S, et al. Gait analysis in idiopathic normal pressure hydrocephalus–which parameters respond to the CSF tap test? Clin Neurophysiol Off J Int Fed Clin Neurophysiol. 2000;111:1678–86.
58. Williams MA, Thomas G, de Lateur B, Imteyaz H, Rose JG, Shore WS, et al. Objective assessment of gait in normal-pressure hydrocephalus. Am J Phys Med Rehabil. 2008;87:39–45.
59. Hellström P, Klinge P, Tans J, Wikkelsø C. A new scale for assessment of severity and outcome in iNPH. Acta Neurol Scand. 2012;126:229–37.
60. Kiefer M, Unterberg A. The differential diagnosis and treatment of normal-pressure hydrocephalus. Dtsch Arzteblatt Int. 2012;109:15–25; quiz 26.
61. Skalický P, Mládek A, Bradáč O. Normotenzní hydrocefalus. Cesk Slov Neurol N. 2021;84/117(6):512–34.
62. Bradley WG. Normal pressure hydrocephalus new concepts on etiology and diagnosis. AJNR Am J Neuroradiol. 2000;21:1586–90.
63. Williams MA, Malm J. Diagnosis and treatment of idiopathic normal pressure hydrocephalus. Continuum. 2016;22(2):579–99.
64. Wikkelsø C, Hellström P, Klinge PM, Tans JT. The European iNPH multicentre study on the predictive values of resistance to CSF outflow and the CSF tap test in patients with idiopathic normal pressure hydrocephalus. European iNPH multicentre study group. J Neurol Neurosurg Psychiatry. 2013;84(5):562–8.
65. Grasso G, Torregrossa F, Leone L, Frisella A, Landi A. Long-term efficacy of shunt therapy in idiopathic normal pressure hydrocephalus. World Neurosurg. 2019;129:e458–63.
66. Raccagni C, Nonnekes J, Bloem BR, Peball M, Boehme C, Seppi K, Wenning GK. Gait and postural disorders in parkinsonism: a clinical approach. J Neurol. 2020;267(11):3169–76.
67. Nürnberger L, Klein C, Baudrexel S, Roggendorf J, Hildner M, Chen S, Kang JS, Hilker R, Hagenah J. Ultrasound-based motion analysis demonstrates bilateral arm hypokinesia during gait in heterozygous PINK1 mutation carriers. Mov Disord. 2015;30(3):386–92.
68. Yokochi F. Lateral flexion in Parkinson's disease and Pisa syndrome. J Neurol. 2006;253(Suppl 7):VII17–20.
69. Doherty KM, van de Warrenburg BP, Peralta MC, Silveira-Moriyama L, Azulay JP, Gershanik OS, Bloem BR. Postural deformities in Parkinson's disease. Lancet Neurol. 2011;10(6):538–49.
70. Pistacchi M, Gioulis M, Sanson F, De Giovannini E, Filippi G, Rossetto F, Zambito Marsala S. Gait analysis and clinical correlations in early Parkinson's disease. Funct Neurol. 2017;32(1):28–34.
71. Borm CDJM, Krismer F, Wenning GK, Seppi K, Poewe W, Pellecchia MT, Barone P, Johnsen EL, Østergaard K, Gurevich T, Djaldetti R, Sambati L, Cortelli P, Petrović I, Kostić VS, Brožová H, Růžička E, Marti MJ, Tolosa E, Canesi M, Post B, Nonnekes J, Bloem BR. European MSA study group (EMSA-SG). Axial motor clues to identify atypical parkinsonism: a multicentre European cohort study. Parkinsonism Relat Disord. 2018;56:33–40.

72. Giladi N, Nieuwboer A. Understanding and treating freezing of gait in parkinsonism, proposed working definition, and setting the stage. Mov Disord. 2008;23(Suppl 2):S423–5.

73. Falla M, Cossu G, Di Fonzo A. Freezing of gait: overview on etiology, treatment, and future directions. Neurol Sci Adv Neurol. 2022;43(3):1627–39.

74. Fahn S. The freezing phenomenon in parkinsonism. 1995;67:53–63.

75. Schaafsma JD, Balash Y, Gurevich T, Bartels AL, Hausdorff JM, Giladi N. Characterization of freezing of gait subtypes and the response of each to levodopa in Parkinson's disease. Eur J Neurol. 2003;10(4):391–8.

76. Vercruysse S, Gilat M, Shine JM, Heremans E, Lewis S, Nieuwboer A. Freezing beyond gait in Parkinson's disease: a review of current neurobehavioral evidence. Neurosci Biobehav Rev. 2014;43:213–27.

77. Espay AJ, Fasano A, van Nuenen BF, Payne MM, Snijders AH, Bloem BR. "On" state freezing of gait in Parkinson disease: a paradoxical levodopa-induced complication. Neurology. 2012;78(7):454–7.

78. Kim SM, Kim DH, Yang IS, Ha SW, Han JH. Gait patterns in Parkinson's disease with or without cognitive impairment. Dement Neurocogn Disord. 2018;17(2):57–65.

79. Chelban V, Bocchetta M, Has sanein S et al. An update on advances in magnetic resonance imaging of multiple system atrophy. J Neurol. 2019;266(4):1036–45.

80. van de Warrenburg BP, Cordivari C, Ryan AM, Phadke R, Holton JL, Bhatia KP, Hanna MG, Quinn NP. The phenomenon of disproportionate antecollis in Parkinson's disease and multiple system atrophy. Mov Disord. 2007;22(16):2325–31.

81. Sławek J, Derejko M, Lass P, Dubaniewicz M. Camptocormia or Pisa syndrome in multiple system atrophy. Clin Neurol Neurosurg. 2006;108(7):699–704.

82. Köllensperger M, Geser F, Seppi K, Stampfer-Kountchev M, Sawires M, Scherfler C, Boesch S, Mueller J, Koukouni V, Quinn N, Pellecchia MT, Barone P, Schimke N, Dodel R, Oertel W, Dupont E, Østergaard K, Daniels C, Deuschl G, Gurevich T, Giladi N, Coelho M, Sampaio C, Nilsson C, Widner H, Sorbo FD, Albanese A, Cardozo A, Tolosa E, Abele M, Klockgether T, Kamm C, Gasser T, Djaldetti R, Colosimo C, Meco G, Schrag A, Poewe W, Wenning GK. European MSA study group. Red flags for multiple system atrophy. Mov Disord. 2008;23(8):1093–9.

83. Sidoroff V, Raccagni C, Kaindlstorfer C, Eschlboeck S, Fanciulli A, Granata R, Eskofier B, Seppi K, Poewe W, Willeit J, Kiechl S, Mahlknecht P, Stockner H, Marini K, Schorr O, Rungger G, Klucken J, Wenning G, Gaßner H. Characterization of gait variability in multiple system atrophy and Parkinson's disease. J Neurol. 2021;268(5):1770–9.

84. Spildooren J, Vercruysse S, Desloovere K, Vandenberghe W, Kerckhofs E, Nieuwboer A. Freezing of gait in Parkinson's disease: the impact of dual-tasking and turning. Mov Disord. 2010;25(15):2563–70.

85. Gassner H, Raccagni C, Eskofier BM, Klucken J, Wenning GK. The diagnostic scope of sensor-based gait analysis in atypical Parkinsonism: further observations. Front Neurol. 2019;22(10):5.

86. Picillo M, Ricciardi C, Tepedino MF, Abate F, Cuoco S, Carotenuto I, Erro R, Ricciardelli G, Russo M, Cesarelli M, Barone P, Amboni M. Gait analysis in progressive supranuclear palsy phenotypes. Front Neurol. 2021;10(12): 674495.

87. Lopez G, Bayulkem K, Hallett M. Progressive supranuclear palsy (PSP): Richardson syndrome and other PSP variants. Acta Neurol Scand. 2016;134(4):242–9.

88. Ali F, Josephs K. The dia¬gnosis of progressive supranuclear palsy: current opinions and challenges. Expert Rev Neurother. 2018;18(7):603–16.

89. Nonnekes J, Goselink RJM, Růžička E, Fasano A, Nutt JG, Bloem BR. Neurological disorders of gait, balance and posture: a sign-based approach. Nat Rev Neurol. 2018;14(3):183–9.

90. Litvan I. Progressive supranuclear palsy revisited. Acta Neurol Scand. 1998;98(6):73–84.

91. Panyakaew P, Anan C, Bhidayasiri R. Posturographic abnormalities in ambulatory atypical parkinsonian disorders: differentiating characteristics. Parkinsonism Relat Disord. 2019;66:94–9.

92. Ondo W, Warrior D, Overby A, et al. Computerized posturography analysis of progressive supranuclear palsy: a case-control comparison with Parkinson's disease and healthy controls. Arch Neurol. 2000;57(10):1464–9.
93. Ebersbach G, Moreau C, Gandor F, Defebvre L, Devos D. Clinical syndromes: Parkinsonian gait. Mov Disord. 2013;28(11):1552–9.
94. Egerton T, Williams DR, Iansek R. Comparison of gait in progressive supranuclear palsy, Parkinson's disease and healthy older adults. BMC Neurol. 2012;2(12):116.
95. Dale ML, Horak FB, Wright WG, et al. Impaired perception of surface tilt in progressive supranuclear palsy. PLoS ONE. 2017;12(3): e0173351.
96. Kammermeier S, Maierbeck K, Dietrich L et al. Qualitative postural control differences in idiopathic Parkinson's disease versus progressive supranuclear palsy with dynamic-on-static platform tilt. Clin Neurophysiol. 2018;129(6):1137–47.
97. Sheridan PL, Solomont J, Kowall N, Hausdorff JM. Influence of executive function on locomotor function: divided attention increases gait variability in Alzheimer's disease. J Am Geriatr Soc. 2003;51(11):1633–7.
98. van Iersel MB, Hoefsloot W, Munneke M, Bloem BR, Olde Rikkert MG. Systematic review of quantitative clinical gait analysis in patients with dementia. Z Gerontol Geriatr. 2004;37(1):27–32.
99. McKeith IG, Galasko D, Kosaka K, et al. Consensus guidelines for the clinical and pathologic diagnosis of dementia with Lewy bodies (DLB): report of the consortium on DLB international workshop. Neurology. 1996;47(5):1113–24.
100. Gnanalingham K, Byrne E, Thornton A, Sambrook M, Bannister P. Motor and cognitive function in Lewy body dementia: comparison with Alzheimer's and Parkinson's diseases. J Neurol Neurosurg Psychiatry. 1997;62:243–52.
101. Waite LM, Broe GA, Grayson DA, Creasey H. Motor function and disability in the dementias. Int J Geriatr Psychiatry. 2000;15:897–903.
102. Merory JR, Wittwer JE, Rowe CC, Webster KE. Quantitative gait analysis in patients with dementia with Lewy bodies and Alzheimer's disease. Gait Posture. 2007;26(3):414–9.
103. Mc Ardle R, Del Din S, Galna B, Thomas A, Rochester L. Differentiating dementia disease subtypes with gait analysis: feasibility of wearable sensors? Gait Posture. 2020;76:372–6.
104. Mc Ardle R, Galna B, Donaghy P, Thomas A, Rochester L. Do Alzheimer's and Lewy body disease have discrete pathological signatures of gait? Alzheimers Dement. 2019;15(10):1367–77.
105. Mathias K, Pinto A, Matar E, Phillips J, Lewis S, Ehgoetz Martens K. Differentiating gait impairments in early Parkinson's disease and early dementia with Lewy bodies [abstract]. Mov Disord. 2021;36(suppl 1).
106. Saranza GM, Whitwell JL, Kovacs GG. Lang AE corticobasal degeneration. Int Rev Neurobiol. 2019;149:87–136.
107. Bluett B, Pantelyat AY, Litvan I, Ali F, Apetauerova D, Bega D, Bloom L, Bower J, Boxer AL, Dale ML, Dhall R, Duquette A, Fernandez HH, Fleisher JE, Grossman M, Howell M, Kerwin DR, Leegwater-Kim J, Lepage C, Ljubenkov PA, Mancini M, McFarland NR, Moretti P, Myrick E, Patel P, Plummer LS, Rodriguez-Porcel F, Rojas J, Sidiropoulos C, Sklerov M, Sokol LL, Tuite PJ, VandeVrede L, Wilhelm J, Wills AA, Xie T, Golbe LI. Best practices in the clinical management of progressive supranuclear palsy and corticobasal syndrome: a consensus statement of the CurePSP centers of care. Front Neurol. 2021;1(12): 694872.
108. Rossor MN, Tyrrell PJ, Warrington EK, Thompson PD, Marsden CD, Lantos P. Progressive frontal gait disturbance with atypical Alzheimer's disease and corticobasal degeneration. J Neurol Neurosurg Psychiatry. 1999;67(3):345–52.
109. Chahine LM, Rebeiz T, Rebeiz JJ, Grossman M, Gross RG. Corticobasal syndrome: five new things. Neurol Clin Pract. 2014;4(4):304–12.
110. Rektor I, Bohnen NI, Korczyn AD, Gryb V, Kumar H, Kramberger MG, de Leeuw FE, Pirtošek Z, Rektorová I, Schlesinger I, Slawek J, Valkovič P, Veselý B. An updated diagnostic approach to subtype definition of vascular parkinsonism—Recommendations from an expert working group. Parkinsonism Relat Disord. 2018;49:9–16.

111. Zijlmans JC, Daniel SE, Hughes AJ, Révész T, Lees AJ. Clinicopathological investigation of vascular parkinsonism, including clinical criteria for diagnosis. Mov Disord. 2004;19(6):630–40.
112. Demirkiran M, Bozdemir H, Sarica Y. Vascular parkinsonism: a distinct, heterogeneous clinical entity. Acta Neurol Scand. 2001;104(2):63–7.
113. Gupta D, Kuruvilla A. Vascular parkinsonism: what makes it different? Postgrad Med J. 2011;87(1034):829–36.
114. Thompson PD, Marsden CD. Gait disorder of subcortical arteriosclerotic encephalopathy: Binswanger's disease. Mov Disord. 1987;2(1):1–8.
115. Giladi N, Kao R, Fahn S. Freezing phenomenon in patients with parkinsonian syndromes. Mov Disord. 1997;12(3):302–5.

Cognitive and Neuropsychiatric Features of Idiopathic Normal Pressure Hydrocephalus

Hana Horáková, Martin Vyhnálek, and Vendula Tegelová

Abstract Progressive cognitive impairment is one of the major symptoms of idiopathic normal pressure hydrocephalus (iNPH), present in about 80% of patients. Together with gait disturbance and urinary incontinence, cognitive impairment constitutes a part of the clinical triad. Cognitive deficit is commonly accompanied by neuropsychiatric symptoms (NPS), observed in up to 85% of the patients. Both cognitive deficits and neuropsychiatric symptoms are thought to result from frontal-subcortical dysfunction. The neuropsychological profile of iNPH is characterised by psychomotor slowing, reduced information processing speed, attention, working memory and executive deficit. The predominant NPS is apathy. Depending on the duration of symptoms, the cognitive continuum ranges from subtle selective cognitive decline to generalised dementia. In this chapter, we summarise the typical cognitive and neuropsychiatric profile associated with iNPH and describe the current cognitive and neuropsychiatric assessment standards. Implementation of a shunt is a treatment option to improve symptoms and slow progression. We describe the evolution of cognitive and neuropsychiatric symptoms after shunting and the power of neuropsychological tests to predict the response to shunting. Finally, we discuss the role of neuropsychological assessment in differential diagnostics of iNPH.

Keywords Normal pressure hydrocephalus · Cognition · Dementia · Frontal-subcortical dysfunction · Apathy · Neuropsychological evaluation · Response to shunting

Hana Horáková and Martin Vyhnálek contributed equally to this work and share first authorship.

H. Horáková · M. Vyhnálek (✉)
Department of Neurology, Second Faculty of Medicine, Charles University and Motol University Hospital, Prague, Czech Republic
e-mail: martin.vyhnalek@fnmotol.cz

H. Horáková
Department of Clinical Psychology, Motol University Hospital, Prague, Czech Republic

V. Tegelová
Department of Neurosurgery, Second Faculty of Medicine, Charles University and Motol University Hospital, Prague, Czech Republic

© The Author(s), under exclusive license to Springer Nature Switzerland AG 2023
O. Bradac (ed.), *Normal Pressure Hydrocephalus*,
https://doi.org/10.1007/978-3-031-36522-5_10

Abbreviations

ACC	Anterior Cingulate Cortices
AD	Alzheimer's Disease
AES	Apathy Evaluation Scale
AS	Apathy Scale
AVLT	Auditory Verbal Learning Test
BAI	Beck Anxiety Inventory
BDI-II	Beck Depression Inventory–II
BNT	Boston Naming Test
BVMT-R	Brief Visual Spatial Memory Test—Revised
CDT	Clock Drawing Test
CNS	Central Nervous System
COWAT	Controlled Oral Word Association Test
CSF	Cerebrospinal Fluid
CVD	Cerebrovascular Disorders
CVLT-II	California Verbal Learning Test—Second Edition
CT	Computed Tomography
D	Dementia
FAB	Frontal Assessment Battery
FCSRT	Free and Cued Selective Reminding Test
FCSRT-IR	Free and Cued Selective Reminding Test—Immediate Recall
FTLD	Frontotemporal Lobar Degeneration
GDS	Geriatric Depression Scale
iNPH	Idiopathic Normal Pressure Hydrocephalus
ISHCSF	International Society for Hydrocephalus and CSF Disorders
JLO	Judgement of Line Orientation
MBI-C	The Mild Behavioral Impairment Checklist
MCI	Mild Cognitive Impairment
MMSE	Mini Mental State Examination
MoCA	Montreal Cognitive Assessment
MRI	Magnetic Resonance Imaging
NPI	Neuropsychiatric Inventory
OFC	Orbitofrontal Cortices
PD	Parkinson's Disease
PSP	Progressive Supranuclear Palsy
P(r)VLT	Philadelphia (repeatable) Verbal Learning Test
RAVLT	Rey Auditory Verbal Learning Test
ROCF	Rey–Osterrieth Complex Figure
SCWT	Stroop Colour and Word Test
SRT	Selective Reminding Test
TMT A	Trail Making Test part A
TMT B	Trail Making Test part B
ToL	Tower of London

VCI	Vascular Cognitive Impairment
VPS	Ventriculoperitoneal Shunt
WAIS-III	Wechsler Intelligence Scale for Adults, Third Edition
WCST	Wisconsin Card Sorting Test

1 Introduction

Progressive cognitive impairment is one of the major symptoms of idiopathic normal pressure hydrocephalus (iNPH), present in about 80% of patients [1]. Together with gait disturbance and urinary incontinence, cognitive impairment constitutes a part of clinical triad. It has been estimated that between 2 and 6% of dementia cases are caused by iNPH, and the prevalence increases with age [2–4]. Although cognitive difficulties in iNPH are not typically the reason for seeking medical help, they can be the initial symptom, and the careful examination of this feature should be an integral part of the initial workup and subsequent monitoring [5].

This chapter focuses on the cognitive and neuropsychiatric features of iNPH. The aim is to characterise the neuropsychological and neuropsychiatric profile of iNPH, its presumed underlying neural dysfunction, and to describe the neuropsychological tests and neuropsychiatric scales commonly used in patients with iNPH. Further, we summarise the evidence about the evolution of cognitive and neuropsychiatric symptoms after shunting, including the power of neuropsychological tests to predict response to ventriculoperitoneal shunting (VPS). Finally, we outline the contribution of cognitive and neuropsychiatric symptoms to the differential diagnosis of iNPH.

2 Stages of Cognitive Deficit

Similar to conditions leading to dementia, the cognitive impairment in iNPH manifests in three stages.

In the first **"cognitively asymptomatic"** stage, patients have no objective cognitive impairment on neuropsychological testing. At this stage, patients or their informants report no or only subtle cognitive changes that do not have any objective cognitive correlation on the formal neuropsychological testing. The preclinical (or clinically asymptomatic) stage is a term widely used in the field of neurodegenerative diseases, particularly in Alzheimer's disease, to describe the fact that neuropathological changes precede the clinical signs by many years. During the preclinical stage, the neurodegenerative disease can be diagnosed by biomarkers [6, 7]. The diagnosis of cognitively asymptomatic stage in iNPH is more problematic, as no reliable markers of iNPH exist in the preclinical stage. We propose the term "cognitively asymptomatic" to designate cognitively normal patients with iNPH in whom the diagnosis of iNPH was made on the basis of other clinical symptoms of iNPH (gait and/or urinary impairment), together with the results of other paraclinical tests (MRI, spinal tap, etc.).

The second (prodromal) stage is called "**mild cognitive impairment**" **(MCI)** and designates patients with cognitive difficulties reported by themselves or by their informants, who score pathologically on neuropsychological testing, but who are still self-sufficient [8].

Dementia stage designates patients who are no longer self-sufficient because of cognitive deficit.

3 Neuropsychological and Neuropsychiatric Profile in iNPH

Cognitive deficit in patients with iNPH has been typically described as a result of frontal-subcortical circuitry dysfunction. Depending on the duration of symptoms, it ranges from more subtle and selective cognitive decline to more generalised cognitive impairment leading to dementia. The early cognitive decline may often remain undetected, which may delay the correct diagnosis.

The frontal-subcortical circuitry dysfunction predominantly refers to **psychomotor slowing, reduced information processing speed, and attention and executive deficit** [9–12]. These cognitive symptoms usually develop early during the iNPH condition. Psychomotor slowing and reduced information processing speed are typically striking, especially in later stages of the condition, although they are usually unnoticed by the patients.[1] Due to the executive deficit, the ability to regulate behaviour to complete activities and reach goals is typically compromised. Specifically, difficulties in the ability to plan and initiate tasks, maintain focus and flexibility in thinking were the most often impaired executive processes in previous studies [9–12]. Judgement is usually preserved for a long time according to the previous literature [13], though, to the best of our knowledge, no study has empirically shown it yet. In later stages, a complex dysexecutive syndrome is typically present, i.e., commonly accompanied by anosognosia when patients are unaware of their cognitive deficit and sometimes gait disturbance and incontinence. Thus, the clinician should not be surprised that a patient who is unstable in walking denies any difficulties. In that situation, a close informant is needed to get reliable and valid information about the development of symptoms over time.

Memory may also be impaired. However, memory deficit is often secondary to attention difficulties, inefficient information processing, or ineffective retrieval due to frontal-subcortical dysfunction. This leads primarily to impaired learning and recall, while retention of information usually remains preserved until later stages of the iNPH condition. The learning phase may be facilitated using semantic cues (the so-called controlled encoding). They help to eliminate the negative influence of

---

[1] On the contrary, the patients report feeling like the world is speeding up around them (clinical experience).

attention and structure the encoding process. Similarly, the retrieval deficits in the free recall may be normalised using the same semantic cues (the so-called cued recall). The efficiency of the controlled encoding and cued recall to normalise the memory performance is the primary feature distinguishing secondary memory deficit due to frontal-subcortical dysfunction from pure memory deficit due to medial temporal lobe (MTL) dysfunction [typical for Alzheimer's disease (AD)]. Recognition was shown to be disproportionally preserved relative to free recall in patients with iNPH [14, 15]. This is not surprising since this measure has been considered to be linked to MTL function [16]. However, another study found that both free recall and recognition were similarly impaired in patients with iNPH [11], suggesting that memory impairment in iNPH may not be entirely ascribable to frontal-subcortical dysfunction. This was further supported by a neuroimaging study in which a reduction in MTL volume was shown in patients with iNPH [17]. In both studies [17, 18], authors aimed to exclude patients with probable AD comorbidity; however, AD biomarkers were not analysed, so the AD comorbidity and its possible effect on memory performance could not be completely ruled out.

Beyond the pure frontal-subcortical circuitry dysfunction, deficits in **visuoperceptual and visuospatial function** have been also observed [11, 19]. In particular, the impairment in visual discrimination, visual counting and visuoconstruction were reported [11, 19], referring to posterior cortical dysfunction, predominantly in the parietal lobes. These findings are in line with previous neuroimaging studies in which a parietal regional cerebral blood flow reduction was shown in patients with iNPH [20, 21]. Still, the current knowledge on the profile of visuoperceptual and visuospatial deficit in iNPH is scant since these functions have not been routinely assessed.

The typical neuropsychological profile in iNPH is summarised in Table 1.

Cognitive deficit in iNPH is often accompanied by **neuropsychiatric symptoms** [22]. The prevalence may vary according to the clinical setting in which the patient

Table 1 Typical neuropsychological profile in iNPH

Cognitive domain	Typical finding in iNPH
Orientation	• Preserved, or only mildly impaired
Speed of processing*	• Impaired
Attention and working memory*	• Impaired
Executive functions*	• Impaired (impairment ranges between the selective deficit of individual executive processes and complex dysexecutive syndrome)
Visuoperceptual and visuospatial functions	• May be impaired
Learning and memory	• Impaired learning and recall, both can be normalised by controlled learning/cued recall/recognition; • Relatively preserved retention;
Language and speech	• Usually preserved

Note *Cognitive domains most commonly and profoundly impaired is evaluated, and the severity depends on the stage of the iNPH condition, with more severe neuropsychiatric symptoms in later stages [23, 24]. In a multicentre study [23], neuropsychiatric symptoms were observed in 85.7% of patients in a psychiatry clinic, 52.6% of patients in two neurosurgery clinics and 79.2% of patients in a dementia centre. According to the previous studies [23, 24], the most prominent neuropsychiatric symptom in iNPH is apathy, followed by anxiety. Other less prevalent neuropsychiatric symptoms were agitation, irritability, depression, or aberrant motor activity. Psychotic symptoms, such as delusions or hallucinations, were the least observed. The prevalence of the neuropsychiatric symptoms observed according to the clinical setting is summarised in Table 2.

It has been suggested that the typical profile of neuropsychiatric symptoms in iNPH predominantly arises from frontal-subcortical circuitry dysfunction [25] involving a series of parallel neural pathways linking orbitofrontal (OFC), medial, dorsolateral prefrontal and anterior cingulate (ACC) cortices to the striatum, globus pallidus and thalamus [26]. Specifically, ACC and its subcortical circuit mediate motivate behaviour; thus, dysfunction in this area may lead to apathy. Hypoperfusion in both the ACC and thalamus was previously shown in iNPH [27–29], which could explain the presence of apathy in these patients. Further, OFC and its subcortical circuit mediate behaviour and emotional regulation; thus, dysfunction in this area may lead to behavioural disinhibition and emotional lability. In functional imaging studies [27, 28], hypofunction in the OFC and ACC was found in iNPH, which could explain anxiety, irritability and aberrant motor activity or stereotyped behaviour in these patients.

Table 2 Typical neuropsychiatric profile in iNPH

Neuropsychiatric symptoms*	Prevalence according to the clinical setting (%)**		
	Psychiatric clinic	Neurosurgical clinic	Dementia centre
Apathy	76	53	79
Anxiety	38	26	13
Irritability	0	16	17
Agitation	19	11	21
Aberrant motor activity	19	11	13
Depression	14	16	13
Delusions	14	5	17
Hallucinations	10	5	0

Note *sorted by the usual prevalence in general; **Kito et al. [23]

4 Neuropsychological and Neuropsychiatric Tests for iNPH Diagnostics

Two main approaches may be applied to assess cognition: cognitive screening or more comprehensive neuropsychological evaluation.

Cognitive screening is usually employed by neurologists or neurosurgeons to quickly assess global cognitive functioning since it is feasible to perform this during a time-limited consultation and its administration and interpretation usually do not require any special professional qualification. Overall, cognitive screening measures are sensitive and specific to detect more advanced stages of cognitive deficit and to monitor the course of cognitive deficit in these stages since more comprehensive and detailed neuropsychological evaluation may represent too much burden for the patient and may bring only little additional information. However, they may not be sensitive enough to capture early and more subtle cognitive decline especially if only some cognitive processes are selectively impaired. They cannot be used for differential diagnostics either. Comprehensive neuropsychological evaluation with a neuropsychological test battery enables us to get a detailed cognitive profile of the patient.

In addition, evaluation of the presence and severity of neuropsychiatric symptoms and their potential impact on cognition should be an integral part of neuropsychological assessment.

4.1 Cognitive Screening

The most commonly used cognitive screening measures cover the majority of cognitive domains [e.g. Mini Mental State Examination (MMSE) [30] and Montreal Cognitive Assessment (MoCA) [31]], or they are focused on a specific cognitive domain [e.g. Clock Drawing Test (CDT) [32] and Frontal Assessment Battery (FAB) [33]].

MMSE was initially developed to detect later stages of cognitive deficit (dementia), while **MoCA** was originally designed to detect earlier and more subtle stages [mild cognitive impairment (MCI)]. MCI is a clinical stage that often precedes dementia [34]. MMSE and MoCA both evaluate orientation, attention, working memory, memory, language and visuoconstruction. Contrary to MoCA, MMSE lacks evaluation of executive function [35]. Further, in comparison with MMSE, MoCA is more difficult in memory since it includes more words to be learned (5 vs. 3). At the same time, there are fewer trials to encode them (2 vs. up to 3), and a longer delay between learning and retrieval.

As for discrimination accuracy, according to a detailed meta-analysis, the MMSE had a pooled sensitivity of 79%, and a pooled specificity of 81% to differentiate an individual with dementia (regardless of aetiology) from cognitively normal older adults [36]. In contrast, the pooled sensitivity and specificity to distinguish individuals with MCI from cognitively normal adults were only 63% and 65%, respectively. Most studies showed MoCA to be superior to MMSE to discriminate patients with MCI (regardless of aetiology) from cognitively normal older adults [37]. The area under the curve (AUC) varied from 0.71 to 0.99 for MoCA and from 0.43 to 0.94 for MMSE. Although both MMSE and MoCA were often used to measure global cognitive function in patients with iNPH [38–40], data about their discrimination accuracy to identify whether the cognitive deficit is specifically due to iNPH are lacking. Based on the knowledge of the typical cognitive profile of iNPH and differences in the item content in MMSE and MoCA, it can be assumed that MoCA is more accurate compared to MMSE, especially in early stages of the cognitive deficit.

Frontal assessment battery (FAB) was originally designed as a screening measure of frontal functions, feasible to be administered even during a bed-side cognitive assessment [33]. It includes items that cover several processes tapping into both cognitive and behavioural executive functions. Its ability to discriminate patients with a prevalent executive deficit (e.g. due to frontotemporal dementia, Parkinson's or Huntington's disease) from cognitively normal controls with good values of sensitivity and specificity was shown in several previous studies [33, 41–43]. Unfortunately, data about its discrimination accuracy for cognitive deficit due to iNPH are not available yet. Although it was initially meant to be used as a stand-alone screening measure, in previous studies it was usually administered as a part of a more extensive neuropsychological battery [11, 38, 44, 45].

Neither MMSE nor MoCA are detailed enough to bring reliable information about the cognitive profile, and FAB is limited to the assessment of executive functions only. Thus, these measures usually do not allow detailed neuropsychological differential diagnosis which is essential, especially in the early stages of cognitive decline. For this purpose, a detailed neuropsychological evaluation is recommended. For the comparison of MMSE, MoCA and FAB, refer to Table 3.

4.2 Comprehensive Neuropsychological Evaluation

So far, no guidelines have been introduced for the neuropsychological test battery to be used for detailed assessment of patients with suspected iNPH and for monitoring the change in their cognitive performance. Usually, flexible test batteries enable the neuropsychologist to adapt the test battery's difficulty to the individual's global cognitive functioning. With respect to the typical profile of frontal-subcortical type of cognitive deficit due to iNPH, it is essential to include tests that measure psychomotor speed, attention and working memory, executive function and memory. Because of the evidence of parietal lobe dysfunction, visuoperceptual and visuospatial function measures should be included, as well. And finally, even though language is usually well preserved until the later stages of iNPH, language and speech measures should be also used since performance may provide important information for differential diagnosis. To evaluate the change in cognitive performance, the tests should not suffer

Table 3 Comparison of selected cognitive screening measures in iNPH

Cognitive domain	Cognitive screening		
	MMSE	MoCA	FAB
Orientation	✔	✔	✗
Executive function	✗	✔	✔
Attention and working memory	✔	✔	✗
Memory	✔	✔	✗
Language	✔	✔	✗
Visuoconstruction	✔	✔	✗
Recommended use			
Stand-alone screening measure*	✔	✔	✗
Part of a more comprehensive neuropsychological battery**	✔	✔	✔

Note MMSE, Mini Mental Stale Examination; MoCA, Montreal Cognitive Assessment; FAB, Frontal Assessment Battery. * To be used as a global measure of cognitive functioning and a basis for deciding whether a comprehensive neuropsychological assessment is valuable or not. ** To be used to monitor development of cognitive function globally and/or to decide on the level of difficulty of the comprehensive neuropsychological battery (MMSE/MoCA); as a specific measure of a cognitive domain (FAB)

from ceiling or floor effects.[2] A summary of the widely used tests according to the cognitive domains is listed below. Still, validation studies for the iNPH population are lacking and should be performed.

Measures that were most commonly used in previous studies to evaluate **psychomotor speed, attention and working memory** include *Trail Making Test (TMT) Part A* [46], any version of the *Stroop Test* (the first subtest, this is reading names of colours or naming the colour of dots according to the version used) [47], *Digit Symbol Substitution Test* [48] and *Forward and Backward Digit Span subtests* [48].

Executive functions in iNPH have been previously evaluated *with TMT Part B* [46], *phonemic verbal fluency* and *Stroop test (the colour word subtest)* [47]. These measures of executive function also include psychomotor speed, attention, and working memory component. There are numerous other tests for the assessment of executive functions, since there are several processes that comprise the executive cognitive domain. In general, *Tower of London (ToL)* [49] and *Wisconsin Card Sorting Test (WCST)* [50] are among the most frequently used. ToL measures the ability to plan, while WCST is a comprehensive measure of abstract reasoning, set shifting and problem solving. To the best of our knowledge, neither ToL nor WCST has been used in any study on patients with iNPH yet, however, they might have a good potential

---

[2] Ceiling effect occurs when the test is too easy and most people are close or achieve the maximum score. The opposite of ceiling effect is floor effect where the test is too difficult and large proportion of participants scores close to the minimum level. In both situations, the variance in the score is low and the tests do not allow to well stratify the patients.

to detect more subtle executive dysfunction in iNPH patients. Further research is needed to verify this assumption.

Several measures were used to evaluate **memory** function. The most commonly used test was the *Rey Auditory Verbal Learning Test (RAVLT)*, a word-list test employing uncontrolled learning over several trials, free recall and recognition measures [51]. There are other word-list tests, such as *California Verbal Learning Test-Second Edition (CVLT-II)* [52], or *Philadelphia (repeatable) Verbal Learning Test (P(r)VLT)* [53]. These tests also employ uncontrolled learning; however, unlike RAVLT, they employ not only free but also cued recall. Another often used test was *Logical memory* [54], a story recall test that evaluates immediate and delayed free recall and recognition. In some studies, not only verbal but also visual memory was tested. Reproduction of the *Rey–Osterrieth Complex Figure (ROCF)* [55] was the most commonly used visual memory test. It is also possible to use the *Brief Visual Spatial Memory Test-Revised (BVMT-R)* [56], which is considered a non-verbal alternative to word-list tasks since it also employs several learning trials, delayed free recall and recognition. Still, to the best of our knowledge, BVMT-R has not yet been used in any study on iNPH.

With respect to the usual memory deficit profile associated with iNPH (see above), the inclusion of a memory test employing controlled encoding/cued recall paradigm seems particularly useful. It was recommended to use this type of test in patients with suspected AD [57]; however, they have not been widely used in patients with (suspected) iNPH despite their supposed value for differential diagnosis purposes. The original test was *Selective Reminding (SRT)* [58]. It was further developed and modified. *Free and Cued Selective Reminding Test (FCSRT)* [59] and *FCSRT with Immediate Recall (FCSRT-IR)* [61] were validated and can be used, too.

To evaluate the **visuoperceptual** and **visuospatial function**, the most often used tests include *ROCF copy* [55], *Clock Drawing Test (CDT)* [61], *Block Design* [54] and *Judgement of Line Orientation (JLO)* [62]. JLO is a traditional measure of visuospatial perception and reasoning. For use in patients with iNPH, its main advantage is that it requires only minimal motor skills in comparison with ROCF copy, CDT or Block Design.

Finally, *semantic verbal fluency* and *Boston Naming Test* [63] were commonly used to evaluate **language**.

Evaluation of **intelligence** was a traditional way to assess cognition and a potential decline from premorbid cognitive level. Historically, cognitive activity was attributed to a single function, usually termed as intelligence. The most common instrument traditionally used for its evaluation in the clinical environment is the Wechsler Adult Intelligence Scale (WAIS, WAIS-IV is the latest edition; [54]). However, the current knowledge of brain organisation makes the concept of intelligence irrelevant for neuropsychological assessment [13] and we do not recommend using WAIS-IV as the main method for cognitive evaluation in iNPH patients.

The summary of neuropsychological tests with a good potential to be used in patients with iNPH is presented in Table 4.

Table 4 Neuropsychological tests with a good potential to be used in patients with (suspected) iNPH

Cognitive domain	Test	Specification of cognitive processes
Psychomotor speed, attention and working memory	Trail Making Test A	Psychomotor speed, visual attention, visual search
	Stroop Test (reading names of colours/naming the colour of dots)	Psychomotor speed, visual attention
	Digit Symbol Substitution Test	Psychomotor speed, visual attention, working memory
	Forward and Backward Digit Span	Auditory attention, working memory
Executive functions	Trail Making Test B	Set shifting, maintenance
	Phonemic verbal fluency	Initiation, maintenance, inhibition
	Stroop Test (colour word subtest)	Inhibition
	Tower of London	Planning
	Wisconsin Card Sorting Test	Abstract reasoning, set shifting, problem solving
Memory	Rey Auditory Verbal Learning Test	Uncontrolled learning over 5 trials, immediate and delayed free recall, recognition
	California Verbal Learning Test-Second Edition	Uncontrolled learning over 5 trials, immediate and delayed free recall, cued recall, recognition
	Philadelphia (repeatable) Verbal Learning Test	
	Rey–Osterrieth Complex Figure Task reproduction	Delayed free recall, recognition
	Brief Visual Spatial Memory Test-Revised	Uncontrolled learning over 3 trials, delayed free recall, recognition
	Selective Reminding Test	Controlled learning, free and cued recall
	Free and Cued Selective Reminding Test	
Visuoperceptual and visuospatial function	Rey–Osterrieth Complex Figure Task copy	Visuoconstruction, planning
	Clock Drawing Test	
	Block Design	

(continued)

Table 4 (continued)

Cognitive domain	Test	Specification of cognitive processes
	Judgement of Line Orientation	Visuospatial perception, visuospatial reasoning
Language	Semantic verbal fluency	Search of words from semantic lexicon, initiation, maintenance, set shifting
	Boston Naming Test	Confrontation naming

4.3 Evaluation of Neuropsychiatric Symptoms

So far, no guidelines have been introduced to evaluate neuropsychiatric symptoms. One of the methods in which clinical neuropsychologists are routinely trained is the clinical interview. It is a type of semi-structured interview in which all the necessary areas of neuropsychiatric symptoms are covered. With respect to the cognitive deficit and anosognosia, which may be present in patients with iNPH, not only the patients but also their close informants should be routinely interviewed. Clinical interview is a standard method to get a comprehensive picture of the neuropsychiatric difficulties of the patient. Its main disadvantage is that it does not yield a quantitative outcome, and thus evaluation of change may be more challenging. This is why standardised instruments should be administered as well.

Numerous standard self-report measures are used for the evaluation of apathy, depressive and anxiety symptoms. **Apathy Evaluation Scale (AES)** was developed to quantify and characterise apathy in adult patients with neuropsychiatric disorders [64]. It consists of 18 items scored on a 4-point scale with a lower total score indicating greater level of apathy and addresses behavioural, cognitive and emotional components of apathy. Except for the self-report version, AES also provides informant, and clinician-rated versions. **Apathy Scale (AS)** is an abbreviated and slightly modified version of the AES [65]. It includes only 14 items scored on a 3-point scale, with higher scores indicating higher level of apathy. It also has not only the self-report but also the informant-report version. **Beck Depression Inventory, second revision (BDI-II),** has been widely used for the evaluation of the severity of depressive symptoms in adult patients [66]. It covers the affective, cognitive, and somatic symptoms of depression. It includes 21 questions with each answer scored on a scale of 0 to 3 in reference to the past two weeks. Higher total scores indicate higher severity of depressive symptoms. However, the clinical presentation of depressive symptoms is different in old age in comparison with earlier periods of life [67]. In older adults, **Geriatric Depression Scale (GDS)** has been extensively used [68]. It covers the affective and behavioural symptoms of depression, while it excludes somatic symptoms not to confound depression with somatic conditions. The full form includes 30 questions, and the short form consists of 15 questions (**GDS-15**) [69] with each answer being scored as yes or no in reference to the past week. Higher total scores also indicate higher severity of depressive symptoms. Both GDS versions are possible to administer to patients with cognitive deficits. However, validation studies in patients with mild to moderate dementia brought ambiguous conclusions [70, 71]. The **Beck Anxiety Inventory (BAI)** is a well-established self-report instrument for measuring the severity of anxiety based on cognitive and somatic symptoms [72, 73]. It includes 21 items, with each of them being scored on a scale value of 0 to 3. Higher total score indicates a higher severity of anxiety symptoms. BAI has been extensively used in older adults, and several studies have documented its good psychometric properties in clinical and nonclinical cohorts of older patients [74]. There are other self-report measures of depressive and anxiety symptoms validated for use in older adults and potentially useful for patients with iNPH that were not mentioned here, for review see work by Balsamo and colleagues [74, 75].

The **Neuropsychiatric Inventory (NPI)** is a well-established instrument to assess dementia-related behavioural symptoms based on a structural interview conducted by a clinician with a close informant of the patient [76]. It covers the following 12 domains of behavioural symptoms: delusions, hallucinations, agitation/aggression, depression/dysphoria, anxiety, euphoria, apathy, disinhibition, irritability/lability, aberrant motor activity, night-time behavioural disturbances, and appetite and eating abnormalities. The frequency and severity of the symptoms and the distress the symptoms cause to the caregiver are evaluated. Although NPI is considered the gold standard among the informant-report measures of neuropsychiatric symptoms in patients with dementia of any aetiology, a recent review showed that its validity needs to be further verified [77]. The neuropsychiatric symptoms may develop before the onset of dementia. Recently, **Mild Behavioural Impairment Checklist (MBI-C)** has been introduced to address the need for a more sensitive and specific neuropsychiatric scale [78]. It is an informant-based questionnaire and includes 34 items evaluating the following behavioural domains: decreased motivation, affective dysregulation, impulse dyscontrol, social inappropriateness, and abnormal perception and thought content. It evaluates the presence and severity of the symptoms over the last six months. The MBI-C was initially developed and validated in the field of prodromal stages of neurodegenerative diseases [79]. Based on those findings, it might also provide a more sensitive alternative to the routinely used NPI in the earlier stages of the iNPH condition. Still, its validity for use in the population of these patients needs to be verified.

With respect to anosognosia, which is common in patients with dementia due to iNPH condition [80], reliability and validity of self-report measures may be compromised, and the presence and severity of neuropsychiatric symptoms may be undervalued. Thus, we recommend using informant-based instruments to assess neuropsychiatric symptoms in iNPH patients, especially in later stages of cognitive deficit.

5 Evolution of Cognition and Neuropsychiatric Features After Shunting, Prediction of Response to Shunting Based on Cognitive Performance

As already mentioned in the previous chapter, approximately 70%–90% of all correctly diagnosed patients with iNPH improve significantly after the VPS implementation [80]. The majority of studies assess the outcome only several months after the intervention. Data from longer follow-up are available in a retrospective study describing excellent clinical results in 59% of patients with iNPH even six years after surgery [82]. Interestingly, the majority of cognitive improvement did not appear until two months after surgery, which contrasted with the improvement of the urinary incontinence and gait that occurred one week and two months after surgery, respectively.

Assessment of cognitive improvement is hampered by methodological differences between studies, mainly due to inconsistencies in diagnostic criteria used for iNPH. Studies also differed in the choice of neuropsychological tests and the different testing intervals after the VPS implementation. Regarding the global cognitive performance measured by the MMSE [30], most studies found significant improvements [84, 85]. In a large meta-analysis, MMSE was one of the tests in which cognitive performance improved considerably after VPS. Interestingly, meta-regressions revealed no statistically significant effect of age, sex or follow-up interval on performance improvement in this test [86]. On the other hand, several studies failed to find any change in MMSE performance after VPS [11, 87, 88]. MMSE is susceptible to the ceiling effect, particularly in high-functioning patients. Thus, selective and subtle cognitive deficits may be missed which might explain these negative findings. It was suggested that MoCA, which is more sensitive to deficit in attention, working memory and executive function compared to MMSE, could be more suitable for screening of the VPS effect. Several studies showed that MoCA was sensitive to changes in cognitive function after lumbar drainage and VPS implementation, regardless of the level of cognitive functioning [39, 89]. In a recent study [40], a 5-point increase in MoCA was reported to be a reliable threshold to determine cognitive improvement after cerebrospinal fluid drainage at an individual level in patients who scored less than 26 points at baseline.

There is a consensus that cognitive assessment should include a battery of neuropsychological tests in addition to screening tests as the latter can fail to recognise selective and more subtle cognitive deficits. When a more comprehensive neuropsychological battery was used, improvements were demonstrated in most cognitive domains, primarily in verbal learning [86], verbal [84, 90–93] and spatial memory [14]. The improved performance was often demonstrated in the Backward Digit Span [85, 93, 94], a measure primarily evaluating working memory and attention. Improvement was also evident in psychomotor speed [84, 95, 96]. The data about improvement in executive functions are contradictory: few studies found improvement on TMT B and FAB [11, 97], still, the major body of previous research reported no significant improvement [84, 85, 87, 88, 96].

Improvement after VPS implementation has been demonstrated also in memory. The RAVLT was the only test in a study by McGovern and colleagues [98] that showed statistically significant improvement after both lumbar drainage and VP shunting. Post-lumbar drain improvement in RAVLT performance predicted further post-shunt improvement on this test. Several other studies also reported improvement in performance on RAVLT [90–92, 95]. Thus, RAVLT may be another useful preoperative predictor of post-operative cognitive improvement [98].

Most studies focused on the domains described above and omitted the tests of visuoperceptual and visuospatial functions. In one study that included tests of visuo-construction improvement in this domain was also found [99] but occurred later (between 2 months and 1 year) compared to the improvement in other cognitive domains. Finally, in one study, no improvement in any cognitive domain was reported [87].

A meta-analysis of 23 studies found evidence for improved performance in global cognitive function, verbal learning and memory and psychomotor speed following shunt surgery [86]. They did not find any strong evidence for improvement in tests of executive functions. Due to the lack of data, visuoconstruction was not analysed in this study. The authors concluded that MMSE, RAVLT, phonemic verbal fluency and TMT A may be useful for the assessment of cognitive outcomes following the iNPH treatment. The heterogeneity of the cognitive protocols and a short monitoring time in some of the included studies were the major limitations of this meta-analysis [86]. Despite the observed cognitive improvement, most patients remained cognitively impaired and performed poorer than healthy controls in tests of psychomotor speed, memory and executive function at both three and twelve months post-shunt [94, 95].

Not only cognition but also the quality of life improved after the VPS [83]. In 86% of the patients, it was almost comparable to the quality of life reported by the normal population. Patients described higher independence in physical and cognitive activities and improvement in autonomy and participation in activities of daily living. In addition, the caregiver burden decreased among caregivers of male patients but remained unchanged in the overall group.

A large proportion of patients with iNPH also manifest other **coexistent patholo-gies**. Studies have shown that 40% to 75% of patients with iNPH have histological findings of AD, while 60% have evidence of cerebrovascular disease [100–102]. **AD pathology** was present in cortical biopsy of 75% of iNPH patients who had dementia at the time of shunt surgery [102]. It was demonstrated that VPS implan-tation mainly improved gait in those cases, while cognitive improvement was less pronounced [101, 103]. According to a study by Kamohara et al. (2020), the group of patients with iNPH and AD comorbidity performed significantly worse than those with "pure" iNPH on memory tests, but otherwise showed improvement in most of the neuropsychological tests after the VPS implantation. In another study, the iNPH patients with positive AD pathology on brain biopsy were cognitively more impaired at the baseline, but their cognitive improvement after shunting did not differ from the AD negative group [102]. Similarly, the positivity of AD biomarkers in cerebrospinal fluid (CSF) predicted the positivity of AD pathology in subsequent biopsy but did not influence the cognitive outcome of patients with iNPH [98]. In another study, CSF levels of total tau (T-tau) but not beta amyloid (1–42; $A\beta_{1-42}$) were predictive of the cognitive outcome, however, the levels showed high interindividual variability. The authors concluded that raised T-tau and shunt responsiveness were not mutually exclusive and such patients should not be necessarily excluded from having a VPS [104]. Finally, a meta-analysis of 13 biomarker studies did not find any influence of CSF biomarkers on shunt response [105]. Altogether, it seems that AD comorbidity in iNPH is common, however, it does not strongly influence the clinical response to shunt surgery if the diagnosis of iNPH is correct [102].

Among **cerebrovascular disorders (CVD),** subcortical arteriosclerotic encephalopathy is the most challenging for iNPH differential diagnosis since these disorders often show similar clinical and radiological signs. In addition, subcortical CVD frequently coexists with iNPH. Patients with CVD often have vascular white matter changes on brain magnetic resonance images (MRI), and they may also present with focal neurological signs or show a profile of cognitive impairment corresponding to the localization of vascular changes on MRI. The iNPH patients with evidence of CVD may also significantly improve in cognitive performance after shunting [106], but this improvement is less favourable than in iNPH without vascular changes [107]. A large amount of attention has been concentrated on the role of cerebrovascular risk factors in the clinical outcome in iNPH patients. Interestingly their presence without an established CVD did not influence the outcome of VPS [107].

A recent study focused on the influence of comorbidities on clinical status [90]. Forty-nine patients with possible iNPH were classified using CSF biomarkers and DAT scan into three groups: iNPH without comorbidities, iNPH with AD pathology and iNPH with Parkinson's disease (PD) pathology. In that study, iNPH patients with AD pathology scored lower in a memory test (RAVLT) and iNPH patients with PD pathology scored lower mainly in an executive function test (Stroop test) compared to iNPH patients without comorbidities [90].

6   Differential Diagnosis of Cognitive Impairment in iNPH

The cognitive impairment in iNPH can be easily mistaken for other conditions leading to dementia. As mentioned previously, the diagnosis is complicated because a large proportion of patients with iNPH also have coexistent cerebrovascular or AD pathology. Thus, the cognitive impairment in iNPH can be the result of several pathologies.

Alzheimer's disease (AD) patients are characterised by a reduction in overall cognitive performance and disproportionately significant deficits in short- and long-term memory, orientation, construction, and executive functions [19, 108]. Contrary to iNPH, the main dysfunction in **AD** originates in the MTL causing memory impairment, which is considered one of the earliest clinical hallmarks of AD, detectable already several years before the dementia onset [109]. Severe memory impairment with preserved psychomotor speed is not typical for cognitive deficit due to iNPH condition. In a study by Saito and colleagues [11], frontal lobe dysfunction accounted for more than 50% of the total cognitive deficit in patients with iNPH. In comparison with that, memory impairment accounted for more than 50% of the cognitive deficit in patients with AD. iNPH patients achieved considerably lower scores in attention and executive functions tests than those with AD (TMT A, phonemic verbal fluency, FAB). Interestingly, their scores in category fluency and memory did not differ [11]. A different pattern of memory impairment was expected for patients with AD and iNPH. The manifestation of the "frontal type of memory impairment" with impaired free recall but relatively preserved cued recall and recognition was expected to be found in patients with iNPH [38, 109]. However, only one study addressed this issue and did not find any difference between AD and iNPH patients in free recall or recognition scores [11]. Only a few studies explored the discriminatory potential of visuoperceptual and visuospatial functions. The iNPH patients were surprisingly more impaired in visual discrimination tasks than AD patients [11].

The typical sequence of development of clinical symptoms in iNPH is different from the course of AD. In iNPH, urinary incontinence and gait disturbances are among the earliest signs, while in AD, these symptoms typically develop in the stages of severe dementia, and the memory deficit is one the earliest signs and predominates the clinical picture in this disease [14]. On the other hand, in iNPH patients with comorbid AD, cognitive deficits also often precede the development of gait disturbance [110].

To the best of our knowledge, no previous study performed a head-to-head comparison of cognitive profiles of patients with iNPH and **vascular cognitive impairment, progressive supranuclear palsy (PSP) or frontotemporal lobar degeneration (FTLD)**. It is well known that these conditions share a similar cognitive profile with prevailing psychomotor slowing, dysexecutive syndrome, and attention and working memory deficit [13]. Thus, we can presume that these diseases cannot be reliably distinguished from iNPH solely based on their cognitive profile. Still, further evidence is needed.

FTLD and iNPH share a high prevalence of neuropsychiatric features. Apathy is a particularly frequent symptom in both diseases. Inappropriate social behaviour, disinhibition, loss of self-control and empathy are the hallmarks of the behavioural variant of FTD (bvFTD), and it was suggested that they could serve as a differential marker [111]. As already mentioned, both iNPH and FTLD share a similar cognitive profile with prevailing dysexecutive syndrome and attentional deficit. On the other hand, aphasias, which are the hallmark of language variants of the FTLD, are not commonly seen in iNPH. Despite some differences, there is an important overlap in neuropsychiatric and cognitive profiles of FTLD and iNPH, and differential diagnosis should also integrate evaluation of neurological and other clinical symptoms and brain imaging.

A comparison of de novo diagnosed patients with iNPH and **Parkinson's disease** demonstrated that iNPH patients showed a more severe cognitive impairment with respect to the PD patients and the cognitively normal controls [10]. Within one year from the onset of the motor symptoms, only 35% of the iNPH patients were cognitively unimpaired in contrast to 74.5% of early PD. iNPH patients showed diffuse cognitive impairment, including memory, visuospatial abilities, frontal-executive functioning and attention, whereas cognitively impaired PD patients showed mainly executive dysfunction [10]. However, the differences in cognitive profile are probably less striking than other clinical signs. As written in Chap. 9, similarly to PD, patients with iNPH may develop gait disturbances; gait tends to be shuffling with short strides. On the other hand, resting tremor and unilateral symptoms (the core features of PD) are uncommon in iNPH. The lack of response to antiparkinsonian drugs in iNPH patients may also help in differential diagnosis.

The differential diagnosis of cognitive impairment in iNPH is challenging since the cognitive profile overlaps with several other common conditions leading to dementia and comorbidity with other neuropathologies is common. The neuropsychological and neuropsychiatric profile should be always interpreted in the context of all other clinical symptoms. An effective differential diagnosis can be achieved by combining neuropsychological and neuropsychiatric markers with other clinical tests.

Cognitive and neuropsychiatric features of the most common diseases considered in differential diagnostics of iNPH are summarised in Table 5.

Table 5 Neuropsychological and neuropsychiatric features useful for differential diagnosis

	Main features of cognitive impairment	Common symptoms shared with iNPH	Difference from iNPH
AD	Global cognitive deficit with prevailing memory impairment	Executive and memory dysfunction	Contrary to iNPH, the psychomotor slowing is mild in AD and the hippocampal type of memory impairment predominates the clinical picture Absence of gait impairment in AD except the stage of severe dementia
FTLD	Executive dysfunction, significant behavioural changes Aphasia in language variants	Executive dysfunction Apathy	Unlike iNPH, disinhibition and socially inappropriate behaviour is typical for FTLD Aphasia is rare in iNPH
PD	Attention deficits, dysexecutive syndrome Possible visual hallucinations	Attention deficit	In iNPH, more profound psychomotor slowing and absence of visual hallucinations
PSP	Dysexecutive syndrome with psychomotor slowing	Psychomotor slowing, apathy	The cognitive profile can be the same. Differential diagnosis should be based on other neurological features

(continued)

Table 5 (continued)

	Main features of cognitive impairment	Common symptoms shared with iNPH	Difference from iNPH
CVD	Often dysexecutive syndrome, psychomotor slowing The clinical picture is variable—depends on the localization of vascular lesions	Dysexecutive syndrome, psychomotor slowing	The cognitive profile can be the same. Differential diagnosis should be based on medical history and brain MRI

Note AD, Alzheimer's disease; FTLD, Frontotemporal lobar degeneration; PD, Parkinson's disease; PSP, Progressive supranuclear palsy; CVD, cerebrovascular disorders; MRI, magnetic resonance imaging

7 Conclusion

Cognitive impairment and neuropsychiatric symptoms constitute major clinical symptoms in iNPH. Their accurate evaluation and monitoring are essential for differential diagnosis, and it may help identify patients who will benefit most from the shunting. In addition, accurate evaluation of neuropsychiatric symptoms can allow the initiation of early treatment which may also improve the quality of life of patients and their caregivers.

8 Key Points

- Cognitive impairment is an important part of iNPH symptomatology, present in 80% of patients with iNPH.
- The typical profile of cognitive impairment is characterised by fronto-subcortical involvement with predominant attention and working memory deficit, psychomotor slowing and dysexecutive syndrome.
- Memory impairment is also common—mainly due to the deficit in learning and recall with relatively preserved retention. Visuospatial impairment including deficits in visuoperception and visuoconstruction is more common than previously reported.
- Speech and language are usually spared.
- Cognitive deficit is often accompanied by neuropsychiatric symptoms. Among them, the most common is apathy. Depression, anxiety, irritability and agitation are also prevalent, while hallucinations and delusions are rare.
- The clinical picture can be blurred by comorbidity with other conditions leading to dementia (vascular cognitive impairment, Alzheimer's disease) present in more than half of patients with iNPH.

- Screening tests such as MMSE or MoCA can be used to monitor patients in the dementia stage. The use of a comprehensive neuropsychological test battery is needed to diagnose the cognitive deficit in cognitively self-sufficient patients or for differential diagnostics of cognitive impairment.
- Most patients improve after shunting, although the improvement of cognition occurs later (even several months after the procedure), contrasting with the rapid improvement in urinary incontinence and gait. The major improvement occurs in global cognitive functions, verbal learning, memory and psychomotor speed.
- The presence of comorbidities such as AD or CVD can limit the cognitive improvement after shunting, but even patients with significant comorbidities benefit from VPS.
- Differential diagnosis of cognitive impairment is challenging as the neuropsychological profile overlaps with numerous neurodegenerative and non-neurodegenerative disorders in old age. The proper differential diagnosis should take into account the whole clinical picture together with the results of brain MRI.

Funding This work was supported by project nr. LX22NPO5107 (MEYS): Financed by EU – Next Generation EU, the EEA/ Norway Grants 2014–2021 and the Technology Agency of the Czech Republic - project number TO01000215, and by the Czech Science Foundation (GAČR) registration number 22-33968S.

References

1. Hashimoto M, Ishikawa M, Mori E, Kuwana N. Diagnosis of idiopathic normal pressure hydrocephalus is supported by MRI-based scheme: a prospective cohort study. Cerebrospinal Fluid Res. 2010;7:18. https://doi.org/10.1186/1743-8454-7-18.
2. Jaraj D, Rabiei K, Marlow T, Jensen C, Skoog I, Wikkelsø C. Prevalence of idiopathic normal-pressure hydrocephalus. Neurology. 2014;82:1449–54. https://doi.org/10.1212/wnl.0000000000000342.
3. Martin-Laez R, Caballero-Arzapalo H, Lopez-Menendez LA, Arango-Lasprilla JC, Vazquez-Barquero A. Epidemiology of idiopathic normal pressure hydrocephalus: a systematic review of the literature. World Neurosurg. 2015;84:2002–9. https://doi.org/10.1016/j.wneu.2015.07.005.
4. Andersson J, Rosell M, Kockum K, Lilja-Lund O, Soderstrom L, Laurell K. Prevalence of idiopathic normal pressure hydrocephalus: a prospective, population-based study. PLoS One. 2019;14:e0217705. https://doi.org/10.1371/journal.pone.0217705.
5. Ravdin LD, Katzen HL. Idiopathic normal pressure hydrocephalus. In: Casebook of clinical neuropsychology. New York: Oxford University Press; 2010.
6. Sperling RA, Aisen PS, Beckett LA, Bennett DA, Craft S, Fagan AM, Iwatsubo T, Jack CR, Jr., Kaye J, Montine TJ, et al. Toward defining the preclinical stages of Alzheimer's disease: recommendations from the National Institute on Aging-Alzheimer's Association workgroups on diagnostic guidelines for Alzheimer's disease. Alzheimers Dement. 2011;7:280–92. https://doi.org/10.1016/j.jalz.2011.03.003.
7. Jack CR, Jr., Bennett DA, Blennow K, Carrillo MC, Dunn B, Haeberlein SB, Holtzman DM, Jagust W, Jessen F, Karlawish J, et al. NIA-AA Research Framework: Toward a biological

definition of Alzheimer's disease. Alzheimers Dement. 2018;14:535–62. https://doi.org/10.1016/j.jalz.2018.02.018.

8. Petersen RC. Clinical practice. Mild cognitive impairment. N Engl J Med. 2011;364:2227–34. https://doi.org/10.1056/NEJMcp0910237.

9. Picascia M, Minafra B, Zangaglia R, Gracardi L, Pozzi NG, Sinforiani E, Pacchetti C. Spectrum of cognitive disorders in idiopathic normal pressure hydrocephalus. Funct Neurol. 2016;31:143–7. https://doi.org/10.11138/fneur/2016.31.3.143.

10. Picascia M, Pozzi NG, Todisco M, Minafra B, Sinforiani E, Zangaglia R, Ceravolo R, Pacchetti C. Cognitive disorders in normal pressure hydrocephalus with initial parkinsonism in comparison with de novo Parkinson's disease. Eur J Neurol. 2019;26:74–9. https://doi.org/10.1111/ene.13766.

11. Saito M, Nishio Y, Kanno S, Uchiyama M, Hayashi A, Takagi M, Kikuchi H, Yamasaki H, Shimomura T, Iizuka O, et al. Cognitive profile of idiopathic normal pressure hydrocephalus. Dement Geriatr Cogn Dis Extra. 2011;1:202–11. https://doi.org/10.1159/000328924.

12. Sindorio C, Abbritti RV, Raffa G, Priola SM, Germano A, Visocchi M, Quattropani MC. Neuropsychological assessment in the differential diagnosis of idiopathic normal pressure hydrocephalus. An important tool for the maintenance and restoration of neuronal and neuropsychological functions. Acta Neurochir Suppl. 2017;124:283–8. https://doi.org/10.1007/978-3-319-39546-3_41.

13. Lezak MD, Howieson DB, Bigler ED, Tranel D. Neuropsychological assessment. New York: Oxford University Press; 2012.

14. Iddon JL, Pickard JD, Cross JJ, Griffiths PD, Czosnyka M, Sahakian BJ. Specific patterns of cognitive impairment in patients with idiopathic normal pressure hydrocephalus and Alzheimer's disease: a pilot study. J Neurol Neurosurg Psychiatry. 1999;67:723–32. https://doi.org/10.1136/jnnp.67.6.723.

15. Walchenbach R, Geiger E, Thomeer RT, Vanneste JA. The value of temporary external lumbar CSF drainage in predicting the outcome of shunting on normal pressure hydrocephalus. J Neurol Neurosurg Psychiatry. 2002;72:503–6. https://doi.org/10.1136/jnnp.72.4.503.

16. Squire LR, Wixted JT, Clark RE. Recognition memory and the medial temporal lobe: a new perspective. Nat Rev Neurosci. 2007;8:872–83. https://doi.org/10.1038/nrn2154.

17. Ishii K, Kawaguchi T, Shimada K, Ohkawa S, Miyamoto N, Kanda T, Uemura T, Yoshikawa T, Mori E. Voxel-based analysis of gray matter and CSF space in idiopathic normal pressure hydrocephalus. Dement Geriatr Cogn Disord. 2008;25:329–35. https://doi.org/10.1159/000119521.

18. Jackson GR, Jessup NS, Kavanaugh BL, Moats VL, Daum KM, Marsh-Tootle WL, Rutstein RP. Measuring visual acuity in children using preferential looking and sine wave cards. Optom Vis Sci. 1990;67:590–4. https://doi.org/10.1097/00006324-199008000-00006.

19. Ogino A, Kazui H, Miyoshi N, Hashimoto M, Ohkawa S, Tokunaga H, Ikejiri Y, Takeda M. Cognitive impairment in patients with idiopathic normal pressure hydrocephalus. Dement Geriatr Cogn Disord 2006;21:113–9. https://doi.org/10.1159/000090510.

20. Takaya M, Kazui H, Tokunaga H, Yoshida T, Kito Y, Wada T, Nomura K, Shimosegawa E, Hatazawa J, Takeda M. Global cerebral hypoperfusion in preclinical stage of idiopathic normal pressure hydrocephalus. J Neurol Sci. 2010;298:35–41. https://doi.org/10.1016/j.jns.2010.09.001.

21. Sasaki H, Ishii K, Kono AK, Miyamoto N, Fukuda T, Shimada K, Ohkawa S, Kawaguchi T, Mori E. Cerebral perfusion pattern of idiopathic normal pressure hydrocephalus studied by SPECT and statistical brain mapping. Ann Nucl Med. 2007;21:39–45. https://doi.org/10.1007/BF03033998.

22. Mega MS, Cummings JL. Frontal-subcortical circuits and neuropsychiatric disorders. J Neuropsychiatry Clin Neurosci. 1994;6:358–70. https://doi.org/10.1176/jnp.6.4.358.

23. Kito Y, Kazui H, Kubo Y, Yoshida T, Takaya M, Wada T, Nomura K, Hashimoto M, Ohkawa S, Miyake H, et al. Neuropsychiatric symptoms in patients with idiopathic normal pressure hydrocephalus. Behav Neurol. 2009;21:165–174. https://doi.org/10.3233/BEN-2009-0233.

24. Mathew R, Pavithran S, Byju P. Neuropsychiatric manifestations of cognitively advanced idiopathic normal pressure hydrocephalus. Dement Geriatr Cogn Dis Extra. 2018;8:467–75. https://doi.org/10.1159/000493914.

25. Micchia K, Formica C, De Salvo S, Muscarà N, Bramanti P, Caminiti F, Marino S, Corallo F. Normal pressure hydrocephalus: neurophysiological and neuropsychological aspects: a narrative review. Medicine (Baltimore). 2022;101:e28922. https://doi.org/10.1097/md.000 0000000028922.

26. Tekin S, Cummings JL. Frontal-subcortical neuronal circuits and clinical neuropsychiatry: an update. J Psychosom Res. 2002;53:647–54. https://doi.org/10.1016/s0022-3999(02)00428-2.

27. Klinge PM, Brooks DJ, Samii A, Weckesser E, van den Hoff J, Fricke H, Brinker T, Knapp WH, Berding G. Correlates of local cerebral blood flow (CBF) in normal pressure hydrocephalus patients before and after shunting—a retrospective analysis of [(15)O]H(2)O PET-CBF studies in 65 patients. Clin Neurol Neurosurg. 2008;110:369–75. https://doi.org/10.1016/j.clineuro. 2007.12.019.

28. Murakami M, Hirata Y, Kuratsu JI. Predictive assessment of shunt effectiveness in patients with idiopathic normal pressure hydrocephalus by determining regional cerebral blood flow on 3D stereotactic surface projections. Acta Neurochir (Wien). 2007;149:991–7. https://doi. org/10.1007/s00701-007-1259-1.

29. Steinberg M, Corcoran C, Tschanz JT, Huber C, Welsh-Bohmer K, Norton MC, Zandi P, Breitner JC, Steffens DC, Lyketsos CG. Risk factors for neuropsychiatric symptoms in dementia: the cache county study. Int J Geriatr Psychiatry. 2006;21:824–30. https://doi.org/ 10.1002/gps.1567.

30. Folstein MF, Folstein SE, McHugh PR. "Mini-mental state". A practical method for grading the cognitive state of patients for the clinician. J Psychiatr Res. 1975;12:189–198. https://doi. org/10.1016/0022-3956(75)90026-6.

31. Nasreddine ZS, Phillips NA, Bedirian V, Charbonneau S, Whitehead V, Collin I, Cummings JL, Chertkow H. The Montreal cognitive assessment, MoCA: a brief screening tool for mild cognitive impairment. J Am Geriatr Soc. 2005;53:695–9. https://doi.org/10.1111/j.1532-5415.2005.53221.x.

32. Ehreke L, Luppa M, König H, Riedel-Heller S. Is the clock drawing test a screening tool for the diagnosis of mild cognitive impairment? A systematic review. Int Psychogeriatr. 2010;22:56–63. https://doi.org/10.1017/S1041610209990676.

33. Dubois B, Slachevsky A, Litvan I, Pillon B. The FAB: a frontal assessment battery at bedside. Neurology. 2000;55:1621–6. https://doi.org/10.1212/wnl.55.11.1621.

34. Petersen RC. Mild cognitive impairment as a diagnostic entity. J Intern Med. 2004;256:183–94. https://doi.org/10.1111/j.1365-2796.2004.01388.x.

35. Jones RN, Gallo JJ. Dimensions of the mini-mental state examination among community dwelling older adults. Psychol Med. 2000;30:605–18. https://doi.org/10.1017/s00332917990 01853.

36. Mitchell AJ. A meta-analysis of the accuracy of the mini-mental state examination in the detection of dementia and mild cognitive impairment. J Psychiatr Res. 2009;43:411–31. https://doi.org/10.1016/j.jpsychires.2008.04.014.

37. Pinto TCC, Machado L, Bulgacov TM, Rodrigues-Júnior AL, Costa MLG, Ximenes RCC, Sougey EB. Is the Montreal cognitive assessment (MoCA) screening superior to the mini-mental state examination (MMSE) in the detection of mild cognitive impairment (MCI) and Alzheimer's disease (AD) in the elderly? Int Psychogeriatr. 2019;31:491–504. https://doi.org/ 10.1017/s1041610218001370.

38. Picascia M, Zangaglia R, Bernini S, Minafra B, Sinforiani E, Pacchetti C. A review of cognitive impairment and differential diagnosis in idiopathic normal pressure hydrocephalus. Funct Neurol. 2015;30:217–28. https://doi.org/10.11138/fneur/2015.30.4.217.

39. Matsuoka T, Kawano S, Fujimoto K, Kawahara M, Hashimoto H. Characteristics of cognitive function evaluation using the Montreal cognitive assessment in a cerebrospinal fluid tap test in patients with idiopathic normal pressure hydrocephalus. Clin Neurol Neurosurg. 2019;186:105524. https://doi.org/10.1016/j.clineuro.2019.105524.

40. Wesner E, Etzkorn L, Bakre S, Chen J, Davis A, Zhang Y, Yasar S, Rao A, Luciano M, Wang J, et al. The clinical utility of the MOCA in iNPH assessment. Front Neurol. 2022;13:887669 https://doi.org/10.3389/fneur.2022.887669.

41. Rodrigues GR, Souza CP, Cetlin RS, de Oliveira DS, Pena-Pereira M, Ujikawa LT, Marques W, Jr., Tumas V. Use of the frontal assessment battery in evaluating executive dysfunction in patients with Huntington's disease. J Neurol. 2009;256:1809–15. https://doi.org/10.1007/s00 415-009-5197-0.

42. Bezdicek O, Růžička F, Fendrych Mazancova A, Roth J, Dušek P, Mueller K, Růžička E, Jech R. Frontal assessment battery in Parkinson's disease: validity and morphological correlates. J Int Neuropsychol Soc. 2017;23:675–84. https://doi.org/10.1017/s1355617717000522.

43. Slachevsky A, Villalpando JM, Sarazin M, Hahn-Barma V, Pillon B, Dubois B. Frontal assessment battery and differential diagnosis of frontotemporal dementia and Alzheimer disease. Arch Neurol. 2004;61:1104–7. https://doi.org/10.1001/archneur.61.7.1104.

44. Miyoshi N, Kazui H, Ogino A, Ishikawa M, Miyake H, Tokunaga H, Ikejiri Y, Takeda M. Association between cognitive impairment and gait disturbance in patients with idiopathic normal pressure hydrocephalus. Dement Geriatr Cogn Disord. 2005;20:71–6. https://doi.org/ 10.1159/000085858.

45. Missori P, Currà A. Progressive cognitive impairment evolving to dementia parallels Parieto-occipital and temporal enlargement in idiopathic chronic hydrocephalus: a retrospective cohort study. Front Neurol. 2015;6:15. https://doi.org/10.3389/fneur.2015.00015.

46. Tombaugh TN. Trail making test A and B: normative data stratified by age and education. Arch Clin Neuropsychol. 2004;19:203–14. https://doi.org/10.1016/s0887-6177(03)00039-8.

47. Troyer AK, Leach L, Strauss E. Aging and response inhibition: Normative data for the Victoria Stroop Test. Neuropsychol Dev Cogn B Aging Neuropsychol Cogn. 2006;13:20–35. https:// doi.org/10.1080/138255890968187.

48. Wechsler D. Wechsler adult intelligence scale-Fourth Edition (WAIS-IV). APA PsycTests; 2008.

49. Shallice T. Specific impairments of planning. Philos Trans R Soc Lond B Biol Sci. 1982;298:199–209. https://doi.org/10.1098/rstb.1982.0082.

50. Stuss DT, Levine B, Alexander MP, Hong J, Palumbo C, Hamer L, Murphy KJ, Izukawa D. Wisconsin card sorting test performance in patients with focal frontal and posterior brain damage: effects of lesion location and test structure on separable cognitive processes. Neuropsychologia. 2000;38:388–402. https://doi.org/10.1016/s0028-3932(99)00093-7.

51. Schoenberg MR, Dawson KA, Duff K, Patton D, Scott JG, Adams RL. Test performance and classification statistics for the Rey auditory verbal learning test in selected clinical samples. Arch Clin Neuropsychol. 2006;21:693–703. https://doi.org/10.1016/j.acn.2006.06.010.

52. Delis DC, Kramer JH, Kaplan E, Ober BA. California verbal learning test-Second Edition (CVLT –II) [Database record]. APA PsycTests 1987–2000.

53. Gifford KA, Liu D, Neal JE, Babicz MA, Thompson JL, Walljasper LE, Wiggins ME, Turchan M, Pechman KR, Osborn KE, Acosta LMY, Bell SP, Hohman TJ, Libon DJ, Blennow K, Zetterberg H, Jefferson AL. The 12-word Philadelphia verbal learning test performances in older adults: brain MRI and cerebrospinal fluid correlates and regression-based normative data. Dement Geriatr Cogn Dis Extra. 2018;8:476–91. https://doi.org/10.1159/000494209.

54. Wechsler D. Wechsler memory scale IV (WMS-IV). Psychological Corporation; 2009.

55. Kasai M, Meguro K, Hashimoto R, Ishizaki J, Yamadori A, Mori E. Non-verbal learning is impaired in very mild Alzheimer's disease (CDR 0.5): normative data from the learning version of the Rey-Osterrieth Complex Figure Test. Psychiatry Clin Neurosci. 2006;60:139–46. https://doi.org/10.1111/j.1440-1819.2006.01478.x.

56. Benedict RHB, Schretlen D, Groninger L, Dobraski M, Shpritz B. Revision of the brief visuospatial memory test: studies of normal performance, reliability, and validity. Psychol Assess. 1996;8:145–53. https://doi.org/10.1037/1040-3590.8.2.145.

57. Dubois B, Feldman HH, Jacova C, Dekosky ST, Barberger-Gateau P, Cummings J, Delacourte A, Galasko D, Gauthier S, Jicha G, et al. Research criteria for the diagnosis of Alzheimer's disease: revising the NINCDS-ADRDA criteria. Lancet Neurol. 2007;6:734–46. https://doi. org/10.1016/s1474-4422(07)70178-3.

58. Buschke H. Selective reminding for analysis of memory and learning. J Verbal Learn Verbal Behav. 1973;12:543–50. https://doi.org/10.1016/S0022-5371(73)80034-9.

59. Buschke H. Cued recall in amnesia. J Clin Neuropsychol. 1984;6:433–40. https://doi.org/10.1080/01688638408401233.

60. Buschke H, Grober E. Free and cued selective reminding test with immediate recall. New York: Albert Einstein College of Medicine; 2012.

61. Ehreke L, Luppa M, König HH, Riedel-Heller SG. Is the clock drawing test a screening tool for the diagnosis of mild cognitive impairment? A systematic review. Int Psychogeriatr. 2010;22:56–63. https://doi.org/10.1017/s1041610209990676.

62. Benton AL, Sivan A, Hamsher K, Varney N, Spreen O. Contributions to neuropsychology assessment: a clinical manual. 2nd ed. New York: Oxford University Press; 1994.

63. Kaplan E, Goodglass H, Weintraub S. Boston naming test. 2nd ed. Philadelphia: Lippincott Williams & Wilkins; 2000.

64. Marin RS, Biedrzycki RC, Firinciogullari S. Reliability and validity of the apathy evaluation scale. Psychiatry Res. 1991;38:143–62. https://doi.org/10.1016/0165-1781(91)90040-v.

65. Starkstein SE, Mayberg HS, Preziosi TJ, Andrezejewski P, Leiguarda R, Robinson RG. Reliability, validity, and clinical correlates of apathy in Parkinson's disease. J Neuropsychiatry Clin Neurosci. 1992;4:134–9. https://doi.org/10.1176/jnp.4.2.134.

66. Beck AT, Steer RA, Brown G. Beck depression inventory–II (BDI-II) [Database record]. APA PsycTests; 1996.

67. de la Torre-Luque A, Ayuso Mateos JL. The course of depression in late life: a longitudinal perspective. Epidemiol Psychiatr Sci. 2020;29:e147. https://doi.org/10.1017/s2045796020000058x.

68. Yesavage JA, Brink TL, Rose TL, Lum O, Huang V, Adey M, Leirer VO. Development and validation of a geriatric depression screening scale: a preliminary report. J Psychiatr Res. 1982;17:37–49. https://doi.org/10.1016/0022-3956(82)90033-4.

69. Yesavage J, Sheikh J. Geriatric depression scale (GDS): recent evidence and development of a shorter version. Vol. 5: Routledge; 1986. https://doi.org/10.1300/J018v05n01_09.

70. Li Z, Jeon YH, Low LF, Chenoweth L, O'Connor DW, Beattie E, Brodaty H. Validity of the geriatric depression scale and the collateral source version of the geriatric depression scale in nursing homes. Int Psychogeriatr. 2015;27:1495–504. https://doi.org/10.1017/s1041610215000721.

71. Kørner A, Lauritzen L, Abelskov K, Gulmann N, Marie Brodersen A, Wedervang-Jensen T, Marie Kjeldgaard K. The geriatric depression scale and the cornell scale for depression in dementia. A validity study. Nord J Psychiatry. 2006;60:360–4. https://doi.org/10.1080/08039480600937066.

72. Beck AT, Epstein N, Brown G, Steer RA. An inventory for measuring clinical anxiety: psychometric properties. J Consult Clin Psychol. 1988;56:893–7. https://doi.org/10.1037//0022-006x.56.6.893.

73. Kabacoff RI, Segal DL, Hersen M, Van Hasselt VB. Psychometric properties and diagnostic utility of the beck anxiety inventory and the state-trait anxiety inventory with older adult psychiatric outpatients. J Anxiety Disord. 1997;11:33–47. https://doi.org/10.1016/s0887-6185(96)00033-3.

74. Balsamo M, Cataldi F, Carlucci L, Fairfield B. Assessment of anxiety in older adults: a review of self-report measures. Clin Interv Aging. 2018;13:573–93. https://doi.org/10.2147/cia.S114100.

75. Balsamo M, Cataldi F, Carlucci L, Padulo C, Fairfield B. Assessment of late-life depression via self-report measures: a review. Clin Interv Aging. 2018;13:2021–4. https://doi.org/10.2147/CIA.S178943.

76. Cummings JL. The neuropsychiatric inventory: assessing psychopathology in dementia patients. Neurology. 1997;48:S10–16. https://doi.org/10.1212/wnl.48.5_suppl_6.10s.

77. Saari T, Koivisto A, Hintsa T, Hänninen T, Hallikainen I. Psychometric properties of the neuropsychiatric inventory: a review. J Alzheimers Dis. 2022;86:1485–99. https://doi.org/10.3233/jad-200739.

78. Ismail Z, Agüera-Ortiz L, Brodaty H, Cieslak A, Cummings J, Fischer CE, Gauthier S, Geda YE, Herrmann N, Kanji J, et al. The mild behavioral impairment checklist (MBI-C): a rating scale for neuropsychiatric symptoms in pre-dementia populations. J Alzheimers Dis. 2017;56:929–38. https://doi.org/10.3233/jad-160979.

79. Mallo SC, Ismail Z, Pereiro AX, Facal D, Lojo-Seoane C, Campos-Magdaleno M, Juncos-Rabadán O. Assessing mild behavioral impairment with the mild behavioral impairment-checklist in people with mild cognitive impairment. J Alzheimers Dis. 2018;66:83–95. https://doi.org/10.3233/jad-180131.

80. Lakhan S, Gross K. The triad of idiopathic normal-pressure hydrocephalus a clinical practice case report. Libyan J Med. 2008;3:54–7. https://doi.org/10.4176/071112.

81. Kiefer M, Unterberg A. The differential diagnosis and treatment of normal-pressure hydrocephalus. Dtsch Arztebl Int. 2012;109:15–25; quiz 26 https://doi.org/10.3238/arztebl.2012.0015.

82. Gölz L, Ruppert FH, Meier U, Lemcke J. Outcome of modern shunt therapy in patients with idiopathic normal pressure hydrocephalus 6 years postoperatively. J Neurosurg. 2014;121:771–5. https://doi.org/10.3171/2014.6.Jns131211.

83. Petersen J, Hellström P, Wikkelsø C, Lundgren-Nilsson A. Improvement in social function and health-related quality of life after shunt surgery for idiopathic normal-pressure hydrocephalus. J Neurosurg. 2014;121:776–84. https://doi.org/10.3171/2014.6.Jns132003.

84. Thomas G, McGirt MJ, Woodworth G, Heidler J, Rigamonti D, Hillis AE, Williams MA. Baseline neuropsychological profile and cognitive response to cerebrospinal fluid shunting for idiopathic normal pressure hydrocephalus. Dement Geriatr Cogn Disord. 2005;20:163–8. https://doi.org/10.1159/000087092.

85. Mataro M, Matarin M, Poca MA, Pueyo R, Sahuquillo J, Barrios M, Junque C. Functional and magnetic resonance imaging correlates of corpus callosum in normal pressure hydrocephalus before and after shunting. J Neurol Neurosurg Psychiatry. 2007;78:395–8. https://doi.org/10.1136/jnnp.2006.096164.

86. Peterson KA, Savulich G, Jackson D, Killikelly C, Pickard JD, Sahakian BJ. The effect of shunt surgery on neuropsychological performance in normal pressure hydrocephalus: a systematic review and meta-analysis. J Neurol. 2016;263:1669–77. https://doi.org/10.1007/s00415-016-8097-0.

87. Savolainen S, Hurskainen H, Paljärvi L, Alafuzoff I, Vapalahti M. Five-year outcome of normal pressure hydrocephalus with or without a shunt: predictive value of the clinical signs, neuropsychological evaluation and infusion test. Acta Neurochir (Wien). 2002;144:515–23; discussion 523. https://doi.org/10.1007/s00701-002-0936-3.

88. Poca MA, Mataró M, Del Mar Matarín M, Arikan F, Junqué C, Sahuquillo J. Is the placement of shunts in patients with idiopathic normal-pressure hydrocephalus worth the risk? Results of a study based on continuous monitoring of intracranial pressure. J Neurosurg. 2004;100:855–66. https://doi.org/10.3171/jns.2004.100.5.0855.

89. Macki M, Mahajan A, Shatz R, Air EL, Novikova M, Fakih M, Elmenini J, Kaur M, Bouchard KR, Funk BA, et al. Prevalence of alternative diagnoses and implications for management in idiopathic normal pressure hydrocephalus patients. Neurosurgery. 2020;87:999–1007. https://doi.org/10.1093/neuros/nyaa199.

90. Kamohara C, Nakajima M, Kawamura K, Akiba C, Ogino I, Xu H, Karagiozov K, Arai H, Miyajima M. Neuropsychological tests are useful for predicting comorbidities of idiopathic normal pressure hydrocephalus. Acta Neurol Scand. 2020;142:623–31. https://doi.org/10.1111/ane.13306.

91. Duinkerke A, Williams MA, Rigamonti D, Hillis AE. Cognitive recovery in idiopathic normal pressure hydrocephalus after shunt. Cogn Behav Neurol. 2004;17:179–84. https://doi.org/10.1097/01.wnn.0000124916.16017.6a.

92. Chaudhry P, Kharkar S, Heidler-Gary J, Hillis AE, Newhart M, Kleinman JT, Davis C, Rigamonti D, Wang P, Irani DN, et al. Characteristics and reversibility of dementia in normal pressure hydrocephalus. Behav Neurol. 2007;18:149–58. https://doi.org/10.1155/2007/456281.

93. Solana E, Poca MA, Sahuquillo J, Benejam B, Junqué C, Dronavalli M. Cognitive and motor improvement after retesting in normal-pressure hydrocephalus: a real change or merely a learning effect? J Neurosurg. 2010;112:399–409. https://doi.org/10.3171/2009.4.Jns081664.

94. Hellström P, Edsbagge M, Blomsterwall E, Archer T, Tisell M, Tullberg M, Wikkelso C. Neuropsychological effects of shunt treatment in idiopathic normal pressure hydrocephalus. Neurosurgery. 2008;63:527–35; discussion 535–526. https://doi.org/10.1227/01.NEU.000 0325258.16934.BB.

95. Hellström P, Klinge P, Tans J, Wikkelsø C. The neuropsychology of iNPH: findings and evaluation of tests in the European multicentre study. Clin Neurol Neurosurg. 2012;114:130–4. https://doi.org/10.1016/j.clineuro.2011.09.014.

96. Mataró M, Poca MA, Del Mar Matarín M, Catalan R, Sahuquillo J, Galard R. CSF galanin and cognition after shunt surgery in normal pressure hydrocephalus. J Neurol Neurosurg Psychiatry. 2003;74:1272–7. https://doi.org/10.1136/jnnp.74.9.1272.

97. Gleichgerrcht E, Cervio A, Salvat J, Loffredo AR, Vita L, Roca M, Torralva T, Manes F. Executive function improvement in normal pressure hydrocephalus following shunt surgery. Behav Neurol. 2009;21:181–5. https://doi.org/10.3233/ben-2009-0249.

98. McGovern RA, Nelp TB, Kelly KM, Chan AK, Mazzoni P, Sheth SA, Honig LS, Teich AF, McKhann GM. Predicting cognitive improvement in normal pressure hydrocephalus patients using preoperative neuropsychological testing and cerebrospinal fluid biomarkers. Neurosurgery. 2019;85:E662-e669. https://doi.org/10.1093/neuros/nyz102.

99. Raftopoulos C, Deleval J, Chaskis C, Leonard A, Cantraine F, Desmyttere F, Clarysse S, Brotchi J. Cognitive recovery in idiopathic normal pressure hydrocephalus: a prospective study. Neurosurgery. 1994;35:397–404; discussion 404–395. https://doi.org/10.1227/000 06123-199409000-00006.

100. Bech-Azeddine R, Høgh P, Juhler M, Gjerris F, Waldemar G. Idiopathic normal-pressure hydrocephalus: clinical comorbidity correlated with cerebral biopsy findings and outcome of cerebrospinal fluid shunting. J Neurol Neurosurg Psychiatry. 2007;78:157–61. https://doi.org/10.1136/jnnp.2006.095117.

101. Shprecher D, Schwalb J, Kurlan R. Normal pressure hydrocephalus: diagnosis and treatment. Curr Neurol Neurosci Rep. 2008;8:371–6. https://doi.org/10.1007/s11910-008-0058-2.

102. Golomb J, Wisoff J, Miller DC, Boksay I, Kluger A, Weiner H, Salton J, Graves W. Alzheimer's disease comorbidity in normal pressure hydrocephalus: prevalence and shunt response. J Neurol Neurosurg Psychiatry. 2000; 68:778–81. https://doi.org/10.1136/jnnp.68.6.778.

103. Kiefer M, Eymann R. Gravitational shunt complications after a five-year follow-up. Acta Neurochir Suppl. 2010;106:107–12. https://doi.org/10.1007/978-3-211-98811-4_18.

104. Craven CL, Baudracco I, Zetterberg H, Lunn MPT, Chapman MD, Lakdawala N, Watkins LD, Toma AK. The predictive value of T-tau and AB1–42 levels in idiopathic normal pressure hydrocephalus. Acta Neurochir (Wien). 2017;159:2293–2300. https://doi.org/10.1007/s00701-017-3314-x.

105. Pfanner T, Henri-Bhargava A, Borchert S. Cerebrospinal fluid biomarkers as predictors of shunt response in idiopathic normal pressure hydrocephalus: a systematic review. Canadian J Neurol Sci/J Canadien Des Sci Neurologiques. 2018;45(1):3–10. https://doi.org/10.1017/cjn.2017.251.

106. Malm J, Graff-Radford NR, Ishikawa M, Kristensen B, Leinonen V, Mori E, Owler BK, Tullberg M, Williams MA, Relkin NR. Influence of comorbidities in idiopathic normal pressure hydrocephalus—research and clinical care. A report of the ISHCSF task force on comorbidities in INPH. Fluids Barriers CNS. 2013;10:22. https://doi.org/10.1186/2045-8118-10-22.

107. Boon AJ, Tans JT, Delwel EJ, Egeler-Peerdeman SM, Hanlo PW, Wurzer HA, Hermans J. Dutch normal-pressure hydrocephalus study: the role of cerebrovascular disease. J Neurosurg. 1999;90:221–6. https://doi.org/10.3171/jns.1999.90.2.0221.

108. Sindorio C, Abbritti RV, Raffa G, Priola SM, Germanò A, Visocchi M, Quattropani MC. Neuropsychological assessment in the differential diagnosis of idiopathic normal pressure hydrocephalus. An important tool for the maintenance and restoration of neuronal and

neuropsychological functions. Acta Neurochir Suppl. 2017;124:283–8. https://doi.org/10.1007/978-3-319-39546-3_41.

109. Vyhnálek M, Marková H, Laczó J, De Beni R, Di Nuovo S. Assessment of memory impairment in early diagnosis of Alzheimer's disease. Curr. Alzheimer Res. 2019; 16:975–85. https://doi.org/10.2174/1567205016666191113125303.

110. Luikku AJ, Hall A, Nerg O, Koivisto AM, Hiltunen M, Helisalmi S, Herukka SK, Sutela A, Kojoukhova M, Mattila J, et al. Multimodal analysis to predict shunt surgery outcome of 284 patients with suspected idiopathic normal pressure hydrocephalus. Acta Neurochir (Wien). 2016;158:2311–9. https://doi.org/10.1007/s00701-016-2980-4.

111. Rusina R, Matěj R, Cséfalvay Z, Keller J, Franková V, Vyhnálek M. Frontotemporal dementia. Cesk Slov Neurol N. 2021;84/117(1):9–29. https://doi.org/10.48095/cccsnn20219.

Normal Pressure Hydrocephalus from the Urologist's Point of View

Klára Havlová

Abstract Bladder impairment is a common clinical feature in the elderly, in both men and women. The aetiology of bladder dysfunction in the aged population is mostly multifactorial, closely linked to possible neurodegenerative comorbidities or intake of medications. However, the differential diagnosis of the cause of urinary problems is essential in order to deliver the best therapeutic approach. Patients with normal pressure hydrocephalus (NPH) share similar clinical signs of urinary incontinence, including frequency, urgency and urge incontinence, features often interpreted as "overactive bladder". Once the diagnosis of NPH is defined and adequate treatment is indicated, the vast majority of patients improve in their symptoms, and thus in their overall quality of life. This chapter discusses the urinary dysfunction in NPH, including the pathophysiology, diagnosis, treatment, and outcome.

Keywords Urinary incontinence · Normal pressure hydrocephalus · Overactive bladder

Abbreviations

iNPH	Idiopathic normal pressure hydrocephalus
IPSS	International prostate symptom score
LUTS	Lower urinary tract symptoms
NPH	Normal pressure hydrocephalus
OABSS	Overactive bladder symptoms score
PMC	Pontine micturition centre
QoL	Quality of Life
UUI	Urge urinary incontinence
VP	Ventriculoperitoneal

K. Havlová (✉)
Department of Urology, 2nd Faculty of Medicine of Charles University, University Hospital Motol, Prague, Czech Republic
e-mail: klara.havlova@fnmotol.cz

© The Author(s), under exclusive license to Springer Nature Switzerland AG 2023   197
O. Bradac (ed.), *Normal Pressure Hydrocephalus*,
https://doi.org/10.1007/978-3-031-36522-5_11

1 Introduction

Normal pressure hydrocephalus (NPH) is a specific form of communicating hydrocephalus defined by dilatation of the ventricular system without elevation of cerebrospinal fluid pressure. It manifests with a clinical triad consisting of gait disturbance, dementia and urge incontinence [1]. Up to 50% of patients experience all symptoms. The urological data on this topic alone are based on a relatively small number of published retrospective studies with a limited number of cases [2].

From a urological point of view, symptoms, such as frequency, urgency and urge incontinence, dominate in the clinical picture. These fall under the umbrella term "overactive bladder". A conservative approach is preferred in the diagnosis and treatment of urological symptoms. Thus, a detailed medical history, physical examination and ultrasound examination are sufficient to initiate treatment, and validated questionnaires are helpful to verify difficulties. Invasive urodynamic examination methods are indicated only in patients with unclear findings or when other aetiologies are suspected. The treatment then proceeds from non-pharmacological behavioural therapy aimed at restoring the micturition reflex, that is, bladder training, to pharmacological therapy with anticholinergics or beta3-mimetics. However, despite the above-mentioned therapeutic modalities, neurosurgical treatment is the basis of therapy and improvement of micturition difficulties can be achieved in 80–90% of patients [3, 4].

2 Physiology of Micturition

The storage and emptying of the urinary bladder is controlled by peripheral parasympathetic, sympathetic and somatic nerves, which are controlled by the central nervous system. Parasympathetic efferent (motor) nerve pathways arise from the sacral spinal cord (S2–S4 segments), continuing through the pelvic plexus into the urinary bladder. Nerve endings are found throughout the urinary bladder, with their greatest concentration is in the fundus. In this case, the neurotransmitter is acetylcholine which acts on muscarinic receptors, the stimulation of which results in muscular contraction. There are five known subtypes of muscarinic receptors (M1–M5), which are also found in other parts of the body, including the central nervous system. M2 and M3 subtypes are present in the urinary bladder [5].

Sympathetic nerve fibres arise from the thoracic and lumbar spinal cord, from Th11–L2 segments, and continue to the sympathetic paravertebral ganglia. Through the hypogastric nerve and pelvic plexus, they innervate primarily the trigone area, a neck of the urinary bladder, and proximal urethra. They act on the alpha-adrenergic receptors which, when stimulated, cause contraction of the musculature in this area and thus contraction of the sphincter. Beta-adrenergic receptors are located in the fundus of the urinary bladder and their stimulation results in the relaxation of musculature. Somatic nerve pathways arise from S3–S4 sacral segments from the so-called

Onuf's nucleus and innervate the pelvic floor muscles and the external sphincter through pudendal nerves [6, 7]. Put simply, the sympathetic nervous system is responsible for the filling phase and the parasympathetic nervous system for the micturition phase.

The actual process of micturition is controlled by three important centres – the cortical micturition centre, the pontine micturition centre and the sacral micturition centre. The sacral micturition centre, located in the S2–S4 region, is considered the basic, so-called reflex centre of micturition. Through volume receptors in the urinary bladder wall, afferent nerve pathways inform about the filling of the urinary bladder. With increasing urinary bladder filling, the intensity of afferent stimuli increases, which are further conducted to the supraspinal centres. This leads to a pressure increase in the urethral sphincter region via the pathway of the Onuf's nucleus [8]. In the micturition phase, the efferent nerve pathways cause contraction of the urinary bladder musculature via the parasympathetic nervous system; thus, if the sacral segments or peripheral nerves are injured by a so-called subsacral lesion, the basal micturition reflex is interrupted. The patient is not capable of spontaneous or reflex micturition. The pontine micturition centre (PMC) is responsible for the coordination of the storage and micturition phases, or the synergy between the detrusor muscle contraction and sphincter relaxation. The excitatory activity towards the spinal centres dominates here. In the case of suprasacral (infrapontine) lesions, detrusor muscle hyperactivity is present, often associated with detrusor-sphincter dyssynergia.

The cortical micturition centre is responsible for the free ability to delay the actual micturition process [6]. Under physiological conditions, it effectively inhibits the pontine centre to prevent the initiation of the micturition reflex. If the micturition phase is initiated, the inhibitory effect on the PMC is weakened and the pathway towards the spinal centre is activated. In the case of a suprapontine lesion, there is a reduction in cortical inhibition of the micturition reflex, leading to the manifestation of an overactive bladder, which is also the case in NPH [9, 10].

3 Epidemiology of Urological Difficulties in Normal Pressure Hydrocephalus

Lower urinary tract symptoms (LUTS) are very common in patients with NPH. Typical symptoms included storage symptoms in 90% of patients, nocturia affecting more than half of patients to varying degrees, urgency and urge incontinence (UUI) which, according to some sources, are experienced by more than 70% of patients [11]. Evacuation symptomatology (e.g. weak stream, post-void residual) is present in 71% of patients [3].

Urge incontinence itself, as one component of the NPH-defining triad, represents a significant socioeconomic problem. It greatly impairs quality of life and affects daily activities. At the same time, patients face a variety of health complications, such as urinary tract infections and dermatoses. Despite media awareness, the issue is still taboo, patients do not talk about the problem and avoid social life. It is reported that only 5% of women and 16% of men address their difficulties with doctors. Therefore, accurate epidemiological data are missing. The overall prevalence of incontinence, regardless of type, increases with age worldwide and is higher in women than in men. According to a review of population studies, its prevalence ranges between 5–70%. The prevalence of urge incontinence is the same in both men and women, and ranges between 1.7–36%. It is estimated that up to 60–70% of urge incontinence cases in the elderly population is caused by a suprapontine lesion [12]. In comparison, stress incontinence is more common in women and the number of patients increases with age, with a reported prevalence of up to 40% in women older than 70 years. Another interesting finding is the difference in prevalence in people over 65 years of age living at home (10–30%) or in social care facilities (36–45%) [13–20]. From an economic point of view, UUI represents an enormous burden on the healthcare system. €7 billion was estimated cost-of-illness in Canada, Germany, Italy, Spain, Sweden, and the United Kingdom in 2005. And $66 billion was estimated cost-of-illness in the United States in 2007 [21].

4   Aetiopathogenesis

The aetiology of micturition dysfunction in patients with NPH is not well understood. Given the nature of the difficulty, it is thought to be a combination of cognitive deficits together with frontal lobe hypoperfusion, often caused by alterations in CNS cell metabolism, microinfarctions or microhaemorrhages [4, 22, 23]. In view of this, we approach micturition difficulties as a lesion above the level of the pontine micturition centre and call it a suprapontine lesion. In such patients, the micturition remains coordinated but the inhibition to the lower micturition centres is reduced. Clinically, it manifests as a detrusor muscle hyperactivity which causes the symptoms mentioned above. Typically, the patient perceives a sudden urge to urinate that can no longer be delayed by will.

5   Diagnostics

Diagnostics of micturition dysfunction in patients with normal pressure hydrocephalus has its specifics. Similarly to elderly patients or patients with cognitive deficits, we are satisfied with non-invasive investigative methods that allow us to initiate adequate therapy in up to 80% of cases [24].

In terms of medical history, it is important to search for the aetiology of the difficulties, for the presence and severity of individual symptoms. We check the frequency of micturition, the number of urges, the occurrence of urge incontinence and nocturia. We ask about the stream of urine, the strength of the stream, the sensation of complete or incomplete emptying after micturition, and the need to engage the abdominal muscles during micturition. In addition to the urological history, we do not forget to ask about associated neurological, psychiatric or internal comorbidities, such as diabetes mellitus or cardiac insufficiency, which are associated with a higher prevalence of LUTS. A pharmacological history is also important because many drug groups affect urinary tract function. Symptomatology may be exacerbated by diuretics. Antipsychotics, antidepressants, anxiolytics and anti-Parkinsonian drugs deserve attention, as they often have a hypnosedative effect in addition to an anticholinergic effect.

When taking the medical history itself, we can use a number of validated questionnaires, for example, Overactive Bladder Questionnaire OAB-q, Incontinence Impact Questionnaire—IIQ. Kings Health Questionnaire, which also has good statistical properties for different groups of patients of both sexes with stress and urge incontinence [25]. Another possible questionnaire is the Urge Impact Scale (URIS), which measures the impact of urge incontinence on quality of life in elderly patients. It contains 24 questions assessing the difficulties (impact on psychological well-being, coping with daily life and sense of self-confidence) during the last month [26]. Additionally, the International Consultation on Incontinence Questionnaire-Urinary Incontinence Short Form (ICIQ-UI SF) [27] is frequently used due to for evaluation of the frequency, severity and overall impact on quality of life (QoL) in patients with urinary incontinence. It contains four main question domains: (1) frequency of urinary incontinence, (2) amount of leakage, (3) overall impact of urinary incontinence, and (4) a self-diagnostic item. The main advantage of this questionnaire is the simplicity, as general practitioners and clinicians in various health institutions are able to screen for incontinence with comprehensive results and level of evidence, which helps to enhance active and early therapy. There are also four other models suggested to use in conjunction with ICIQ-UI SF, namely the International Consultation on Incontinence Questionnaire Male Lower Urinary Tract Symptoms Module (ICIQ-MLUTS) and the same for female patients (ICIQ-FLUTS), if there is a need for gender-specific symptoms. The two remaining were built to assess gender-specific sexual matters modules (ICIQ-MLUTSsex for males and ICIQ-FLUTSsex for females).

The classical physical examination of patients includes, among others, a neurological examination of the perineum, during which we evaluate the sensation in S2–S5 segments, anal reflex, bulbocavernosus reflex and free sphincter contraction. In men, we should not omit the examination of the prostate. In women, we focus on the examination of trophic characteristics of vaginal entrance and vagina. We look for pelvic organ prolapse and urethral hypermobility.

6 Accompanying Examinations

Urinalysis can help us to diagnose another primary cause of micturition difficulties, and the detection of any leukocyturia, erythrocyturia, glycosuria or proteinuria requires further investigation. Basic completion of a micturition diary, which ideally consists of 48–72 h of systematic recording of the time and volume of fluid intake, frequency of micturition, volume of micturition portions, and frequency of urine leakage, is also useful to objectify lower urinary tract dysfunction. We can rule out polyuria, or excesses in fluid intake. From this information, we can get an idea of the functional capacity of the urinary bladder. Depending on the cognitive status, either the patient or the attending staff keeps a record. In addition to diagnosis, the micturition diary allows assessment of response to treatment and is part of behavioural therapy. In diagnostics, ultrasound examination is of particular importance to determine post-void residual. Of course, we do not neglect ultrasound imaging of the upper urinary tract.

7 Invasive Examination

We use complete urodynamic examination and cystoscopy in patients after failure of primary therapy or in strictly selected patients and only in situations when the obtained results will change the current course of therapy. During invasive urodynamic examination—a functional examination of the lower urinary tract using a catheter inserted into the urinary bladder and rectum to measure intravesical and abdominal pressure during filling and voiding—the most common finding is detrusor overactivity (70–95%) [3, 4]. Although studies have been performed on small cohorts of several dozen patients, this finding is consistent with a presumed suprapontine lesion. Secondary findings included reduced urinary bladder capacity in 57% of patients and urodynamically confirmed subvesical obstruction in almost half of the male patients [28].

Cystoscopy should be indicated in patients with verified microscopic or macroscopic haematuria, and it should be considered in patients with refractory overactive bladder unresponsive to treatment. The aim is to evaluate the urinary bladder mucosa and exclude its pathology, such as malignancy, foreign body, etc.

8 Treatment

The basic treatment of lower urinary tract symptoms is the early establishment of a correct diagnosis of NPH. Improvement in all clinical symptoms after surgical treatment of NPH occurs in about 60% of patients, with improvement in micturition difficulties occurring in up to 80–90% of patients [3, 4]. Patients with a good response include those with a shorter time from onset of symptoms to initiation of treatment and those without pathological findings during urodynamic examination [29, 30]. Urological treatment must respect the limitations imposed by the patient's cognitive status, general condition, mobility, and ideally should be carried out in collaboration with family or medical staff. More detailed results of urinary incontinence outcomes following shunt surgery is described in Chap. 28, dedicated to overall prognosis and outcomes in NPH treatment.

9 Behavioural Therapy

The aim of behavioural therapy is to restore cortical control of the micturition reflex, the so-called bladder training/bladder drill. This involves the patient keeping a micturition card to get a clear idea of micturition intervals and portions. This is followed by prolonging the intervals between micturitions "micturitions by the clock", maintaining regular micturitions and trying to suppress urges. These intervals are not set at night. Everything is done under control and keeping a micturition diary [31, 32]. Patient motivation and cooperation are important. Behavioural therapy also includes lifestyle changes. This means weight reduction, modification of the drinking regime, and dietary measures, such as limitation of caffeinated drinks, spicy foods, and alcohol. Patients should also be advised to stop smoking.

10 Pharmacotherapy

10.1 Anticholinergics

Pharmacotherapy should play an adjunctive role. Anticholinergics are considered the first-line oral therapy [33]. The urinary bladder is richly supplied with parasympathetic fibres whose mediator at postganglionic muscarinic receptors is acetylcholine. Anticholinergic agents reduce the release of acetylcholine and thus help to increase urinary bladder capacity and reduce detrusor muscle hyperactivity. A limiting factor in the treatment with anticholinergics is their potential adverse effects. The selectivity and tissue affinity for each muscarinic receptor subtype and the ability to cross the blood–brain barrier determine the extent of adverse effects. Adverse effects on central nervous system function and cognitive function are most commonly experienced by elderly patients and those with central nervous system disorders, such as Parkinson's disease, Alzheimer's disease, dementia and NPH. Neurological manifestations include dizziness, memory impairment, confusion, and, rarely, hallucinations or delirious states or sleep disturbances [34, 35]. The most risky agents for these patients are oxybutynin, propiverine, and tolterodine. M1 anticholinergic receptors are further located in the salivary glands. In non-selective anticholinergics, they result in drying of the mucous membranes. Dry mouth (xerostomia) and dry eye syndrome (xerophthalmia) as adverse effects are generally the most poorly tolerated by patients. In addition to the positive, desirable effect on the urinary bladder, they may impair bowel motility and promote the development of obstipation. Absolute contraindication is severe renal or hepatic insufficiency or myasthenia gravis.

First-generation anticholinergics include oxybutynin, trospium chloride, propiverine, which have the advantage of high efficacy. Unfortunately, due to their non-selectivity, they exhibit a higher incidence of adverse effects. Of the first-generation anticholinergics, trospium chloride is suitable for elderly patients as it does not cross the blood–brain barrier and, therefore, has no negative side effects on the central nervous system and does not affect cognitive function [36].

Second-generation anticholinergics (tolterodine, solifenacin, fesoterodine) are better tolerated by patients as they are selective to M2 and M3 receptors. Fesoterodine is a good choice for elderly patients because of its low permeability across the blood–brain barrier. In studies, fesoterodine administration had no significant effect on cognitive function in healthy older adults. Overall, it was well tolerated by patients over 65 years of age with overactive bladder [37]. Of note is clinical trial form 2012 [38] with the aim to evaluate the efficacy and safety of solifenacin to treat voiding symptoms caused by iNPH following the VP shunt insertion. Overall urinary outcome was assessed according to Prostate Symptom Score (IPSS), QoL Score, Overactive Bladder Symptom Score (OABSS), maximal urine flow rate, voided volume and post-voiding residual urine volume. Afore-described variables were measured before VP shunt insertion, and then at 4-week and 12-week follow-up examinations. The mean voided volume significantly increased from 147.18 ± 61.84 ml before surgery solifenacin administration to 160.03 ± 62.59 ml at last follow-up at 12 weeks solifenacin intake ($p < 0.001$). Post-voiding residual urine volume was similarly improved at last follow-up ($p = 0.009$). Finally, upon administering 5 mg of solifenacin to patients with iNPH after surgery showed improvement in symptoms including frequency, urgency and urge incontinence with only minor adverse effects (oral hydration or supplemental laxative agents).

10.2 Beta3-Sympathomimetics

Another treatment option is beta3-sympathomimetics. By activating beta3-adrenoceptors in the detrusor muscle, the concentration of cyclic adenosine monophosphate is increased via the enzyme adenylate cyclase and the detrusor muscle is subsequently relaxed. This results in improved storage function of the urinary bladder [39–41]. Compared with anticholinergics, beta3-sympathomimetics have a lower incidence of adverse effects. The most common side effects include headache, hypertension, and gastrointestinal distress [42]. In contrast, no negative effect on cognitive function has been demonstrated in patients over 65 years of age [43, 44].

In practice, pharmacological therapy is discontinued due to adverse effects in 30% of patients and due to lack of treatment effect in up to 39% of patients [45, 46].

11 Conclusion

Frequency, urgency and urge incontinence are the most commonly seen features in the iNPH clinical profile. For the majority of patients suffering from urinary dysfunction, conservative treatment is indicated, although invasive urodynamic examination methods may be beneficial, especially in patients with contradictory findings in cases of unclear aetiology of urinary symptoms. Neurosurgical treatment is the golden standard in iNPH urinary impairment management with good outcomes achieved in the vast majority of treated patients. Early improvement of urinary dysfunction in shunted NPH patients is well described. However, the improvement for longer follow-ups is less known. Similarly to the worsening of cognitive deficits, symptoms of urinary incontinence tend to decline after longer periods of time, despite the initial improvement in early or short-term follow-up.

12 Key Points

- Symptoms such as frequency, urgency and urge incontinence dominate in the clinical picture of patients with iNPH.
- A conservative approach is preferred in the diagnosis and treatment of urological symptoms.
- Invasive urodynamic examination methods are indicated only in patients with unclear findings or when other aetiologies are suspected.
- Neurosurgical treatment is the basis of therapy and improvement of micturition difficulties can be achieved in 80–90% of patients.

References

1. Hakim S, Adams RD. The special clinical problem of symptomatic hydrocephalus with normal cerebrospinal fluid pressure. Observations on cerebrospinal fluid hydrodynamics. J Neurol Sci. 1965;2(4):307–27. https://doi.org/10.1016/0022-510x(65)90016-x.
2. Adams RD, Fisher CM, Hakim S, Ojemann RG, Sweet WH. Symptomatic occult hydrocephalus with "normal" cerebrospinal-fluid pressure. A treatable syndrome. N Engl J Med. 1965;273:117–26. https://doi.org/10.1056/NEJM196507152730301.
3. Sakakibara R, Kanda T, Sekido T, Uchiyama T, Awa Y, Ito T, Liu Z, Yamamoto T, Yamanishi T, Yuasa T, Shirai K, Hattori T. Mechanism of bladder dysfunction in idiopathic normal pressure hydrocephalus. Neurourol Urodyn. 2008;27(6):507–10. https://doi.org/10.1002/nau.20547.

 4. Campos-Juanatey F, Gutiérrez-Baños JL, Portillo-Martín JA, Zubillaga-Guerrero S. Assessment of the urodynamic diagnosis in patients with urinary incontinence associated with normal pressure hydrocephalus. Neurourol Urodyn. 2015;34(5):465–8. https://doi.org/10.1002/nau.22600.
 5. Abrams P, Andersson KE. Muscarinic receptor antagonists for overactive bladder. BJU Int. 2007;100(5):987–1006. https://doi.org/10.1111/j.1464-410X.2007.07205.x.
 6. Yoshimura N, Chancellor MB (2003) Neurophysiology of lower urinary tract function and dysfunction. Rev Urol. 2003;5(Suppl 8):S3–10.
 7. Consortium for Spinal Cord Medicine. Bladder management for adults with spinal cord injury: a clinical practice guideline for health-care providers. J Spinal Cord Med. 2006;29(5):527–73.
 8. Krhut J, Zachoval R. Neurální kontrola dolních močových cest. Ces Urol. 2011;15(2):69–77.
 9. Krhut J, Doležel J, Doležil D, Zachoval R, Ženíšek J. Neurourologie. 1. vyd. Praha: Galén. 2005;141.
10. de Groat WC. Integrative control of the lower urinary tract: preclinical perspective. Br J Pharmacol. 2006;147(Suppl 2):S25–40. https://doi.org/10.1038/sj.bjp.0706604.
11. Abrams P, Cardozo L, Fall M, Griffiths D, Rosier P, Ulmsten U, van Kerrebroeck P, Victor A, Wein A, Standardisation Sub-committee of the International Continence Society. The standardisation of terminology of lower urinary tract function: report from the Standardisation Sub-committee of the International Continence Society. Neurourol Urodyn. 2002;21(2):167–78. https://doi.org/10.1002/nau.10052.
12. Madersbacher H, Awad S, Fall M, et al. Urge Inkontinenz beim älteren Menschen—supraspinale Reflexinkontinenz. Der Urologe B. 1998;38:S10–8. https://doi.org/10.1007/s001310050363.
13. Milsom I, Gyhagen M. The prevalence of urinary incontinence. Climacteric J Int Menopause Soc. 2019;22(3):217–22. https://doi.org/10.1080/13697137.2018.1543263.
14. Temml C, Haidinger G, Schmidbauer J, Schatzl G, Madersbacher S. Urinary incontinence in both sexes: prevalence rates and impact on quality of life and sexual life. Neurourol Urodyn. 2000;19(3):259–71. https://doi.org/10.1002/(sici)1520-6777(2000)19:3%3c259::aid-nau7%3e3.0.co;2-u.
15. Milsom I, Altman D, Cartwright R, Lapitan MC, Nelson R, Sillén U, Tikkinen K. Epidemiology of urinary incontinence (UI) and other lower urinary tract symptoms (LUTS), pelvic organ prolapse (POP) and anal incontinence (AI). In: Abrams P, Cardozo L, Khoury S, Wein AJ, editors. Incontinence: 5th international consultation on incontinence. 5th ed. Paris: ICUD-EAU; 2012. p. 15–107. https://www.ics.org/Publications/ICI_5/INCONTINENCE.pdf.
16. Vaughan CP, Goode PS, Burgio KL, Markland AD. Urinary incontinence in older adults. Mount Sinai J Med New York. 2011;78(4):558–70. https://doi.org/10.1002/msj.20276.
17. Irwin DE, Milsom I, Hunskaar S, Reilly K, Kopp Z, Herschorn S, Coyne K, Kelleher C, Hampel C, Artibani W, Abrams P. Population-based survey of urinary incontinence, overactive bladder, and other lower urinary tract symptoms in five countries: results of the EPIC study. Eur Urol. 2006;50(6):1306–15. https://doi.org/10.1016/j.eururo.2006.09.019.
18. Campbell AJ, Reinken J, McCosh L. Incontinence in the elderly: prevalence and prognosis. Age Ageing. 1985;14(2):65–70. https://doi.org/10.1093/ageing/14.2.65.
19. Drennan VM, Rait G, Cole L, Grant R, Iliffe S. The prevalence of incontinence in people with cognitive impairment or dementia living at home: a systematic review. Neurourol Urodyn. 2013;32:314–24. https://doi.org/10.1002/nau.22333.
20. Junqueira JB, Santos V. Urinary incontinence in hospital patients: prevalence and associated factors. Rev Lat Am Enfermagem. 2018;25:e2970. https://doi.org/10.1590/1518-8345.2139.2970.
21. Milsom I, Coyne KS, Nicholson S, Kvasz M, Chen CI, Wein AJ. Global prevalence and economic burden of urgency urinary incontinence: a systematic review. Eur Urol. 2014;65(1):79–95. https://doi.org/10.1016/j.eururo.2013.08.031.
22. Sasaki H, Ishii K, Kono AK, Miyamoto N, Fukuda T, Shimada K, Ohkawa S, Kawaguchi T, Mori E. Cerebral perfusion pattern of idiopathic normal pressure hydrocephalus studied by SPECT and statistical brain mapping. Ann Nucl Med. 2007;21(1):39–45. https://doi.org/10.1007/BF03033998.

23. Sakakibara R, Uchida Y, Ishii K, Kazui H, Hashimoto M, Ishikawa M, Yuasa T, Kishi M, Ogawa E, Tateno F, Uchiyama T, Yamamoto T, Yamanishi T, Terada H. Correlation of right frontal hypoperfusion and urinary dysfunction in iNPH: a SPECT study. Neurourol Urodyn. 2012;31:50–5. https://doi.org/10.1002/nau.21222.
24. Krhut MUDJ, Mainer MUDK. INKONTINENCE VE STÁŘÍ–ZVLÁŠTNOSTI DIAGNOS-TIKY A LÉČBY. Urologie pro praxi. 56–61.
25. DuBeau CE, Kiely DK, Resnick NM. Quality of life impact of urge incontinence in older persons: a new measure and conceptual structure. J Am Geriatr Soc. 1999;47(8):989–94. https://doi.org/10.1111/j.1532-5415.1999.tb01295.x.
26. Patrick DL, Martin ML, Bushnell DM, Yalcin I, Wagner TH, Buesching DP. Quality of life of women with urinary incontinence: further development of the incontinence quality of life instrument (I-QOL). Urology. 1999;53(1):71–6. https://doi.org/10.1016/s0090-4295(98)004 54-3.
27. Avery K, Donovan J, Peters T, Shaw C, Gotoh M, Abrams P. ICIQ: a brief and robust measure for evaluating the symptoms and impact of urinary incontinence. Neurourol Urodyn. 2004;23(4):322–30.
28. Jonas S, Brown J. Neurogenic bladder in normal pressure hydrocephalus. Urology. 1975;5(1):44–50. https://doi.org/10.1016/0090-4295(75)90300-3. PMID: 1114545.
29. Hebb AO, Cusimano MD. Idiopathic normal pressure hydrocephalus: a systematic review of diagnosis and outcome. Neurosurgery. 2001;49(5):1166–86. https://doi.org/10.1097/000 06123-200111000-00028.
30. Ahlberg J, Norlén L, Blomstrand C, Wikkelsö C. Outcome of shunt operation on urinary incontinence in normal pressure hydrocephalus predicted by lumbar puncture. J Neurol Neurosurg Psychiatry. 1988;51(1):105–8. https://doi.org/10.1136/jnnp.51.1.105.
31. Wallace SA, Roe B, Williams K, Palmer M. Bladder training for urinary incontinence in adults. Cochrane Database Syst Rev. 2004;2004(1):CD001308. https://doi.org/10.1002/146 51858.CD001308.pub2..
32. Fantl JA, Wyman JF, McClish DK, Harkins SW, Elswick RK, Taylor JR, Hadley EC. Efficacy of bladder training in older women with urinary incontinence. JAMA. 1991;265(5):609–13.
33. Samuelsson E, Odeberg J, Stenzelius K, Molander U, Hammarström M, Franzen K, Andersson G, Midlöv P. Pharmacotherapy of geriatric incontinence. Geriatr Gerontol Int. 2015;15:521–34. https://doi.org/10.1111/ggi.12451.
34. Desmarais JE, Beauclair L, Annable L, Bélanger MC, Kolivakis TT, Margolese HC. Effects of discontinuing anticholinergic treatment on movement disorders, cognition and psychopathology in patients with schizophrenia. Therapeutic Adv Psychopharmacol. 2014;4(6):257–67. https://doi.org/10.1177/2045125314553611.
35. López-Álvarez J, Llewellyn-Jones J, Agüera L. Anticholinergic drugs in geriatric psychopharmacology. Front Neurosci. 2019;13. https://doi.org/10.3389/fnins.2019.01309.
36. Chapple C. New once-daily formulation for trospium in overactive bladder. Int J Clin Pract. 2010;64:1535–40. https://doi.org/10.1111/j.1742-1241.2010.02493.x.
37. Nitti VW, Dmochowski R, Appell RA, Wang JT, Bavendam T, Guan Z. Efficacy and tolerability of tolterodine extended-release in continent patients with overactive bladder and nocturia. BJU Int. 2006;97:1262–6. https://doi.org/10.1111/j.1464-410X.2006.06146.x.
38. Chung JH, Lee JY, Kang DH, et al. Efficacy and safety of solifenacin to treat overactive bladder symptoms in patients with idiopathic normal pressure hydrocephalus: an open-label, multi-center, prospective study. Neurourol Urodyn. 2012;31(7):1175–80. https://doi.org/10.1002/ nau.22234.
39. Kuei Ch, Peng Ch, Liao Ch. Perspectives on mirabegron in the treatment of overactive bladder syndrome: a new beta-3 adrenoceptor agonist. Urol Sci. 2015;26(1):17–23.
40. Chapple C, Khullar V, Nitti VW, Frankel J, Herschorn S, Kaper M, Blauwet MB, Siddiqui E. Efficacy of the β3-adrenoceptor agonist mirabegron for the treatment of overactive bladder by severity of incontinence at baseline: a post hoc analysis of pooled data from three randomised phase 3 trials. Eur Urol. 2015;67(1):11–4. https://doi.org/10.1016/j.eururo.2014.06.052.

41. Wagg A, Staskin D, Engel E, Herschorn S, Kristy RM, Schermer CR. Efficacy, safety, and tolerability of mirabegron in patients aged ≥65yr with overactive bladder wet: a phase IV, double-blind, randomised, placebo-controlled study (PILLAR). Eur Urol. 2020;77(2):211–20. https://doi.org/10.1016/j.eururo.2019.10.002.
42. Abrams P, Kelleher C, Staskin D, Rechberger T, Kay R, Martina R, Newgreen D, Paireddy A, van Maanen R, Ridder A. Combination treatment with mirabegron and solifenacin in patients with overactive bladder: efficacy and safety results from a randomised, double-blind, dose-ranging, phase 2 study (Symphony). Eur Urol. 2015;67(3):577–88. https://doi.org/10.1016/j.eururo.2014.02.012.
43. Griebling TL, Campbell NL, Mangel J, Staskin D, Herschorn S, Elsouda D, Schermer CR. Effect of mirabegron on cognitive function in elderly patients with overactive bladder: MoCA results from a phase 4 randomized, placebo-controlled study (PILLAR). BMC Geriatr. 2020;20(1):109. https://doi.org/10.1186/s12877-020-1474-7.
44. Kalder M, Pantazis K, Dinas K, Albert US, Heilmaier C, Kostev K. Discontinuation of treatment using anticholinergic medications in patients with urinary incontinence. Obstet Gynecol. 2014;124(4):794–800. https://doi.org/10.1097/AOG.0000000000000468. PMID: 25198276.
45. Tijnagel MJ, Scheepe JR, Blok BF. Real life persistence rate with antimuscarinic treatment in patients with idiopathic or neurogenic overactive bladder: a prospective cohort study with solifenacin. BMC Urol. 2017;17(1):30. https://doi.org/10.1186/s12894-017-0216-4.
46. Chen SF, Kuo HC. Therapeutic efficacy of low-dose (25 mg) mirabegron therapy for patients with mild to moderate overactive bladder symptoms due to central nervous system diseases. Low Urin Tract Symptoms. 2019;11(2):O53–8. https://doi.org/10.1111/luts.12215. Epub 2018 Jan 30 PMID: 29380517.

Extended Lumbar Drainage: Supplementary Test to Diagnose Shunt Responsive iNPH

Ahmed K. Toma

Abstract Predicting shunt responsiveness in patients with suspected normal pressure hydrocephalus can be a challenging task. A number of supplementary tests have been used to help in this process. Extended lumbar drainage is the most accurate of these tests. In essence, it represents temporary shunting for few days. Not only it helps in predicting who would benefit from shunt insertion, but it will also help in estimating the extent of improvement. However, this test does require hospitalisation for few days, with resulting cost implications and is associated with risk of complications.

Keywords External lumbar drainage · Normal pressure hydrocephalus · Diagnostics · Cerebrospinal fluid · Functional test · Drainage · Shunt system · Shunt responsiveness

Abbreviations

CSF	Cerebrospinal fluid
DESH	Disproportionately enlarged subarachnoid space hydrocephalus
ELD	Extended lumbar drainage
iNPH	Idiopathic normal pressure hydrocephalus
MRI	Magnetic resonance imaging

A. K. Toma (✉)
National Hospital for Neurology and Neurosurgery, UCLH and Queen Square Institute of Neurology, UCL London, London, UK
e-mail: ahmedtoma@nhs.net

© The Author(s), under exclusive license to Springer Nature Switzerland AG 2023
O. Bradac (ed.), *Normal Pressure Hydrocephalus*,
https://doi.org/10.1007/978-3-031-36522-5_12

1 Introduction

There is no single test that can diagnose shunt responsive idiopathic normal pressure hydrocephalus (iNPH). If shunt placement was offered solely on the basis of patient history, examination, and the presence of ventriculomegaly on neuroimaging, about 50% of patients with suspected iNPH would benefit from surgery. The difficulty with iNPH diagnosis is that there are no generally accepted neuropathological criteria for post-mortem confirmation of a diagnosis of iNPH, pathophysiology is not fully understood and the natural history of untreated iNPH has not been well characterised. iNPH can resemble, or occur in combination with, various disorders that are prevalent in the elderly; such as cerebrovascular disease, Alzheimer's or Parkinson's disease. Furthermore, epidemiological imaging studies of elderly population have shown that enlarged cerebral ventricles with typical iNPH features like Disproportionately enlarged subarachnoid space hydrocephalus (DESH sign), could occur in asymptomatic patients, indicating a possible subclinical phase of this condition.

To improve these odds, clinicians have used tests to supplement clinical and radiological findings, based on physiological testing (such as the determination of cerebrospinal fluid (CSF) outflow resistance) or functional testing (such as the CSF tap test and extended lumbar drainage [ELD]) [1, 2].

In essence, ELD acts as a temporary shunt. Haan and Thomeer first described ELD as supplementary test to predict shunt responsiveness in iNPH, based on the principle that the larger CSF volume drained through tap test, the better is the sensitivity of predicting shunt responsiveness [3].

There are relatively few published case series that specifically looked into the value of ELD in predicting shunt responsiveness [3–7]. A recent review by Nunn et al. [1] identified four small prospective cohort studies with 84 patients in total. Most of the included studies conducted ELD for 5 days (range 4–5) and the mean CSF drainage rate was 11.6 ml/hr (range 5.3–16.5). The summary estimates for sensitivity and specificity were 94% (CI 41–100%) and 85% (CI 33–100%), respectively. The summary estimates of positive and negative predictive value were both 90% (CIs 65–100% and 48–100%, respectively). This review confirms the generally accepted concept that ELD is the most accurate test in predicting shunt responsiveness in iNPH patients.

The America–European guidelines for iNPH management published in 2005 stated that prolonged external lumbar drainage in excess of 300 ml is associated with high sensitivity (50–100%) and high positive predictive value (80–100%). The authors highlighted that the advantage of lumbar drainage is the increased sensitivity compared with the CSF tap test, even though sensitivities are underestimated because those patients improving with tap test were excluded from drainage protocols in most studies. These guidelines recognise the main restrictions of this technique is the expense, as hospital admission is required. Reported complication rates with ELD are generally low but may be significant in terms of added morbidity [2].

The Japanese Society of Normal Pressure Hydrocephalus (Third Edition) Guidelines for Management of Idiopathic Normal Pressure Hydrocephalus published in

2021 place more emphasis on clinical and radiological picture. It does not, however, dismiss the value of ELD completely, and reserve it to patients with atypical imaging features, who fail to respond to tap test. It does state however that in these patients, there is controversy about whether to repeat the tap test, perform continuous drainage, or perform shunt intervention if a false-negative response to the CSF tap test is suspected [8].

2 Patient Selection

Patients with possible diagnosis of iNPH should be counselled in outpatient clinic regarding options of management. The options for most patients include continuing with conservative treatment and observation, proceeding directly to shunt insertion, or to start with a prognostic test.

Conservative treatment is not recommended in the context of iNPH, unless the patient has no significant symptoms and only incidental imaging features. Typical imaging features of iNPH (DESH sign) has been shown in epidemiological studies to be incidental, indicating a likely (pre-clinical) stage of the condition.

Proceeding directly to shunt surgery has the advantage of reaching a conclusion quicker with less need for hospital and clinic attendance. The main disadvantage, as mentioned above, is that not all patients will have a positive response to shunt insertion and that shunt surgery has risk of complications. Should patients fail to improve following direct shunt surgery, questions will be raised about shunt proper placement and patency or need for shunt valve adjustment aiming to achieve benefit. That is, patient might still need to attend clinics and undergo procedures. Having said that, it is not unreasonable to proceed directly to shunt insertion in patients with typical clinical and imaging features (DESH positive scan), particularly if the patient or healthcare system circumstances favour such approach.

ELD, in essence, is a trial of a shunt on temporary basis. The results of this trial will inform clinicians, patients, and patients' family and carers, about the likelihood of benefit from shunt surgery, as well as the likely extent of improvement with shunt surgery. Most patients who improve following lumbar drainage, will continue to exhibit this improvement for a week or two following drain removal. Patients and carers will be able to experience the change in functional status in patients own environment. The delayed decline in a couple of weeks following drain removal, will further confirm CSF drainage responsiveness. This will provide a solid base for making an informed decision about proceeding to shunt surgery, particularly in patients with atypical imaging features, other underlying neurological conditions (e.g. Parkinson's disease), or significant medical comorbidities. Extended lumbar drainage is often regarded by sceptical clinicians, as well as patients and carers, as an acceptable procedure that will help in accepting or refuting future shunt surgery. The degree of improvement with lumbar drainage will also help in guiding post-shunt insertion care. For instance, should the improvement with the shunt be less than that recorded with drainage, shunt proper placement and patency need to be checked and optimal valve setting need to be questioned.

This is a major advantage of lumbar drainage compared with tap test. Although tap test is simple and quick, the negative predictive value is relatively low and, in majority of patients, the improvement will be short-lived. Many published case series of lumbar drainage in iNPH have selected only patients who had negative response to tap test. This approach will result in less patients requiring lumbar drainage to confirm the diagnosis, will save resources and potentially shorten the patient management journey.

Infusion studies are useful diagnostic tests that also have the advantage of not requiring hospital admission. However, it's negative- and positive-predictive value are not as high as lumbar drainage. Furthermore, it does require local expertise with measurement and interpretation of results [2].

Ultimately, management decisions of iNPH patients are multifactorial and involves careful discussion between clinician, patients, and family or carers to agree what is suitable to that particular patient's condition and needs and taking into consideration the local healthcare facilities.

3 Contraindications

Patients with contraindications for lumbar CSF drainage include those with intracranial mass lesion, obstructive hydrocephalus or spinal lesion causing spinal canal obstruction, for example, large intradural tumour. In these patients, CSF shift could result in harm.

In bed-bound patients, it is often not possible to conduct pre- and post-drainage mobility and balance assessment, making the test futile. Furthermore, risk of infection is likely to be higher, particularly in incontinent patients. Therefore, it might be more appropriate in these patients to proceed directly to shunt insertion, knowing that the results will not be guaranteed. Example of this group of patients include those with advanced NPH process or those with femoral fracture. It is not advisable to delay surgical intervention for possible NPH patients by more than three months, as published studies have shown that outcome will be worse.

4 Pre-procedure Preparation

Medical assessment of this elderly often frail group of patients is essential. Although lumbar drain insertion could be done under local anaesthetics, those with positive response will need to have the shunt insertion under general anaesthetics; therefore, the sooner the medical assessment is done, the less likely ultimate shunt surgery will be delayed. This is often related to cardiac assessment or haematological assessment for those on anticoagulation. Patients should be seen in pre-admission clinic with routine blood testing including clotting assessment. Recent brain imaging is needed. Patients who had a fall following date of most recent scan would need a new one to exclude subdural haematoma that could be exacerbated by lumbar drainage. Magnetic resonance imaging (MRI) scan of the lumbar spine is also advisable. It will help guiding the optimal level to place needle during lumbar drain insertion. Many patients will have severe degenerative spinal changes and severe canal stenosis. The presence of previous lumbar decompression surgery, or even metallic fixation, is not a contraindication. In fact, it might make needle placement easier by identifying a bone-free window from previous decompression. In the presence of previous spinal fixation, patients would need to be counselled about risk of infection. Stopping antiplatelet is advisable, but not essential. Communications with treating physicians to understand risk of stopping antiplatelet would facilitate decision making, not only for drain insertion, but also for potential future shunt surgery.

5 Baseline Assessment

iNPH tetrad includes gait and balance, urinary control and cognitive impairment. Ideally, patients should have baseline assessment of all these elements, with view to repeat those after drainage period to confirm if the drainage resulted in an objective improvement or not.

Gait and balance are most widely assessed in published studies. Ideally, a walking test should be performed by an independent assessor, with same assessor, if possible, conducting both pre and post drainage assessment. Various methods of assessment are used in different hospitals. These include walking speed tests supervised by physiotherapists or video assessments with or without semiautomated systems to provide objective walking speed measures. Increasingly, wearable technologies are being explored for this purpose.

The 2 main walking tests used are:

- Ten meters walking test: Patients will be asked to walk ten meters distance twice, with normal pace and with fast pace. Walking speed and number of steps are calculated. Use of walking aids or help with one or even two people are allowed, as long as same is used in post drainage test.
- Up and go three meters test: This test will take into account the ability of the patient to sit, stand and turn.

Numbers of steps needed to make a 360° turn is also used. There is no clear advantage of any of these tests compared with others. The preferred method of use depends on local unit expertise and preference.

Most neurosurgeons and neurologists will consider 20% improvement in walking speed as an objective evidence of improvement. Some consider 10% as sufficient threshold.

There is a variety of methods of testing cognitive function pre- and post-drainage with less clear evidence of validity compared with walking tests. Questionnaires are often used to assess change with urinary control symptoms.

Patient subjective impression of change is not as reliable in comparison with objective assessment; however, there is some evidence that family and carers subjective impression of change with drainage is often in line with the objective assessment results.

6　Insertion Techniques

Lumbar drain insertion could be done bedside; however, placement in operating theatre is advisable, if feasible. This might reduce the risk of infection. More importantly, it will facilitate the process given the available space and personnel support. The other advantage of having lumbar drain insertion in operating theatre, is ability to perform procedure under sedation. This will reduce degree of patients' discomfort, particularly those with severe degenerative changes that could render needle insertion difficult, particularly in patients with a degree of cognitive impairment.

Procedure could be done with patient in left lateral or sitting position. Doing the procedure in sitting position will make it significantly easier, particularly in patients with a degree of degenerative scoliosis, which is not uncommon in this age group. There are commercially available epidural positioning frames that will help supporting patients having lumbar drain in sitting position. These have support for legs, trunk and upper limb that not only make patient positioning easier and safer but will also alleviate NPH patients fear of fall and retropulsion by allowing them to hold to the frame.

Needless to say, that procedure should be done under strictly aseptic technique preparing the lumbar spine area with suitable antiseptic and using suitable drapes. Local anaesthetics is infiltrated. Different lumbar drains sets are available commercially. Most include 14G Tuohy needle, through which a five French external lumbar catheter is introduced. The author prefers using External Silverline (Spiegelberg GmbH & Co. KG) lumbar catheters as they have the theoretical advantage of less risk of infection. Use of prophylactic antibiotics according the local hospital policy is advisable.

Unless the MRI scan findings dictate otherwise, Tuohy needle is introduced at L3/L4 level and advanced to the spinal canal. Paramedian approach is often needed in patients in this age group, given the degenerative changes affecting the spine. Operator will need to negotiate bony landmarks, reaching a small window into the canal, with CSF space entrance evident on withdrawing the Tuohy obturator. Fluoroscopic guidance could be useful in difficult cases.

Once the needle in within the right space, careful withdrawal of obturator and introduction of catheter is done. In sitting position, care should be taken to avoid sudden large loss of CSF, as this could result in over-drainage headache and risk of subdural hygroma or even haematoma formation.

Commonly, catheter will not progress beyond the tip of the needle. In these occasions, rotating the Tuohy needle by 90° increment in each direction, could often allow the catheter advance by bypassing bony or ligamentous obstacles. If catheter still fails to advance, careful withdrawal of the needle by one or two millimetres would allow the catheter to advance if the needle tip is against an obstacle. Care should be taken to avoid shearing the catheter against the sharp end of the needle. A guidewire is used only if catheter advancement is difficult. Once a sufficient length of the catheter is introduced, needle could be withdrawn over the remaining distal part of the catheter and disposed off securely. Catheter is then connected to port. Different operators prefer to leave different length of tubing into the spinal canal. There is no evidence this makes any difference. It is advisable at this stage to withdraw enough CSF to reach a total of 40–50 ml of CSF (accounting for the amount lost during the insertion process). The rational of this additional aspiration, is to achieve at least a lumbar tap test outcome, should the drain get disconnected or blocked inadvertently early post-procedure, which would allow for a degree of diagnostic yield.

Suitable dressing is applied to secure the drain. (Tegaderm; 3M Health Care, St. Paul, MN). Various sets have different securing attachments that often require suturing to skin. There are special epidural catheters dressings available, which could avoid need for suturing. These could serve the same purpose with lumbar drains. The distal catheter is then tapped to patient skin (Mefix Mölnlycke Health Care AB) all the way to the tip of right shoulder and then connected to drainage system catheter. The rational of this is to facilitate patient movement post-procedure during hospital stay and reduce risk of inadvertent catheter disconnection.

7　Drainage

Traditionally, simple bags using gravity to assist in drainage (e.g. The Becker® External Drainage and Monitoring System, Medtronic) are connected to external lumbar drains and are mounted on an intravenous fluid carrying pole. These could be set to allow for volume or pressure led drainage. Various operators use different ways draining over 3–5 days up to 500 or 700 ml. Some aim to have continuous drainage, with nurses adjusting the height of the drainage bag in relation to the patient external auditory meatus, to achieve desired drainage. Some simply drain certain volume per hour and then clamp the drain. There is no evidence that a particular volume or number of days would have an advantage. There is no evidence that CSF sampling during drainage would have a benefit, if anything, it might increase risk of infection.

The main problem with traditional drainage bags is that, every time patient changes position, there will be a need to re-adjust bag position or stop drainage. This requires frequent nursing observations, particularly with non-compliant patients who have impaired cognitive function, where sudden changes in patient position could result in large and rapid CSF loss.

The author now routinely uses automated drainage system (Liquoguard® 7) that allows accurate volume and pressure adjusted CSF drainage continuously. It has been shown to be highly accurate in draining the required volume with no need to restrict patient's mobility or stop drainage on changing position. It has also been shown to reduce severity of headache symptoms associated with CSF drainage in some patients. The parameters are set to drain up to ten millilitre per hour unless the intracranial pressure is very low. In the majority of iNPH patients, this translates into more than 500 ml drained over 72 hours. If patients develop severe over-drainage symptoms, drainage volume is reduced or even stopped for few hours until patient is symptomatically improved.

Patients are encouraged to ask for nursing assistance to transfer from bed to chair or to walk to toilets. Particular considerations are needed to reduce risk of falls as well as tube disconnection. This include careful nursing, bed rails elevation and using bed alarms when available to alert nursing staff to patients trying to leave bed.

Graded compression stockings and pneumatic boots are used to reduce risk of deep venous thrombosis. Administration of low molecular weight heparin should be considered after discussing with treating team and in accordance with local policy.

In the event of drain blockage, drain dressing is exposed to exclude presence of tube kink. If there is no clear external kink, careful flushing of the drain is attempted under aseptic technique. If this fails in achieving drainage, drain would be removed and walking test is repeated. If tube gets accidentally disconnected or snapped, drain is clamped and, if the event is discovered soon after occurrence, reconnection is done under aseptic technique. Low threshold should be adopted for drain removal if there is any concern of contamination, or if drain is discovered to have significant amount of CSF over significant amount of time. This is important to reduce risk of infection, which could have serious consequences in this group of patients.

In patients were drainage is interrupted soon after insertion with no significant drainage, and where walking test shows no clear change, no attempt is made of reinserting the drain in the same setting. Patients are discharged home and reassessed as outpatient to discuss options again.

Patients who report clear improvement in their mobility would undergo repeat walking assessment with drain in place. Those who achieve more than 20% improvement in walking speed will have drain removed at that stage without the need to complete the 72 hours. In the absence of that, drain is removed at 72 hours and post-drain assessment is conducted after a couple of hours.

Drain removal is done in the ward with patient on lateral position. Under aseptic technique, dressings are removed, and tube is pulled out ensuring that all parts are removed. Choice of inserting a stich or simple compression dressing is dependant on local team preference.

Patients are then be assessed by occupational therapist to assess for suitability to be discharged home, with clear advice regarding post-operative care, removal of stich if inserted, and need to seek medical help should signs of infection are noticed.

In patients who achieve satisfactory drainage and complete assessments as planned, post-operative review in outpatient clinic is conducted in about 3–4 weeks. Those who have objective improvement in walking speed are advised to have shunt surgery. A gap of few weeks is left between the two procedures to reduce risk of central nervous system and systemic infection. Those patients who have no objective or subjective improvement are advised against shunt surgery, as it would be unlikely to result in improvement. Occasionally, patients and family notice delayed subjective improvement following discharge with no objective improvement in mobility or cognitive assessment. Careful consideration of options should be discussed as chances of improvement would be low. However, in the author experience, some patients who developed low pressure symptoms during admission did notice improvement in their mobility after few days, indicating that the low pressure symptoms have masked the modest benefit with drainage. In these circumstances, it would not be unreasonable to proceed to shunting, aiming, if anything, to reduce chances of future deterioration.

8 Complications

Although lumbar drain insertion and external drainage are deemed to be simple, these are not without risk. The chance of having a complication is often underestimated. The majority of complications are simple and reversible but in a small percentage, the complication could be major.

El Ahmadieh et al. [7] recently published a large single-centre retrospective cohort of 254 patients reporting 5.5% had complications, which was minor in majority of 14 affected patients but included three patients developing meningitis and one developing epidural abscess. Governale et al. [6] also reported a large retrospective cohort complications rate of There were significant complications in 3.0% of patients, including symptomatic subdural or subarachnoid haemorrhage in 1.7%, meningitis in 0.8%, and retained catheter in 0.4%. Another 5.2% of patients had minor problems, including nerve root irritation in 2.6%, low-pressure headache substantial enough to warrant premature removal of the drain in 1.7%, and local infection in 0.8%.

Over-drainage: Headache and nausea should be managed by reducing drainage volume. In a minority of patients, these could be significant, even after complete drainage cessation, and might last for few weeks. Management is by adhering to bed rest, increase fluid intake, in particular, drinks with caffeine and prescribing anti sickness. Subdural hygromas or even haematomas are infrequent occurrence. Intraventricular or subarachnoid haemorrhage are rare reported complications. Use of automated drainage systems (like Liquoguard 7) is likely to reduce the likelihood of such occurrence.

Spinal nerve root irritations: This is often mild and settles with time. Some patients report numbness. Management with analgesia is often enough to control symptoms. In patients where symptoms are severe, shortening of the intradural part of the catheter could resolve the problem. These symptoms are usually resolved when drain is removed. Persistent symptoms after drain removal would need investigation with MRI scan to exclude subdural empyema or haematoma.

Leak at the insertion site: This often happens if multiple puncture sites are used due to difficulty entering spinal canal during drain insertion, in patients with marked degenerative changes. Pressure dressing is likely to stop the leak.

Infection: Inserting a lumbar drain under aseptic technique would reduce this occurrence but would not eliminate it. Bed-bound frail patients are more at risk. Drain disconnection and CSF leak is likely to increase the risk. Low threshold to treat with antibiotics would reduce risk of superficial infection spreading to cause meningitis or epidural empyema.

Retained (sheared) catheter: This is likely to be caused during insertion on withdrawing a catheter caught on sharp edge of Tuohy needle. Upon removal of every lumbar drain, inspection to ensure complete removal is needed. In the event of catheter retention, no specific intervention is needed apart from informing patient and caring team. There will be a need, however, to surgically retrieve the catheter tip, should patient develop infection, as the retained piece of tube will prevent elimination of the infection.

Prolonged hospital length of stay: Elderly frail patients could be judged by occupational therapists not fit for discharge home, particularly in patients who have negative results from the drain or those who have severe over drainage symptoms. Careful preadmission assessment by occupational therapist could prevent this by allowing for provision of necessary support at home settings.

9 Conclusion

Extended lumbar drainage is the most accurate supplementary test that could help clinicians, patients and carers, in accepting or refuting shunt surgery for management of possible normal pressure hydrocephalus. In essence, it is a temporary shunt. It does require hospital admission for few days; hence, it does have implications on costs. It is also associated with risk of complications. It can be done under local anaesthetic, with or without sedation. Best outcome could be achieved if it is done by a team familiar in managing this elderly often co morbid and frail group of patients, and with expertise in conducting necessary assessments aiming to detect objective change in baseline clinical parameters. Attention to details during drain insertion and subsequent drainage by trained team is essential to produce good outcome.

Key Points

- Extended lumbar drainage is, in essence, temporary shunting.
- ELD is the most accurate test in predicting shunt responsiveness in patients with normal pressure hydrocephalus.
- ELD is often regarded by sceptical clinicians, as well as patients and carers, as an acceptable procedure that will help in accepting or refuting future shunt surgery.
- Lumbar drain insertion requires hospitalisation, with costs implications.
- Common ELD complications includes infection, over drainage and prolonged hospital stay.

- Risk of complications can be mitigated by careful preadmission preparation, attention to details in insertion and connection to drainage system as well as good nursing care and therapist's assessment. That is, it requires team approach.

References

1. Nunn AC, Jones HE, Morosanu CO, Singleton WGB, Williams MA, Nagel SJ, Luciano MG, Zwimpfer TJ, Holubkov R, Wisoff JH, McKhann GM 2nd, Hamilton MG, Edwards RJ. Extended lumbar drainage in idiopathic normal pressure hydrocephalus: a systematic review and meta-analysis of diagnostic test accuracy. Br J Neurosurg. 2021 Jun;35(3):285–91. https://doi.org/10.1080/02688697.2020.1787948. Epub 2020 Jul 9. PMID: 32643967.
2. Marmarou A, Bergsneider M, Klinge P, Relkin N, Black PM. The value of supplemental prognostic tests for the preoperative assessment of idiopathic normal-pressure hydrocephalus. Neurosurgery. 2005 Sep;57(3 Suppl):S17–28; discussion ii-v. https://doi.org/10.1227/01.neu.0000168184.01002.60. PMID: 16160426.
3. Haan J, Thomeer RT. Predictive value of temporary external lumbar drainage in normal pressure hydrocephalus. Neurosurgery. 1988 Feb;22(2):388–91. https://doi.org/10.1227/00006123-198802000-00020. PMID: 3352890.
4. Walchenbach R, Geiger E, Thomeer RT, Vanneste JA. The value of temporary external lumbar CSF drainage in predicting the outcome of shunting on normal pressure hydrocephalus. J Neurol Neurosurg Psychiatry. 2002 Apr;72(4):503–6. https://doi.org/10.1136/jnnp.72.4.503. PMID: 11909911; PMCID: PMC1737811.
5. Williams MA, Razumovsky AY, Hanley DF. Comparison of Pcsf monitoring and controlled CSF drainage diagnose normal pressure hydrocephalus. Acta Neurochir Suppl. 1998;71:328–30. https://doi.org/10.1007/978-3-7091-6475-4_95. PMID: 9779221.
6. Governale LS, Fein N, Logsdon J, Black PM. Techniques and complications of external lumbar drainage for normal pressure hydrocephalus. Neurosurgery. 2008 Oct;63(4 Suppl 2):379–84; discussion 384. https://doi.org/10.1227/01.NEU.0000327023.18220.88. PMID: 18981847.
7. El Ahmadieh TY, Wu EM, Kafka B, Caruso JP, Neeley OJ, Plitt A, Aoun SG, Olson DM, Ruchinskas RA, Cullum CM, Barnett S, Welch BG, Batjer HH, White JA. Lumbar drain trial outcomes of normal pressure hydrocephalus: a single-center experience of 254 patients. J Neurosurg. 2019 Jan 4;132(1):306–12. https://doi.org/10.3171/2018.8.JNS181059. PMID: 30611143.
8. Nakajima M, Yamada S, Miyajima M, Ishii K, Kuriyama N, Kazui H, Kanemoto H, Suehiro T, Yoshiyama K, Kameda M, Kajimoto Y, Mase M, Murai H, Kita D, Kimura T, Samejima N, Tokuda T, Kaijima M, Akiba C, Kawamura K, Atsuchi M, Hirata Y, Matsumae M, Sasaki M, Yamashita F, Aoki S, Irie R, Miyake H, Kato T, Mori E, Ishikawa M, Date I, Arai H; research committee of idiopathic normal pressure hydrocephalus. Guidelines for Management of Idiopathic Normal Pressure Hydrocephalus (Third Edition): Endorsed by the Japanese Society of Normal Pressure Hydrocephalus. Neurol Med Chir (Tokyo). 2021 Feb 15;61(2):63–97. https://doi.org/10.2176/nmc.st.2020-0292. Epub 2021 Jan 15. PMID: 33455998; PMCID: PMC7905302.

Spinal Tap Test

Uwe Kehler

Abstract The spinal tap test (STT) is a clinical functional test used to diagnose normal pressure hydrocephalus (NPH). Although the STT is widely accepted to serve as a credible test in the diagnosis of NPH, negative STT does not completely rule out a definite NPH diagnosis and it does not serve as a single determinant of surgical candidates. So far, there is no existing consent about the time of clinical examination following the cerebrospinal fluid-tapping. Some NPH patients may improve immediately after the STT but only for a very short time, others may show delayed gait improvements within the following days. Continuous observation after STT is therefore necessary in order to prevent unwanted omission of patients with NPH who experience short-term improvements in between the clinical examinations. The positive tap test with objective clinical improvement correlates with a good shunt outcome, and a subjective improvement after lumbar drainage has the same predictive value as an objective improvement itself. Additionally, since the clinical tests for NPH after STT are not sensitive enough to detect objective clinical improvement, subjective improvement after STT seems to be a reliable diagnostic factor as good as an objective improvement for predicting shunt responsiveness.

Keywords Spinal tap test · Hydrocephalus · Neurofunctional testing · Normal pressure hydrocephalus · Clinical tests

Abbreviations

CSF   Cerebrospinal fluid
ICP   Intracranial pressure
NPH   Normal pressure hydrocephalus
STT   Spinal tap test

U. Kehler (✉)
Department of Neurosurgery, Asklepios Klinik Altona, 22763 Hamburg, Germany

© The Author(s), under exclusive license to Springer Nature Switzerland AG 2023   221
O. Bradac (ed.), *Normal Pressure Hydrocephalus*,
https://doi.org/10.1007/978-3-031-36522-5_13

1   Introduction

The spinal tap test is probably the most common test to verify the diagnosis of NPH. However, the reliability is controversial, and a subject of ongoing discussion. There is general consent that a temporary clinical improvement after the tap test predicts a positive outcome of shunting. But the predictive value of the negative tap test is low and remains a topic of discussion [1, 2].

2   How to Perform a Spinal Tap Test

The patient with the suspected NPH is laid in the lateral position (if you want to determine ICP as well) or in the sitting position (easier to puncture). After disinfection of the skin, the lumbar subarachnoid space is punctured with a 'traumatic' lumbar puncture needle caudal of the spinal cord—most often in the levels L4/5, L3/4 and L5/S1 (Fig. 1). The puncture can be done with or without local anaesthesia.

Around 40 ml of CSF should be collected, if the patient starts complaining of a headache, further tapping should be stopped in order not to provoke severe over drainage/low-pressure discomfort. However, in NPH, a post-punctional headache is rare.

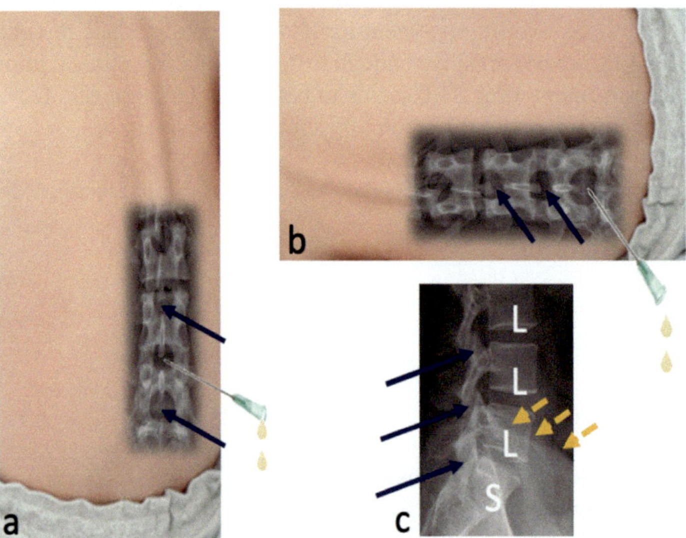

Fig. 1 The puncture for the tap test can be done in sitting (**a**) or lateral position (**b**). Most often the levels L3/4, L4/5 or L5/S1 are used for puncture. L4/5 is located approximately at the level of the iliac crest—image (**c**) yellow arrows. In the lateral position (**b**) the puncture needle can be connected to a riser tube, to measure ICP—the zero level is the spine

A traumatic needle is recommended for the tap test because the chance of a longer lasting hole in the dura may facilitate CSF drainage to the muscle and subcutaneous tissue even after removing the needle. This may result in a clearer and prolonged improvement of symptoms.

Optionally, in the lateral position, before collecting CSF, a riser tube can be connected to the lumbar puncture needle to measure the ICP and even determine the pulse amplitude, getting additional information to confirm the diagnosis.

No consensus exists about the time of clinical examination after the CSF-tapping [3]. Several patients may improve immediately after the tap test but only for a very short time, others may show delayed gait improvements over the following days. Figure 2 shows the clinical course of different patients after tapping. Each colour represents a different patient. Patients show different clinical courses after tapping with immediate distinct but short improvements, others with delayed improvements or with only slight improvements, which may be recognized by the patients themselves but not shown by the insensitive gait tests. Figure 2 also shows, if a clinical examination is done only once after 3, 6 or 24 h after the tapping, the temporary improvement might be missed—which easily might result in a false-negative tap test.

In our department, no bed rest is recommended after the puncture and observation starts immediately. Due to the different courses after tapping and the lack of manpower (for examining the patients every hour), an observation sheet (Fig. 3) is handed over to the patients, where they have to log in the noticed gait changes every hour and from the second day on once a day for a whole week. They are also asked to write a diary about changes in bladder function (especially regarding urgency) and

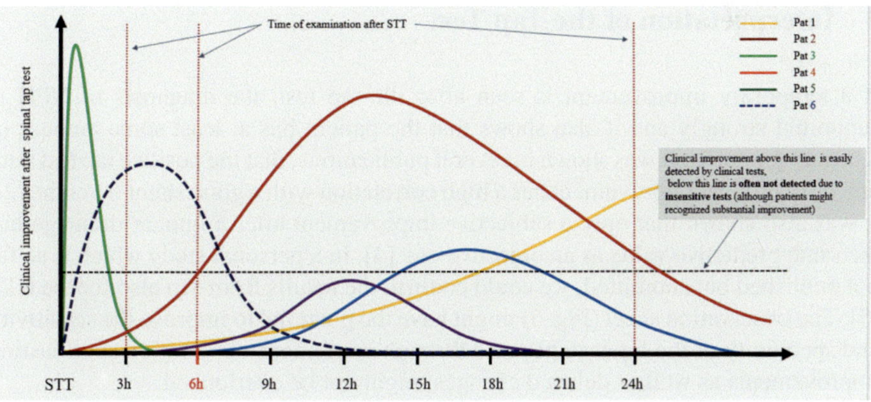

Fig. 2 Different clinical courses after STT. Each colour represents a different patient. The courses show a large variety with short-term distinct improvement (green), intermediate slight improvement (purple) or delayed substantial improvement (yellow). If the curves exceed the dotted line, the improvement could be demonstrated with objective tests. Curves below show only slight improvement—noticed by the patients—but not detected by the low sensitivity of the objective tests. The figure also shows that if only one or two clinical examinations are done there is a chance that the improvements can be missed

224 U. Kehler

Spinal-Tap-Test (STT) – Observation Sheet

Name:

Lumbar puncture (LP) date: xx.xx.20xx   Time: xx:xx   Volume tapped: xx ml

Gait:

Pre STT	Changes after STT		LP		0.5 hour	1 hour	2 hours	3 hours	4 hours	5 hours	6 hours	12 hours	1 day	2 days	3 days	4 days	5 days	6 days	7 days
	massive improvement	😊😊😊😊	LP				X	X											
	marked improvement	😊😊😊	LP			X			X										
Gait pre STT	slight improvement	😊😊	LP	X						X	X								
	very slight improvement	😊	LP									X	X						
X	no change	😐	LP											X	X	X	X	X	X
	deterioration	🙁	LP																

Fig. 3 An observation sheet completed by a patient after the spinal tap test that shows a temporary gait improvement in the first hours. Patients (and their families) should document in a diary as well about bladder function (frequency and urgency) and cognitive changes

about the cognitive changes together with the family members. So, we do get a more or less continuous impression from the clinical course after the tap test. Additionally, the same day and the following day a clinical objective gait examination is done by the attending physicians.

3 Interpretation of the Tap Test

If a temporary improvement is seen after the tap test, the diagnosis of NPH is supported strongly and it also shows that the patient has at least some amount of recovery potential. It was shown in several publications, that the positive tap test with objective clinical improvement has a high correlation with a good shunt outcome [2]. It was also shown that only a subjective improvement after a lumbar drainage has the same predictive value as an objective one [4]. In a personal study which is so far not published but submitted, we could confirm the results from Wu also for the STT [5]. The observation sheet (Fig. 3) might have the potential to improve the sensitivity and specificity of the tap test, because through continuous observation short lasting improvements as well as delayed changes might not be overlooked.

If there is no temporary improvement at all, it does not rule out a diagnosis of normal pressure hydrocephalus [2]. A repeated tap test the following day might show a clearer result. In negative results, the tap test should be repeated after 6–12 weeks or complemented by a temporary lumbar drainage, infusion tests, etc.

The aim is to not overlook any NPH patient and consequently to not withhold beneficial shunt surgery. On the other hand, no patient should be shunted if NPH is not the cause of the clinical symptoms.

4 Conclusion

The spinal tap test is easy to perform and can be used to prove the diagnosis of suspected NPH. However, because of individual variable clinical responses, frequent gait testing is necessary, so that an improvement is not overseen. The observation sheet completed by the patients can be very helpful in realizing almost continuous monitoring, which also detects short-term improvements. Subjective improvements after STT seems to be as good as an objective improvements for the diagnosis of NPH and for shunt responsiveness. In cases of no clinical improvement after STT, patients should undergo a repeated STT or additional testing with more invasive procedures as with lumbar drain or infusion tests.

5 Key Points

- STT is easy to perform and widely accepted to prove the diagnosis of NPH.
- Negative STT does not completely rule out NPH.
- Continuous observation after STT is necessary—otherwise several patients with short-time improvements in-between the clinical examinations are missed.
- Clinical tests for NPH after STT are not sensitive enough to detect improvement despite improvements noticed by the patients and relatives.
- Subjective improvement after STT seems to be as good as objective improvement for predicting shunt responsiveness.

References

1. Gallia GL, Rigamonti D, Williams MA. The diagnosis and treatment of idiopathic normal pressure hydrocephalus. Nat Clin Pract Neurol. 2006;2(7):375–81. https://doi.org/10.1038/ncp neuro0237.
2. Wikkelsø C, Hellström P, et al. European iNPH multicentre study group: study on the predictive values of resistance to CSF outflow and the CSF tap test in patients with idiopathic normal pressure hydrocephalus the European iNPH multicentre. Neurol Neurosurg Psychiatry. 2013;84(5):562–8. https://doi.org/10.1136/jnnp-2012-303314.
3. Caiyan L, Liling D, Jie L, et al. A pilot study of multiple time points and multidomain assessment in cerebrospinal fluid tap test for patients with idiopathic normal pressure hydrocephalus. Clin Neurol Neurosurg. 2021;210:107012. https://doi.org/10.1016/j.clineuro.2021. 107012. Epub 2021 Nov 2.

4. Wu EM, et al. Clinical outcomes of normal pressure hydrocephalus in 116 patients: objective versus subjective assessment. J Neurosurg. 2019;12:1–7.
5. Greiner-Perth M, Mersch M, Kehler U: NPH—Subjective improvement after STT predicts good outcome after shunting. Submitted.

Lumbar Infusion Test

**Petr Skalický, Arnošt Mládek, Adéla Bubeníková, Aleš Vlasák,
Helen Whitley, and Ondřej Bradáč**

Abstract The lumbar infusion test (LIT) is one of the most commonly used functional tests clinically useful for the diagnostic examination of normal pressure hydrocephalus (NPH). During the test, intracranial pressure (ICP) is measured while a cerebrospinal fluid substitute (commonly Ringer's solution) is infused into the subarachnoid space in the lumbar region. Within the evaluation of the results, the resistance of the system is determined. One of the most evaluated parameters is resistance to outflow (Rout). Autoregulation is better preserved in patients with increased Rout, most likely thanks to greater cerebrovascular load in patients with normal or low resistance. The most used cut-off value for iNPH diagnosis is 12 mmHg/ml/min. The tests' measurements can be affected by various factors, including different needle(s) diameters, length and types of connecting tubes, but also compliance of the patient which can significantly affect the validity of the test results. This chapter discusses the physical principles of the LIT, the procedure itself, and further demonstrates the results of this test in NPH diagnosis.

Keywords Lumbar infusion test · Cerebrospinal fluid · Hydrocephalus · Normal pressure hydrocephalus · Cerebral blood flow · Intracranial pressure

P. Skalický · A. Mládek · A. Bubeníková · A. Vlasák · O. Bradáč (✉)
Department of Neurosurgery, 2nd Medical Faculty, Charles University and Motol University Hospital, Prague, Czech Republic
e-mail: ondrej.bradac2@fnmotol.cz

A. Mládek
Department of Cognitive Systems and Neurosciences, Czech Institute of Informatics, Robotics and Cybernetics, Czech Technical University, Prague, Czech Republic

A. Bubeníková · H. Whitley · O. Bradáč
Department of Neurosurgery and Neurooncology, 1st Medical Faculty, Charles University and Military University Hospital, Prague, Czech Republic

227

O. Bradac (ed.), *Normal Pressure Hydrocephalus*,
https://doi.org/10.1007/978-3-031-36522-5_14

Abbreviations

AMP   Amplitude
CaBV   Cerebral arterial blood volume
CBF   Cerebral blood flow
CSF   Cerebrospinal fluid
E   Elastance coefficient
ECG   Electrocardiogram
FV   Flow velocity
ICP   Intracranial pressure
iNPH   Idiopathic normal pressure hydrocephalus
LIT   Lumbar infusion test
NIRS   Near-infrared spectroscopy
NPH   Normal pressure hydrocephalus
RAP   Pressure-volume compensatory reserve
VP   Ventriculoperitoneal

1   Introduction

Normal pressure hydrocephalus (NPH) is a clinical syndrome characterised by a clinical triad of gait apraxia, urinary incontinence and cognitive impairment, associated with dilation of cerebral ventricles and normal cerebrospinal fluid (CSF) pressure. It is classified either as idiopathic or secondary to certain processes such as subarachnoid haemorrhage, traumatic brain injury or meningitis. The treatment is the placement of a shunt system to derive the cerebrospinal fluid mainly from the lateral ventricles of the brain elsewhere, mainly to the peritoneal cavity. The diagnosis is based on a combination of clinical symptoms, radiological findings and results of functional tests using invasive methods.

One of the functional tests is the lumbar infusion test (LIT). The basic technique of the LIT was described by Katzman and Hussey as early as 1970 [1]. During the test, intracranial pressure (ICP) is measured while a cerebrospinal fluid substitute (usually Ringer's solution) is infused into the lumbar subarachnoid space. The course of the test can be complicated by reduced compliance of the patient, which affects the validity of the result [2]. However, the test can usually be performed without sedation of the patient with or without the use of local anaesthesia. For the validity and evaluation of the results, the resistance of the system must be determined, which is different when using different diameters of the needle or needles, length and type of connecting tubes. The infusion rate is usually 1.5 ml per minute. From the change in the character of the pressure curve and its values, parameters about the dynamics of the cerebrospinal fluid circulation can be determined. Most often, the outflow resistance, (Rout) [3], is calculated, which corresponds to the difference in the resulting pressure in the phase when the ICP does not increase further during constant infusion (the so-called plateau phase), from the initial pressure values minus the system resistance, divided by the infusion rate [4]. An alternative assessment that is also widely used, despite lower evidence, is the modification according to Nelson and Goodman in 1971, which only calculates the average increase in ICP over a certain period of time (usually 10–15 min) [5]. The most accepted cut-off value for LIT positivity is a Rout value greater than 12 mmHg/ml/min [6]. In healthy volunteers, it was shown that the value of Rout did not exceed 10 mmHg/ml/min [7]. Another study [8] in iNPH patients showed that if Rout was less than 6 mmHg/ml/min, no improvement after shunt insertion was observed. Other indicators within LIT were weakly associated with the outcome of shunting. Although an association of degree of symptom improvement after ventriculoperitoneal (VP) shunt implantation with Rout value in a European multicentre study was not found [9], when resistance higher than 8 mmHg/ml/min was used, accuracy was higher than for Tap test.

Autoregulation is better preserved in patients with more increased Rout—probably due to greater cerebrovascular load in patients with normal or low resistance. Despite all the debate over this feature, resistance is the main indicator of impaired cerebrospinal fluid circulation. However, it cannot be used as the sole indicator when deciding on surgery. The negative-predictive value is low too. The result after surgery is multifactorial and it is probably naive to associate it with a single parameter [10]. In the recommendation from the American guidelines at level B [11], it follows that as Rout increases, the probability of response to VP shunt increases. Compared to expert evaluation, when machine learning and artificial intelligence methods were used to calculate and process 48 scalar characteristics of the ICP and electrocardiogram (ECG) signal, this was able to better differentiate patients who responded to the lumbar drainage test. The best method combined eight characteristics by XGBoost classifier, which increased the sensitivity and specificity of the test by more than 21% [12]. LIT is simple to perform, inexpensive, and the diagnostic accuracy is considerable.

2 Introduction to the ICP/CSF Dynamics

According to the Monro-Kellie (M-K) doctrine, assuming an intact and absolutely rigid cranium, the sum of the volumes of the individual intracranial compartments—the brain, cerebrospinal fluid and blood—is constant. Since the compartments are considered to be practically incompressible, an increase in the volume of one compartment must thus be compensated by a corresponding decrease in one or more of the remaining compartments. Changes in volumes are manifested by variations in intracranial pressure.

ICP represents the pressure in the shared intracranial space that acts on individual compartments. Physiological ICP changes periodically with respiration and the cardiac cycle. Transient fluctuations in ICP may occur with a change in body position relative to the gravitational field, coughing or the Valsalva manoeuver [13]. The physiological ICP value in an adult in the supine position is approximately in the range of 7–15 mmHg [14]. If the ICP is persistently elevated above approximately 15 mmHg, intracranial hypertension occurs and the decreasing CBP, the pressure gradient maintaining cerebral perfusion, gradually leads to focal and subsequently global ischemia. In addition, organic lesions, underlying the increase in ICP (more precisely its gradient), may cause a shift of brain structures up to the image of herniation (subfalcine, transtentorial, temporal, occipital). This is the most serious complication of intracranial hypertension.

ICP is more than a number. It is a complex, time-varying biosignal with distinctive properties [15]. The ICP waveform consists of three components that overlap in the time domain, but in the frequency domain, their separation is possible (Fig. 1).

The pulse waveform has fundamental and higher harmonic components. The frequency of the fundamental component corresponds to the heart rate, and the magnitude of its amplitude is important for the evaluation of intracranial physiology. The respiratory waveform is generated by respiratory movements, with a frequency maximum of around 8–20 1/min. The so-called 'slow waves' described in Lundberg's original work [16] (also called B-waves) are not precisely defined, and all contributions corresponding to a period of 20 s to 3 min (0.005–0.05 Hz) fall into this category. Using near-infrared spectroscopy (NIRS), Lundberg's B-waves have been shown to be coherent with fluctuations in cerebral arterial blood volume (CaBV; Fig. 2).

In the time domain, the ICP waveform is characterised by three peaks at P1, P2 and P3 [17]. The first P1 maximum, the so-called percussive peak, is probably associated

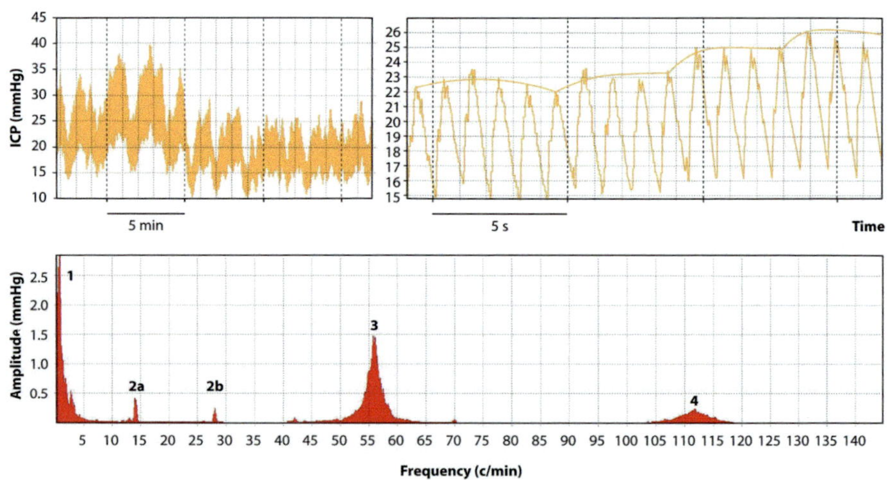

Fig. 1 ICP components observed in the time (yellow) and frequency (red) domains. Upper left panel: slow vasogenic waves (0.005–0.05 Hz) associated with continuous vasomotor activity regulate cerebrovascular resistance, CBF and CBV. Upper right panel: pulse waveform of ICP and respiratory waves. Lower panel: frequency domain of the ICP signal. 1: slow waves, 2a, 2b: respiratory waves (2a) and respiratory higher harmonics (2b), 3, 4: pulse waves (3) and pulse higher harmonics (4). Picture adapted from Czosnyka et al. [15]

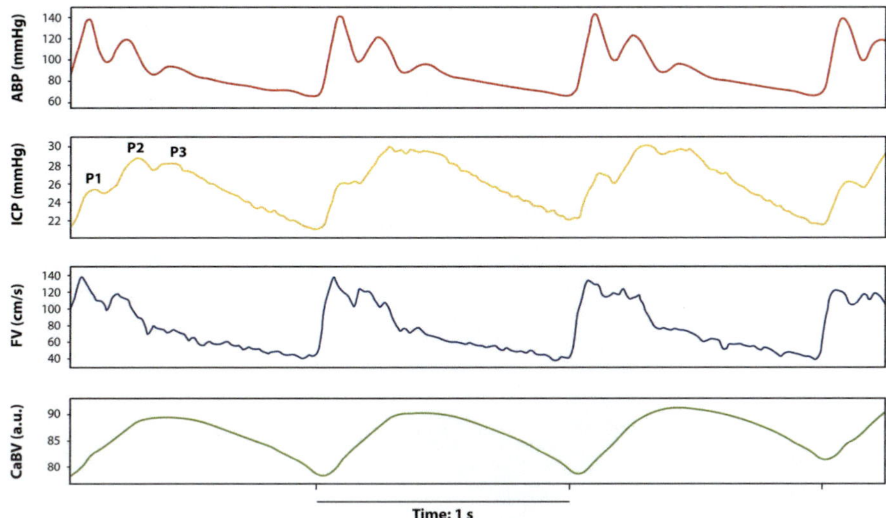

Fig. 2 ABP: arterial blood pressure waveform (red); ICP: intracranial pressure waveform (yellow); FV: flow velocity (blue); CaBV: cerebral arterial blood volume (green). Picture adapted from Czosnyka et al. [15]

with rapid distension of the arterial walls at the moment when arterial pressure reaches its systolic maximum. The late peaks P2 and P3 are probably related to the increase in arterial blood volume and its transport from large, high-flow cerebral arterioles to arterioles of higher resistance. The position and size of P2 and P3 are influenced by intracranial compliance, among other factors. According to some studies [15], P3 is related to the dicrotic notch and the secondary peak in arterial pressure and thus indirectly to the aortic valve closure (Fig. 2).

M–K homoeostasis represents a complex physiological mechanism compensating for the transient increase in CBV during cardiac systole. The goal of M–K homoeostasis is to minimise ICP dispersion during the cardiac cycle and to reduce systolic–diastolic pressure differences at the level of the cerebral microvasculature. Minimization of pressure changes is also maintained by arterial wall elasticity, which dampens the pressure wave amplitude and thus ensures constant blood flow through the capillaries (Windkessel effect, see Chap. 6 for more details regarding this effect). Figure 3 shows a schematic representation of the M–K homeostasis model, which can be used to describe the fluid dynamics for different phases of the cardiac cycle:

During ventricular systole, the cerebral arteries dilate and propagate a pressure wave through the CSF. The fluid is pushed through the foramen magnum in a caudal direction, and the venous outflow increases. During the filling of the ventricles, CSF returns from the extracranial subarachnoidal spaces in a rostral direction back into the intracranial space, venous outflow decreases.

Pathological or physiological increase in the volume of one or more compartments is initially 'buffered' by displacement of an equivalent volume of venous blood

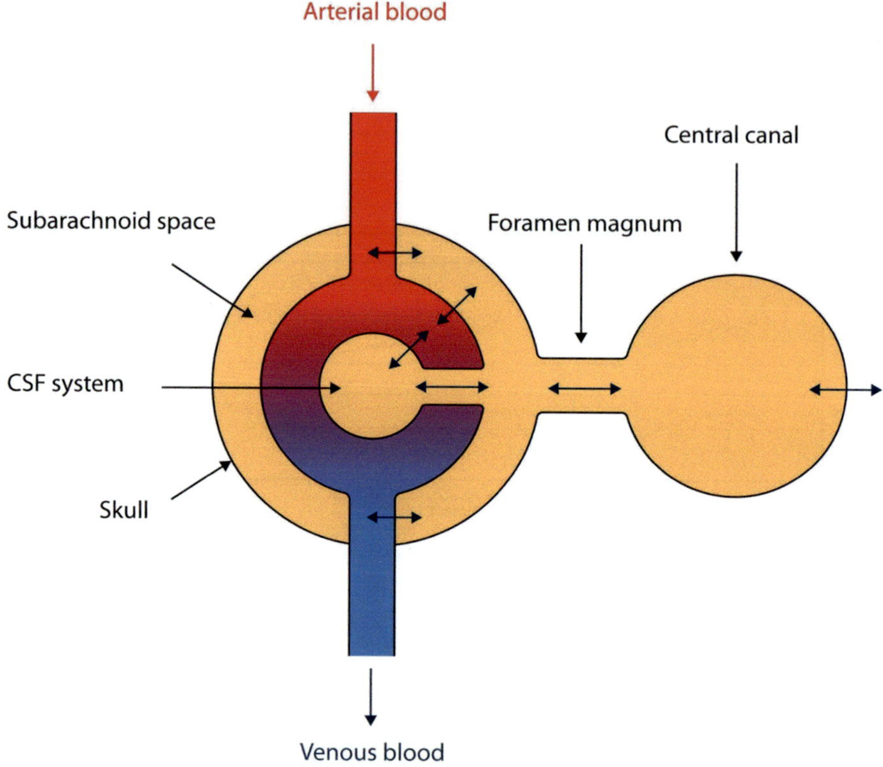

Fig. 3 Schematic model of M–K homoeostasis. Bidirectional arrows across compartments symbolise compliance (possible change of volume of one compartment at the expense of the other), bidirectional arrows within one compartment symbolise liquor communication between extra- and intracranial space

and/or of venous fluid outside the intracranial space. This compensatory mechanism prevents or significantly limits the increase in ICP. The volume of venous blood and CSF responds to the change in intracranial first, as their respective compartments (venous sinuses and subarachnoid space) are very compliant (compliance $\sim$ dV/dp). The state of the system is at the interval of moderate linear increase on the pressure–volume (pV) curve with a good compensatory margin; the correlation coefficient between the change in pulse amplitude and the mean ICP value (RAP coefficient) is equal to 0, the pulse amplitude of ICP does not change with intracranial pressure. The upper limit of ICP to maintain good compensatory reserve is the exponential growth threshold (Fig. 4).

In case of further increase in intraluminal volume, ICP increases exponentially and the system reaches the area of weak compensatory reserve. Compliance decreases rapidly, the RAP coefficient is equal to 1. The pulse amplitude of ICP increases linearly with the mean value of ICP.

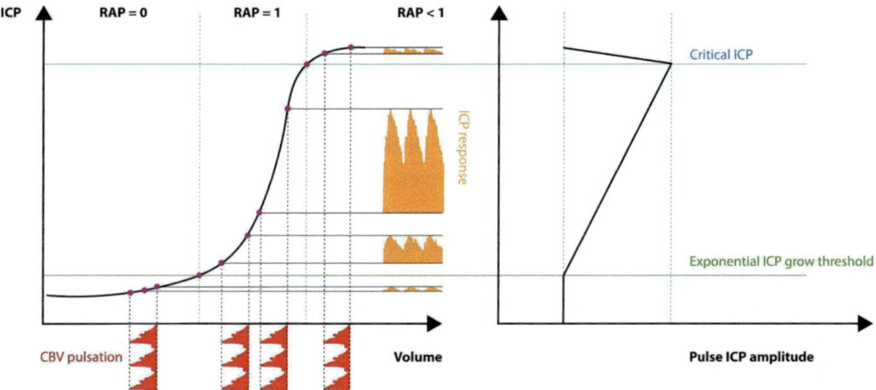

Fig. 4 Intracranial pressure-volume diagram (left) and the relationship between the mean ICP value and the amplitude of its pulse component (right). RAP: correlation coefficient between the change in pulse amplitude and the mean ICP value. The pulsations of CBV are shown in red, and the pulsatile response of ICP is in yellow. System elastance is proportional to the dp/dV. Picture adapted from Czosnyka et al. [15]

If the ICP exceeds a critical value, regulatory mechanisms fail and cerebral arterioles become active. ICP pulse amplitude decreases rapidly, although mean ICP continues to increase; RAP < 1. ICP and mean arterial pressure (MAP) gradually equilibrate, and perfusion pressure is low.

The Monro-Kellie doctrine of intracranial volume compensations leads to interactions of the CSF dynamics and hemodynamics related to the ICP pulsations with cardiac frequency caused by the transient increase in arterial blood occurring with each stroke [18]. The pulse amplitude of ICP pulsations depends on the compliance of the system, or from the opposite point of view the outflow resistance (Rout) as the major aspect of CSF dynamics. One of the approaches to functional testing is to investigate CSF dynamics with a lumbar infusion test.

Some of the theories of the pathophysiology of idiopathic normal pressure hydrocephalus (iNPH) favour a decrease in intracranial compliance as an important underlying principle. Di Rocco et al. [19] stressed the role of pulsations, demonstrating how CSF pulsatility can lead to ventricular dilation. The ICP fluctuation of waves consists of those reflecting arterial pulsations, with other vasogenic components and elevations with breathing. Cough and movements can influence the process. Lundberg identified slow waves—spontaneous rhythmic oscillations of ICP from 0.5 to 2 cycles per minute with variable amplitude [16]. The relatively high frequency of slow waves is indicative of reduced craniospinal compliance [20]. However, cut-offs for the frequency and amplitude vary widely [21].

In a study group of 35 patients, the authors demonstrated a change in blood flow velocity in the middle cerebral artery during the infusion test. The observation resulted in a decrease in the mean blood flow velocity by 4 cm/s, which did not correlate with CSF pressure [22]. A study on 40 NPH patients showed that mean cerebral blood flow is maintained despite a significant increase in ICP within the limits of the infusion test. A relative increase in the pulsatility indices of cerebral blood flow (CBF) was noted, which may indicate preserved cerebrovascular reactivity [23].

The classic theory of CSF dynamics describes a CSF pathway. This consists of compartments that produce resistance to outflow (Rout) as CSF circulates. NPH patients have normal CSF pressure, however, abnormalities in the outflow may be involved [6].

The measures are extracted from the recorded pressure curves. The initial baseline pressure is extracted as the mean at the start of the infusion. The plateau pressure is derived from the mean pressure in a pressure-stable phase during the infusion [24]. These results can be used for the determination of various cerebrospinal fluid dynamics variables. The most frequently used is the outflow resistance (Rout) or outflow conductance (Cout). Rout is the difference between the plateau and baseline pressure minus system resistance divided by the infusion rate. The other comprises the pressure curve characteristics devoted mainly to the amplitude. Baseline amplitude is the mean of the difference between systolic and diastolic pressure before starting the infusion. Plateau amplitude is the mean of the difference between systolic and diastolic pressure during the plateau phase (Fig. 5) [25]. The resistance of Rout correlates with the magnitude of slow vasogenic components of ICP—respiratory waves and slow waves in the spectrum similar to Lundberg's 'B' waves. All vasogenic components increase during CSF volume load [26].

Change of Rout has been seen to occur with time in hydrocephalus after subarachnoid haemorrhage [27] and with increasing age [28]. Changes in Rout and other physiological parameters probably also occur in iNPH patients. The exact mechanisms are unknown but might be due to increased time of transparenchymal drainage [29].

One may also calculate the elastance coefficient (E). The exact meaning of E is not yet fully understood. It describes the stiffness of the cerebrospinal system determined by the ability to displace a volume of cerebrospinal blood. Tans and Poortvliet [30] showed a weak correlation of Rout and E, though no further studies exploring this

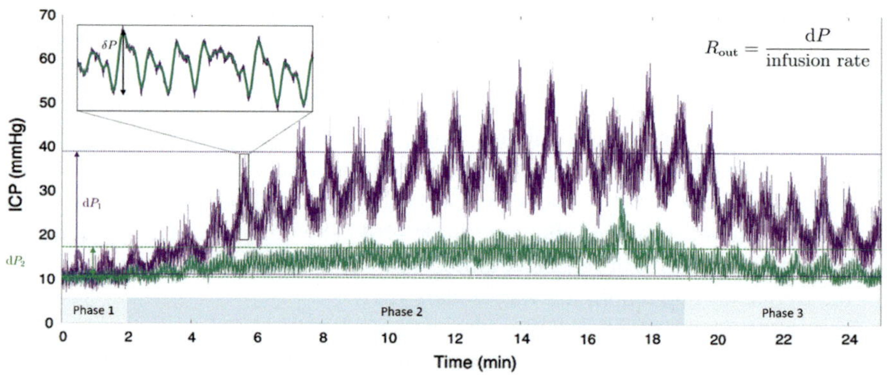

Fig. 5 Illustration of a positive (purple) and negative (green) LIT recording. The pressure difference dP is denoted by the dashed lines. The amplitude difference deltaP is shown in the inlet figure

concept have followed. Tisell et al. [31] demonstrated that elevated E correlated positively with the result of a third ventriculostomy in primary aqueductal stenosis. Thus, E is a parameter that is not widely used for iNPH evaluation.

From the derived parameters, the pressure–volume compensatory reserve (RAP) index may be assessed. It is a correlation coefficient [R] between the amplitude (AMP) [A] and the mean intracranial pressure [P]) and is derived by the linear correlation between 40 consecutive, time-averaged data points of AMP of ICP and mean ICP, acquired within a 6-s-wide time-window. RAP describes the degree of correlation between AMP and mean ICP over short periods of time (4 min). RAP coefficient close to 0 indicates a lack of coupling between the changes in AMP and the mean ICP. This relates to good pressure–volume compensatory reserve, i.e. the working range is still in the horizontal part of the curve. When the pressure–volume curve starts to increase exponentially, AMP co-varies directly with ICP and consequently RAP rises to +1. This indicates a low compensatory reserve [32].

3   Procedure

During infusion, the infused CSF will increase the intracranial CSF volume. This volume will eventually decrease the venous volume and during arterial pulsations the delivered blood is compensated by compression of the venous pool by the same amount. The increased venous outflow resistance causes an increase in intracranial pressure [33].

To perform the lumbar infusion test, you need a monitoring device that could measure the pressure curve via a connected system, often a device which is used for invasive blood pressure monitoring. During the test, the pressure monitor will be connected through the same system with an infusion pump or with a second lumbar cannula. Contemporary ECG measurement could be used to calculate special parameters for novel methods. The lumbar cannula could be 14G Tuohy needle to end the test with lumbar drain insertion or narrower as f.e. 22G needle, but the system resistance will increase and needs to be calculated.

The patient is lying on the side in a horizontal position with head support in order to align the proper position of the inion and spine parallel to the bed or floor. The infusion is usually a Ringer solution (NaCl 6.6 g/l, KCl 0.3 g/l, CaCl 0.33 g/l; 290 mosm/kg). The test starts with a lumbar puncture that could be done only in local or with no anaesthesia in the majority of patients. The system is calibrated, and connected and opening pressure could be taken from the recording device. In normal pressure hydrocephalus, the opening pressure is of maximal 20 mmHg.

Typically, LIT is divided into three phases. The first phase is short for approximately 2 min just to balance the initial value which could be prolonged by bad compliance of the patient. The stable baseline is superimposed by pulse waves— transient pressure increases caused by the arterial blood volume of each pulse stroke. The basal points define the basal pressure amplitude. Mean pressure is used for the calculation of major parameters.

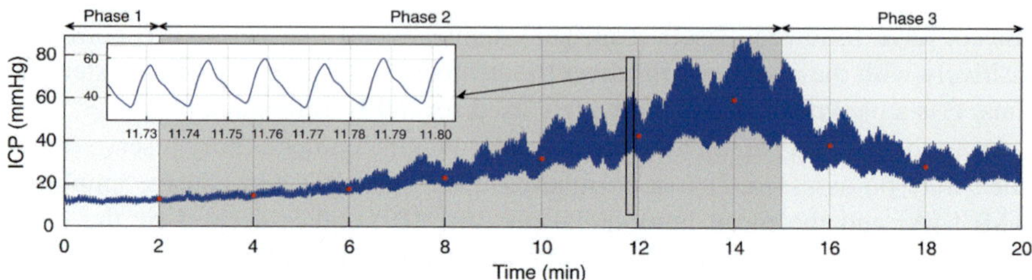

Fig. 6 LIT. ICP measured during LIT

The second phase is usually 10–20 min long. The infusion of Ringer solution is constant at the rate of 1.5 ml/min. The phase stops when the pressure approaches a plateau value which coincides with the maximal outflow resistance (Rout) and is stable for around 3 min or if the mean pressure exceeds 50 mmHg. After the infusion is interrupted the third phase starts which is 5 min long. This measures how the pressure decreases after the interruption of infusion (Fig. 6). After the test the infusion system is disconnected lumbar drain could be inserted or a tap test could be performed and lumbar cannula is extracted and the system resistance is calculated.

4 Results

Cordero Tous et al. [34] found an improvement in 64% of patients after 12 months with the criteria based on having a Rout of more than 12 mmHg/ml/min. They achieved a specificity of 35% and sensitivity of 89%. Another study [25] of 80 patients presented 69% sensitivity and 75% specificity. The positive predictive value of Rout of more than 15 mmHg/ml/min was 91.7%. Another study [35] found a global improvement in 60 (88.2%) patients. The positive predictive value of Rout of more than or equal to 14 mmHg/ml/min was 90%. The Dutch Normal Pressure Hydrocephalus Study [36] reported that improvement in patients selected according to the CSF dynamics test (Ro) reached 74% against 55% in those selected just according to clinical and radiological criteria. According to Albeck et al. [7], in healthy subjects the normal values are 6–10 mmHg/ml/min. Eide et al. [37] calculated the upper limits of normal between 8.33 and 13 mmHg/ml/min in children. Malm et al. [38] found a mean Rout of 8.6 mmHg/ml/min in healthy elderly subjects over 60 years of age.

Another study by Mahr et al. presented 51% specificity and 79% sensitivity of LIT when using a cut-off value of Rout of 12 mmHg/ml/min. ROC analysis showed 13 mmHg/ml/min as an optimal value based on Youden's index. If the Rout was more than 10 mmHg/ml/min the sensitivity was 96%.

A meta-analysis by Kim et al. [6] has shown that a LIT with a Rout > 12 mmHg/mL/min seems to be the most suitable threshold for predicting shunt responsiveness in NPH patients with high accuracy (72.95%), high sensitivity (80.26%), and moderate specificity (46.79%). In a recent overview of diagnostic methods [40] a sensitivity of LIT between 56 and 100% and specificity between 50 and 90% were found. The positive predictive value of LIT was 80% and the occurrence of false negatives was up to 16%. Furthermore, Czosnyka et al. [27] suggested that the threshold for normal Rout should be adjusted according to the duration of symptoms considering a tendency to decrease with time when lasting longer than 2–3 years.

The lumbar infusion test can determine not only the Rout but also the mean amplitudes. Amplitudes tend to be greater in responders versus non-responders, which might reflect a change in the compliance of the system [25]. It was considered abnormal if the mean wave amplitude exceeded 5 mmHg during the night intracranial monitoring [41]. Eide et al. [42] found elevated baseline amplitude higher than 2 mmHg with a positive predictive value of 89%. Kahlon et al. [2] found that 92% of patients with plateau amplitudes of more than 20 mmHg or Rout of more than 18 mmHg/ml/min improved following shunt placement. A study by Santamarta et al. [43] found that the combined use of ICP monitoring and lumbar infusion to forecast the response to shunting in patients with suspected iNPH did not improve the accuracy provided by any of them alone. Meier and Bartels [3] reported that 19% of 107 patients developed headaches after lumbar infusion studies and 2 patients developed meningismus without signs of inflammation in the CSF. Kahlon et al. [44] reported no complications related to the infusion test.

The results of lumbar infusion testing are probably not related to the severity of iNPH. Comparably, the results of lumbar infusion testing probably do not associate with ventricular size as assessed by the Evan's index [1, 45].

Lumbar infusion test can also be used for shunt patency testing. Rout should not be elevated with a proper functioning VP shunt [24, 46, 47].

It was shown in a study of 4473 infusion tests [48] that CSF infusion studies are safe, with the incidence of infection at less than 1%. They presented that raised resistance to CSF outflow positively correlates (p < 0.014) with improvement after shunting and is associated with the disturbance of CBF and its autoregulation (p < 0.02). With the methods of artificial intelligence and machine learning the classificator increased the accuracy of LIT by more than 20% [12]. Such advanced methods could bring new approaches to LIT evaluation to increase its diagnostic yield.

5 Conclusion

Lumbar infusion test is one of the functional tests used in the evaluation of normal pressure hydrocephalus. One of the most evaluated parameters is resistance to outflow (Rout). Autoregulation is better preserved in patients with more increased Rout— probably due to greater cerebrovascular load in patients with normal or low resistance. The most used cut-off value for iNPH diagnosis is 12 mmHg/ml/min. Meta-analysis showed high accuracy (72.95%), high sensitivity (80.26%), and moderate specificity (46.79%). The procedure is straightforward and the technical and operational requirements are low. The knowledge of dynamic CSF parameters may give valuable information for shunt implantation candidates—as Rout increases, the probability of response to VP shunt increases.

6 Key Points

- ICP is more than a number. It is a complex, time-varying biosignal with distinctive properties. During LIT ICP is measured during a constant infusion of artificial CSF. The results can describe basic CSF dynamic parameters.
- The classic theory of CSF dynamics describes a CSF pathway. This consists of compartments that produce resistance to outflow (Rout) as CSF circulates. NPH patients have normal CSF pressure, however, abnormalities in the outflow may be involved.
- Rout corresponds to the difference in the resulting pressure in the phase when the ICP does not increase further during constant infusion (the so-called plateau phase), from the initial pressure values minus the system resistance, divided by the infusion rate.
- Rout > 12 mmHg/ml/min seems to be the most suitable threshold for predicting shunt responsiveness in NPH patients with high accuracy (72.95%), high sensitivity (80.26%), and moderate specificity (46.79%)
- LIT can give valuable information for shunt candidate selection.

Funding This chapter was supported by the Ministry of Health of the Czech Republic institutional grant no. NU23-04-00551.

References

1. Brean A, Eide PK. Assessment of idiopathic normal pressure patients in neurological practice: the role of lumbar infusion testing for referral of patients to neurosurgery. Eur J Neurol. 2008;15(6):605–12. https://doi.org/10.1111/j.1468-1331.2008.02134.x.
2. Kahlon B, Sundbärg G, Rehncrona S. Lumbar infusion test in normal pressure hydrocephalus. Acta Neurol Scand. 2005;111(6):379–84. https://doi.org/10.1111/j.1600-0404.2005.00417.x.
3. Meier U. The importance of the intrathecal infusion test in the diagnostics of normal pressure hydrocephalus. Biomed Tech (Berl). 2001;46(7–8):191–9. https://doi.org/10.1515/bmte.2001.46.7-8.191.
4. Børgesen SE, Gjerris F. Relationships between intracranial pressure, ventricular size, and resistance to CSF outflow. J Neurosurg. 1987;67(4):535–9. https://doi.org/10.3171/jns.1987.67.4.0535.
5. Nelson JR, Goodman SJ. An evaluation of the cerebrospinal fluid infusion test for hydrocephalus. Neurology. 1971;21(10):1037–53. https://doi.org/10.1212/wnl.21.10.1037.
6. Kim DJ, Kim H, Kim YT, Yoon BC, Czosnyka Z, Park KW, et al. Thresholds of resistance to CSF outflow in predicting shunt responsiveness. Neurol Res. 2015;37(4):332–40. https://doi.org/10.1179/1743132814y.0000000454.

7. Albeck MJ, Børgesen SE, Gjerris F, Schmidt JF, Sørensen PS. Intracranial pressure and cerebrospinal fluid outflow conductance in healthy subjects. J Neurosurg. 1991;74(4):597–600. https://doi.org/10.3171/jns.1991.74.4.0597.

8. Nabbanja E, Czosnyka M, Keong NC, Garnett M, Pickard JD, Lalou DA, et al. Is there a link between ICP-derived infusion test parameters and outcome after shunting in normal pressure hydrocephalus? Acta Neurochir Suppl. 2018;126:229–32. https://doi.org/10.1007/978-3-319-65798-1_46.

9. Wikkelsø C, Hellström P, Klinge PM, Tans JT. The European iNPH multicentre study on the predictive values of resistance to CSF outflow and the CSF tap test in patients with idiopathic normal pressure hydrocephalus. J Neurol Neurosurg Psychiatry. 2013;84(5):562–8. https://doi.org/10.1136/jnnp-2012-303314.

10. Lalou AD, Czosnyka M, Donnelly J, Pickard JD, Nabbanja E, Keong NC, et al. Cerebral autoregulation, cerebrospinal fluid outflow resistance, and outcome following cerebrospinal fluid diversion in normal pressure hydrocephalus. J Neurosurg. 2018;130(1):154–62. https://doi.org/10.3171/2017.7.Jns17216.

11. Halperin JJ, Kurlan R, Schwalb JM, Cusimano MD, Gronseth G, Gloss D. Practice guideline: Idiopathic normal pressure hydrocephalus: Response to shunting and predictors of response: Report of the Guideline Development, Dissemination, and Implementation Subcommittee of the American Academy of Neurology. Neurology. 2015;85(23):2063–71. https://doi.org/10.1212/wnl.0000000000002193.

12. Mládek A, Gerla V, Skalický P, Vlasák A, Zazay A, Lhotská L, et al. Prediction of shunt responsiveness in suspected patients with normal pressure hydrocephalus using the lumbar infusion test: a machine learning approach. Neurosurgery. 2022;90(4):407–18. https://doi.org/10.1227/neu.0000000000001838.

13. Oswal A, Toma AK. Intracranial pressure and cerebral haemodynamics. Anaesth Intensive Care Med. 2017;18(5):259–63. https://doi.org/10.1016/j.mpaic.2017.03.002.

14. Steiner LA, Andrews PJ. Monitoring the injured brain: ICP and CBF. Br J Anaesth. 2006;97(1):26–38. https://doi.org/10.1093/bja/ael110.

15. Czosnyka M, Pickard JD, Steiner LA. Principles of intracranial pressure monitoring and treatment. Handb Clin Neurol. 2017;140:67–89. https://doi.org/10.1016/b978-0-444-63600-3.00005-2.

16. Lundberg N. Continuous recording and control of ventricular fluid pressure in neurosurgical practice. Acta Psychiatr Scand Suppl. 1960;36(149):1–193.

17. Cardoso ER, Rowan JO, Galbraith S. Analysis of the cerebrospinal fluid pulse wave in intracranial pressure. J Neurosurg. 1983;59(5):817–21. https://doi.org/10.3171/jns.1983.59.5.0817.

18. Mokri B. The Monro-Kellie hypothesis: applications in CSF volume depletion. Neurology. 2001;56(12):1746–8. https://doi.org/10.1212/wnl.56.12.1746.

19. Pettorossi VE, Di Rocco C, Mancinelli R, Caldarelli M, Velardi F. Communicating hydrocephalus induced by mechanically increased amplitude of the intraventricular cerebrospinal fluid pulse pressure: Rationale and method. Exp Neurol. 1978;59(1):30–9. https://doi.org/10.1016/0014-4886(78)90198-X.

20. Sahuquillo J, Rubio E, Codina A, Molins A, Guitart JM, Poca MA, et al. Reappraisal of the intracranial pressure and cerebrospinal fluid dynamics in patients with the so-called? Normal pressure hydrocephalus? Syndrome. Acta Neurochir. 1991;112(1–2):50–61. https://doi.org/10.1007/bf01402454.

21. Krauss JK, Halve B. Normal pressure hydrocephalus: survey on contemporary diagnostic algorithms and therapeutic decision-making in clinical practice. Acta Neurochir (Wien). 2004;146(4):379–88; discussion 88. https://doi.org/10.1007/s00701-004-0234-3.

22. Czosnyka ZH, Czosnyka M, Whitfield PC, Donovan T, Pickard JD. Cerebral autoregulation among patients with symptoms of hydrocephalus. Neurosurgery. 2002;50(3):526–32; discussion 32–3. https://doi.org/10.1097/00006123-200203000-00018.

23. Adv Clin Exp Med. 2012;21(1):55–61. ISSN 1899-5276.

24. Czosnyka M, Whitehouse H, Smielewski P, Simac S, Pickard JD. Testing of cerebrospinal compensatory reserve in shunted and non-shunted patients: a guide to interpretation based on an observational study. J Neurol Neurosurg Psychiatry. 1996;60(5):549–58. https://doi.org/10.1136/jnnp.60.5.549.

25. Otero Rodríguez Á, Arandia Guzmán D, García Martín A, Torres Carretero L, Garrido Ruiz A, Sousa Casasnovas P, et al. Prognostic value of the pulse pressure amplitudes, time to reach the plateau and the slope obtained in the lumbar infusion test for the study of idiophatic normal pressure hydrocephalus. Neurocirugia (Astur: Engl Ed). 2021. https://doi.org/10.1016/j.neucir.2021.02.004.

26. Momjian S, Czosnyka Z, Czosnyka M, Pickard J. Link between vasogenic waves of intracranial pressure and cerebrospinal fluid outflow resistance in normal pressure hydrocephalus. Br J Neurosurg. 2004;18(1):56–61. https://doi.org/10.1080/02688690410001660481.

27. Czosnyka Z, Owler B, Keong N, Santarius T, Baledent O, Pickard JD, et al. Impact of duration of symptoms on CSF dynamics in idiopathic normal pressure hydrocephalus. Acta Neurol Scand. 2011;123(6):414–8. https://doi.org/10.1111/j.1600-0404.2010.01420.x.

28. Albeck MJ, Skak C, Nielsen PR, Olsen KS, Børgesen SE, Gjerris F. Age dependency of resistance to cerebrospinal fluid outflow. J Neurosurg. 1998;89(2):275–8. https://doi.org/10.3171/jns.1998.89.2.0275.

29. Weller RO, Kida S, Zhang E-T. Pathways of fluid drainage from the brain—morphological aspects and immunological significance in rat and man. Brain Pathol. 1992;2(4):277–84. https://doi.org/10.1111/j.1750-3639.1992.tb00704 x.

30. Tans JT, Poortvliet DC. Relationship between compliance and resistance to outflow of CSF in adult hydrocephalus. J Neurosurg. 1989;71(1):59–62. https://doi.org/10.3171/jns.1989.71.1.0059.

31. Tisell M, Edsbagge M, Stephensen H, Czosnyka M, Wikkelsø C. Elastance correlates with outcome after endoscopic third ventriculostomy in adults with hydrocephalus caused by primary aqueductal stenosis. Neurosurgery. 2002;50(1):70–7. https://doi.org/10.1097/00006123-200201000-00013.

32. Kim DJ, Czosnyka Z, Keong N, Radolovich DK, Smielewski P, Sutcliffe MP, et al. Index of cerebrospinal compensatory reserve in hydrocephalus. Neurosurgery. 2009;64(3):494–501; discussion-2. https://doi.org/10.1227/01.Neu.0000338434.59141.89.

33. Marmarou A, Shulman K, Rosende RM. A nonlinear analysis of the cerebrospinal fluid system and intracranial pressure dynamics. J Neurosurg. 1978;48(3):332–44. https://doi.org/10.3171/jns.1978.48.3.0332.

34. Cordero Tous N, Román Cutillas AM, Jorques Infante AM, Olivares Granados G, Saura Rojas JE, Iañez Velasco B, et al. Hidrocefalia crónica del adulto: diagnóstico, tratamiento y evolución. Estudio Prospectivo Neurocirugía. 2013;24(3):93–101. https://doi.org/10.1016/j.neucir.2011.12.007.

35. Raneri F, Zella MAS, Di Cristofori A, Zarino B, Pluderi M, Spagnoli D. Supplementary tests in idiopathic normal pressure hydrocephalus: a single-center experience with a combined lumbar infusion test and tap test. World Neurosurg. 2017;100:567–74. https://doi.org/10.1016/j.wneu.2017.01.003.

36. Boon AJ, Tans JT, Delwel EJ, Egeler-Peerdeman SM, Hanlo PW, Wurzer HA, et al. Dutch normal-pressure hydrocephalus study: prediction of outcome after shunting by resistance to outflow of cerebrospinal fluid. J Neurosurg. 1997;87(5):687–93. https://doi.org/10.3171/jns.1997.87.5.0687.

37. Eide P, Due-Tønnessen B, Helseth E, Lundar T. Assessment of intracranial pressure volume relationships in childhood: the lumbar infusion test versus intracranial pressure monitoring. Childs Nerv Syst. 2001;17(7):382–90. https://doi.org/10.1007/s003810000437.

38. Malm J, Jacobsson J, Birgander R, Eklund A. Reference values for CSF outflow resistance and intracranial pressure in healthy elderly. Neurology. 2011;76(10):903–9. https://doi.org/10.1212/WNL.0b013e31820f2dd0.

39. Mahr CV, Dengl M, Nestler U, Reiss-Zimmermann M, Eichner G, Preuß M, et al. Idiopathic normal pressure hydrocephalus: diagnostic and predictive value of clinical testing, lumbar drainage, and CSF dynamics. J Neurosurg. 2016;125(3):591–7. https://doi.org/10.3171/2015.8.Jns151112.

40. Skalický P, Mládek A, Vlasák A, De Lacy P, Beneš V, Bradáč O. Normal pressure hydrocephalus—an overview of pathophysiological mechanisms and diagnostic procedures. Neurosurg Rev. 2020;43(6):1451–64. https://doi.org/10.1007/s10143-019-01201-5.

41. Czosnyka Z, Czosnyka M. Long-term monitoring of intracranial pressure in normal pressure hydrocephalus and other CSF disorders. Acta Neurochir. 2017;159(10):1979–80. https://doi.org/10.1007/s00701-017-3282-1.

42. Eide PK, Brean A. Cerebrospinal fluid pulse pressure amplitude during lumbar infusion in idiopathic normal pressure hydrocephalus can predict response to shunting. Cerebrospinal Fluid Res. 2010;7(1):5. https://doi.org/10.1186/1743-8454-7-5.

43. Santamarta D, González-Martínez E, Fernández J, Mostaza A. The prediction of shunt response in idiopathic normal-pressure hydrocephalus based on intracranial pressure monitoring and lumbar infusion. Acta Neurochir Suppl. 2016;122:267–74. https://doi.org/10.1007/978-3-319-22533-3_53.

44. Kahlon B, Sundbärg G, Rehncrona S. Comparison between the lumbar infusion and CSF tap tests to predict outcome after shunt surgery in suspected normal pressure hydrocephalus. J Neurol Neurosurg Psychiatry. 2002;73(6):721–6. https://doi.org/10.1136/jnnp.73.6.721.

45. Sorteberg A, Eide PK, Fremming AD. A prospective study on the clinical effect of surgical treatment of normal pressure hydrocephalus: the value of hydrodynamic evaluation. Br J Neurosurg. 2004;18(2):149–57. https://doi.org/10.1080/02688690410001681000.

46. Malm J, Lundkvist B, Eklund A, Koskinen LOD, Kristensen B. CSF outflow resistance as predictor of shunt function. A long-term study. Acta Neurol Scand. 2004;110(3):154–60. https://doi.org/10.1111/j.1600-0404.2004.00302.x.

47. Woodford J, Saunders RL, Sachs E Jr. Shunt system patency testing by lumbar infusion. J Neurosurg. 1976;45(1):60–5. https://doi.org/10.3171/jns.1976.45.1.0060.

48. Czosnyka ZH, Czosnyka M, Smielewski P, Lalou AD, Nabbanja E, Garnett M, et al. Single center experience in cerebrospinal fluid dynamics testing. Acta Neurochir Suppl. 2021;131:311–3. https://doi.org/10.1007/978-3-030-59436-7_58.

Laboratory Findings of NPH

**Adéla Bubeníková, Ludmila Máčová, Petr Skalický, Arnošt Mládek,
and Ondřej Bradáč**

Abstract Considering the high occurrence of neurodegenerative comorbidities, it is rather challenging to clearly determine the precise diagnosis of normal pressure hydrocephalus (NPH), as well as to predict treatment responsiveness in these patients. Detailed investigation of cerebrospinal fluid (CSF) biomarkers potentially applicable in clinical practice might be particularly useful in the NPH diagnostic battery, together with clinical and radiological findings characteristic of the disease itself. Research has revealed a range of reliable information on the overall CSF profile in iNPH patients, although it is so far impossible to determine a single biomarker specific to NPH. The CSF profile of NPH seems to be easily differentiated from healthy controls; however, the differentiation from other neurodegenerative disorders based only on these parameters remains a challenge. The comorbidities frequently share similar (abnormally raised or abnormally decreased) concentrations of biomarkers in the CSF when compared to iNPH. Although laboratory findings of NPH are not used in current clinical practice, further research may be of great importance to better predict the NPH progression and therefore also to deliver better treatment outcomes and improved prognosis in NPH patients. This chapter summarizes up-to-date conceptions of the topic and provides relevant information discussing and introducing laboratory findings of NPH.

A. Bubeníková · P. Skalický · O. Bradáč (✉)
Department of Neurosurgery, 2nd Medical Faculty, Charles University and Motol University
Hospital, Prague, Czech Republic
e-mail: ondrej.bradac2@fnmotol.cz

A. Bubeníková · A. Mládek · O. Bradáč
Department of Neurosurgery and Neurooncology, 1st Medical Faculty, Charles University and
Military University Hospital, Prague, Czech Republic

L. Máčová
Department of Steroid Hormones and Proteofactors, Institute of Endocrinology, Prague, Czech
Republic

A. Mládek
Department of Cognitive Systems and Neurosciences, Czech Institute of Informatics, Robotics
and Cybernetics, Czech Technical University, Prague, Czech Republic

© The Author(s), under exclusive license to Springer Nature Switzerland AG 2023   243
O. Bradac (ed.), *Normal Pressure Hydrocephalus*,
https://doi.org/10.1007/978-3-031-36522-5_15

Keywords Normal pressure hydrocephalus · Cerebrospinal fluid biomarkers · Amyloid beta · Aquaporin · Glymphatic system · Leucine-rich glycoprotein · Alzheimer's disease · Parkinson's disease

Abbreviations

5-HT	5-Hydroxytryptamine
Aβ	Amyloid beta
ABC	ATP-binding cassette
AMPA	α-Amino-3-hydroxy-5-methyl-4-isoxazolepropionic acid
AQP	Aquaporin
APP	Amyloid precursor protein
AD	Alzheimer's disease
AUC	Area under curve
BBB	Blood-brain barrier
CNS	Central nervous system
CSF	Cerebrospinal fluid
CTF	C-terminal fragments
CYP450scc	Cytochrome P450 cholesterol side-chain cleavage enzyme
DHEA/DHEAS	Dehydroepiandrosterone/dehydroepiandrosteronesulphate
FTLD	Frontotemporal lobe degeneration
GABA-A	γ-Aminobutyric acid receptor type A
HC	Healthy controls
HSD11B1	Hydroxysteroid dehydrogenase 11-beta type 1
IDE	Insulin degrading enzyme
IL	Interleukin
iNPH	Idiopathic normal pressure hydrocephalus
LRG	Leucine-rich-α2-glycoprotein
LRR	Leucine-rich repeats
MAP	Microtubule-associated protein
MAPT	Microtubule-associated protein tau
MBP	Myelin based protein
MCI	Mild cognitive impairment
MCP-1	Monocyte chemoattractant protein 1
MS	Multiple sclerosis
MSA	Multiple system atrophy
MTB	Microtubule-binding
NAS	Neuroactive neurosteroids
NFL	Neurofilament protein light
NMDA	N-methyl-D-aspartate
NPH	Normal pressure hydrocephalus
p-tau	Hyperphosphorylated tau
PD	Parkinson's disease

PREG/PREGS	Pregnenolone/pregnenolonesulphate
PSP	Progressive supranuclear palsy
ROC	Receiver operating characteristic
sAPP	Soluble amyloid precursor protein
SD	Standard deviation
SIVD	Subcortical ischemic vascular disease
SLC	Solute carrier
SMD	Standardized mean difference
sNPH	Secondary normal pressure hydrocephalus
t-tau	Total tau
TGF-β	Transforming growth factor beta
TNF-α	Tumor necrosis factor alpha
TNF-β	Tumor necrosis factor beta
VD	Vascular dementia
VDR	Vitamin D receptor
VEGF	Vascular endothelial growth factor
YKL-40	Chitinase-3-like protein

1 Introduction

Normal pressure hydrocephalus (NPH) is one form of treatable dementia primarily present in the elderly [1, 2]. It is crucial to clearly differentiate two primary subgroups of NHP: (1) idiopathic NPH (iNPH) and (2) secondary NPH (sNPH). The latter may evolve at any age due to its cause by prior events and additional factors such as meningitis, subarachnoid haemorrhage, and tumours [3–7].

Nowadays, many diagnostic approaches are available for NPH, including clinical evaluation, brain imaging, and invasive tests [8–14], while the clinical responses to the third option remain to be the most precise and accurate method for NPH diagnosis [15]. Nevertheless, there is a demand for more precise diagnostic measures of NPH as a significant number of patients, despite all progress in the field that has been made, are still underdiagnosed or misdiagnosed and are therefore undertreated [16–19]. One of the potential solutions arises from laboratory examinations of molecular indicators which are particularly specific for NPH. The aim is to effectively distinguish NPH from other neurodegenerative disorders, such as vascular dementia (VD), Alzheimer's (AD), Parkinson's disease (PD), or progressive supranuclear palsy (PSP) and to more clearly predict shunt responsiveness in NPH patients [4, 20–27]. Accordingly, further investigation of cerebrospinal fluid (CSF) biomarkers potentially applicable in clinical practice might contribute to a more definite diagnosis of NPH [26, 28–32].

Several scientific publications [30–36] defined promising candidates suitable for relevant clinical use in NPH identification. However, there is still no evidence of such application in current medical practice [28, 31, 37]. CSF biomarkers are already successfully used in the clinic as diagnostic indicators for AD [25, 38, 39] and have revealed results, which encouraged attempts to do so for NPH as well. In this chapter, we describe the most up-to-date knowledge of the topic and provide a brief overview of the laboratory findings in NPH.

2　Amyloid β-Related Proteins

Amyloids are a diverse group of proteins characteristic with β-sheet secondary structure (so-called cross-β) [40]. They are best known for their pathological influence when released abnormally in the human body, subsequently leading to their extracellular deposition and the subsequent onset of amyloidosis [41]. Amyloid precursors proteins (APPs) are single transmembrane proteins with a short cytoplasmic tail and a long N-terminal domain, particularly present in neural tissues where they are involved in axonogenesis, neurite growth, and synaptogenesis [42, 43]. There are two major cleavage pathways accomplished by α-, β-, and γ-secretases, which are fundamental for APP's repairment mechanisms [44]. The first, also known as the non-amyloidogenic pathway, is driven by the enzymatic activity of α- and γ-secretases. It inhibits the generation of amyloid beta (Aβ) and simultaneously releases soluble APP alpha protein (aAPPα), the N-terminal ectodomain. Polypeptide Aβ, which is found in cellular membranes, plasma, and CSF [45, 46], contains 37–49 amino acid residues and is primarily produced through the proteolytic process of APP performed by β- and γ-secretases—the so-called amyloidogenic pathway. This generates soluble APP beta protein (sAPPβ) and Aβ [47–50]. Both pathways generate membrane-tethered α- or β-C-terminal fragments (CTFs), which are separated within the intramembrane space by γ-secretase. This leads to the emancipation of Aβ (molecular weight of 4 kDa) and P3 (3 kDa) peptides [49]. The abnormal accumulation and subsequent deposition of Aβ in the form of amyloid plaques is a well-known fundamental step in the development of AD [42, 51–53]. The toxic plaque's fibrils can be partly enzymatically cleaved, mainly by neprilysin, insulin-degrading enzyme (IDE) or endothelin-converting enzymes, or they can be exported via the blood–brain barrier (BBB) [49, 54]. Still, there is approximately 10% of Aβ left that is subsequently cleared through the interstitial fluid (ISF) and the glymphatic system into CSF [55, 56]. Among all isoforms of Aβ, three are the most important for CSF evaluation purposes: (1) Aβ38, (2) Aβ40 (Fig. 1), and (3) Aβ42 [57, 58]. Extra alanine and isoleucine in Aβ42 C-terminus present a unique difference among other Aβ proteins; still, this seemingly small structural change significantly modifies physiology, toxicity, and the overall metabolism of the protein. When compared to its shorter isoforms, Aβ42 is not only more amyloidogenic but also able to faster configure pathological insoluble fibrils and is more neurotoxic with subsequent increased inflammatory activity [50, 57, 59]. Aβ is in lower concentrations (which do not allow the formation of toxic fibrils) present in healthy brain tissue where it plays a role in depressing the synaptic activity [60–62], providing the protection of mature neurons from excitotoxic cell death [63], or even enhancing the survival of the hippocampal neurons in vitro [64].

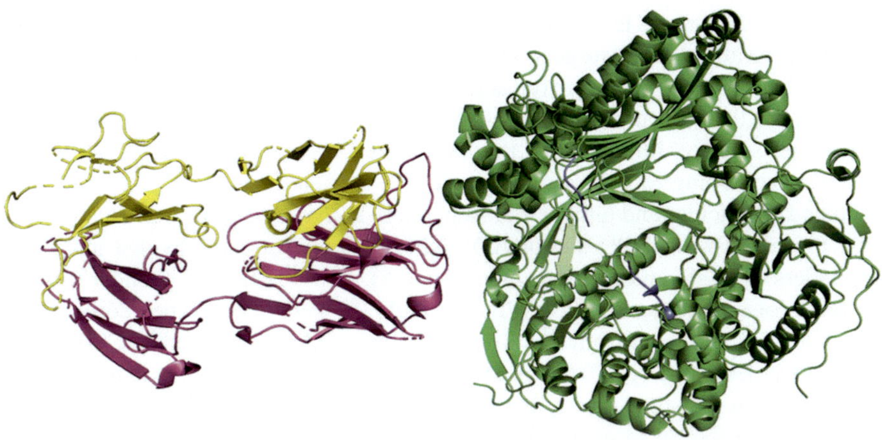

Fig. 1 Crystal structure of amyloid beta (Aβ40) in complex with fab-bound insulin-degrading enzyme (IDE). PDB ID: 4M1C [65]. On the left, the light chain of fab-bound IDE is depicted in yellow, the heavy chain of fab-bound IDE is in pink. The IDE is outlined in green colour, with Aβ40 protein in dark purple

In a recent analysis of the differential diagnosis of iNPH, Schirinzi et al. [30] published results on CSF levels of Aβ42 among 56 patients presenting with iNPH, AD, PSP, and the rest who were entered into the control group. All subjects underwent lumbar puncture, MRI imaging, and possible NPH patients additionally received a CSF tap test for more precise evaluation of their clinical status. The levels of CSF Aβ42, measured in pg/ml, were higher in iNPH patients compared to the AD group ([mean ± standard deviation, SD], iNPH [477.5 ± 223.10], AD [308.43 ± 91.38]; $p = 0.01$) and lower when compared to the controls (HC [862 ± 230.40]; $p < 0.01$). The authors, however, could not confirm a statistically significant difference between iNPH and PSP group (PSP [482.77 ± 209.35]; $p = 0.509$). The presence of reduced Aβ42 in iNPH patients compared to healthy individuals was similarly verified by other authors [36, 66–68] who defined several probable causes of such a state. Biochemical metabolic changes in periventricular tissue, decreased generation of Aβ and other amyloid derivatives, and their accumulation or disruption of their clearance within the extracellular fluid are the most frequently mentioned possible explanations [30, 36]. According to such findings, it has been proposed that iNPH pathophysiology, in terms of molecular pathways\leading to amyloidopathy, differs from the mechanisms present in AD patients [29, 36, 68, 69]. A recent report [70] evaluated different biochemical variants of Aβ among patients with iNPH and AD. They have proposed that studying specific molecular variants obtained from brain biopsies may be useful in predicting potential AD onset in iNPH patients.

Jeppsson et al. [36] disclosed convincing results on shunt responsiveness in iNPH patients with respect to the measured levels of Aβ42 and analogous APP derivatives (namely Aβ38, Aβ40, sAPPα, and sAPPβ) in comparison with healthy controls. In this study, ventricular CSF was examined pre- and postoperatively in order to exclusively evaluate the levels of CSF biomarkers. Besides indisputably raised levels of APP derivatives after surgery in iNPH patients, subjects who postoperatively presented with an overall improved status had apparently higher concentration rates of Aβ and APP derivatives than those who worsened or did not perform notably better after surgery. Interestingly, the measured levels of Aβ and APP derivatives may vary according to CSF sampling sites. In a related study, Pyykko et al. [71] evaluated ventricular and lumbar CSF separately in the same groups of patients who were presented with iNPH and/or AD. iNPH patients were subdivided into shunt responders (n = 48) and non-responders (n = 5). In iNPH shunt responder's group, the levels of ventricular Aβ42, sAPPα, and sAPPβ were higher when compared to the same CSF extracted from the lumbar puncture. Moreover, lumbar CSF sAPPα levels were decreased (p < 0.05) in iNPH shunt responder's group when compared to iNPH shunt non-responders, but the levels of sAPPβ were similar (p = 0.06). It has been proposed in a recent meta-analysis [72] of 39 studies yielding 5000 patients that the accuracy of measured CSF levels of Aβ42 for distinguishing AD from other neurodegenerative disorders (including NPH) remains to be imperfect, mirroring the close relationship and high concurrence of these abnormalities. It has been verified in numerous studies [27, 36] that the reduction of amyloid β-related proteins and analogous APP derivatives is present in both iNPH and AD, and the final measurements may therefore reveal conflicting results. An illustrative example is a meta-analysis from Chen et al. [73] as they confirmed that the concentrations of CSF Aβ42 were significantly lower in iNPH when compared to healthy individuals (the standardized mean difference (SMD) was –1.14 and the levels decreased within 95% confidence interval (CI) from –1.74 to –0.55; p = 0.0002) but were only slightly increased when compared to AD (SMD = 0.32, the measured levels decreased within 95% CI from 0.00 to –0.63; p = 0.05).

3   Tau Proteins

A family of microtubule-associated proteins (MAPs), identified by Weingarten et al. in 1975 for the first time [74], consists of three subgroups: MAP1, MAP2, and tau proteins (also known with the starting Greek tau letter as τ proteins). MAPs are playing a fundamental role in microtubular stabilization as they support kinesin, dynein-based anterograde, and retrograde transport, and they are therefore involved in cargo packages trafficking from the neuronal perikaryon to axons and dendrites. Tau proteins are composed of amino-terminal projection domain, microtubule-binding (MTB) repeats, and a short carboxyl-terminal tail sequence [75]. They are encoded by microtubule-associated protein tau (*MAPT*) located on chromosome 17q21, has a size of over 100 kb, and contains 16 exons [76, 77]. Six major isoforms consisting of 352–441 amino acids are known, with the molecular weight ranging from 45 to 65 kDa [78]. The differentiation among these isoforms is based on the presence of either three or four repeat regions in the C-terminus or the presence/absence of one or two inserts (29 or 58 amino acids) in the N-terminus of the protein [79, 80].

Their presence at dendrites, where they are involved in postsynaptic scaffolding, is relatively low [81]; they are primarily active at providing microtubule stabilization and flexibility in the distal proportions of axons [82]. Tau isoforms have prespecified functions related to their structural architecture and may not be expressed in neurons equally. Namely, no tau mRNAs containing exon 10 were found in granular cells in the dentate gyrus [79]. Besides their neuronal occurrence, tau mRNA can be detected in peripheral tissue such as lung, muscle, pancreas, testis, heart, or kidney [78, 83, 84]. The major pathological influence of tau in several neurodegenerative disorders is the intraneuronal aggregation of tau isoforms in a form of fibrillar polymers [78, 79, 82, 85, 86]. There are several types of post-translational modifications important for modulation of tau function including phosphorylation as the most common, ubiquitination, deamidation, glycosylation, nitration, oxidation, and others. The regulation pathways are managed developmentally by a spectrum of kinases and phosphatases [82]. Under pathological conditions, tau's phosphorylation and dephosphorylation are not equally regulated. The resulting hyperphosphorylation subsequently leads to tauopathies [87, 88].

Findings on tau CSF levels within scientific publications are heterogeneous. The most attention with respect to the neurodegenerative and pathological mechanisms was paid to hyperphosphorylated tau (known as P-tau) and total tau (T-tau) proteins. Lim et al. [89] conducted enzyme-linked immunosorbent assay analyses for CSF biomarkers in order to evaluate the coexistence of AD and iNPH. Tau proteins (both T- and P-tau) were measured among three patient groups: iNPH, AD, and controls. Significant differences between the measured tau levels were recognized only between iNPH and AD (in both tau proteins). Comparisons of tau levels in iNPH and healthy individuals or AD and healthy controls were not statistically significant. The low tau concentrations may be attributed to reduced neuronal activity or impaired cortical metabolism. Other studies presented similarly reduced tau levels [24, 27, 66], or unchanged/non-significant differences of CSF tau concentrations between iNPH and healthy control groups [29, 30], and only a study by Kapaki et al. [68] measured slight increase of tau biomarkers in iNPH patients.

Interestingly, in a meta-analysis [73] of 413 patients with, the iNPH, 186 with AD and 147 healthy controls (HC), CSF levels of tau proteins (T- and P-tau) were significantly decreased in iNPH when compared to AD ($p = 0.0004$ and $p = 0.0002$, respectively) and also lower compared to HC ($p < 0.0001$). In 2020, Manniche et al. [90] evaluated CSF biomarker concentrations in patients with iNPH, subcortical ischemic vascular disease (SIVD), AD, and healthy individuals. The levels of T- and P-tau were lowest (T-tau [155 ± 63]; P-tau [28 ± 12] pg/ml) in iNPH group and highest (T-tau [453 ± 211]; P-tau [72 ± 27] pg/ml) in patients suffering from AD. The differences between the iNPH versus SIVD group were considered as statistically significant only in T-tau concentrations ($p = 0.0017$). P-values of T- and P-tau in iNPH versus AD and iNPH versus healthy controls were equalized at $p < 0.0002$ (Fig. 2).

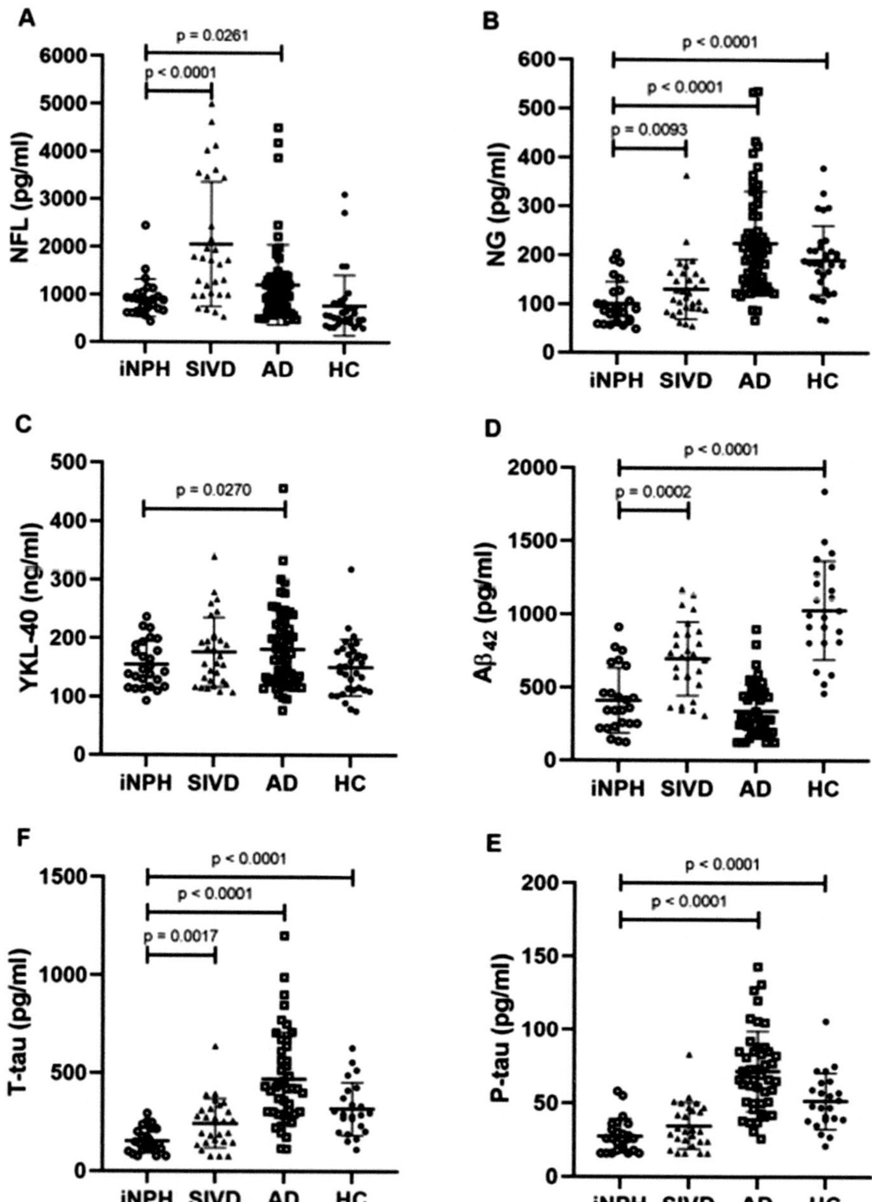

Fig. 2 Scatter plots depicting the CSF levels of six analysed biomarkers in patients experiencing iNPH, SIVD, AD, and healthy individuals who were entered into the control group (HC). The error bars show median and interquartile ranges. The abbreviation NG refers to neurogranin. Reprinted from the Journal of Alzheimer's disease, Volume 75, Manniche et al., Cerebrospinal Fluid Biomarkers to Differentiate Idiopathic Normal Pressure Hydrocephalus from Subcortical Ischemic Vascular disease, Page No. 28, Copyright (2020) [90], with permission from IOS Press

4 Aquaporins

Transmembrane polypeptides, so-called aquaporins, play a fundamental role in permitting water molecules across the cellular membrane in response to an osmotic gradient [90]. As already described above, although most of the Aβ particles are cleared through enzymatic activity or trans-BBB migration, there is a minor amount left which is erased through the glymphatic system—a complex network of fluid interchange which plays a vital role in eliminating toxic molecules and aggregated compounds from the CNS as well as in distributing indispensable metabolites within the brain. Its adequate functioning depends on several factors, such as intracranial respiration pressure and arterial pulsatile flow [31, 56]. However, impaired glymphatic function has been found in both iNPH and AD in correlation with disfigurement of astrocytic aquaporin-4 (AQP4). Such a state is typically present not only in these two conditions [92–94], but also in other pathologies including mesial temporal lobe epilepsy [95], neuromyelitis optica [96], and ischemic stroke [97]. In the brain, AQP4 is bound to astrocytes and ependymal cells, and its occurrence is particularly enriched in the astrocytic perivascular region where it is involved in endfoot biochemical processes. AQP4 is primarily important in maintaining water homeostasis within the brain as the cerebral function is directly dependent on adequately regulated water transport via protein channels located in the intraneuronal plasma membranes [98, 99]. Glymphatic system disfigurement has been already broadly discussed in cases of both AD and iNPH patients when considering the accumulation of Aβ as a result of the reduced glymphatic efficacy and associated loss of perivascular astrocytic endfeet membranes secondary leading to amyloidopathy or abnormal Aβ metabolism [94, 100, 101]. The loss of AQP4 has been confirmed in a recent study [93] in iNPH patients who were compared to surgically managed patients with completely different clinical anamnesis (epilepsy, subarachnoid haemorrhage, tumour). However, explicit differences among AQP4 profile in iNPH and other neurodegenerative disorders still remain unclear and continue to be crucial for any potential clinical application.

Gastaldi et al. [102] investigated a predictive correlation between the loss of AQP4 and aquaporin antibodies in patients with iNPH. From 43 enrolled iNPH patients, only one 79-year-old woman with a characteristic iNPH presentation tested positive for AQP4-IgM. The evidence for a link between aquaporin antibodies and iNPH is not strong. Nevertheless, the authors proposed that the levels of aquaporin antibodies may be detectable in the early disease onset but difficult to identify in later stages.

Another member of the transmembrane water channels family is aquaporin 1 (AQP1), localized at the apical plasma membrane within the choroid plexus ependymal cells [103]. Its CFS concentrations were investigated by Ruiz et al. [104] in patients experiencing a mild cognitive impairment (MCI) and those with iNPH, in comparison with controls. Although the measured levels of AQP1 between patients with MCI and the controls did not significantly differ, nor with the tiNPH patients, the concentrations of AQP1 were slightly increased in the iNPH group. To date, there is still a very limited number of reports dedicated to AQP1 and most of them are devoted to animal models [103–105]. Therefore, further research is needed if any consensus on its specificity for iNPH is to be made.

5 Inflammatory Biomarkers

Inflammation itself is in most cases a beneficial response of an organism to a range of infections but may sometimes be detrimental. Most neurodegenerative diseases are accompanied by inflammatory processes, and released mediators typically contribute to disease progression. Such mediators are predominantly cytokines, protein-like molecules that are involved in cell signalling, and inflammation pathways in the human body [106]. Based on their targets, cytokines can be further classified into (1) anti-inflammatory, which consist predominantly of interleukin (IL)-1 receptor antagonist, IL-4, IL-6, IL-10, IL-11, and IL-13 and (2) pro-inflammatory cytokines, consisting of the well-known IL-1 and tumour necrosis factor-alpha (TNF-α). The latter is a mediator primarily produced by macrophages and further released by microglia and astrocytes within the process of acute inflammation [107]. TNF-α is responsible for signalling events leading to cellular apoptosis and necrosis [107]; however, numerous other functions generally accompanied by IL-1 and IL-6 are defined in various organ systems. Based on two studies [108, 109], the levels of CSF TNF-α were higher in iNPH patients when compared to the controls, but these findings were subsequently rejected by several publications [71, 109]. TNF-α is considered to be unreliable as a diagnosis indicator and predictor of shunt responsiveness [28], but it is typically present in higher concentrations in chronic obstructive hydrocephalus [110]. Interestingly, it is believed that TNF-α is directly associated with sulfatide, i.e., 3-O-sulfogalactosylceramide, synthesized from ceramide involved in various biochemical pathways in the human body [31, 111]. Sulfatide itself was measured in various studies as a potential biomarker for iNPH; however, the results rejected its possible clinical application as the differences among patients with iNPH, other neurodegenerative comorbidities, and healthy individuals were generally statistically non-significant [27, 108, 112]. However, Tullberg et al. [113] consider sulfatide to be a biomarker distinguishing iNPH and subcortical arteriosclerotic encephalopathy. The concentrations of IL-1β, known as an important determinant of CNS inflammation pathways [114], and IL-6 are upregulated by TNF-α, and increased levels have been identified in numerous neurodegenerative disorders [32]. Although raised levels of these neuroinflammatory mediators are also present in iNPH, the differentiation may be rather challenging due to the high concurrence of other pathologic conditions.

In an analysis of 24 adult patients with various types of hydrocephalus [110], Lee et al. compared their TNF-α and TNF-β levels with healthy controls, but the authors could not confirm any difference between these two groups. Other publications including exclusively patients with iNPH [36, 71, 115] which measured an even larger number of inflammatory biomarkers could not confirm any results on specific iNPH indicators. According to Sosvorova et al. [32], CSF levels of IL-1β and IL-6 were significantly increased on the first day of LD in the NPH group compared to controls ($p < 0.01$). However, the levels afterwards equalized with the controls. IL-10 levels were significantly higher within the first day of LD, but on the third day both NPH and controls levels decreased and remained the same. The levels of IL-33 and soluble CD40-ligand were notably higher in NPH, but on the second day of LD the levels of cytokines increased in controls and remained increased for the whole duration of LD. The levels of CSF IL-4, IL-17A, IL-21, IL-22, IL-31, and TNF-α were decreased for the entire duration of the LD. Unfortunately, this study did not further investigate associations of mediators among NPH and other neurodegenerative diseases, since neuroinflammation of this type is typically present in AD and PD as well [31].

5.1 Transforming Growth Factors (TGF)

Another example of cytokines derived from the same diverse group of inflammatory mediators, also released from astrocytes and microglia, is transforming growth factors beta (TGFs-β) [116]. These proteins constitute a family of pleiotropic cytokine mediators developmentally involved in cell differentiation and tissue modelling but are also partly responsible for neuroinflammatory and neurodegenerative cascades accompanied by fibrosis, neuronal apoptosis, or vascular hypertrophy [117, 118]. There are three defined isoforms (TGF-β1, -β2, and -β3), considered to be 25 kDa homodimers [31]. The number of studies dedicated to TGF-β functioning in iNPH remains low, but according to recently published analysis [119], the levels of TGF-β1 (Fig. 3) and TGF-type II receptor were found to be significantly higher in iNPH subjects when compared to controls. The levels of TGF-β1 were 1439.3 ± 149.2 in iNPH and 492.1 ± 34.7 pg/ml in controls ($p < 0.001$). TGF-type II receptor CSF concentrations were 1992.3 ± 134.1 in iNPH and 1065.7 ± 87.8 pg/ml in controls ($p < 0.001$). This result further mirrored the association of TGF-β1 and TGF-type II receptor with leucine-rich-α2-glycoprotein (LRG)—a characteristic biomarker of cerebral damage present in some iNPH patients, introduced more in detail below. The levels of LRG in this study were 1047.2 ± 63.4 in iNPH and 520.4 ± 49.5 pg/ml in controls, which was found to be statistically significant ($p < 0.001$) [119].

5.2 Monocyte Chemoattractant Protein 1 (MCP-1)

Firstly identified in 1977 [121], chemokines are heparin-binding proteins consisting of 60–100 amino acids structurally similar to cytokines. CXC, also known as α-chemokines, and CC, so-called β chemokines, are the two primary chemokines-related families. α-chemokines, regulators of cell trafficking, are encoded by genes for CXC located on chromosome 4 and can be further differentiated based on the localization and a total number of cysteine residues at the N-terminal tail [122]. The

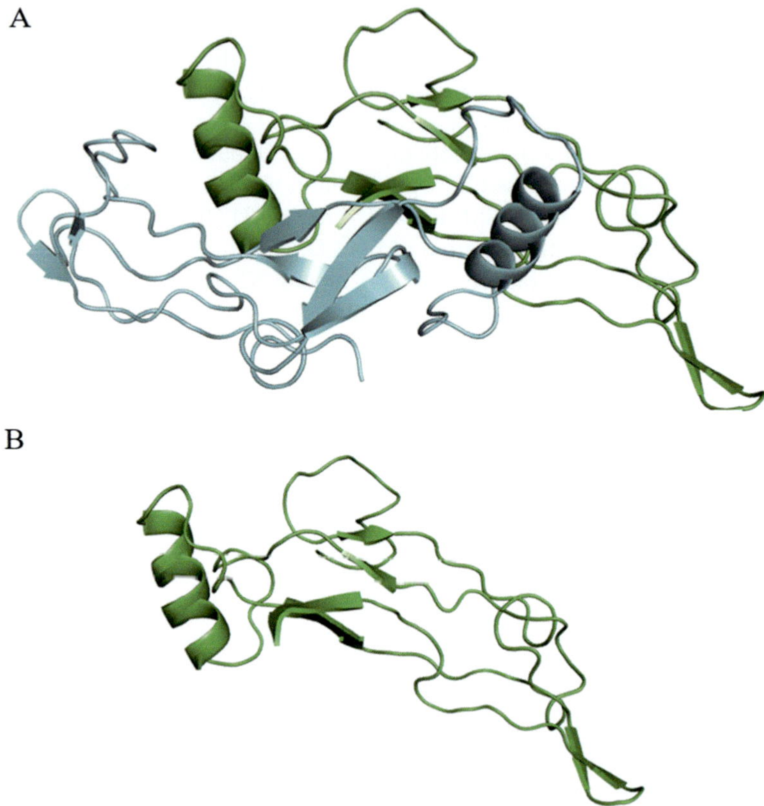

Fig. 3 Geometric structure of transforming growth factor beta (TGF-β). PDB ID: 1KLA [119]. In picture A, TGF-β is depicted as a dimer, in picture B as a monomer

genes encoding the latter are localized on chromosome 17 and include a monocyte chemoattractant protein 1 (MCP-1), a protein consisting of 76 amino acid residues secreted in two forms with different molecular weights—the first with 9 and the second with 19 kDa [123]. So far the research dedicated to CSF MCP-1 levels either could not measure the MCP-1 levels as the used samples were above the lower limit of detection [71], revealed results proposing the fact that MCP-1 needs to be measured with other accompanying biomarkers, namely T-tau and Aβ40 [26], or suggest that MCP-1 is related to a less favourable shunting outcome, thus indicating a non-beneficial immunologic reaction [36]. Based on such findings, the role of MCP-1 in iNPH diagnosis seems to be of little importance.

5.3 *Chitinase-3-Like Protein 1 (YKL-40)*

A promising inflammatory biomarker, chitinase-3-like protein 1 (YKL-40) [124], has been investigated in several studies. Its potential use for iNPH diagnosis remains unclear due to the absence of relevant data. It is believed that the protein's expression located in astrocytes and microglia may be associated with neuroinflammation and reactive gliosis [125]. CSF YKL-40 levels seem to be increased in patients experiencing cognitive decline when compared to healthy individuals and thus may predict dementia progression [125]. Higher concentrations were also identified in post-stroke brain tissue and brains associated with other neurological disorders [126]. These findings support the hypothesis that YKL-40 is not unique in AD, where it may play a key role in predicting the disease progression but is presented as a more universal inflammatory biomarker [126, 127] (see the comparison with other biomarkers in Fig. 4). Interestingly, the plasma concentrations of YKL-40 were increased in iNPH patients when compared to healthy controls in a statistically significant manner in a recent study by Ko et al. [128].

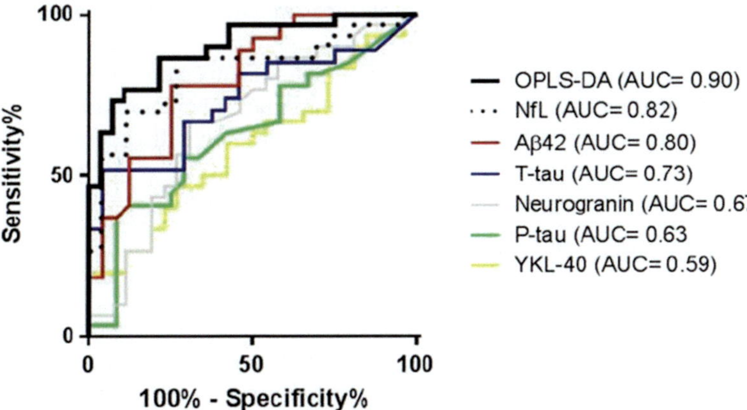

Fig. 4 Diagnostic accuracy of each biomarker and the above-mentioned combination of all six proteins together based on the orthogonal projections to latent structures discriminant analysis (OPLS-DA). Reprinted from the Journal of Alzheimer's disease, Volume 75, Manniche et al., Cerebrospinal Fluid Biomarkers to Differentiate Idiopathic Normal Pressure Hydrocephalus from Subcortical Ischemic Vascular disease, Page No. 30, Copyright (2020) [90], with permission from IOS Press

6 Biomarkers of Subcortical Damage

6.1 Neurofilament Protein Light

Neurofilaments play a fundamental role in the neuronal cytoskeleton structure and the maintenance of axonal architecture [31]. These proteins are further differentiated by three composing chains: light, medium, and heavy units. The first, neurofilament protein light (NFL), encoded by the *NEFL* gene, consists of 543 amino acids with a molecular weight of 68 kDa. It has recently been the subject of a lot of research dedicated to axonal architecture degeneration and inflammatory and dementia-related disorders [129]. In the presence of axonal damage, NFL is released into the CSF and blood plasma [130]. Higher levels of NFL, therefore, serve as indicators of cerebral axonal degeneration and are typically present in some neurodegenerative disorders (namely AD [131], Huntington's disease [132], PD [133], FTLD [134], amyotrophic lateral sclerosis [135], multiple sclerosis (MS) [136], and atypical parkinsonian disorders). Although a recent study could not confirm increased CSF NFL concentrations in iNPH, various publications have reported contradictory findings [27, 36, 71, 137, 138]. More details about the NFL CSF levels measured in several studies are depicted in Table 1.

It is important to note that statistically significant results were measured between iNPH and control groups and therefore cannot further elucidate NFL's role in the differential diagnosis of iNPH from other neurodegenerative disorders.

6.2 Myelin Basic Protein

The oligodendroglial structural protein of myelin, myelin basic protein (MBP), is a biomarker typical for many neurodegenerative disorders, as it is a characteristic of periventricular white matter damage [139]. MBP plays an important role in the adhesion of cytosolic surfaces of compact myelin, interactions with the cellular cytoskeleton, binding to the membrane surfaces, and in the transmission of extracellular signals [140]. MBP is also one of the most abundant components of CNS myelin [141]. Unfortunately, the results so far are consistent in revealing the fact of significant coexistence of MBP in numerous cerebral disorders including MS, other neurodegenerative or cerebrovascular disorders, and iNPH [139, 140]. High levels of MBP are present in many other pathologies, and no clarification on possible specificity for iNPH has been made [36, 71]. Jeppsson et al. [36] disclosed results comparing CSF MBP levels between iNPH and healthy controls. The measured concentrations were seemingly the same, 1.5 (1.1 − 1.9) pg/ml in iNPH and 1.3 (1.0 − 1.5) pg/ml in control patients, which are findings without any statistical significance. Similar results were verified by other authors as well [71, 142].

Table 1 Overview of ventricular and lumbar CSF NFL levels

Study	Groups	N	Males (%)	Age (range), year	CSF sampling site	NFL (pg/ml), mean ± SD	p-value
Agren-Wilsson et al. [27]	iNPH	62	39 (63)	72 (55–83)	Lumbar	854 ± 917	p < 0.01
	HC	23	10 (43)	73 (59–88)		1268 ± 1134	
Jeppsson et al. [36]	iNPH	28	15 (54)	69	Lumbar	1260	p < 0.05
	HC	20	11 (55)	70		825	
Jeppsson et al. [26]	iNPH	82	53 (65)	73 (52–89)	Lumbar	1717 ± 1963	Not statistically significant
	AD	50	21 (37)	71 (51–81)		1977 ± 2508	
	FTLD	19	5 (16)	69 (55–84)		2089 ± 1401	
	VD	75	30 (40)	79 (58–88)		2646 ± 3475	
	PD	70	47 (67)	60 (26–87)		839 ± 622	
	MSA	34	14 (41)	65 (49–83)		2322 ± 987	
	PSP	34	14 (41)	70 (54–82)		2219 ± 2761	
	non-iNPH	295	134 (45)	73 (52–89)		2137 ± 1178	
	HC	54	22 (41)	71 (53–93)		1170 ± 896	
Pyykko et al. [71]	iNPH 1	48	25 (52)	73	Ventricular	886 ± 681	No significant relation of NFL CSF levels*
	iNPH 2	5	2 (40)	83		6692 ± 9723	
	AD	16	6 (38)	78		1567 ± 2152	
	The same patients within the same groups				Lumbar	2511 ± 1798	
						6545 ± 6242	
						2007 ± 867	

*The p-value of 0.05 was measured for lower ventricular CSF values in iNPH 2. iNPH 1—shunt responders; iNPH2—shunt non-responders

6.3 Leucine-Rich-A2-Glycoprotein

Haupt and Baundner isolated in 1977 [143] one of the most discussed candidates for the biomarker of iNPH, extracellular leucine-rich-α2-glycoprotein (LRG). LRG consists of 66 leucines in a total of 312 amino acids encoded by the LRG gene, located on chromosome 19, the short arm p, at position p13.3. The protein is built up of eight repeating consensus sequences, so-called leucine-rich repeats (LRR) with a periodic occurrence of leucine, proline, and asparagine, while each sequence consists of 24 amino acid residues [144, 145]. The increased levels of LRG in CSF are in direct association with ageing and dementia-related disorders [146]. Although it has been proposed that LRG is iNPH specific [35], there is a lack of reliable data to prove such a statement. It is certain that raised CSF LRG levels in patients with an unclear diagnosis of iNPH or some neurodegenerative comorbidities may be significantly misleading and hard to clearly elucidate. However, Nakajima et al. [147] performed a detailed analysis of evaluating symptom improvement after shunting in 52 patients with proved iNPH. Subsequently, results certainly indicated LRG as a biomarker of positive shunt response and verifications by other authors have been disclosed [35, 148].

7 Steroids in CSF

7.1 Neuroactive Steroids and Neurosteroids

To date, there is an interesting amount of evidence about the application of steroids and neurosteroid in serving as biomarkers in the diagnosis of many disorders. The French physiologist Etienne Baulieu coined the term "neurosteroids" in the second half of the twentieth century, to mean steroids synthesized de novo within the brain [149]. Since then, both neurosteroid and neuroactive steroids (NAS)—steroids that affect neurological functions regardless of the place of production—have been considered in the treatment of many neurodegenerative conditions such as depression, schizophrenia, dementia [150], multiple sclerosis [151], and others. Neurosteroids are produced notably in the hippocampus, cortex, basal ganglia, or amygdala either de novo from their hormonal precursors through the functioning of glial cells and neurons, or are directly derived from cholesterol [152–154]. Neurosteroids synthesis requires a similar enzymatic apparatus known from adrenal steroid synthesis, but these steroidogenic enzymes are not equally expressed in all neurosteroid-secreting cells (i.e., glia vs. neurons) nor are they present at all stages of the developing brain. The de novo production through the activity of astrocytes and neurons are dependent on cytochrome P450 cholesterol side-chain cleavage enzyme (CYP450scc), which is responsible for the conversion of cholesterol to pregnenolone (PREG), a metabolite involved in further neurosteroidogenesis [155]. To date, many neurosteroids have been described as involved in the regulation of neurological functions.

Based on their structural characteristics, neurosteroids can be classified into pregnane (e.g., pregnanolone, allopregnanolone, corticosterone, allo tetrahydrodeoxycorticosterone), androstane (dehydroepiandrosterone, testosterone, androstanediol, and etiocholanolone), oestrogen (estradiol), and the conjugated group (pregnenolone sulphate, PREGS; dehydroepiandrosterone sulphate, DHEAS, or estradiol sulphate).

In the brain, neurosteroids act mainly in autocrine and/or paracrine ways. They exert biological action via both genomic and non-genomic effects. "Classical" genomic effects (in the order of hours to days) act through nuclear receptors, which serve as modulators of gene transcription. In contrast, rapid non-genomic effects of neurosteroids modulate numerous neural signalling pathways and brain excitability via interactions with ion channels and neurotransmitter receptors found within neuronal plasma membranes [156]. It has been observed that neurosteroids directly inflect the activity of ligand-ion channels, especially GABA-A, NMDA, AMPA, kainite, glycine 5-HT3 (serotonin), sigma type I, nicotinic acetylcholine, oxytocin receptors, and others [157–159].

The BBB is an important regulator of NAS levels in the brain. Not all neuroactive steroids cross the BBB in the same way, thus the BBB regulates hormonal communication between the brain and the body. While lipophilic free and loosely bound steroids can pass the BBB rapidly via bidirectional and non-saturable transmembrane diffusion [160], the steroids bounded to transport proteins (selective transport proteins—sex hormone-binding globulin and transcortin) are not transported across the BBB [161]. By this mechanism, plasma steroid-binding proteins can alter the degree and rate of BBB penetration of their free ligands. On the opposite side, transport of conjugated NASs (esp. PREGS and DHEAS), across the BBB, involves the use of transmembrane transporters, specifically the ATP-binding cassette (ABC)- and solute carrier (SLC)-type membrane proteins, or transport along a high concentration gradient [162]. Although steroids in the brain are usually several times lower than steroids in the circulating bloodstream, some NASs, such as DHEA/S, pregnenolone, or allopregnanolone, can reach even higher concentrations in the CSF than in plasma [163].

DHEA and its sulphate DHEAS, characterized by antioxidant, anti-inflammatory, and neuroprotective functions [33, 164], are so far the most promising candidates for clinical use as biomarkers particularly specific for iNPH, although there is still a lack of studies dedicated to the topic. Hence, DHEA/S stimulates neurite growth, neurogenesis and neuronal survival, apoptosis, catecholamine synthesis, and secretion [163]. The DHEA metabolic pathways include the formation of its derivatives, namely 7α-OH-DHEA, 7β-OH-DHEA, 7-oxo-DHEA, and finally also 16α-OH-DHEA DHEA metabolites [33, 165]. This requires the enzymatic activity of type 11-beta-hydroxysteroid dehydrogenase type 1 (HSD11B1), 7α- and 16α-hydroxylases. These derivatives are showing functions similar to DHEA itself, especially in the area of neuroprotection and anti-inflammation. According to a recent analysis of steroids in CSF [33], 7α-OH-DHEA, 7β-OH-DHEA, 7-oxo-DHEA, aldosterone, and cortisone together with ratios 7α-OH-DHEA/DHEA, 7-oxo-DHEA/7α-OH-DHEA, 7β-OH-DHEA/7-oxo-DHEA, and 16α-OH-DHEA/DHEA were found to be specific predictors of NPH with both 100% sensitivity and specificity determined by the predictive model of orthogonal projections (OPLS). The CSF levels of aldosterone were significantly higher in NPH when compared to the control group, and conversely, concentrations of cortisone, 7α-OH-DHEA, 7β-OH-DHEA, and 7-oxo-DHEA were significantly decreased in NPH patients. The levels of DHEA, 16α-OH-DHEA, and cortisol did not correlate with statistically significant differences between the two studied groups. Unfortunately, Sosvorova et al. [33, 34] are so far the only authors who evaluated DHEA and its metabolites as specific for NPH, and thus the role of DHEA and its derivatives in NPH diagnosis is far from complete. The above-mentioned authors further studied CSF steroids, neurosteroids, and their concentration changes with respect to shunt insertion in NPH patients [33, 34, 166, 167]. Their results should be implemented in future research.

7.2 *Vitamin D as a Neurosteroid*

Vitamin D is an essential micronutrient with pleiotropic effects in humans. In addition to calcium/phosphate metabolism, vitamin D also regulates many other physiologic processes in the human body and interacts with the immune, endocrine, cardiovascular, and nervous system. Moreover, the vitamin D receptor (VDR) and the enzymes necessary for vitamin D synthesis have been observed in more than 35 types of tissues throughout the human organism including the brain tissue [168–170]. Since vitamin D is a secosteroid, it acts like other steroids with both "classical" genomic and "alternative" non-genomic effects. The long-term genomic effects cause alteration in expression of more than 1500 genes, whereas short-term effects are manifested by the opening of ion channels, the induction of second messengers, and the control of adenylate cyclase, phosphatase, kinase, phospholipase activity, and others.

Studies confirmed that vitamin D can be synthesized and metabolized in the brain [168] and is subject to autocrine and paracrine regulation. The onset of VDR expression highly corresponds with the dopaminergic neurons within the mesencephalon and especially in substantia nigra, which highlights the role of vitamin D in dopaminergic pathways [171]. Vitamin D metabolites can cross the blood–brain barrier [172], but the levels of biologically active form—1,25(OH)2D3—do not correlate between plasma and the CNS [173], supporting the thesis of local vitamin D synthesis in the brain.

A growing body of evidence shows that vitamin D has a significant effect on both the developing and adult brain, consisting primarily of calcium signalling regulation, neurotrophic factors release, neuroprotection against toxicity and neuroinflammation, regulation of neurotransmission, and altering synaptic plasticity [174].

Recently, several studies have reported that the elderly with low vitamin D levels have significantly similar clinical symptoms to NPH. Low serum vitamin D has been associated with dementia and mild cognitive impairment. Conversely, increased serum vitamin D has predicted a lower risk for cognitive decline and better cognitive performance [175–177]. Moreover, low serum vitamin D concentrations were related to gait disturbance [178, 179] and brain morphological changes [175, 180]. Another study focused on the clinical significance of vitamin D in NPH and showed that significantly lower concentrations of vitamin D may be related to lower preoperative cognition, urinary incontinence, and brain changes [181].

8 Vascular Biomarkers

One of the most notoriously known chemical mediators responsible for several physiological as well as pathophysiological modifications of vascular architecture or inflammation proangiogenic vascular endothelial growth factor (VEGF) increases the BBB permeability and is an important component of neuroprotective substances in the CNS, as it is upregulated after the injury of CNS [182]. It has been demonstrated [183] that CSF VEGF concentrations correlate with subsequent clinical outcomes of iNPH patients—higher VEGF concentrations are associated with the poorer clinical status of analysed patients. Additionally, VEGF has been proved to play a role in diseases such as stroke or hydrocephalus-induced hypoxia [182, 184]. It should be noted that the concentrations of cerebral metabolites are dynamic, dependent on many factors including blood flow, and thus are changeable over time. Longer follow-up and monitoring of these changes are crucial determinants for a decision about potential applicability in iNPH diagnosis.

9 Approach and Guidelines

In practice, it is rather challenging to identify a biomarker particularly specific for NPH that would be simultaneously reliable in the prediction of shunt responsiveness and related diagnostic measures. In the study [90], which was already mentioned with respect to the very similar measurement of P-tau CSF levels, the authors subsequently conducted the diagnosis accuracy analysis by performing receiver operating characteristics (ROC) curves in each biomarker within the predefined patient's groups (iNPH, AD, SIVD, and healthy individuals). Based on its results, the combination of NFL, Aβ42, and T- and P-tau resulted in the area under the curve (AUC) value of 0.9 which is considered as a convincing outcome worth further investigation (Fig. 4). Good diagnostic sensitivity and specificity of distinguishing patients with iNPH and movement or cognitive conditions were evaluated [26] within the combination of T-tau, Aβ40, and MCP-1 (the AUC equalized at the value of 0.86 when comparing overall CSF biomarker levels in patients with iNPH and non-iNPH diagnosis). Therefore, searching for combinations and mixed settings of CSF and other biomarkers may be helpful for their potential applicability in ongoing clinical practice.

According to recently disclosed guidelines for iNPH management [185], CSF levels of both T- and P-tau, Aβ42, NFL, and LRG may be effective in predicting the shunt response which is a statement awarded with the recommendation grade 2 and C-level of evidence, further mirroring the fact of inadequate research dedicated to the topic. Amyloid β-related and tau proteins were disclosed as useful in separating iNPH (or AD) from healthy individuals, but they are not specific for iNPH (recommendation grade 2, level of evidence B). The widely discussed LRG has been found to be increased not only in iNPH, but also in other neurodegenerative disorders and therefore cannot be considered as a characteristic marker of iNPH. However, the authors of the mentioned guidelines did not differentiate the primary classification of iNPH patients according to the algorithm of diagnosis and management of the disease, since they should be divided into possible, probable, and definite iNPH. As we have already interpreted, the measured levels of particular biomarkers in many cases differ among these iNPH groups. Therefore, the findings on the potential applicability of Aβ42, NFL, P- and T-tau proteins, or LRG should be considered individually for prespecified iNPH patients (Fig. 5).

One of the least discussed issues in NPH diagnosis is a potential link among NPH pathophysiology, brain ventricular volume, and changes in the concentrations of CSF biomarkers. In the case of AD, a different pattern of ventricular volume was evaluated in comparison with healthy individuals since the dilatation of cerebral ventricles correlates with impaired CSF clearance mechanisms [186], and thus, it is associated with abnormal CSF composition. In patients experiencing neurodegenerative disorders, the ventricular volume has been considered as a promising determinant of distinguishing individual pathologies in terms of measuring specific levels of CSF markers [187–189]. Unfortunately, there are no available findings of similar research dedicated specifically to NPH, and the majority of studies reporting results on laboratory findings of NPH do not consider the ventricular volume in their calculations.

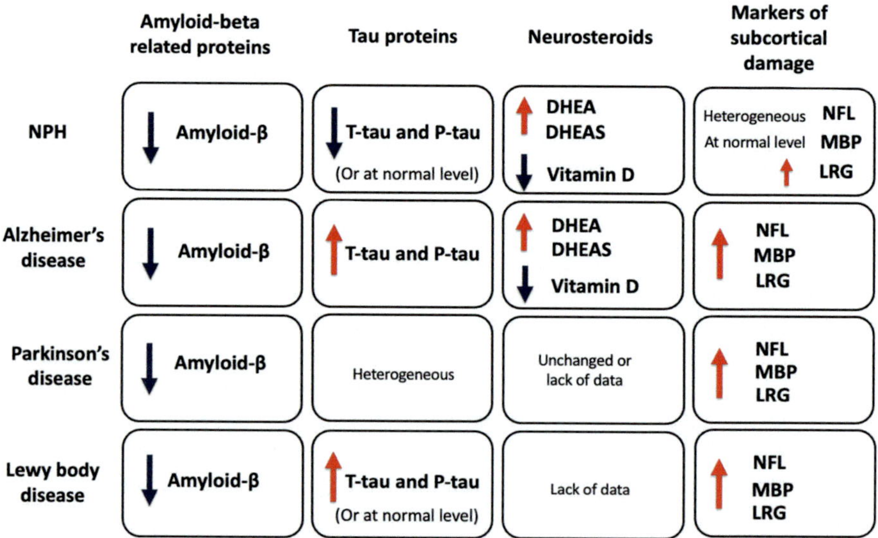

Fig. 5 Summarized results of CSF biomarkers analysed in various neurodegenerative disorders

10   Conclusion

Although the survey of potentially specific biomarkers for NPH is far from being complete, research so far has revealed enormous amounts of reliable information on the overall CSF profile in iNPH patients. Neuropathological and neuropatho-physiological abnormalities which distinguish iNPH from other neurodegenerative disorders are certain, and important findings dedicated to this topic have been identified. Unfortunately, the research does not unequivocally determine a biomarker specific for iNPH, even though many of these have been investigated. Studies with larger patient cohorts are needed for more precise results and better differentiation of iNPH from other neurodegeneration-related disorders. Many studies report results only on measured CSF levels of specific biomarkers between two patient's groups, most commonly iNPH and healthy controls. However, the explicit iNPH diagnosis remains crucial especially between iNPH and other neurodegenerative comorbidities as many of these disorders are present together in a concurrent manner.

11   Key Points

- The most problematic issue of iNPH diagnosis is the high concurrence of iNPH and neurodegenerative disorders and the lack of research dedicated to the topic as many of the results were evaluating the abnormalities only between probable or definite iNPH patients with control subjects.
- Both iNPH and AD are characterized by the reduction of amyloid-β proteins. T-tau and P-tau are increased in AD and conversely reduced or at a normal level in iNPH which makes the differentiation difficult due to frequent concurrence of both pathologies.
- The CSF levels of inflammatory biomarkers (particularly IL-β1, IL-6, IL-10, TGF-β1) may be increased, but up-to-date results are heterogeneous and the consensus on their validity for iNPH diagnosis remains unclear.
- Biomarkers of subcortical damage (NFL, MBP, and LRG) are not disease specific, but their potential purpose in clinical practice may be found in direct reflection of periventricular white matter damage as well as prediction of shunt responsiveness.
- Neurosteroids, particularly DHEA and its derivatives, are promising candidates for clinical use in iNPH diagnosis; however, there is a lack of studies dedicated to the topic.
- The exact role of VEGF in iNPH has not been elucidated, but its higher concentrations are believed to correlate with worse clinical outcome.
- Searching for specific combinations of biomarkers that are associated with characteristic signs of iNPH may be helpful for clearly distinguishing iNPH from other conditions.

- Prospectively held studies evaluating a larger proportion of patients with iNPH and coexisting neurodegenerative disorders are needed in order to clarify currently uncertain and miscellaneous results on specific biomarkers of iNPH and to reveal more definite results on the differentiation of iNPH from other pathologies.
- The ventricular volume may serve as a determinant of neurodegeneration-related impaired CSF clearance, and according to the measured levels of CSF biomarkers, it may help to distinguish comorbidities from in NPH. Research dedicated to the topic is needed.

Funding This chapter was supported by the Ministry of Health of the Czech Republic institutional grant no. NU23-04–00551.

References

1. Akai K, Uchigasaki S, Tanaka U, Komatsu A. Normal pressure hydrocephalus. Neuropathological study. Acta Pathol Jpn. 1987;37:97–110.
2. Kiefer M, Unterberg A. The differential diagnosis and treatment of normal-pressure hydrocephalus. Deutsches Aerzteblatt Online. 2012. https://doi.org/10.3238/arztebl.2012.0015.
3. Daou B, Klinge P, Tjoumakaris S, Rosenwasser RH, Jabbour P. Revisiting secondary normal pressure hydrocephalus: does it exist? A review Neurosurgical Focus. 2016;41:E6. https://doi.org/10.3171/2016.6.focus16189.
4. Hebb AO, Cusimano MD. Idiopathic normal pressure hydrocephalus: a systematic review of diagnosis and outcome. Neurosurgery 2001;49:1166–1184; discussion 1184–1166. https://doi.org/10.1097/00006123-200111000-00028.
5. Wang C, Du HG, Yin LC, He M, Zhang GJ, Tian Y, Hao BL. Analysis of related factors affecting prognosis of shunt surgery in patients with secondary normal pressure hydrocephalus. Chin J Traumatol. 2013;16:221–4.
6. Zemack G, Romner B. Adjustable valves in normal-pressure hydrocephalus: a retrospective study of 218 patients. Neurosurgery 2002;51:1392–1400; discussion 1400–1392.
7. Børgesen SE. Conductance to outflow of CSF in normal pressure hydrocephalus. Acta Neurochir. 1984;71:1–45. https://doi.org/10.1007/bf01401149.
8. Craven CL, Toma AK, Mostafa T, Patel N, Watkins LD. The predictive value of DESH for shunt responsiveness in idiopathic normal pressure hydrocephalus. J Clin Neurosci. 2016;34:294–8. https://doi.org/10.1016/j.jocn.2016.09.004.
9. Skalický P, Vlasák A, Mládek A, Vrána J, Bajaček M, Whitley H, Beneš V, Bradáč O. Role of DESH, callosal angle and cingulate sulcus sign in prediction of gait responsiveness after shunting in iNPH patients. J Clin Neurosci. 2021;83:99–107. https://doi.org/10.1016/j.jocn.2020.11.020.
10. Otero-Rodríguez A, Sousa-Casasnovas P, Cruz-Terrón H, Arandia-Guzmán DA, García-Martín A, Pascual-Argente D, Muñoz-Martín MC. Utility of radiologic variables to predict the result of lumbar infusion test in the diagnosis of idiopathic normal pressure hydrocephalus. World Neurosurg. 2019;127:e957–64. https://doi.org/10.1016/j.wneu.2019.04.009.
11. Vlasák A, Skalický P, Mládek A, Vrána J, Beneš V, Bradáč O. Structural volumetry in NPH diagnostics and treatment—future or dead end? Neurosurg Rev. 2021;44:503–14. https://doi.org/10.1007/s10143-020-01245-y.

12. Mihalj M, Dolić K, Kolić K, Ledenko V. CSF tap test - Obsolete or appropriate test for predicting shunt responsiveness? A Systemic Rev. J Neurol Sci. 2016;362:78–84. https://doi.org/10.1016/j.jns.2016.01.028.

13. Relkin N, Marmarou A, Klinge P, Bergsneider M, Black PM. Diagnosing idiopathic normal-pressure hydrocephalus. Neurosurgery 2005;57:S4–16; discussion ii–v. https://doi.org/10.1227/01.neu.0000168185.29659.c5.

14. Brean A, Eide PK. Assessment of idiopathic normal pressure patients in neurological practice: the role of lumbar infusion testing for referral of patients to neurosurgery. Eur J Neurol. 2008;15:605–12. https://doi.org/10.1111/j.1468-1331.2008.02134.x.

15. Wilson RK, Williams MA. Normal pressure hydrocephalus. Clin Geriatr Med 2006;22:935–951, viii. https://doi.org/10.1016/j.cger.2006.06.010.

16. Brean A, Eide PK. Prevalence of probable idiopathic normal pressure hydrocephalus in a Norwegian population. Acta Neurol Scand. 2008;118:48–53. https://doi.org/10.1111/j.1600-0404.2007.00982.x.

17. Martín-Láez R, Caballero-Arzapalo H, López-Menéndez L, Arango-Lasprilla JC, Vázquez-Barquero A. Epidemiology of idiopathic normal pressure hydrocephalus: a systematic review of the literature. World Neurosurg. 2015;84:2002–9. https://doi.org/10.1016/j.wneu.2015.07.005.

18. Jaraj D, Rabiei K, Marlow T, Jensen C, Skoog I, Wikkelso C. Prevalence of idiopathic normal-pressure hydrocephalus. Neurology. 2014;82:1449–54. https://doi.org/10.1212/wnl.0000000000000342.

19. Brean A, Fredø HL, Sollid S, Müller T, Sundstrøm T, Eide PK. Five-year incidence of surgery for idiopathic normal pressure hydrocephalus in Norway. Acta Neurol Scand. 2009;120:314–6. https://doi.org/10.1111/j.1600-0404.2009.01250.x.

20. Kim DJ, Kim H, Kim YT, Yoon BC, Czosnyka Z, Park KW, Czosnyka M. Thresholds of resistance to CSF outflow in predicting shunt responsiveness. Neurol Res. 2015;37:332–40. https://doi.org/10.1179/1743132814y.0000000454.

21. Williams MA, Malm J. Diagnosis and treatment of idiopathic normal pressure hydrocephalus. CONTINUUM: Lifelong Learning in Neurol. 2016;22:579–599. https://doi.org/10.1212/con.0000000000000305.

22. Allali G, Laidet M, Armand S, Assal F. Brain comorbidities in normal pressure hydrocephalus. Eur J Neurol. 2018;25:542–8. https://doi.org/10.1111/ene.13543.

23. Stolze H. Comparative analysis of the gait disorder of normal pressure hydrocephalus and Parkinson's disease. J Neurol Neurosurg Psychiatry. 2001;70:289–97. https://doi.org/10.1136/jnnp.70.3.289.

24. Tarnaris A, Kitchen ND, Watkins LD. Noninvasive biomarkers in normal pressure hydrocephalus: evidence for the role of neuroimaging. J Neurosurg. 2009;110:837–51. https://doi.org/10.3171/2007.9.17572.

25. Olsson B, Lautner R, Andreasson U, Öhrfelt A, Portelius E, Bjerke M, Hölttä M, Rosén C, Olsson C, Strobel G, et al. CSF and blood biomarkers for the diagnosis of Alzheimer's disease: a systematic review and meta-analysis. The Lancet Neurol. 2016;15:673–84. https://doi.org/10.1016/s1474-4422(16)00070-3.

26. Jeppsson A, Wikkelsö C, Blennow K, Zetterberg H, Constantinescu R, Remes AM, Herukka S-K, Rauramaa T, Nagga K, Leinonen V, et al. CSF biomarkers distinguish idiopathic normal pressure hydrocephalus from its mimics. J Neurol Neurosurg Psychiatry. 2019;90:1117–23. https://doi.org/10.1136/jnnp-2019-320826.

27. Agren-Wilsson A, Lekman A, Sjöberg W, Rosengren L, Blennow K, Bergenheim AT, Malm J. CSF biomarkers in the evaluation of idiopathic normal pressure hydrocephalus. Acta Neurol Scand. 2007;116:333–9. https://doi.org/10.1111/j.1600-0404.2007.00890.x.

28. Pfanner T, Henri-Bhargava A, Borchert S. Cerebrospinal fluid biomarkers as predictors of shunt response in idiopathic normal pressure hydrocephalus: a systematic review. Canadian J Neurol Sci/J Canadien des Sci Neurologiques. 2018;45:3–10. https://doi.org/10.1017/cjn.2017.251.

29. Ray B, Reyes PF, Lahiri DK. Biochemical studies in normal pressure hydrocephalus (NPH) patients: change in CSF levels of amyloid precursor protein (APP), amyloid-beta (Aβ) peptide and phospho-tau. J Psychiatr Res. 2011;45:539–47. https://doi.org/10.1016/j.jpsychires.2010.07.011.

30. Schirinzi T, Sancesario GM, Ialongo C, Imbriani P, Madeo G, Toniolo S, Martorana A, Pisani A. A clinical and biochemical analysis in the differential diagnosis of idiopathic normal pressure hydrocephalus. Front Neurol. 2015;6. https://doi.org/10.3389/fneur.2015.00086.

31. Schirinzi T, Sancesario GM, Di Lazzaro G, D'Elia A, Imbriani P, Scalise S, Pisani A. Cerebrospinal fluid biomarkers profile of idiopathic normal pressure hydrocephalus. J Neural Transm. 2018;125:673–9. https://doi.org/10.1007/s00702-018-1842-z.

32. Sosvorova L, Vcelak J, Mohapl M, Vitku J, Bicikova M, Hampl R. Selected pro- and anti-inflammatory cytokines in cerebrospinal fluid in normal pressure hydrocephalus. Neuro Endocrinol Lett. 2014;35:586–93.

33. Sosvorova L, Hill M, Mohapl M, Vitku J, Hampl R. Steroid hormones in prediction of normal pressure hydrocephalus. J Steroid Biochem Mol Biol. 2015;152:124–32. https://doi.org/10.1016/j.jsbmb.2015.05.004.

34. Sosvorova L, Mohapl M, Hill M, Starka L, Bicikova M, Vitku J, Kanceva R, Bestak J, Hampl R. Steroid hormones and homocysteine in the outcome of patients with normal pressure hydrocephalus. Physiol Res. 2015;S227–S236. https://doi.org/10.33549/physiolres.933072.

35. Li X, Miyajima M, Mineki R, Taka H, Murayama K, Arai H. Analysis of potential diagnostic biomarkers in cerebrospinal fluid of idiopathic normal pressure hydrocephalus by proteomics. Acta Neurochir. 2006;148:859–64. https://doi.org/10.1007/s00701-006-0787-4.

36. Jeppsson A, Zetterberg H, Blennow K, Wikkelsø C. Idiopathic normal-pressure hydrocephalus: pathophysiology and diagnosis by CSF biomarkers. Neurology. 2013;80:1385–92. https://doi.org/10.1212/WNL.0b013e31828c2fda.

37. Skalický P, Mládek A, Vlasák A, De Lacy P, Beneš V, Bradáč O. Normal pressure hydrocephalus—an overview of pathophysiological mechanisms and diagnostic procedures. Neurosurg Rev. 2020;43:1451–64. https://doi.org/10.1007/s10143-019-01201-5.

38. Andreasen N, Minthon L, Davidsson P, Vanmechelen E, Vanderstichele H, Winblad B, Blennow K. Evaluation of CSF-tau and CSF-Aβ42 as diagnostic markers for Alzheimer disease in clinical practice. Archives of Neurol. 2001;58. https://doi.org/10.1001/archneur.58.3.373.

39. Blennow K, Zetterberg H. Biomarkers for Alzheimer's disease: current status and prospects for the future. J Intern Med. 2018;284:643–63. https://doi.org/10.1111/joim.12816.

40. Greenwald J, Riek R. Biology of amyloid: structure, function, and regulation. Structure. 2010;18:1244–60. https://doi.org/10.1016/j.str.2010.08.009.

41. Dogan A. Amyloidosis: insights from proteomics. Annu Rev Pathol. 2017;12:277–304. https://doi.org/10.1146/annurev-pathol-052016-100200.

42. Baumkotter F, Schmidt N, Vargas C, Schilling S, Weber R, Wagner K, Fiedler S, Klug W, Radzimanowski J, Nickolaus S, et al. Amyloid precursor protein dimerization and synaptogenic function depend on copper binding to the growth factor-like domain. J Neurosci. 2014;34:11159–72. https://doi.org/10.1523/jneurosci.0180-14.2014.

43. Chasseigneaux S, Allinquant B. Functions of Aβ, sAPPα and sAPPβ : similarities and differences. J Neurochem. 2012;120:99–108. https://doi.org/10.1111/j.1471-4159.2011.07584.x.

44. Pearson HA, Peers C. Physiological roles for amyloid β peptides. J Physiol. 2006;575:5–10. https://doi.org/10.1113/jphysiol.2006.111203.

45. Mayeux R, Honig LS, Tang MX, Manly J, Stern Y, Schupf N, Mehta PD. Plasma Aβ40 and Aβ42 and Alzheimer's disease. Neurology. 2003;61:1185. https://doi.org/10.1212/01.WNL.0000091890.32140.8F.

46. Shoji M, Kanai M. Cerebrospinal fluid Aβ40 and Aβ42: Natural course and clinical usefulness. J Alzheimers Dis. 2001;3:313–21. https://doi.org/10.3233/JAD-2001-3306.

47. Kojro E, Fahrenholz F. The non-amyloidogenic pathway: structure and function of alpha-secretases. Subcell Biochem. 2005;38:105–27. https://doi.org/10.1007/0-387-23226-5_5.

48. Sun X, Chen W-D, Wang Y-D. β-Amyloid: the key peptide in the pathogenesis of Alzheimer's disease. Frontiers in Pharmacol. 2015;6. https://doi.org/10.3389/fphar.2015.00221.

49. Chen G-F, Xu T-H, Yan Y, Zhou Y-R, Jiang Y, Melcher K, Xu HE. Amyloid beta: structure, biology and structure-based therapeutic development. Acta Pharmacol Sin. 2017;38:1205–35. https://doi.org/10.1038/aps.2017.28.

50. Qiu T, Liu Q, Chen YX, Zhao YF, Li YM. Aβ42 and Aβ40: similarities and differences. J Pept Sci. 2015;21:522–9. https://doi.org/10.1002/psc.2789.

51. O'Brien RJ, Wong PC. Amyloid precursor protein processing and Alzheimer's disease. Annu Rev Neurosci. 2011;34:185–204. https://doi.org/10.1146/annurev-neuro-061010-113613.

52. Masters CL, Beyreuther K. Alzheimer's centennial legacy: prospects for rational therapeutic intervention targeting the A amyloid pathway. Brain. 2006;129:2823–39. https://doi.org/10.1093/brain/awl251.

53. Zirah S, Kozin SA, Mazur AK, Blond A, Cheminant M, Ségalas-Milazzo I, Debey P, Rebuffat S. Structural changes of region 1–16 of the Alzheimer disease amyloid β-peptide upon zinc binding and in vitro aging. J Biol Chem. 2006;281:2151–61. https://doi.org/10.1074/jbc.m504454200.

54. Chander H, Chauhan A, Chauhan V. Binding of proteases to fibrillar amyloid-beta protein and its inhibition by Congo red. J Alzheimers Dis. 2007;12:261–9. https://doi.org/10.3233/jad-2007-12308.

55. Karran E, Mercken M, Strooper BD. The amyloid cascade hypothesis for Alzheimer's disease: an appraisal for the development of therapeutics. Nat Rev Drug Discovery. 2011;10:698–712. https://doi.org/10.1038/nrd3505.

56. Iliff JJ, Wang M, Liao Y, Plogg Benjamin A, Peng W, Gundersen Georg A, Benveniste H, Vates GE, Deane R, Goldman Steven A, et al. A paravascular pathway facilitates CSF flow through the brain parenchyma and the clearance of interstitial solutes, including amyloid β. Sci Translational Med. 2012;4:147ra111–147ra111. https://doi.org/10.1126/scitranslmed.3003748.

57. Murray MM, Bernstein SL, Nyugen V, Condron MM, Teplow DB, Bowers MT. Amyloid β protein: Aβ40 inhibits Aβ42 oligomerization. J Am Chem Soc. 2009;131:6316–7. https://doi.org/10.1021/ja8092604.

58. Schoonenboom NS, Mulder C, Van Kamp GJ, Mehta SP, Scheltens P, Blankenstein MA, Mehta PD. Amyloid β 38, 40, and 42 species in cerebrospinal fluid: more of the same? Ann Neurol. 2005;58:139–42. https://doi.org/10.1002/ana.20508.

59. Cai Z, Hussain MD, Yan LJ. Microglia, neuroinflammation, and beta-amyloid protein in Alzheimer's disease. Int J Neurosci. 2014;124:307–21. https://doi.org/10.3109/00207454.2013.833510.

60. Burdick D, Soreghan B, Kwon M, Kosmoski J, Knauer M, Henschen A, Yates J, Cotman C, Glabe C. Assembly and aggregation properties of synthetic Alzheimer's A4/beta amyloid peptide analogs. J Biol Chem. 1992;267:546–54. https://doi.org/10.1016/s0021-9258(18)48529-8.

61. Gravina SA, Ho L, Eckman CB, Long KE, Otvos L, Younkin LH, Suzuki N, Younkin SG. Amyloid β protein (Aβ) in Alzheimeri's disease brain. J Biol Chem. 1995;270:7013–6. https://doi.org/10.1074/jbc.270.13.7013.

62. Kamenetz F, Tomita T, Hsieh H, Seabrook G, Borchelt D, Iwatsubo T, Sisodia S, Malinow R. APP processing and synaptic function. Neuron. 2003;37:925–37. https://doi.org/10.1016/s0896-6273(03)00124-7.

63. Giuffrida ML, Caraci F, Pignataro B, Cataldo S, De Bona P, Bruno V, Molinaro G, Pappalardo G, Messina A, Palmigiano A, et al. Beta-amyloid monomers are neuroprotective. J Neurosci. 2009;29:10582–7. https://doi.org/10.1523/jneurosci.1736-09.2009.

64. Whitson Janet S, Selkoe Dennis J, Cotman CW. Amyloid β protein enhances the survival of hippocampal neurons in vitro. Science. 1989;243:1488–90. https://doi.org/10.1126/science.2928783.

65. McCord L, Liang W, Farcasanu M, Scherpelz K, Meredith S, Koide S, Tang W. Crystal structure analysis of fab-bound human insulin degrading enzyme (IDE) in complex with amyloid-beta (1–40). 2014. https://doi.org/10.2210/pdb4M1C/pdb.

66. Jingami N, Asada-Utsugi M, Uemura K, Noto R, Takahashi M, Ozaki A, Kihara T, Kageyama T, Takahashi R, Shimohama S, et al. Idiopathic normal pressure hydrocephalus has a different cerebrospinal fluid biomarker profile from Alzheimer's disease. J Alzheimers Dis. 2015;45:109–15. https://doi.org/10.3233/jad-142622.

67. Hall S, Öhrfelt A, Constantinescu R, Andreasson U, Surova Y, Bostrom F, Nilsson C, Widner H, Decraemer H, Nägga K, et al. Accuracy of a panel of 5 cerebrospinal fluid biomarkers in the differential diagnosis of patients with dementia and/or parkinsonian disorders. Arch Neurol. 2012;69:1445. https://doi.org/10.1001/archneurol.2012.1654.

68. Kapaki EN, Paraskevas GP, Tzerakis NG, Sfagos C, Seretis A, Kararizou E, Vassilopoulos D. Cerebrospinal fluid tau, phospho-tau181 and beta-amyloid1-42 in idiopathic normal pressure hydrocephalus: a discrimination from Alzheimer's disease. Eur J Neurol. 2007;14:168–73. https://doi.org/10.1111/j.1468-1331.2006.01593.x.

69. Miyajima M, Nakajima M, Ogino I, Miyata H, Motoi Y, Arai H. Soluble amyloid precursor protein α in the cerebrospinal fluid as a diagnostic and prognostic biomarker for idiopathic normal pressure hydrocephalus. Eur J Neurol. 2013;20:236–42. https://doi.org/10.1111/j.1468-1331.2012.03781.x.

70. Libard S, Walter J, Alafuzoff I. In vivo characterization of biochemical variants of amyloid-β in subjects with idiopathic normal pressure hydrocephalus and Alzheimer's disease neuropathological change. J Alzheimers Dis. 2021;80:1003–12. https://doi.org/10.3233/jad-201469.

71. Pyykkö OT, Lumela M, Rummukainen J, Nerg O, Seppälä TT, Herukka S-K, Koivisto AM, Alafuzoff I, Puli L, Savolainen S, et al. Cerebrospinal fluid biomarker and brain biopsy findings in idiopathic normal pressure hydrocephalus. PLoS ONE 2014;9:e91974. https://doi.org/10.1371/journal.pone.0091974.

72. Kokkinou M, Beishon LC, Smailagic N, Noel-Storr AH, Hyde C, Ukoumunne O, Worrall RE, Hayen A, Desai M, Ashok AH, et al. Plasma and cerebrospinal fluid ABeta42 for the differential diagnosis of Alzheimer's disease dementia in participants diagnosed with any dementia subtype in a specialist care setting. Cochrane Database of Systematic Rev. 2021. https://doi.org/10.1002/14651858.CD010945.pub2.

73. Chen Z, Liu C, Zhang J, Relkin N, Xing Y, Li Y. Cerebrospinal fluid Aβ42, t-tau, and p-tau levels in the differential diagnosis of idiopathic normal-pressure hydrocephalus: a systematic review and meta-analysis. Fluids and Barriers of the CNS 2017;14. https://doi.org/10.1186/s12987-017-0062-5.

74. Weingarten MD, Lockwood AH, Hwo SY, Kirschner MW. A protein factor essential for microtubule assembly. Proc Natl Acad Sci. 1975;72:1858–62. https://doi.org/10.1073/pnas.72.5.1858.

75. Schweers O, Schönbrunn-Hanebeck E, Marx A, Mandelkow E. Structural studies of tau protein and Alzheimer paired helical filaments show no evidence for beta-structure. J Biol Chem. 1994;269:24290–7.

76. Andreadis A, Brown WM, Kosik KS. Structure and novel exons of the human .tau. gene. Biochemistry 1992;31:10626–10633. https://doi.org/10.1021/bi00158a027.

77. Neve RL, Harris P, Kosik KS, Kurnit DM, Donlon TA. Identification of cDNA clones for the human microtubule-associated protein tau and chromosomal localization of the genes for tau and microtubule-associated protein 2. Mol Brain Res. 1986;1:271–80. https://doi.org/10.1016/0169-328X(86)90033-1.

78. Buée L, Bussière T, Buée-Scherrer V, Delacourte A, Hof PR. Tau protein isoforms, phosphorylation and role in neurodegenerative disorders. Brain Res Rev. 2000;33:95–130. https://doi.org/10.1016/S0165-0173(00)00019-9.

79. Goedert M, Spillantini MG, Jakes R, Rutherford D, Crowther RA. Multiple isoforms of human microtubule-associated protein tau: sequences and localization in neurofibrillary tangles of Alzheimer's disease. Neuron. 1989;3:519–26. https://doi.org/10.1016/0896-6273(89)90210-9.

80. Goedert M, Spillantini MG, Potier MC, Ulrich J, Crowther RA. Cloning and sequencing of the cDNA encoding an isoform of microtubule-associated protein tau containing four tandem

repeats: differential expression of tau protein mRNAs in human brain. EMBO J. 1989;8:393–9. https://doi.org/10.1002/j.1460-2075.1989.tb03390.x.

81. Ittner LM, Ke YD, Delerue F, Bi M, Gladbach A, Van Eersel J, Wölfing H, Chieng BC, Christie MJ, Napier IA, et al. Dendritic function of tau mediates amyloid-β toxicity in Alzheimer's disease mouse models. Cell. 2010;142:387–97. https://doi.org/10.1016/j.cell.2010.06.036.

82. Avila J, Lucas JJ, Pérez MAR, Hernández F. Role of tau protein in both physiological and pathological conditions. Physiol Rev. 2004;84:361–84. https://doi.org/10.1152/physrev.00024.2003.

83. Vanier MT, Neuville P, Michalik L, Launay JF. Expression of specific tau exons in normal and tumoral pancreatic acinar cells. J Cell Sci. 1998;111(Pt 10):1419–32.

84. Gu Y, Oyama F, Ihara Y. τ Is Widely Expressed in Rat Tissues. J Neurochem. 1996;67:1235–44. https://doi.org/10.1046/j.1471-4159.1996.67031235.x.

85. Pîrşcoveanu DFV, Pirici I, Tudorică V, Bălşeanu TA, Albu VC, Bondari S, Bumbea AM, Pîrşcoveanu M. Tau protein in neurodegenerative diseases—a review. Rom J Morphol Embryol. 2017;58:1141–50.

86. Lee G, Neve RL, Kosik KS. The microtubule binding domain of tau protein. Neuron. 1989;2:1615–24. https://doi.org/10.1016/0896-6273(89)90050-0.

87. Grundke-Iqbal I, Iqbal K, Tung YC, Quinlan M, Wisniewski HM, Binder LI. Abnormal phosphorylation of the microtubule-associated protein tau (tau) in Alzheimer cytoskeletal pathology. Proc Natl Acad Sci. 1986;83:4913–7. https://doi.org/10.1073/pnas.83.13.4913.

88. Sergeant N, Bussière T, Vermersch P, Lejeune JP, Delacourte A. Isoelectric point differentiates PHF-tau from biopsy-derived human brain tau proteins. NeuroReport 1995;6. https://doi.org/10.1097/00001756-199511000-00028.

89. Lim TS, Choi JY, Park SA, Youn YC, Lee HY, Kim BG, Joo IS, Huh K, Moon SY. Evaluation of coexistence of Alzheimer's disease in idiopathic normal pressure hydrocephalus using ELISA analyses for CSF biomarkers. BMC Neurol. 2014;14:66. https://doi.org/10.1186/1471-2377-14-66.

90. Manniche C, Simonsen AH, Hasselbalch SG, Andreasson U, Zetterberg H, Blennow K, Høgh P, Juhler M, Hejl A-M. Cerebrospinal fluid biomarkers to differentiate idiopathic normal pressure hydrocephalus from subcortical ischemic vascular disease. J Alzheimers Dis. 2020;75:937–47. https://doi.org/10.3233/jad-200036.

91. Rasmussen MK, Mestre H, Nedergaard M. The glymphatic pathway in neurological disorders. The Lancet Neurol. 2018;17:1016–24. https://doi.org/10.1016/s1474-4422(18)30318-1.

92. Yang C, Huang X, Huang X, Mai H, Li J, Jiang T, Wang X, Lü T. Aquaporin-4 and Alzheimer's disease. J Alzheimers Dis. 2016;52:391–402. https://doi.org/10.3233/JAD-150949.

93. Hasan-Olive MM, Enger R, Hansson HA, Nagelhus EA, Eide PK. Loss of perivascular aquaporin-4 in idiopathic normal pressure hydrocephalus. Glia. 2019;67:91–100. https://doi.org/10.1002/glia.23528.

94. Reeves BC, Karimy JK, Kundishora AJ, Mestre H, Cerci HM, Matouk C, Alper SL, Lundgaard I, Nedergaard M, Kahle KT. Glymphatic system impairment in Alzheimer's disease and idiopathic normal pressure hydrocephalus. Trends Mol Med. 2020;26:285–95. https://doi.org/10.1016/j.molmed.2019.11.008.

95. Eid T, Lee TSW, Thomas MJ, Amiry-Moghaddam M, Bjornsen LP, Spencer DD, Agre P, Ottersen OP, De Lanerolle NC. Loss of perivascular aquaporin 4 may underlie deficient water and K+ homeostasis in the human epileptogenic hippocampus. Proc Natl Acad Sci. 2005;102:1193–8. https://doi.org/10.1073/pnas.0409308102.

96. Misu T, Fujihara K, Kakita A, Konno H, Nakamura M, Watanabe S, Takahashi T, Nakashima I, Takahashi H, Itoyama Y. Loss of aquaporin 4 in lesions of neuromyelitis optica: distinction from multiple sclerosis. Brain. 2007;130:1224–34. https://doi.org/10.1093/brain/awm047.

97. Verkman AS, Smith AJ, Phuan P-W, Tradtrantip L, Anderson MO. The aquaporin-4 water channel as a potential drug target in neurological disorders. Expert Opin Ther Targets. 2017;21:1161–70. https://doi.org/10.1080/14728222.2017.1398236.

98. Nagelhus EA, Ottersen OP. Physiological roles of aquaporin-4 in brain. Physiol Rev. 2013;93:1543–62. https://doi.org/10.1152/physrev.00011.2013.

99. Desai B, Hsu Y, Schneller B, Hobbs JG, Mehta AI, Linninger A. Hydrocephalus: the role of cerebral aquaporin-4 channels and computational modeling considerations of cerebrospinal fluid. Neurosurg Focus. 2016;41:E8. https://doi.org/10.3171/2016.7.focus16191.
100. Bradley WG. CSF flow in the brain in the context of normal pressure hydrocephalus. Am J Neuroradiol. 2015;36:831–8. https://doi.org/10.3174/ajnr.a4124.
101. Graff-Radford NR. Alzheimer CSF biomarkers may be misleading in normal-pressure hydrocephalus. Neurology. 2014;83:1573–5. https://doi.org/10.1212/wnl.0000000000000916.
102. Gastaldi M, Todisco M, Carlin G, Scaranzin S, Zardini E, Minafra B, Zangaglia R, Pichiecchio A, Reindl M, Jarius S, et al. AQP4 autoantibodies in patients with idiopathic normal pressure hydrocephalus. J Neuroimmunol. 2020;349. https://doi.org/10.1016/j.jneuroim.2020.577407.
103. Kalani MYS, Filippidis AS, Rekate HL. Hydrocephalus and aquaporins: the role of aquaporin-1. In: Springer Vienna; 2012. p. 51–54. https://doi.org/10.1007/978-3-7091-0923-6_11.
104. Castañeyra-Ruiz L, González-Marrero I, Carmona-Calero EM, Abreu-Gonzalez P, Lecuona M, Brage L, Rodríguez EM, Castañeyra-Perdomo A. Cerebrospinal fluid levels of tumor necrosis factor alpha and aquaporin 1 in patients with mild cognitive impairment and idiopathic normal pressure hydrocephalus. Clin Neurol Neurosurg. 2016;146:76–81. https://doi.org/10.1016/j.clineuro.2016.04.025.
105. Hua Y, Ying X, Qian Y, Liu H, Lan Y, Xie A, Zhu X. Physiological and pathological impact of AQP1 knockout in mice. Biosci. Reports 2019;39:BSR20182303. https://doi.org/10.1042/bsr20182303.
106. Paul L, Madan M, Rammling M, Chigurupati S, Chan SL, Pattisapu JV. Expression of aquaporin 1 and 4 in a congenital hydrocephalus rat model. Neurosurgery 2011;68;462–73. https://doi.org/10.1227/NEU.0b013e3182011860.
107. Levin SG, Godukhin OV. Modulating effect of cytokines on mechanisms of synaptic plasticity in the brain. Biochem Mosc. 2017;82:264–74. https://doi.org/10.1134/s000629791703004x.
108. Idriss HT, Naismith JH. TNF alpha and the TNF receptor superfamily: structure-function relationship(s). Microsc Res Tech. 2000;50:184–95. https://doi.org/10.1002/1097-0029(20000801)50:3%3c184::Aid-jemt2%3e3.0.Co;2-h.
109. Leinonen V, Koivisto AM, Savolainen S, Rummukainen J, Sutela A, Vanninen R, Jääskeläinen JE, Soininen H, Alafuzoff I. Post-mortem findings in 10 patients with presumed normal-pressure hydrocephalus and review of the literature. Neuropathol Appl Neurobiol. 2012;38:72–86. https://doi.org/10.1111/j.1365-2990.2011.01195.x.
110. Lee J-H, Park D-H, Back D-B, Lee J-Y, Lee C-I, Park K-J, Kang S-H, Cho T-H, Chung Y-G. Comparison of cerebrospinal fluid biomarkers between idiopathic normal pressure hydrocephalus and subarachnoid hemorrhage-induced chronic hydrocephalus: A pilot study. Medical Sci. Monitor 2012;18:PR19–PR25. https://doi.org/10.12659/msm.883586.
111. Takahashi T, Suzuki T. Role of sulfatide in normal and pathological cells and tissues. J Lipid Res. 2012;53:1437–50. https://doi.org/10.1194/jlr.r026682.
112. Tisell M, Tullberg M, Månsson JE, Fredman P, Blennow K, Wikkelsø C. Differences in cerebrospinal fluid dynamics do not affect the levels of biochemical markers in ventricular CSF from patients with aqueductal stenosis and idiopathic normal pressure hydrocephalus. Eur J Neurol. 2004;11:17–23. https://doi.org/10.1046/j.1351-5101.2003.00698.x.
113. Tullberg M. CSF sulfatide distinguishes between normal pressure hydrocephalus and subcortical arteriosclerotic encephalopathy. J Neurol Neurosurg Psychiatry. 2000;69:74–81. https://doi.org/10.1136/jnnp.69.1.74.
114. Simi A, Tsakiri N, Wang P, Rothwell NJ. Interleukin-1 and inflammatory neurodegeneration. Biochem Soc Trans. 2007;35:1122–6. https://doi.org/10.1042/BST0351122.
115. Rota E, Bellone G, Rocca P, Bergamasco B, Emanuelli G, Ferrero P. Increased intrathecal TGF-β1, but not IL-12, IFN-γ and IL-10 levels in Alzheimer's disease patients. Neurol Sci. 2006;27:33–9. https://doi.org/10.1007/s10072-006-0562-6.
116. Boyd FT, Cheifetz S, Andres J, Laiho M, Massagué J. Transforming growth factor-β receptors and binding proteoglycans. J Cell Sci. 1990;1990:131–8. https://doi.org/10.1242/jcs.1990.supplement_13.12.

117. Clark DA, Coker R. Molecules in focus transforming growth factor-beta (TGF-β). Int J Biochem Cell Biol. 1998;30:293–8. https://doi.org/10.1016/S1357-2725(97)00128-3.

118. Morikawa M, Derynck R, Miyazono K. TGF-β and the TGF-β Family: context-dependent roles in cell and tissue physiology. Cold Spring Harbor Perspectives in Biol. 2016;8:a021873. https://doi.org/10.1101/cshperspect.a021873.

119. Li X, Miyajima M, Jiang C, Arai H. Expression of TGF-βs and TGF-β type II receptor in cerebrospinal fluid of patients with idiopathic normal pressure hydrocephalus. Neurosci Lett. 2007;413:141–4. https://doi.org/10.1016/j.neulet.2006.11.039.

120. Hinck AP, Archer SJ, Qian SW, Roberts AB, Sporn MB, Weatherbee JA, Tsang MLS, Lucas R, Zhang B-L, Wenker J, et al. Transforming growth factor β1: three-dimensional structure in solution and comparison with the X-ray structure of transforming growth factor β2. Biochemistry. 1996;35:8517–34. https://doi.org/10.1021/bi9604946.

121. Wu V-Y, Walz DA, McCoy LE. Purification and characterization of human and bovine platelet factor 4. Prep Biochem. 1977;7:479–93. https://doi.org/10.1080/00327487708065515.

122. Deshmane SL, Kremlev S, Amini S, Sawaya BE. Monocyte chemoattractant protein-1 (MCP-1): an overview. J Interferon Cytokine Res. 2009;29:313–26. https://doi.org/10.1089/jir.2008.0027.

123. Groves DT, Jiang Y. Chemokines, a family of chemotactic cytokines. Crit Rev Oral Biol Med. 1995;6:109–18. https://doi.org/10.1177/10454411950060020101.

124. Matute-Blanch C, Calvo-Barreiro L, Carballo-Carbajal I, Gonzalo R, Sanchez A, Vila M, Montalban X, Comabella M. Chitinase 3-like 1 is neurotoxic in primary cultured neurons. Scient. Reports 2020;10. https://doi.org/10.1038/s41598-020-64093-2.

125. Kester MI, Teunissen CE, Sutphen C, Herries EM, Ladenson JH, Xiong C, Scheltens P, Van Der Flier WM, Morris JC, Holtzman DM, et al. Cerebrospinal fluid VILIP-1 and YKL-40, candidate biomarkers to diagnose, predict and monitor Alzheimer's disease in a memory clinic cohort. Alzheimer's Res Therapy 2015;7. https://doi.org/10.1186/s13195-015-0142-1.

126. Bonneh-Barkay D, Wang G, Starkey A, Hamilton RL, Wiley CA. In vivo CHI3L1 (YKL-40) expression in astrocytes in acute and chronic neurological diseases. J Neuroinflammation. 2010;7:34. https://doi.org/10.1186/1742-2094-7-34.

127. Hjalmarsson C, Bjerke M, Andersson B, Blennow K, Zetterberg H, Åberg ND, Olsson B, Eckerström C, Bokemark L, Wallin A. Neuronal and glia-related biomarkers in cerebrospinal fluid of patients with acute ischemic stroke. J Central Nervous Syst Disease 2014;6:JCNSD.S13821. https://doi.org/10.4137/jcnsd.s13821.

128. Ko PW, Lee HW, Lee M, Youn YC, Kim S, Kim JH, Kang K, Suk K. Increased plasma levels of chitinase 3-like 1 (CHI3L1) protein in patients with idiopathic normal-pressure hydrocephalus. J Neurol Sci 2021;423:117353. https://doi.org/10.1016/j.jns.2021.117353.

129. Rossi S, Motta C, Studer V, Barbieri F, Buttari F, Bergami A, Sancesario G, Bernardini S, De Angelis G, Martino G, et al. Tumor necrosis factor is elevated in progressive multiple sclerosis and causes excitotoxic neurodegeneration. Mult Scler J. 2013;20:304–12. https://doi.org/10.1177/1352458513498128.

130. Lin Y-S, Lee W-J, Wang S-J, Fuh J-L. Levels of plasma neurofilament light chain and cognitive function in patients with Alzheimer or Parkinson disease. Scientific Reports 2018;8. https://doi.org/10.1038/s41598-018-35766-w.

131. Mattsson N, Andreasson U, Zetterberg H, Blennow K. Association of plasma neurofilament light with neurodegeneration in patients with alzheimer disease. JAMA Neurol. 2017;74:557. https://doi.org/10.1001/jamaneurol.2016.6117.

132. Constantinescu R, Romer M, Oakes D, Rosengren L, Kieburtz K. Levels of the light subunit of neurofilament triplet protein in cerebrospinal fluid in Huntington's disease. Parkinsonism Relat Disord. 2009;15:245–8. https://doi.org/10.1016/j.parkreldis.2008.05.012.

133. Olsson B, Portelius E, Cullen NC, Sandelius Å, Zetterberg H, Andreasson U, Höglund K, Irwin DJ, Grossman M, Weintraub D, et al. Association of cerebrospinal fluid neurofilament light protein levels with cognition in patients with dementia, motor neuron disease, and movement disorders. JAMA Neurol. 2019;76:318. https://doi.org/10.1001/jamaneurol.2018.3746.

134. Rohrer JD, Woollacott IOC, Dick KM, Brotherhood E, Gordon E, Fellows A, Toombs J, Druyeh R, Cardoso MJ, Ourselin S, et al. Serum neurofilament light chain protein is a measure of disease intensity in frontotemporal dementia. Neurology. 2016;87:1329–36. https://doi.org/10.1212/wnl.0000000000003154.

135. Lu CH, Macdonald-Wallis C, Gray E, Pearce N, Petzold A, Norgren N, Giovannoni G, Fratta P, Sidle K, Fish M, et al. Neurofilament light chain: a prognostic biomarker in amyotrophic lateral sclerosis. Neurology. 2015;84:2247–57. https://doi.org/10.1212/wnl.0000000000001642.

136. Varhaug KN, Torkildsen Ø, Myhr K-M, Vedeler CA. Neurofilament light chain as a biomarker in multiple sclerosis. Frontiers in Neurol. 2019;10. https://doi.org/10.3389/fneur.2019.00338.

137. Tullberg M, Rosengren L, Blomsterwall E, Karlsson JE, Wikkelsö C. CSF neurofilament and glial fibrillary acidic protein in normal pressure hydrocephalus. Neurology. 1998;50:1122. https://doi.org/10.1212/WNL.50.4.1122.

138. Tullberg M, Blennow K, Månsson J-E, Fredman P, Tisell M, Wikkelsö C. Cerebrospinal fluid markers before and after shunting in patients with secondary and idiopathic normal pressure hydrocephalus. Cerebrospinal Fluid Res. 2008;5:9. https://doi.org/10.1186/1743-8454-5-9.

139. Lamers KJB, Vos P, Verbeek MM, Rosmalen F, van Geel WJA, van Engelen BGM. Protein S-100B, neuron-specific enolase (NSE), myelin basic protein (MBP) and glial fibrillary acidic protein (GFAP) in cerebrospinal fluid (CSF) and blood of neurological patients. Brain Res Bull. 2003;61:261–4. https://doi.org/10.1016/S0361-9230(03)00089-3.

140. Boggs JM. Myelin basic protein: a multifunctional protein. Cellular and Molecular Life Sci CMLS. 2006;63:1945–61. https://doi.org/10.1007/s00018-006-6094-7.

141. Raasakka A, Ruskamo S, Kowal J, Darker R, Baumann A, Martel A, Tuusa J, Myllykoski M, Bürck J, Ulrich AS, et al. Membrane association landscape of myelin basic protein portrays formation of the myelin major dense line. Scientific Reports 2017;7. https://doi.org/10.1038/s41598-017-05364-3.

142. Sutton LN, Wood JH, Brooks BR, Barrer SJ, Kline M, Cohen SR. Cerebrospinal fluid myelin basic protein in hydrocephalus. J Neurosurg. 1983;59:467–70. https://doi.org/10.3171/jns.1983.59.3.0467.

143. Haupt H, Baudner S. [Isolation and characterization of an unknown, leucine-rich 3.1-S-alpha2-glycoprotein from human serum (author's transl)]. Hoppe Seylers Z Physiol Chem. 1977;358:639–646.

144. Matsushima N, Tanaka T, Enkhbayar P, Mikami T, Taga M, Yamada K, Kuroki Y. Comparative sequence analysis of leucine-rich repeats (LRRs) within vertebrate toll-like receptors. BMC Genomics. 2007;8:124. https://doi.org/10.1186/1471-2164-8-124.

145. Shirai R, Hirano F, Ohkura N, Ikeda K, Inoue S. Up-regulation of the expression of leucine-rich α2-glycoprotein in hepatocytes by the mediators of acute-phase response. Biochem Biophys Res Commun. 2009;382:776–9. https://doi.org/10.1016/j.bbrc.2009.03.104.

146. Akiba C, Nakajima M, Miyajima M, Ogino I, Miura M, Inoue R, Nakamura E, Kanai F, Tada N, Kunichika M, et al. Leucine-rich α2-glycoprotein overexpression in the brain contributes to memory impairment. Neurobiol Aging. 2017;60:11–9. https://doi.org/10.1016/j.neurobiolaging.2017.08.014.

147. Nakajima M, Miyajima M, Ogino I, Watanabe M, Miyata H, Karagiozov KL, Arai H, Hagiwara Y, Segawa T, Kobayashi K, et al. Leucine-rich α-2-glycoprotein is a marker for idiopathic normal pressure hydrocephalus. Acta Neurochir. 2011;153:1339–46. https://doi.org/10.1007/s00701-011-0963-z.

148. Nakajima M, Miyajima M, Ogino I, Watanabe M, Hagiwara Y, Segawa T, Kobayashi K, Arai H. Brain localization of leucine-rich α2-glycoprotein and its role. In: Hydrocephalus. Vienna: Springer Vienna; 2012.

149. Baulieu E-E, Robel P. Neurosteroids: a new brain function? J Steroid Biochem Mol Biol. 1990;37:395–403. https://doi.org/10.1016/0960-0760(90)90490-C.

150. Maninger N, Wolkowitz OM, Reus VI, Epel ES, Mellon SH. Neurobiological and neuropsychiatric effects of dehydroepiandrosterone (DHEA) and DHEA sulfate (DHEAS). Front Neuroendocrinol. 2009;30:65–91. https://doi.org/10.1016/j.yfrne.2008.11.002.

151. Caruso D, Melis M, Fenu G, Giatti S, Romano S, Grimoldi M, Crippa D, Marrosu MG, Cavaletti G, Melcangi RC. Neuroactive steroid levels in plasma and cerebrospinal fluid of male multiple sclerosis patients. J Neurochem. 2014;130:591–7.
152. Mellon SH, Griffin LD, Compagnone NA. Biosynthesis and action of neurosteroids. Brain Res Brain Res Rev. 2001;37:3–12.
153. Reddy DS. Neurosteroids. Elsevier 2010;113–137. https://doi.org/10.1016/B978-0-444-53630-3.00008-7.
154. Akwa Y, Young J, Kabbadj K, Sancho MJ, Zucman D, Vourc'h C, Jung-Testas I, Hu ZY, Le Goascogne C, Jo DH, et al. Neurosteroids: biosynthesis, metabolism and function of pregnenolone and dehydroepiandrosterone in the brain. J Steroid Biochem Mol Biol. 1991;40:71–81. https://doi.org/10.1016/0960-0760(91)90169-6.
155. Vallée M. Neurosteroids and potential therapeutics: focus on pregnenolone. J Steroid Biochem Mol Biol. 2016;160:78–87. https://doi.org/10.1016/j.jsbmb.2015.09.030.
156. Reddy DS. Pharmacology of endogenous neuroactive steroids. Crit Rev Neurobiol. 2003;15:197–234. https://doi.org/10.1615/critrevneurobiol.v15.i34.20.
157. Lambert JJ, Belelli D, Peden DR, Vardy AW, Peters JA. Neurosteroid modulation of GABAA receptors. Prog Neurobiol. 2003;71:67–80. https://doi.org/10.1016/j.pneurobio.2003.09.001.
158. Mellon SH, Griffin LD. Neurosteroids: biochemistry and clinical significance. Trends Endocrinol Metab. 2002;13:35–43. https://doi.org/10.1016/s1043-2760(01)00503-3.
159. Rupprecht R. Neuroactive steroids: mechanisms of action and neuropsychopharmacological properties. Psychoneuroendocrinology. 2003;28:139–68. https://doi.org/10.1016/s0306-4530(02)00064-1.
160. Banks WA. Brain meets body: the blood-brain barrier as an endocrine interface. Endocrinology. 2012;153:4111–9. https://doi.org/10.1210/en.2012-1435.
161. Compagnone NA, Mellon SH. Neurosteroids: biosynthesis and function of these novel neuromodulators. Front Neuroendocrinol. 2000;21:1–56.
162. Grube M, Hagen P, Jedlitschky G. Neurosteroid transport in the brain: role of ABC and SLC transporters. Front Pharmacol. 2018;9:354. https://doi.org/10.1006/frne.1999.0188.
163. Maggio M, De Vita F, Fisichella A, Colizzi E, Provenzano S, Lauretani F, Luci M, Ceresini G, Dall'Aglio E, Caffarra P, Valenti G, Ceda GP. DHEA and cognitive function in the elderly. J Steroid Biochem Mol Biol. 2015;145:281–92. https://doi.org/10.1016/j.jsbmb.2014.03.014.
164. Friess E, Schiffelholz T, Steckler T, Steiger A. Dehydroepiandrosterone—a neurosteroid. Eur J Clin Invest. 2000;30:46–50. https://doi.org/10.1046/j.1365-2362.2000.0300s3046.x.
165. Li A, May MP, Bigelow JC. An LC/MS method for the quantitative determination of 7α-OH DHEA and 7β-OH DHEA: an application for the study of the metabolism of DHEA in rat brain. Biomed Chromatogr. 2010;24:833–7. https://doi.org/10.1002/bmc.1371.
166. Sosvorova L, Vitku J, Chlupacova T, Mohapl M, Hampl R. Determination of seven selected neuro- and immunomodulatory steroids in human cerebrospinal fluid and plasma using LC-MS/MS. Steroids. 2015;98:1–8. https://doi.org/10.1016/j.steroids.2015.01.019.
167. Sosvorová L, Bešťák J, Bičíková M, Mohapl M, Hill M, Kubátová J, Hampl R. Determination of homocysteine in cerebrospinal fluid as an indicator for surgery treatment in patients with hydrocephalus. Physiol Res. 2014:521–527. https://doi.org/10.33549/physiolres.932650.
168. Eyles DW, Smith S, Kinobe R, Hewison M, McGrath JJ. Distribution of the vitamin D receptor and 1 alpha-hydroxylase in human brain. J Chem Neuroanat. 2005;29:21–30. https://doi.org/10.1016/j.jchemneu.2004.08.006.
169. Hewison M, Burke F, Evans KN, Lammas DA, Sansom DM, Liu P, Modlin RL, Adams JS. Extra-renal 25-hydroxyvitamin D3–1alpha-hydroxylase in human health and disease. J Steroid Biochem Mol Biol. 2007;103:316–321. https://doi.org/10.1016/j.jsbmb.2006.12.078.
170. Norman AW. Minireview. vitamin D receptor: new assignments for an already busy receptor. Endocrinology 2006;147:5542–5548. https://doi.org/10.1210/en.2006-0946.
171. Cui X, Pelekanos M, Liu PY, Burne TH, McGrath JJ, Eyles DW. The vitamin D receptor in dopamine neurons; its presence in human substantia nigra and its ontogenesis in rat midbrain. Neuroscience. 2013;236:77–87. https://doi.org/10.1016/j.neuroscience.2013.01.035.

172. Pardridge WM, Sakiyama R, Coty WA. Restricted transport of vitamin D and A derivatives through the rat blood-brain barrier. J Neurochem. 1985;44:1138–41. https://doi.org/10.1111/j.1471-4159.1985.tb08735.x.
173. Spach KM, Hayes CE. Vitamin D3 confers protection from autoimmune encephalomyelitis only in female mice. J Immunol. 2005;175:4119–26. https://doi.org/10.4049/jimmunol.175.6.4119.
174. Groves NJ, McGrath JJ, Burne TH. Vitamin D as a neurosteroid affecting the developing and adult brain. Annu Rev Nutr. 2014;34:117–41. https://doi.org/10.1146/annurev-nutr-071813-105557.
175. Annweiler C, Bartha R, Goncalves S, Karras SN, Millet P, Feron F, Beauchet O. Vitamin D-related changes in intracranial volume in older adults: a quantitative neuroimaging study. Maturitas. 2015;80:312–7. https://doi.org/10.1016/j.maturitas.2014.12.011.
176. Lau H, Mat Ludin AF, Rajab NF, Shahar S. Identification of neuroprotective factors associated with successful ageing and risk of cognitive impairment among malaysia older adults. Curr Gerontol Geriatr Res. 2017;2017:4218756. https://doi.org/10.1155/2017/4218756.
177. Wang R, Wang W, Hu P, Zhang R, Dong X, Zhang D. Association of dietary vitamin D intake, serum 25(OH)D(3), 25(OH)D(2) with cognitive performance in the elderly. Nutrients 2021;13. https://doi.org/10.3390/nu13093089.
178. Beauchet O. Vitamin D insufficiency and mild cognitive impairment: cross-sectional association. Eur J Neurol. 2012;19:1023–9. https://doi.org/10.1111/j.1468-1331.2012.03675.x.
179. Bird ML, El Haber N, Batchelor F, Hill K, Wark JD. Vitamin D and parathyroid hormone are associated with gait instability and poor balance performance in mid-age to older aged women. Gait Posture. 2018;59:71–5. https://doi.org/10.1016/j.gaitpost.2017.09.036.
180. Eyles DW, Feron F, Cui X, Kesby JP, Harms LH, Ko P, McGrath JJ, Burne TH. Developmental vitamin D deficiency causes abnormal brain development. Psychoneuroendocrinology 2009;34 Suppl 1:S247–257. https://doi.org/10.1016/j.psyneuen.2009.04.015.
181. Lee C, Seo H, Yoon SY, Chang SH, Park SH, Hwang JH, Kang K, Kim CH, Hahm MH, Park E, Ahn JY, Park KS. Clinical significance of vitamin D in idiopathic normal pressure hydrocephalus. Acta Neurochir (Wien). 2021;163:1969–77. https://doi.org/10.1007/s00701-021-04849-5.
182. Rosenstein JM, Krum JM, Ruhrberg C. VEGF in the nervous system. Organogenesis 2010;6:107–114.https://doi.org/10.4161/org.6.2.11687.
183. Huang H, Yang J, Luciano M, Shriver LP. Longitudinal metabolite profiling of cerebrospinal fluid in normal pressure hydrocephalus links brain metabolism with exercise-induced VEGF production and clinical outcome. Neurochem Res. 2016;41:1713–22. https://doi.org/10.1007/s11064-016-1887-z.
184. Dombrowski SM, Deshpande A, Dingwall C, Leichliter A, Leibson Z, Luciano MG. Chronic hydrocephalus–induced hypoxia: Increased expression of VEGFR-2+ and blood vessel density in hippocampus. Neuroscience. 2008;152:346–59. https://doi.org/10.1016/j.neuroscience.2007.11.049.
185. Nakajima M, Yamada S, Miyajima M, Ishii K, Kuriyama N, Kazui H, Kanemoto H, Suehiro T, Yoshiyama K, Kameda M, et al. Guidelines for management of idiopathic normal pressure hydrocephalus (Third Edition): endorsed by the Japanese society of normal pressure hydrocephalus. Neurol Med Chir (Tokyo). 2021;61:63–97. https://doi.org/10.2176/nmc.st.2020-0292.
186. Ott BR, Cohen RA, Gongvatana A, Okonkwo OC, Johanson CE, Stopa EG, Donahue JE, Silverberg GD. Brain ventricular volume and cerebrospinal fluid biomarkers of alzheimer's disease. J Alzheimers Dis. 2010;20:647–57. https://doi.org/10.3233/jad-2010-1406.
187. Bjerke M, Jonsson M, Nordlund A, Eckerstrom C, Blennow K, Zetterberg H, Pantoni L, Inzitari D, Schmidt R, Wallin A. Cerebrovascular biomarker profile is related to white matter disease and ventricular dilation in a LADIS substudy. Dementia and Geriatric Cognitive Disorders Extra. 2014;4:385–94. https://doi.org/10.1159/000366119.

188. Kresge HA, Liu D, Gupta DK, Moore EE, Osborn KE, Acosta LMY, Bell SP, Pechman KR, Gifford KA, Mendes LA, et al. Lower left ventricular ejection fraction relates to cerebrospinal fluid biomarker evidence of neurodegeneration in older adults. J Alzheimers Dis. 2020;74:965–74. https://doi.org/10.3233/jad-190813.
189. Kaipainen A, Jääskeläinen O, Liu Y, Haapalinna F, Nykänen N, Vanninen R, Koivisto AM, Julkunen V, Remes AM, Herukka S-K. Cerebrospinal fluid and MRI biomarkers in neurodegenerative diseases: a retrospective memory clinic-based study. J Alzheimers Dis. 2020;75:751–65. https://doi.org/10.3233/jad-200175.

Imaging of NPH

Aleš Vlasák, Vojtěch Sedlák, Adéla Bubeníková, and Ondřej Bradáč

Abstract Since the discovery of normal pressure hydrocephalus, scientists around the world have been trying to find a sufficiently accurate imaging biomarker that would identify shunt-responsive patients. Unlike functional tests, which currently play a fundamental role, the role of imaging methods is only supportive. In its basic form, MRI is the modality of choice. It can detect ventriculomegaly well and at the same time exclude any other pathology. MRI also allows us to perform some measurements, which will be described in more detail in the relevant subsections. It is primarily callosal angle, dilated Sylvian fissures, tight high convexity and focal sulcal dilation. These findings, along with ventriculomegaly, form the basis of the DESH score. Another finding typical for NPH is cingulate sulcus sign. Further MRI examinations already require special sequences. In this chapter, we will describe individual methods, including our personal experience with them. These are volumetric studies, diffusion tensor imaging and the phase contrast method. We will also marginally mention the experimental imaging of the glymphatic pathway.

Keywords Hydrocephalus · Imaging · Normal pressure hydrocephalus · DESH · Ventriculomegaly · Computed tomography · Magnetic resonance imaging

Abbreviations

AdaBoost   Adaptive Boosting
AD   Alzheimer's disease

A. Vlasák · A. Bubeníková · O. Bradáč (✉)
Department of Neurosurgery, 2nd Faculty of Medicine, Charles University and Motol University Hospital, Prague, Czech Republic
e-mail: ondrej.bradac2@fnmotol.cz

A. Bubeníková · O. Bradáč
Department of Neurosurgery and Neurooncology, 1st Faculty of Medicine, Charles University and Military University Hospital, Prague, Czech Republic

V. Sedlák
Department of Radiology, Military University Hospital, Prague, Czech Republic

O. Bradac (ed.), *Normal Pressure Hydrocephalus*,
https://doi.org/10.1007/978-3-031-36522-5_16

AUC   Area under the curve
CSF   Cerebrospinal fluid
CT   Computed tomography
DESH   Disproportionately enlarged subarachnoid space hydrocephalus
DTI   Diffusion tensor imaging
DWI   Diffusion-weighted imaging
FA   Fractional anisotropy
GaussNB   Gaussian Naive Bayes
iNPH   Idiopathic normal pressure hydrocephalus
MD   Mean diffusivity
MRI   Magnetic resonance imaging
NPH   Normal pressure hydrocephalus
ROC   Receiver operating characteristic
VP   Vetriculo-peritoneal

1   Introduction

Normal pressure hydrocephalus was first described in 1957 by Colombian neurosurgeon and scientist Salomón Hakim [1]. It is a disease of the elderly with a typical clinical triad—gait disorder, dementia and continence disorder. Unlike other neurodegenerative diseases, NPH can sometimes be cured. The method of treatment, in this case, is shunt surgery. A fundamental problem is the correct indication of patients for this procedure in the absence of clear criteria. At the same time, early and correct diagnosis brings better treatment results [2]. Imaging methods should play an essential role in the diagnosis of NPH. Patients are usually first examined by CT or MRI which reveals ventriculomegaly. This is a mandatory sign of NPH. Unfortunately, to date, no other sufficiently sensitive and specific imaging biomarker has been found.

   In the following chapter, we summarise the current knowledge of imaging methods from the point of view of NPH diagnostics. The chapter is divided into two main sections—basic and advanced MRI imaging, each with several subsections. In the end, we will try to evaluate the position of imaging methods within the complete set of examinations.

2   Roles of CT and MRI in NPH Workup

Imaging studies, due to their non-invasiveness, are often one of the first studies in NPH workup. Since a large proportion of iNPH patients present with findings suggestive of neurodegenerative disorders (e.g. cognitive deficits, gait disturbances), MRI should be the modality of choice for this group of patients. Advantages of MRI include the absence of ionising radiation and availability of more tissue contrasts (i.e.

various sequences.) which usually provide more information than the single tissue contrast available from non-contrast head CT. For a recommended MRI protocol and further discussion of individual MRI sequences see the chapter "Differential diagnosis of neurodegenerative disorders".

CT on the other hand should not be a primary imaging tool for initial workup. However, in cases where CT is contraindicated, like claustrophobia or MRI-incompatible pacemakers, CT is an excellent alternative, especially if the clinical question is focused mostly on NPH. There are two major reasons for this. The first is that the dominant imaging features of NPH are confined to morphological changes, not tissue composition changes, which manifest as a different MRI signal or a different density on CT. This means that the lack of tissue contrast on CT imaging is not a major issue for the diagnosis of NPH, and modern volumetric CT acquisitions allow for reconstruction in any imaging plane desirable. The second reason why CT is a solid alternative to MRI is the image acquisition duration. Clinical-grade MR exams take anywhere from 10 to 30 min of scanner time, during which the patient must stay still in order not to compromise the image quality. On the other hand, a head CT requires the patient to stay still for less than 10 s, and in case of volumetric acquisitions available on multi-row CT scanners, this time can be shortened to less than 1 s. This means that modern CT scanners are resilient to motion artefacts, which are a common obstacle when imaging an elderly population with cognitive deficits, chronic back pain and/or incontinence, which describes a large proportion of NPH patients. CT is also a modality of choice after shunting when complications are suspected, due to its availability.

3 Imaging Findings of NPH

3.1 Evans Index

The first mandatory sign of NPH is ventricular enlargement. We have several indices available to assess it. The most easy and widespread parameter is the Evans index described in 1942 [3]. It is determined by the ratio of maximal width of the frontal horns to the maximal width of the internal dimension of the skull at the same level. It can be measured on both CT and MRI images with the same results (Fig. 1).

In the classic concept of the index, a ratio of 0.3 or more is considered sufficient for the diagnosis of ventriculomegaly. However, new studies emphasise differences in the size of an individual's ventricular system over the years and suggest a change in the ratio according to age groups [4]. It should be also noted that ventriculomegaly can occur for a variety of reasons other than hydrocephalus. This, among other things, explains why the absolute size of the ventricular system does not correlate with the clinical outcome after VP shunt insertion [5].

Some studies point to the deficiencies of the classic Evans index. Images of iNPH patients are characterised by dilatation of the lateral ventricles in the vertical direction

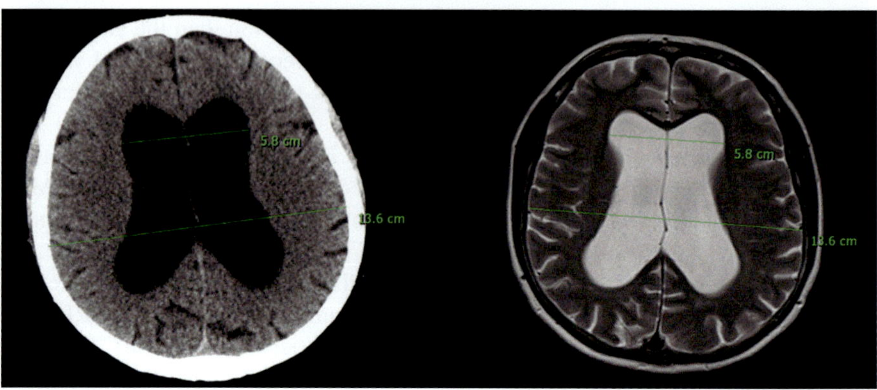

Fig. 1 Evans score gives the same results on CT scan and MRI

in the coronal plane, i.e. the z-axis [6]. This adjustment is called the z-Evans index, which is defined as the ratio of the height of the frontal horns in the direction of the z-axis to the maximum cranial z-axial length. The threshold value of the z-Evans index is set to be > 0.42 (Fig. 2).

There are other scoring systems to determine the size of the ventricles. One is, for example, the distance of the frontal and temporal horns, or the frontal and occipital horns [7]. Although some authors advocate the use of these scores, none have achieved widespread use, despite the fact that the Evans index is only approximate and does not tell us much about the actual size of the ventricular system [8]. In addition, with independent repeated measurements, its value fluctuates and thus its reliability decreases [9]. Nevertheless, the Evans index, due to its simplicity, is still used as a basic measurement for virtually all types of hydrocephalus, including iNPH.

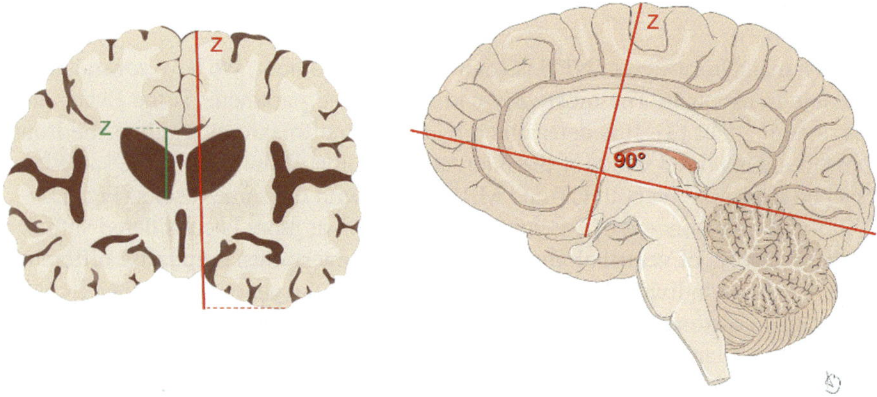

Fig. 2 Measurement of z-Evans index. Z-Evans index is measured on a coronal slice perpendicular to AC-PC line at the level of the anterior commissure by dividing the maximal z-axis dimension of the lateral ventricles (green Z) by a maximal z-axis dimension of brain at the same slice (red Z)

Image segmentation and voxel-based morphometry allow more accurate measurement of the ventricular system. Its disadvantage is the technical and time complexity, which nevertheless decreases over time. Miskin [10] in his article describes the length of the image segmentation process about 8 h, in our study from 2020 the same process took about 15–20 min [11].

3.2 Callosal Angle

Another long-known and frequently measured sign is narrower callosal angle, which was noticed already in the early studies of normal pressure hydrocephalus. Its history stretches back to pneumo-encephalographic imaging. Differences were noted comparing iNPH patients to patients with cerebral atrophy [12]. The methodology for measuring the callosal angle on MRI images was recently revived by the Japanese group for iNPH [13]. The angle is measured on coronal images, between the lateral ventricles at the posterior commissure level, in a plane perpendicular to the anteroposterior commissural plane (Figs. 3 and 4).

The callosal angle has a high predictive value of up to 93% [14]. The smaller the measurement result on preoperative images, the greater the chance for post-operative improvement. Similarly, a better correlation was found with post-operative reduction of the ventricular volume than with the Evans index [15]. Combining the measurements of Evans index and callosal angle has one of the best results in differentiating NPH patients from patients with Alzheimer's disease or from healthy controls. Miskin states in his work accuracy of up to 96% in patients with callosal angle up to 90° and Evans index above 0.3 [10]. Our group also advocates routine measurement of the callosal angle in preoperative diagnosis.

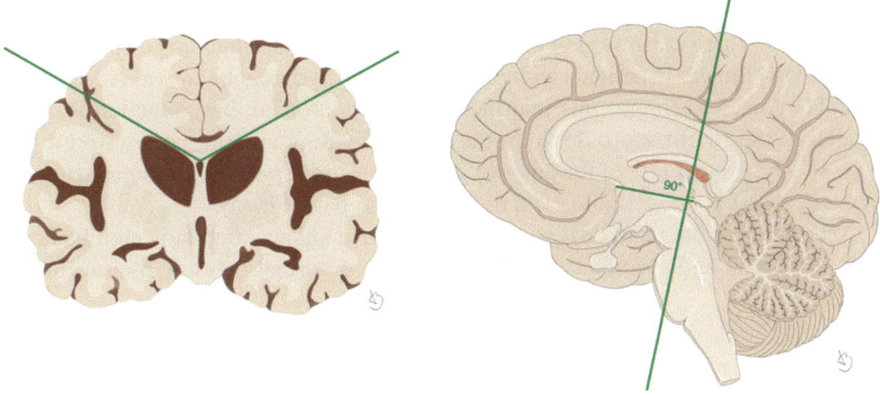

Fig. 3 Callosal angle measurement. Callosal angle is measured on a coronal slice perpendicular to AC-PC line at the level of the posterior commissure

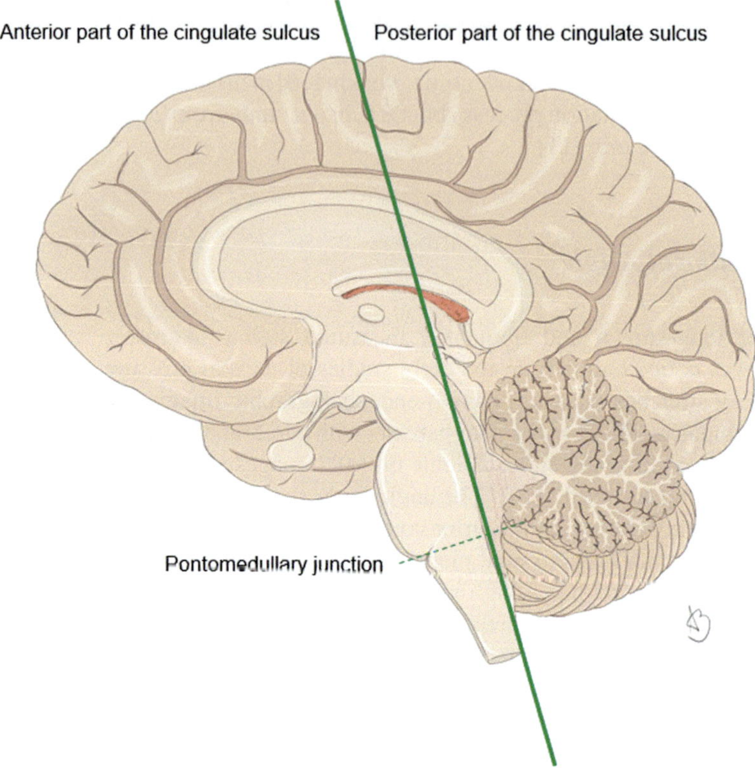

Fig. 4 Line dividing cingulate sulcus into anterior and posterior part

3.3 Cingulate Sulcus Sign

The first to notice a narrowing of the posterior part of sulcus cingularis on paramedian sagittal MRI images in patients with normal pressure hydrocephalus was Adachi et al. [16]. They used a straight line that included the pontomedullary junction and was parallel to the fourth ventricle floor, the sulcus dividing anterior and posterior part (Fig. 4). The same width of the anterior and the posterior part is considered a normal sign. An iNPH positive finding is a tight posterior part (Fig. 5).

According to the published studies, the positive sulcus cingularis sign has both high sensitivity and specificity for the diagnosis of normal pressure hydrocephalus [16].

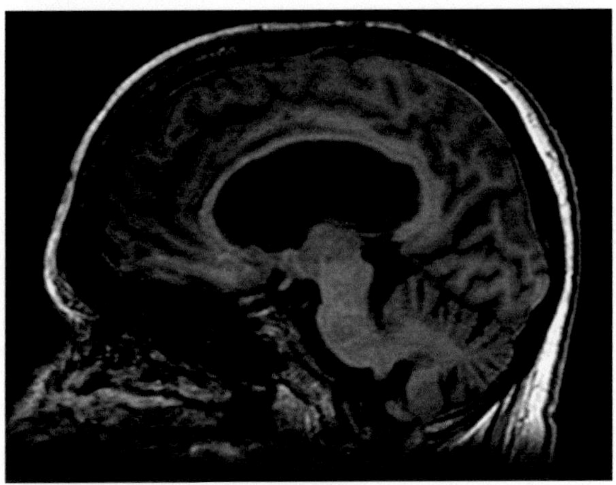

Fig. 5 Positive cingulate sulcus sign. Anterior part of the cingulate sulcus is visibly more spacious than the crowded posterior part

3.4 DESH Score

As mentioned before, various authors have described tight subarachnoid spaces high on the convexity in patients with normal pressure hydrocephalus [17]. The Japanese study SINPHONI (Study of Idiopathic Normal Pressure Hydrocephalus on Neurological Improvement) demonstrated a high predictive value of this sign in identifying patients benefiting from ventriculoperitoneal shunt surgery [18]. Some studies acknowledge that uneven expansion of subarachnoid spaces contributes to the diagnosis of normal pressure hydrocephalus, on the other hand, they emphasise that the absence of these signs does not exclude patients from this diagnosis [19].

Shinoda further developed this concept by introducing a score of 5 scored items—ventriculomegaly, dilated Sylvian fissures, tight subarachnoid spaces on the convexity, callosal angle and focal dilatation of the sulci [20].

Normal pressure hydrocephalus is characterised by an asymmetric distribution of cerebrospinal fluid. While there is a narrowing of the sulci in the area of the apex, they are widening basally and in the area of the Sylvian fissures [21]. Widening of the Sylvian fissures is itself also a diagnostic feature. Virhammar pointed to the inconsistency in the measurement methodology and set the level of measurement to the line leading through the central part of the brainstem [14], (Figs. 6 and 7).

The presence of focally widened sulci has been repeatedly observed in normal pressure hydrocephalus [22]. The disappearance of this sign after a ventriculoperitoneal shunt insertion operation has also been described. As part of the DESH score, we also evaluate the presence or absence of widened sulci on axial and coronal planes (Fig. 8).

According to some authors [23], high-convexity tightness has the highest predictive value of all the listed graphic findings observable on standard MRI imaging (Fig. 9).

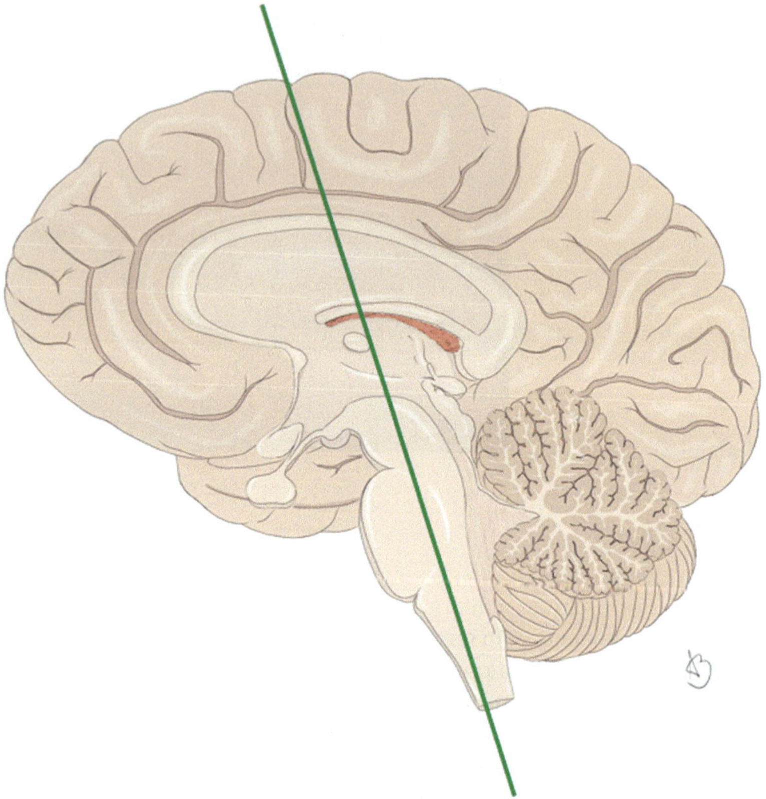

Fig. 6 Identifying the right plane for measurement of the Sylvian fissures

Fig. 7 Widening of the Sylvian fissures

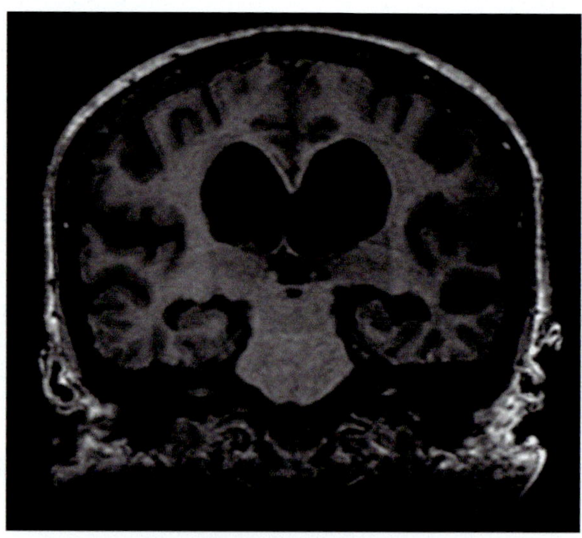

Fig. 8 Focally widened sulcus

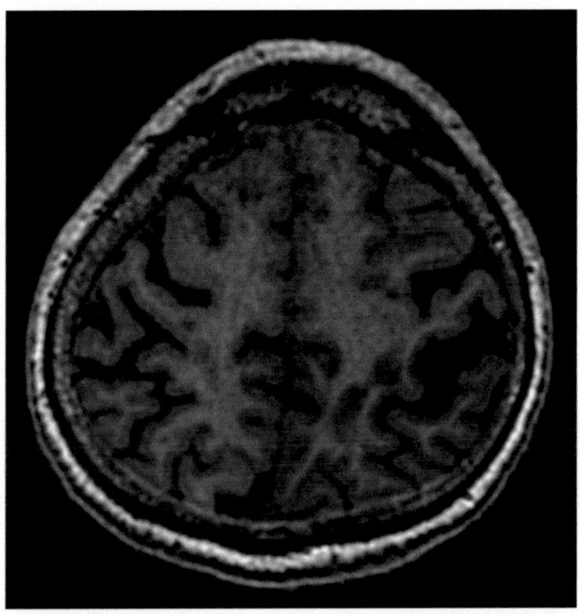

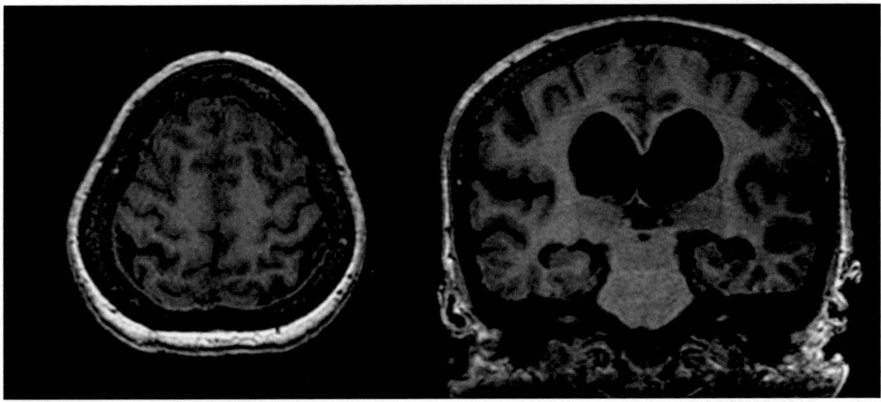

Fig. 9 Tight high convexity

All these 5 above-mentioned prognostic features were summarised by Shinoda [20] into a unified classification scheme (Table 1). A high score in this system has a positive predictive value for neurological improvement after shunt surgery. DESH score is also mentioned in the latest iNPH guidelines as important in identifying shunt responsive patients, but it should not be the sole determinant of a treatment course [24]. Our own research in this field supports this finding [25].

Table 1 DESH score introduced by Shinoda

Ventriculomegaly	Normal (Evans' index < 0.3)	0
	Slight dilatation (Evans' index $\geq$ 0.3 & $\leq$ 0.35)	1
	Dilatation (Evans' index > 0.35)	2
	Normal or narrow	0
Dilated Sylvian fissures	Slight dilatation or unilateral	1
	Bilateral dilatation	2
	Normal or wider than normal	0
Tight high convexity	Slight compression	1
	Definitive compression	2
	Obtuse angle (>100°)	0
Acute callosal angle	Not acute, but not obtuse angle ($\geq$90° & $\leq$ 100°)	1
	Acute angle (<90°)	2
	Not present	0
Focal sulcal dilation	Some present	1
	Many present	2

4 Advanced Imaging of NPH

Diagnosis of NPH is currently based on clinical examination and functional tests. The technique of these examinations and the method of evaluation are part of other chapters of this book. It cannot be denied that these tests are invasive, unpleasant for the examined patient and burdened with a small but significant risk of complications. Great expectations were placed on advanced MRI imaging techniques. Our group has also conducted several larger studies in this area. Unfortunately, we have to state that all these techniques can only play a supporting role in the diagnosis of NPH and cannot be recommended as the only decisive diagnostic modality by themselves.

4.1 Volumetry

The idea behind this method is that NPH can be characterised by specific morphological patterns. The method of volumetric measurement allows us to determine the exact size of individual brain structures. Nevertheless, there are very few volumetric studies of normal pressure hydrocephalus in the literature. This is primarily due to the fact that previously these measurements required manual drawing of the required structures with subsequent calculation of its volume. This process was very time-consuming. Advances in technological development along with discovery of voxel-based morphometry have significantly accelerated this process in the last two decades. Steadily evolving technology-enabled automated, easy-to-use and time-efficient segmentation of more structures at once [11].

The fundamental problem is choosing the right structure for a volumetric study. The ventricular system measured by volumetric methods and its ratio to the brain tissue can detect hydrocephalus itself, more precisely the Evans index and can thus better monitor subtle changes in the ventricular system during treatment. The size of the ventricles is of course related to the size of brain parenchyma implying that the size of grey and white matter could have predictive value in itself. Unfortunately, the predictive value of their size seems to be minimal [26, 27].

Another suspicious structure with respect to the assumed pathophysiology of NPH should be periventricular white matter, especially internal and external capsule and corpus callosum. The internal capsule plays a combined role both in psychiatric [28] and movement disorders [29]. The external capsule connects the prefrontal cortex to the striatum and plays a significant role in social desirable behaviour [30]. Corpus callosum atrophy has already been observed in other neurodegenerative diseases [31]. Other structures that we can focus on during volumetry are the deep structures of the temporal lobe, which play a key role in cognitive [32] and emotional [33] decline. The last group of structures that, with regard to the diagnosis of NPH, encourage volumetric monitoring is the basal ganglia. In this context, the main talk is about a possible role of the putamen [34], caudate [35, 36], pallidum [37] and thalamus [38]. Periaqueductal grey has a paramount role in the control of micturition and its role in NPH [39].

We included all the above-mentioned structures in a large summary study where, thanks to automatic segmentation software, we were able to examine the volumes of all structures in each patient. The measurements were done both in the preoperative diagnostics and post-operative checks [11]. We document the segmentation process in following figures (Figs. 10, 11, 12 and 13).

We observed several statistically significant differences in our study. The most significant was expectedly the size of the ventricles—p < 0.000001 and related to this significant difference in grey and white matter volume. We also observed some changes in the size of the corpus callosum (p-value 0.002), the left hippocampus (p-value 0.02) and the left globus pallidus internus (p-value 0.04). Unfortunately, we have to state that the observed changes were discriminating only the NPH group from the controls; the differences against a group of other neurodegenerative diseases were minimal. In the second phase of the study, we compared changes within the group of NPH patients before the insertion of the VP shunt and 3 months after the procedure. The only significant change was again the expected difference in the size of the ventricular system and the telencephalon. Furthermore, we observed a significant enlargement of the right putamen. We explain this by better drainage of the right hemisphere during the routine introduction of the ventricular end of the shunt into the right lateral ventricle. This hypothesis is supported by other findings of larger structural volumes in the right hemisphere although these were not statistically significant findings.

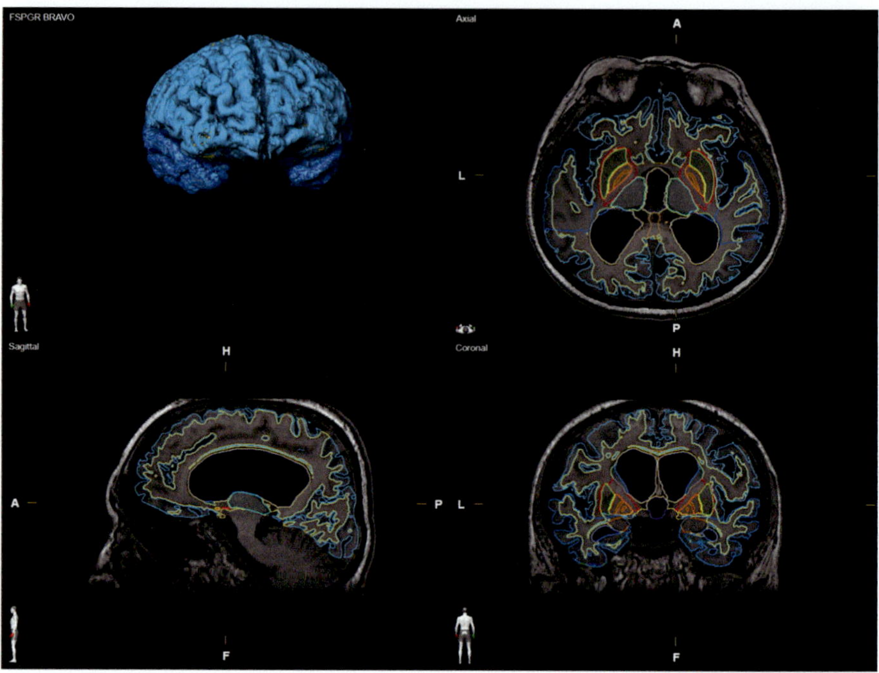

Fig. 10 Segmentation process using Anatomical Mapping Ver. 1.1 as a part of Brainlab Elements neuronavigation software

In view of the inconsistent results of the studies and our above-mentioned results, we must state that, despite the assumptions, volumetry cannot be used for the diagnosis of NPH.

4.2 Diffusion Tensor Imaging

As mentioned earlier in this chapter, assessment of morphological changes in NPH by imaging studies is an integral part of the iNPH workup, with certain studies showing excellent diagnostic accuracy when distinguishing iNPH from healthy controls [40]. However, distinguishing shunt-responders from non-responders is arguably of a higher importance since this distinction vastly alters the course of future management. Unfortunately, to date, there is no single imaging test reliably predicting the outcome of the CSF tap test [41]. Therefore, the search for promising imaging biomarkers continues, and one of the imaging methods under investigation is the diffusion tensor imaging (DTI) (Fig. 14).

DTI is a diffusion technique based on detecting the directional preference of water diffusion in tissues—in the case of iNPH, brain tissue. One of the possible outputs of

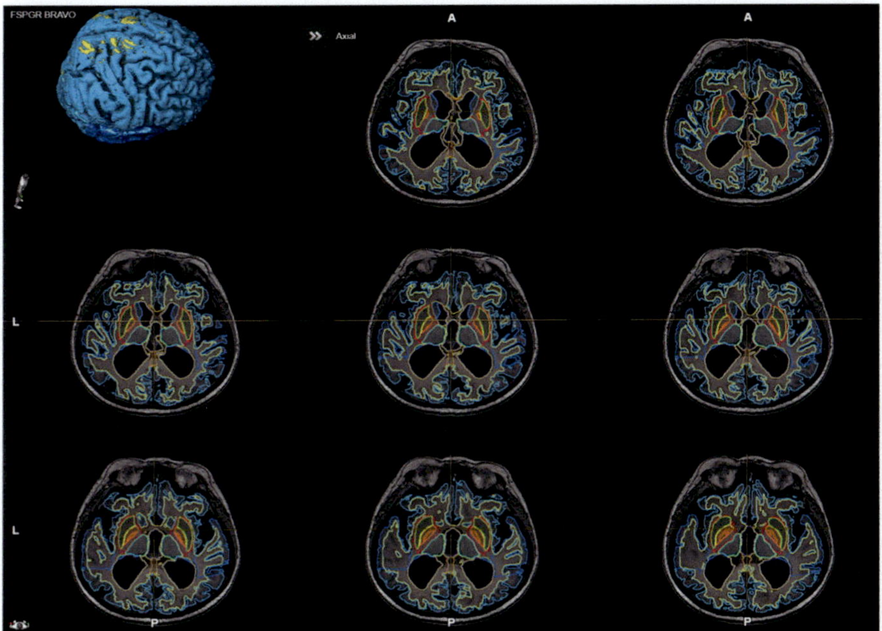

Fig. 11 Volumetric images decomposed into thin axial slices

DTI is the generation of quantitative tissue maps based on four main indices: Fractional anisotropy (FA), mean diffusivity (MD), axial diffusivity and radial diffusivity. These can be viewed as proxies for assessing white matter integrity and are therefore a possible biomarker for the assessment of iNPH, where it is hypothesised, that the morphological changes [42] and/or glymphatic pathway alterations may disturb the integrity and organisation of the white matter [43].

For the assessment of DTI indices, several anatomical areas of interest have been proposed, with the corticospinal tract, internal capsule, corpus callosum, fornices and forceps minor and major being among the most mentioned in the literature. In iNPH patients, for most of the investigated structures the FA decreases, while MD increases [44], which can be a sign of decreased axonal density due to chronic neuronal loss. However, significant overlaps in DTI indices exist between NPH and controls (healthy or AD) [45] as well as between shunt-responders and non-responders. Some authors [46] even propose the possibility of FA of certain regions to transiently increase early in the disease course due to mechanical compression, only to decrease later on as the axons are lost. In addition to these challenges, DTI values for certain regions, like the corticospinal tract, tend to differ between studies, as some report higher FA values in NPH patients compared to controls [47], while other studies report FA values lower [48] in the same context. There are multiple possible reasons for these discrepancies, including scanner and protocol differences,

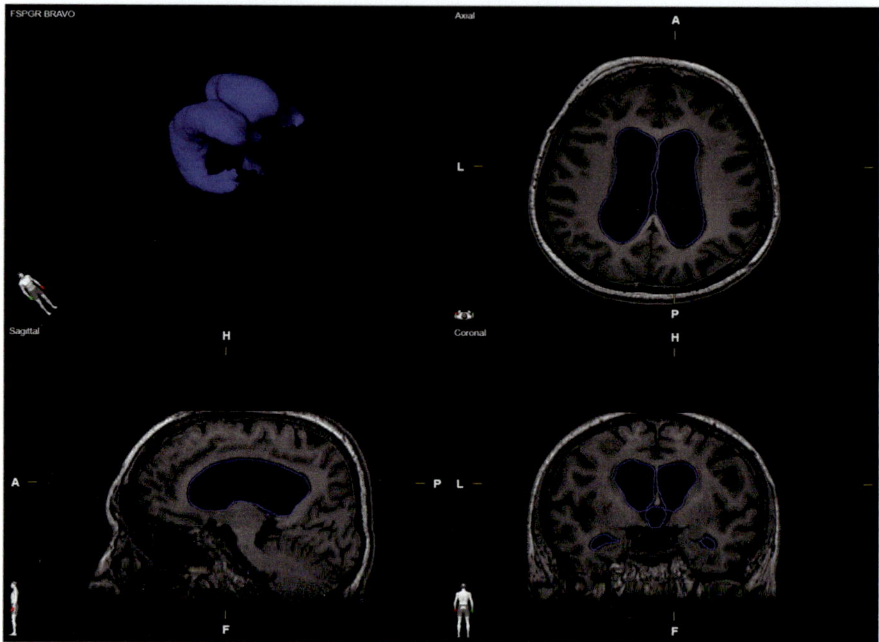

Fig. 12 Volumetry of lateral and 3rd ventricle. The fourth ventricle was manually removed because its volume is not related to NPH diagnosis

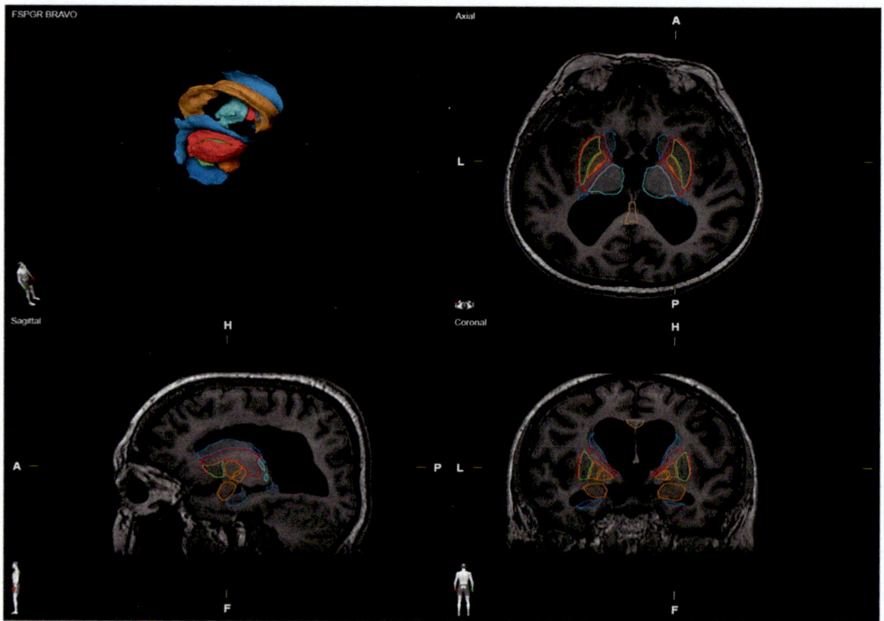

Fig. 13 Volumetry of basal ganglia

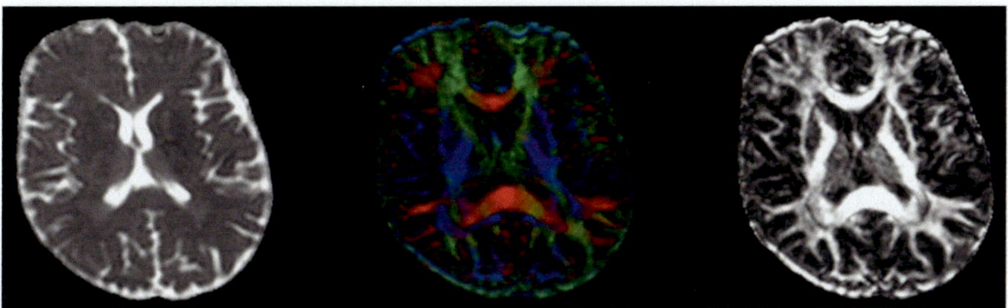

Fig. 14 DTI Indices. Axial slices of a healthy brain showing some of the outputs from DTI modelling: **FA map** (on the right) shows increased anisotropy of water diffusion in white matter compared to grey matter due to differences in their microstructure (increased FA corresponds to higher signal intensity in a voxel). This distinction is less visible on the **MD maps** (on the left), where signal intensity difference depends more on the cellularity and composition of extracellular matrix of these regions. **Colour-coded FA maps** (centre) are created by modulating signal intensity of FA maps by a colour which corresponds to dominant direction of water diffusion in a given voxel—red being x-axis (e.g. splenium of corpus callosum), green y-axis (anterior thalamic radiation) and blue the z-axis (posterior limb of internal capsule)

Table 2 FA values of selected ROI in iNPH patients and healthy controls (adapted from Grazzini et al. 5)

	Motor cortex	Forceps minor	Genu of the CC	Splenium of CC	Genu of CI
iNPH patients	0.36 ± 0.02	0.328 ± 0.03	0.63 ± 0.07	0.61 ± 0.12	0.63 ± 0.07
HC	0.54 ± 0.05	0.475 ± 0.06	0.72 ± 0.7	0.76 ± 0.07	0.618 ± 0.12

CC–corpus callosum. CI–capsula interna

small cohort sizes or different methods used during DTI data modelling [49] (Table 2).

Therefore, while white matter studies by MRI seem to be a promising direction for future investigation, they have not fully proven their clinical potential yet. However, this may change in the future as novel methods of white matter tract analysis are being investigated, including more complex evaluation of DTI outputs [50] or non-DTI-based diffusion techniques [52] (Fig. 15).

4.3 Phase-Contrast MRI

Using phase-contrast imaging we are able to visualise and quantify velocity. It is therefore suitable for describing the flow of cerebrospinal fluid through the ventricular system. Its first use in hydrocephalus diagnostics dates back to 1990 [53].

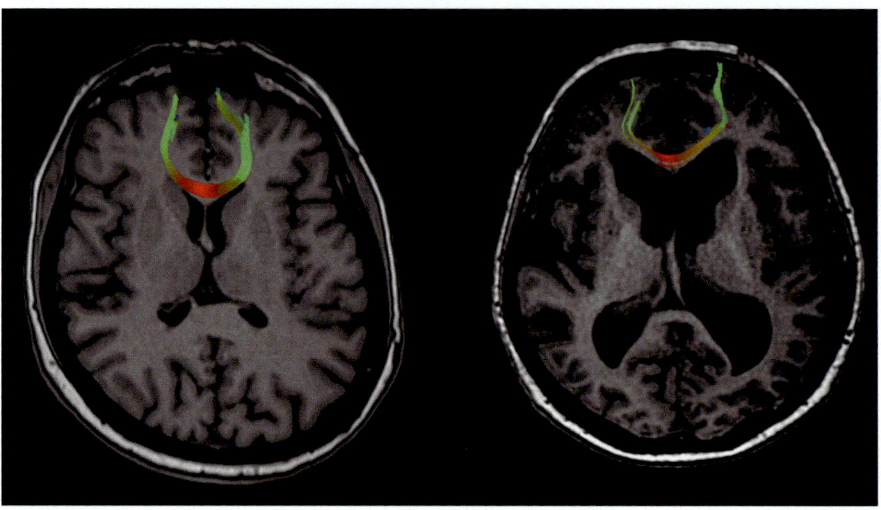

Fig. 15 Tract-based FA analysis of Forceps minor using Brainlab Fibertracking suite. On the left, a healthy individual with Forceps minor FA 0.51. On the right, a patient with DESH and established diagnosis of iNPH with Forceps minor FA 0.36

Bradley described the possibilities of phase-contrast in normal pressure hydrocephalus. He noticed a correlation between the so-called flow void phenomenon and shunt responsiveness [54].

The method is based on the traditional Monro-Kellie doctrine. During systole and diastole, small pulsatile changes occur in the "blood" compartment. Since the cerebrospinal fluid cannot be absorbed this quickly, the pressure is compensated by changes in the size of the brain parenchyma. Brain tissue expands into the ventricles and into the subarachnoid spaces. Internal pressure induces a pressure wave through the aqueduct and other parts of the ventricular system during systole, retrograde flow occurs during diastole [55]. In the case of normal pressure hydrocephalus, the compensatory mechanisms of the brain parenchyma are largely exhausted, which leads to a significantly higher pulse pressure through the aqueduct than in healthy individuals [56].

The most frequently monitored parameter of phase-contrast imaging is the so-called aqueductal CSF stroke volume. It is counted as an average of the flows in the craniocaudal and caudocranial directions in the region of the Sylvian aqueduct at the level of the inferior colliculus. A complicating factor is the considerable variability of results depending on the examining device [56]. Other more frequently studied parameters include peak positive and negative velocity, peak amplitude, average velocity, positive, negative and average flow and aqueductal area.

The results of flow studies are highly variable from great results [57] to no significant difference between the iNPH group and healthy controls [58]. Our recent study using machine learning methods shows promising results [59].

The MRI phase-contrast signal which characterises the flow of cerebrospinal fluid through the aqueduct is made up of 7 vectors—aqueduct area, highest positive velocity, highest negative velocity, average velocity, positive flow, negative flow and average flow. Each vector is made up of 32 points evenly distributed throughout the cardiac cycle. This results in 85 complex features that can be counted for each patient. Such a number of features are difficult to handle (especially with a larger number of patients). Therefore, we used machine learning methods in our study. With their help we managed to achieve an accuracy of 80.4 ± 2.9%, a sensitivity of 72.0 ± 5.6%, a specificity of 84.7 ± 3.8% and an AUC of 0.812 ± 0.047 using the AdaBoost model. In addition, the best sensitivity of 85.7 ± 5.6% was achieved by the GaussNB model and the best AUC of 0.854 ± 0.028 by the ExtraTrees classifier. An ROC curve for every machine learning classifier is shown in the following figure (Fig. 16).

Overall, it can be stated that the results of phase-contrast are very difficult to interpret and are different according to the device used. Our developed feature extraction algorithms combined with machine learning approaches simplify the utilisation of phase-contrast MRI. The results still do not reach the values that would allow using this examination as the only and decisive one, on the other hand, we achieved promising results. Adding more patients to the test population would improve the results even more. Nevertheless, in our opinion, this method will probably play a rather supportive role as part of a mix of several examinations.

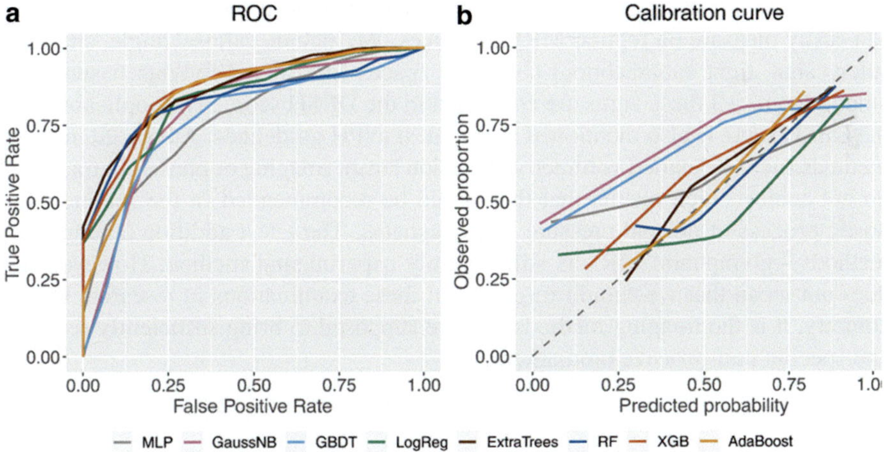

Fig. 16 ROC (left) and calibration (right) curves for all individual machine learning models. The dashed diagonal line represents the performance of an ideal model, where the predicted outcome would correspond perfectly with the actual outcome. Reprinted from the Neurosurgical Focus, Volume 52, Vlasak et al., Boosting phase-contrast MRI performance in idiopathic normal pressure hydrocephalus diagnostics by means of machine learning approach, Page No. 6, Copyright (2022), with permission from Journal of Neurosurgery Press

4.4 Glymphatic MRI

Recent pathophysiological studies describe the role of the glymphatic system in the formation of NPH (for more details on this issue, we refer you to the Pathophysiology chapter). This assumption is based on the work of Ringstadt et al. [60]. They tracked clearance of an intrathecally administered contrast agent. Compared to the control group, iNPH patients showed delayed signal enhancement. However, so far the use of gadobutrol is only experimental and a safe level needs to be established first [61]. Attempts to diagnose NPH patients based on intrathecal administration of contrast are still rather experimental in nature, yet there are studies that show promising results. Further studies are needed in this area before the use of this examination can also be recommended in routine practice.

5 Conclusion

Currently, the diagnostics of NPH are based on clinical examination and functional tests. Imaging plays only an auxiliary role. A mandatory finding is ventriculomegaly, which can be well captured on CT and MRI. This can be described either by the classic Evans index or by a more modern volumetric methodology. Other tests that can successfully discriminate shunt responders include a series of signs that we can easily measure on regular MRI sequences. We include callosal angle, cingulate sulcus sign, tight subarachnoid convexity spaces and dilated Sylvian fissures and among them. All these signs are combined in the DESH score. The applicability of the DESH score is also mentioned in the latest iNPH guidelines. Advanced imaging methods such as detailed volumetry, diffusion tensor imaging or phase-contrast MRI do not achieve such results that they could be recommended in the routine diagnostic process of normal pressure hydrocephalus. The latest addition among these methods—glymphatic MRI, is still a purely experimental method. However, this does not mean that we should forget about these examinations in research. On the contrary, it is the imaging methods that are supposed to bring sufficiently sensitive and specific non-invasive biomarkers.

6 Key Points

- MRI should be the method of choice for NPH diagnosis, however, it can be partially replaced in some respects by modern CT scan.
- Evans index is still the most used parameter for ventricular enlargement.
- The best results in the discrimination of shunt responders are achieved by the set of signs included in DESH score—ventriculomegaly, dilated Sylvian fissures, tight high convexity, acute callosal angle and focal sulcal dilation.

- Volumetry enables a more accurate assessment of the size of the ventricles, but it does not seem to bring any other diagnostic benefit.
- Diffusion tensor imaging seems to show promising results, but still has not proven their clinical potential yet.
- Phase-contrast imaging is difficult to interpret and is device dependent, however, our results point to its potential using machine learning methods.

Funding This chapter was supported by the Ministry of Health of the Czech Republic institutional grant no. NU23-04–00551.

References

1. Adams RD, Fisher CM, Hakim S, Ojemann RG, Sweet WH. symptomatic occult hydrocephalus with "Normal" cerebrospinal-fluid pressure. A treatable syndrome. N Engl J Med. 1965;273:117–26.
2. Vakili S, Moran D, Hung A, Elder BD, Jeon L, Fialho H, et al. Timing of surgical treatment for idiopathic normal pressure hydrocephalus: association between treatment delay and reduced short-term benefit. Neurosurg Focus. 2016;41(3):E2.
3. Evans WA, Jr. An encephalographic ratio for estimating ventricular enlargement and cerebral atrophy. Archives of Neurol Psychiatry. 1942;47(6):931–7.
4. Brix MK, Westman E, Simmons A, Ringstad GA, Eide PK, Wagner-Larsen K, et al. The Evan's index revisited: new cut-off levels for use in radiological assessment of ventricular enlargement in the elderly. Eur J Radiol. 2017;95:28–32.
5. Meier U, Paris S, Grawe A, Stockheim D, Hajdukova A, Mutze S. Is there a correlation between operative results and change in ventricular volume after shunt placement? A study of 60 cases of idiopathic normal-pressure hydrocephalus. Neuroradiology. 2003;45(6):377–80.
6. Yamada S, Ishikawa M, Yamamoto K. Optimal diagnostic indices for idiopathic normal pressure hydrocephalus based on the 3D quantitative volumetric analysis for the cerebral ventricle and subarachnoid space. Am J Neuroradiol. 2015;36(12):2262–9.
7. Radhakrishnan R, Brown BP, Kralik SF, Bain D, Persohn S, Territo PR, et al. Frontal occipital and frontal temporal horn ratios: comparison and validation of head ultrasound-derived indexes with mri and ventricular volumes in infantile Ventriculomegaly. Am J Roentgenol. 2019;213(4):925–31.
8. Ambarki K, Israelsson H, Wahlin A, Birgander R, Eklund A, Malm J. Brain ventricular size in healthy elderly: comparison between Evans index and volume measurement. Neurosurgery. 2010;67(1):94–9; discussion 9.
9. Toma AK, Holl E, Kitchen ND, Watkins LD. Evan's index revisited: the need for an alternative in normal pressure hydrocephalus. Neurosurgery. 2011;68(4):939–44.
10. Miskin N, Patel H, Franceschi AM, Ades-Aron B, Le A, Damadian BE, et al. Diagnosis of normal-pressure hydrocephalus: use of traditional measures in the era of volumetric MR imaging. Radiology. 2017;285(1):197–205.
11. Vlasák A, Skalický P, Mládek A, Vrána J, Beneš V, Bradáč O. Structural volumetry in NPH diagnostics and treatment-future or dead end? Neurosurg Rev. 2020.
12. Benson DF, LeMay M, Patten DH, Rubens AB. Diagnosis of normal-pressure hydrocephalus. N Engl J Med. 1970;283(12):609–15.
13. Ishii K, Kanda T, Harada A, Miyamoto N, Kawaguchi T, Shimada K, et al. Clinical impact of the callosal angle in the diagnosis of idiopathic normal pressure hydrocephalus. Eur Radiol. 2008;18(11):2678–83.

14. Virhammar J, Laurell K, Cesarini KG, Larsson EM. Preoperative prognostic value of MRI findings in 108 patients with idiopathic normal pressure hydrocephalus. AJNR Am J Neuroradiol. 2014;35(12):2311–8.

15. Virhammar J, Laurell K, Cesarini KG, Larsson E-M. Increase in callosal angle and decrease in ventricular volume after shunt surgery in patients with idiopathic normal pressure hydrocephalus. 2018;130(1):130.

16. Adachi M, Kawanami T, Ohshima F, Kato T. Upper midbrain profile sign and cingulate sulcus sign: MRI findings on sagittal images in idiopathic normal-pressure hydrocephalus, Alzheimer's disease, and progressive supranuclear palsy. Radiat Med. 2006;24(8):568–72.

17. Kitagaki H, Mori E, Ishii K, Yamaji S, Hirono N, Imamura T. CSF spaces in idiopathic normal pressure hydrocephalus: morphology and volumetry. AJNR Am J Neuroradiol. 1998;19(7):1277–84.

18. Hashimoto M, Ishikawa M, Mori E, Kuwana N, Improvement SoIoN. Diagnosis of idiopathic normal pressure hydrocephalus is supported by MRI-based scheme: a prospective cohort study. Cerebrospinal Fluid Res. 2010;7(1):18.

19. Agerskov S, Wallin M, Hellström P, Ziegelitz D, Wikkelsö C, Tullberg M. Absence of disproportionately enlarged subarachnoid space hydrocephalus, a sharp callosal angle, or other morphologic MRI markers should not be used to exclude patients with idiopathic normal pressure hydrocephalus from shunt surgery. AJNR Am J Neuroradiol. 2019;40(1):74–9.

20. Shinoda N, Hirai O, Hori S, Mikami K, Bando T, Shimo D, et al. Utility of MRI-based disproportionately enlarged subarachnoid space hydrocephalus scoring for predicting prognosis after surgery for idiopathic normal pressure hydrocephalus: clinical research. J Neurosurg. 2017;127(6):1436–42.

21. Yamada S, Ishikawa M, Yamamoto K. Comparison of CSF distribution between idiopathic normal pressure hydrocephalus and Alzheimer disease. AJNR Am J Neuroradiol. 2016;37(7):1249–55.

22. Holodny AI, George AE, Leon MJd, Golomb J, Kalnin AJ, Cooper PR. Focal dilation and paradoxical collapse of cortical fissures and sulci in patients with normal-pressure hydrocephalus. 1998;89(5):742.

23. Narita W, Nishio Y, Baba T, Iizuka O, Ishihara T, Matsuda M, et al. High-convexity tightness predicts the shunt response in idiopathic normal pressure hydrocephalus. Am J Neuroradiol. 2016;37(10):1831–7.

24. Nakajima M, Yamada S, Miyajima M, Ishii K, Kuriyama N, Kazui H, et al. Guidelines for management of idiopathic normal pressure hydrocephalus (Third Edition): endorsed by the japanese society of normal pressure hydrocephalus. Neurol Med Chir. 2021;61(2):63–97.

25. Skalicky P, Mladek A, Vlasak A, De Lacy P, Benes V, Bradac O. Normal pressure hydrocephalus-an overview of pathophysiological mechanisms and diagnostic procedures. Neurosurg Rev. 2019.

26. Moore DW, Kovanlikaya I, Heier LA, Raj A, Huang C, Chu KW, et al. A pilot study of quantitative MRI measurements of ventricular volume and cortical atrophy for the differential diagnosis of normal pressure hydrocephalus. Neurol Res Int. 2012;2012: 718150.

27. Palm WM, Walchenbach R, Bruinsma B, Admiraal-Behloul F, Middelkoop HA, Launer LJ, et al. Intracranial compartment volumes in normal pressure hydrocephalus: volumetric assessment versus outcome. AJNR Am J Neuroradiol. 2006;27(1):76–9.

28. Spiegelhalder K, Regen W, Prem M, Baglioni C, Nissen C, Feige B, et al. Reduced anterior internal capsule white matter integrity in primary insomnia. Hum Brain Mapp. 2014;35(7):3431–8.

29. Kim MJ, Seo SW, Lee KM, Kim ST, Lee JI, Nam DH, et al. Differential diagnosis of idiopathic normal pressure hydrocephalus from other dementias using diffusion tensor imaging. AJNR Am J Neuroradiol. 2011;32(8):1496–503.

30. Andrejević M, Meshi D, van den Bos W, Heekeren HR. Individual differences in social desirability are associated with white-matter microstructure of the external capsule. Cogn Affect Behav Neurosci. 2017;17(6):1255–64.

31. Wang X-D, Ren M, Zhu M-W, Gao W-P, Zhang J, Shen H, et al. Corpus callosum atrophy associated with the degree of cognitive decline in patients with Alzheimer's dementia or mild cognitive impairment: a meta-analysis of the region of interest structural imaging studies. J Psychiatr Res. 2015;63:10–9.
32. Savolainen S, Laakso MP, Paljärvi L, Alafuzoff I, Hurskainen H, Partanen K, et al. MR imaging of the hippocampus in normal pressure hydrocephalus: correlations with cortical Alzheimer's disease confirmed by pathologic analysis. AJNR Am J Neuroradiol. 2000;21(2):409–14.
33. Poulin SP, Dautoff R, Morris JC, Barrett LF, Dickerson BC. Amygdala atrophy is prominent in early Alzheimer's disease and relates to symptom severity. Psychiatry Res: Neuroimaging. 2011;194(1):7–13.
34. Braak H, Braak E. Alzheimer's disease: striatal amyloid deposits and neurofibrillary changes. J Neuropathol Exp Neurol. 1990;49(3):215–24.
35. Grahn JA, Parkinson JA, Owen AM. The cognitive functions of the caudate nucleus. Prog Neurobiol. 2008;86(3):141–55.
36. Bauer E, Toepper M, Gebhardt H, Gallhofer B, Sammer G. The significance of caudate volume for age-related associative memory decline. Brain Res. 2015;1622:137–48.
37. Draganski B, Kherif F, Klöppel S, Cook PA, Alexander DC, Parker GJM, et al. Evidence for segregated and integrative connectivity patterns in the human basal ganglia. J Neurosci. 2008;28(28):7143–52.
38. Swartz RH, Black SE. Anterior-medial thalamic lesions in dementia: frequent, and volume dependently associated with sudden cognitive decline. J Neurol Neurosurg Psychiatry. 2006;77(12):1307–12.
39. Zare A, Jahanshahi A, Rahnama'i M-S, Schipper S, van Koeveringe GA. The role of the periaqueductal gray matter in lower urinary tract function. Mol Neurobiol. 2019;56(2):920–34.
40. Kockum K, Virhammar J, Riklund K, Söderström L, Larsson E-M, Laurell K. Diagnostic accuracy of the iNPH Radscale in idiopathic normal pressure hydrocephalus. PLoS ONE. 2020;15(4): e0232275.
41. Laticevschi T, Lingenberg A, Armand S, Griffa A, Assal F, Allali G. Can the radiological scale "iNPH Radscale" predict tap test response in idiopathic normal pressure hydrocephalus? J Neurol Sci. 2021;420.
42. Hoza D, Vlasak A, Horinek D, Sames M, Alfieri A. DTI-MRI biomarkers in the search for normal pressure hydrocephalus aetiology: a review. Neurosurg Rev. 2015;38(2):239–44; discussion 44.
43. Tan C, Wang X, Wang Y, Wang C, Tang Z, Zhang Z, et al. The pathogenesis based on the glymphatic system, diagnosis, and treatment of idiopathic normal pressure hydrocephalus. Clin Interv Aging. 2021;16:139–53.
44. Grazzini I, Redi F, Sammartano K, Cuneo GL. Diffusion tensor imaging in idiopathic normal pressure hydrocephalus: clinical and CSF flowmetry correlations. Neuroradiol J. 2019;33(1):66–74.
45. Kang K, Yoon U, Choi W, Lee H-W. Diffusion tensor imaging of idiopathic normal-pressure hydrocephalus and the cerebrospinal fluid tap test. J Neurol Sci. 2016;364:90–6.
46. Osuka S, Matsushita A, Ishikawa E, Saotome K, Yamamoto T, Marushima A, et al. Elevated diffusion anisotropy in gray matter and the degree of brain compression: clinical article. J Neurosurgery JNS. 2012;117(2):363–71.
47. Hattori T, Yuasa T, Aoki S, Sato R, Sawaura H, Mori T, et al. Altered microstructure in corticospinal tract in idiopathic normal pressure hydrocephalus: comparison with Alzheimer disease and Parkinson disease with dementia. AJNR Am J Neuroradiol. 2011;32(9):1681–7.
48. Koyama T, Marumoto K, Domen K, Ohmura T, Miyake H. Diffusion tensor imaging of idiopathic normal pressure hydrocephalus: a voxel-based fractional anisotropy study. Neurol Med Chir. 2012;52(2):68–74.
49. Grazzini I, Venezia D, Cuneo GL. The role of diffusion tensor imaging in idiopathic normal pressure hydrocephalus: a literature review. Neuroradiol J. 2020;34(2):55–69.
50. Keong NC, Pena A, Price SJ, Czosnyka M, Czosnyka Z, DeVito EE, et al. Diffusion tensor imaging profiles reveal specific neural tract distortion in normal pressure hydrocephalus. PLoS ONE. 2017;12(8): e0181624.

51. Irie R, Tsuruta K, Hori M, Suzuki M, Kamagata K, Nakanishi A, et al. Neurite orientation dispersion and density imaging for evaluation of corticospinal tract in idiopathic normal pressure hydrocephalus. Jpn J Radiol. 2017;35(1):25–30.
52. Ciraolo L, Mascalchi M, Bucciolini M, Dal Pozzo G. Fast multiphase MR imaging of aqueductal CSF flow: 1. Study of healthy subjects. AJNR Amer J Neuroradiol. 1990;11(3):589–96.
53. Bradley WG Jr, Whittemore AR, Kortman KE, Watanabe AS, Homyak M, Teresi LM, et al. Marked cerebrospinal fluid void: indicator of successful shunt in patients with suspected normal-pressure hydrocephalus. Radiology. 1991;178(2):459–66.
54. Bradley WG Jr, Kortman KE, Burgoyne B. Flowing cerebrospinal fluid in normal and hydrocephalic states: appearance on MR images. Radiology. 1986;159(3):611–6.
55. Motl RW, Hubbard EA, Sreekumar N, Wetter NC, Sutton BP, Pilutti LA, et al. Pallidal and caudate volumes correlate with walking function in multiple sclerosis. J Neurol Sci. 2015;354(1):33–6.
56. Bradley WG Jr. Magnetic resonance imaging of normal pressure hydrocephalus. Semin Ultrasound CT MR. 2016;37(2):120–8.
57. Tawfik AM, Elsorogy L, Abdelghaffar R, Naby AA, Elmenshawi I. Phase-contrast MRI CSF flow measurements for the diagnosis of normal-pressure hydrocephalus: observer agreement of velocity versus volume parameters. AJR Am J Roentgenol. 2017;208(4):838–43.
58. Shanks J, Markenroth Bloch K, Laurell K, Cesarini KG, Fahlström M, Larsson EM, et al. Aqueductal CSF stroke volume is increased in patients with idiopathic normal pressure hydrocephalus and decreases after shunt surgery. AJNR Am J Neuroradiol. 2019;40(3):453–9.
59. Vlasák A, Gerla V, Skalický P, Mládek A, Sedlák V, Vrána J, et al. Boosting phase-contrast MRI performance in idiopathic normal pressure hydrocephalus diagnostics by means of machine learning approach. Neurosurg Focus. 2022;52(4):E6.
60. Ringstad G, Vatnehol SAS, Eide PK. Glymphatic MRI in idiopathic normal pressure hydrocephalus. Brain: A J Neurol. 2017;140(10):2691–705.
61. Eide PK, Lashkarivand A, Hagen-Kersten Å A, Gjertsen Ø, Nedregaard B, Sletteberg R, et al. Intrathecal contrast-enhanced magnetic resonance imaging of cerebrospinal fluid dynamics and glymphatic enhancement in idiopathic normal pressure hydrocephalus. Frontiers in Neurol. 2022;13:857328.

Imaging Differential Diagnosis of Adult-Onset Hydrocephalus

Vojtěch Sedlák, Aleš Vlasák, Petr Skalický, Adéla Bubeníková, and Ondřej Bradáč

Abstract As clinical presentation of adult-onset hydrocephalus varies, imaging modalities often provide the first evidence of its presence. Features of increased intraventricular pressure can be subtle, especially early on in the disease course, and knowledge of radiologically relevant anatomy is important. When the presence of hydrocephalus is established, the next step is to determine its aetiology. This includes the assessment of which parts of the CSF spaces are involved, whether there is an obstruction and where it is located, if there are other signs of altered CSF hydrodynamics, or if there are secondary complications related to hydrocephalus. For optimal evaluation of hydrocephalus, a standardised protocol including flow-sensitive and high-resolution imaging should be employed.

Keywords Adult-onset hydrocephalus · Differential diagnosis · Imaging · Cerebrospinal fluid flow · Magnetic resonance imaging · Normal pressure hydrocephalus

Abbreviations

BRAVO	Brain Volume Imaging
bSSFP	Balanced steady-state free precession
CISS	Constructive Interference in the Steady State
CSF	Cerebrospinal fluid
CT	Computed tomography

V. Sedlák
Department of Radiology, Military University Hospital, Prague, Czech Republic

A. Vlasák · P. Skalický · A. Bubeníková · O. Bradáč (✉)
Department of Neurosurgery, 2nd Faculty of Medicine, Charles University and Motol University Hospital, Prague, Czech Republic
e-mail: ondrej.bradac2@fnmotol.cz

A. Bubeníková · O. Bradáč
Department of Neurosurgery and Neurooncology, 1st Faculty of Medicine, Charles University and Military University Hospital, Prague, Czech Republic

DESH	Disproportionately Enlarged Subarachnoid space Hydrocephalus
DWI	Diffusion-weighted imaging
EDH	Epidural hematoma
ETL	Echo train length
FIESTA	Fast Imaging Employing Steady State Acquisition
FIESTA-C	Fast Imaging Employing Steady State Acquisition-Constructive Interference
FLAIR	Fluid attenuated inversion recovery
FSE	Fast spin echo
iNPH	Idiopathic Normal Pressure Hydrocephalus
LIAS	Late-onset idiopathic aqueductal stenosis
LOVA	Long-standing Overt Ventriculomegaly in Adults
MPR	MultiPlanar Reconstruction
MPRAGE	Magnetization Prepared RApid Gradient Echo
MR	Magnetic Resonance
MRI	Magnetic Resonance Imaging
PC	Phase Contrast
PROPELLER	Periodically Rotated Overlapping ParallEL Lines with Enhanced Reconstruction
ROI	Region of Interest
SDH	Subdural hematoma
SNR	Signal to noise ratio
SPACE	Sampling Perfection with Application optimized Contrasts using different flip angle Evolution
SSFP	Steady-state free precession
SWI	Susceptibility weighted imaging
TE	Echo time
TSE	Turbo spin echo

1 Introduction

Hydrocephalus (literally "water head" from Greek) is an increase in the volume of the ventricular system as a result of altered production, flow or resorption of the CSF. In keeping with the topic of this book, we will focus mostly on non-acute adult-onset hydrocephalus. This chapter is split into 4 sections: *Section one* is dedicated to optimising the MRI protocol in order to get the most information out of your scans for the correct diagnosis while keeping the imaging time within feasible limits. *Section two* contains comments on ventricular anatomy, its normal variants and physiological imaging findings to avoid potential pitfalls when evaluating for hydrocephalus. *Section three* breaks down individual imaging signs and features of hydrocephalus and the last section; *section four* discusses the most notable examples of adult-onset hydrocephalus.

Table 1 Recommended MR protocol for investigation of adult-onset hydrocephalus

Pulse sequence	Estimated time [3 T]
Mandatory sequences	
2D Ax DWI	< 1 min
3D T1 [MPRAGE OR BRAVO]	3–4 min
2D Ax T2	2 min
2D or 3D FLAIR	2–3 min
3D Sag T2	2–3 min
3D Ax SWI (or T2* GRE)	4 (2) mins
Optional sequences	
3D Sag SSFP (CISS, FIESTA…)	3 min
CSF Flow study	4 min

2 Recommended MRI Protocol

Table 1 outlines a recommended MRI protocol for evaluation of adult-onset hydrocephalus. It is a standard, run-of-the-mill non-contrast brain protocol with some additions—a mandatory, **flow-sensitive sagittal T2 sequence** and optional **sagittal SSFP sequence** and **CSF flow study**. These three additions are further discussed below.

Sagittal T2 sequences are ideal for assessment of the aqueduct, third ventricle, foramina of monro and the outflow foramina of the 4th ventricle. However, there are few caveats. The above-mentioned structures can get exceedingly thin for usual 2D imaging, with volume-averaging becoming an issue. In order to remedy this, a thin-section acquisition is preferred, a 3 mm thickness or less, with no inter-slice gap. What you also require from this sequence is clear and reliable visualisation of flow-voids[1] in the aqueduct and other foramina. This means thin-section imaging, with no flow-compensation and moderate to long TE (all improve the conspicuity of flow-voids). While this can be achieved with 2D acquisition (i.e. T2 TSE/FSE), probably a better alternative is **3D T2 sagittal acquisition** (e.g. T2 CUBE or SPACE), where all 3 stated requirements are fulfilled by the standard pulse sequence design that comes by default with any modern MRI system. Ucar et al. compared 2D T2 TSE and 3D T2 SPACE pulse sequences in their study [1] and 3D T2 SPACE provided excellent diagnostic accuracy (100% sensitivity and specificity) for determining aqueductal patency and was superior to 2D T2 TSE (which yielded 80.7% sensitivity, 100% specificity and 50% negative predictive value). If time is an issue, setting the slice thickness of the 3D sequence to 2–2.5 mm will decrease the acquisition time (under 2 min with phase and/or slice acceleration techniques), improve SNR for evaluation of brain parenchyma, and will maintain all the necessary properties of the sequence.

---

[1] A phenomenon of flow-related signal loss in MRI due to time-of-flight and spin-phase effects. While disliked by some authors, the term "flow-voids" is in widespread clinical use and for the sake of conciseness, we will use the term in this book as well.

Avoid using T2 sequences with radial readout[2] (e.g. BLADE, PROPELLER) as these have inherent flow-compensation that cannot be turned off. This will lead to false interpretation of CSF flow via aqueduct and especially other foramina, where flow-voids tend to be less conspicuous.

Using flow-sensitive sequences is mandatory to increase the sensitivity to CSF flow and therefore is needed to reliably prove obstruction. This comes at a cost of decreased visualisation of ventricular anatomy due to intervening flow-voids, but this is usually not an issue since you will have axial T2 (with flow-compensation) and sagittal bSSFP which will provide a clear picture inside the ventricular system.

If you prove to flow through all the ventricles, foramina and the aqueduct, then the hydrocephalus is unlikely to be of the non-communicating type and further search for macroscopic obstruction is unnecessary. However, if you do prove a functional obstruction (e.g. no flow-void through aqueduct), high-resolution anatomical information might be needed. In these cases, a **3D sagittal bSSFP sequence** (e.g. CISS, FIESTA-C) is an excellent option for detection of subtle causes of obstruction, for example, an aqueductal web. Sometimes a resolution under 0.5 mm isotropic is needed to visualise this subtle pathology reliably. Beware of in-console post-processing steps (e.g. filtering, interpolation), as these might decrease the conspicuity of thin aqueductal webs, so a conservative approach to post-processing is recommended.

Some institutions use phase contrast **CSF flow studies** in the sagittal plane to assess the flow through the aqueduct (Fig. 1). While this is a valid approach and might provide useful information on its own, it rarely brings anything new to the table if a flow-sensitive T2 sequence has been performed as well, with the notable exception of a dedicated iNPH workup. In addition, acquiring CSF flow data is logistically more difficult (pulse oximeter or ECG gating is required), more expensive (CSF flow studies are usually a purchasable add-on option to the MRI system), somewhat time consuming (expect 4 min long acquisition, longer if the patient has arrhythmia) and assessing non-midline structures requires additional acquisitions. Therefore, CSF flow studies should be reserved for special cases, like iNPH.

3 Ventricular System Anatomy and Variants

This section is not a detailed anatomical description of the ventricular system, as there is plenty of available literature on the topic. Instead, it focuses on radiologically relevant anatomy for assessment of hydrocephalus and its normal variants. For reference, a diagram of the ventricular system can be seen in Fig. 2 of the "CSF physiology" chapter and Fig. 4 of this chapter demonstrates important anatomy of the third and fourth ventricle on a midsagittal high-resolution MR image.

---

[2] As opposed to cartesian readout, employed in the standard T2 FSE/TSE sequences.

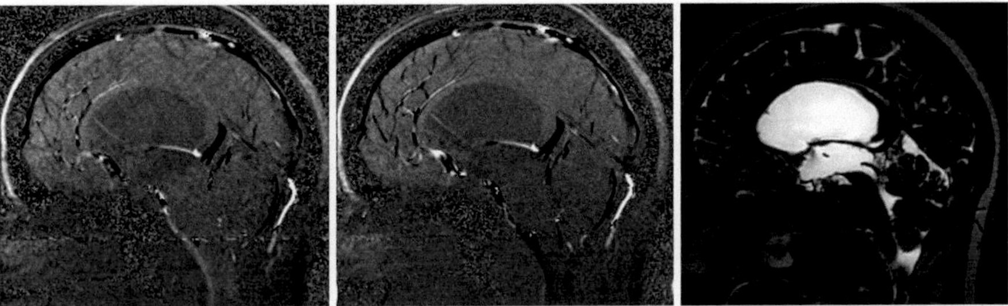

Fig. 1 CSF flow studies. CSF flow study using phase contrast imaging through the aqueduct shows pulsatile CSF flow during systole (left) and diastole (centre), but no CSF movement through the aqueduct. Notice that 3D flow-sensitive T2 acquisition (right) can detect the absence of CSF flow through aqueduct as well, but also proves flow through foramen of Monro which the CSF study did not show

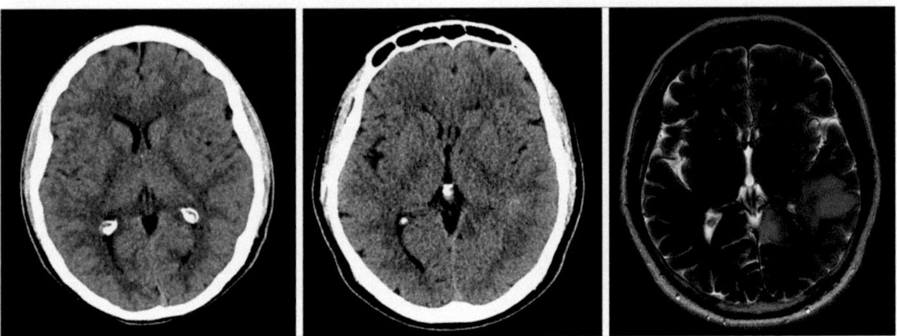

Fig. 2 Asymmetry of lateral ventricles. Asymmetric lateral ventricles are usually a normal finding (left) and common amongst healthy individuals. In certain cases, however, it can be the first clue to pathology as of certain cases (e.g. lymphomas, grade III gliomas) mass effect of a lesion may be more conspicuous than its density changes on CT. Notice the compression of the antrum and occipital horn of lateral ventricles in a patient with mixed grade 2 and 3 gliomas (centre and left)

3.1 Lateral Ventricles

Each lateral ventricle, apart from its body and antrum, has three recesses—the frontal, occipital and temporal horns, which need to be carefully assessed in any individual. They also contain choroid plexus, which is often a source of incidental findings, like small choroid plexus cysts or xanthogranulomas, both of which are usually without any clinical significance. The walls of lateral ventricles also commonly give rise to other inconsequential findings, like for example ring-shaped lateral ventricular nodules. The most common anatomical variants of lateral ventricles include their asymmetry (Fig. 2) [2] and cavum septi pellucidi et vergae.

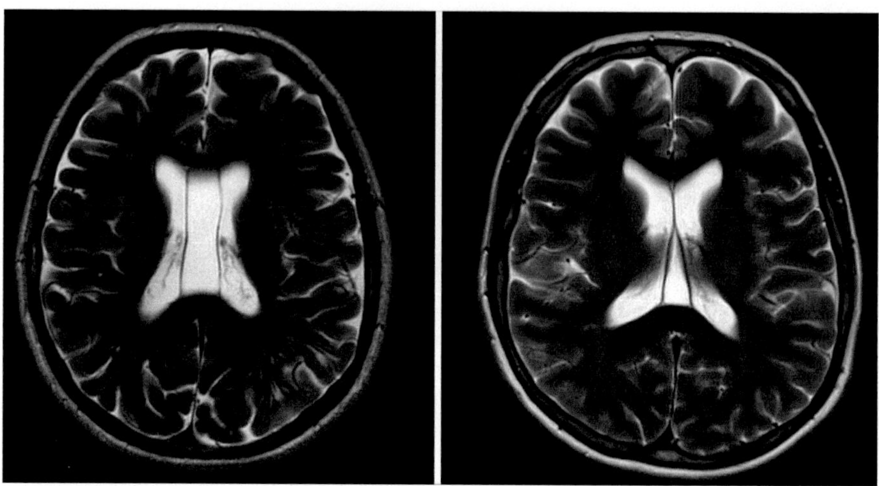

Fig. 3 Cavum septi pellucidi et vergae and cavum veli interpositi. CSF-filled space between the leaflets of septum pellucidum is usually cavum septi pellucidi, with or without cavum vergae (seen on the left is the combination of the two). CSF-filled space between the antra of the lateral ventricles is more commonly cavum veli interpositi (on the right) as isolated cavum vergae is somewhat rare. None of the shown findings has any mass effect, therefore can be considered as inconsequential normal variant

3.2 Cavum Septi Pellucidi et Vergae

During embryonic development, the septum pellucidum is split into two leaflets, with CSF filling the spaces in between. In the majority of the population, these leaflets fuse within the first year of life in postero-anterior direction, but often incompletely [3] and this incomplete fusion creates normal anatomical variants called **cavum septi pellucidi** (anterior to forniceal columns) and **cavum vergae** (posteriorly) (Fig. 3). In adulthood, these do not have significant association with any pathology and should not have any clinical impact whatsoever. The exception is an abnormally enlarged cavum vergae with convex margins and mass effect, called **cavum vergae cyst**. While usually asymptomatic, in rare cases, it can push on the aqueduct and cause obstructive hydrocephalus [4]. Since the leaflets of septum pellucidum fuse from posterior to anterior, cavum vergae rarely, if ever, occurs without accompanying cavum septi pellucidi, so before diagnosing solitary cavum vergae, carefully rule out other possibilities.

3.3 Cavum Veli Interpositi and Cyst of Velum Interpositum

Velum interpositum is a thin membrane located between the bodies of the fornices and internal cerebral veins, dorsally to the foramina of Monro. If distended by fluid, it contains **cavum veli interpositi**, which is an incidental finding with no clinical significance. If, however, distended beyond 1 cm and/or exerting substantial mass effect, this formation is called a **cyst of velum interpositum**. As with cavum vergae cyst, this can in rare cases compress the aqueduct and cause hydrocephalus, or cause symptoms via pressure on nearby structures e.g. fornices [5].

3.4 Foramina of Monro

Foramina of Monro (also known as interventricular foramina) connect lateral ventricles to the third ventricle and along with the neighbouring part of the third ventricle form a **Y-shaped** conduit for CSF, which can be obstructed along any of its arms. This can result in the development of either unilateral or bilateral hydrocephalus depending on the exact location of obstruction. The foramina of Monro contain parts of the choroid plexus, which should not be mistaken for pathology. Another potential pitfall is caused by flow of CSF in and out of the foramina during cardiac revolution which can cause round **defects of CSF suppression** on FLAIR sequences and mimic a preforaminal mass. These artefacts can arise at any location with turbulent flow of CSF but are most common here, around foramina of Monro. A true lesion is usually easily ruled out by examining other available sequences.

3.5 Third Ventricle

The third ventricle has four recesses that are vital when assessing for the possibility of hydrocephalus—the **supraoptic** and **infundibular** recesses anteriorly, which are usually well seen on thin-section MR imaging and **pineal** and **suprapineal** recesses posteriorly, which can be more difficult to appreciate. In their physiologic state, these recesses are sharp and thin with flat or concave borders on sagittal imaging. As pressure in the third ventricle builds up, they become distended and bulge outward. Similar pattern is seen with the floor of the third ventricle and lamina terminalis as well. Normal morphology of the third ventricle including its recesses can be seen in Fig. 4.

3.6 Interthalamic Adhesion

Interthalamic adhesion is a variably present structure (75–96% of population) [6], with variable volume and so far without any established clinical significance. Because of its variable proportions, its diameter should not be used to approximate third ventricular dilation and in the majority of cases can be ignored.

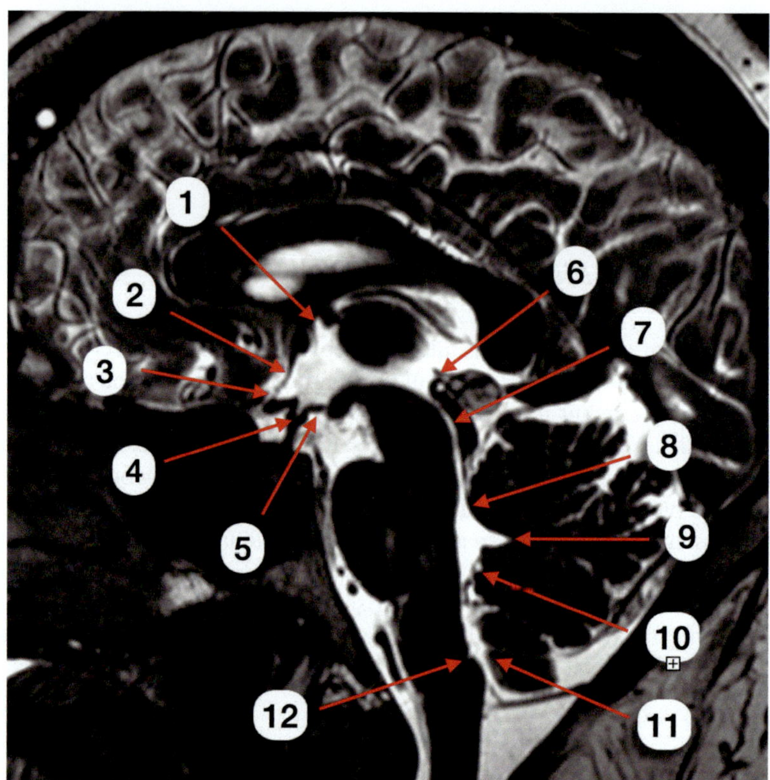

Fig. 4 Normal midline anatomy of the ventricular system. 1-Foramina of Monro orifice. 2-Lamina terminalis. 3-Supraoptic recess. 4-Infundibular recess. 5-Floor of the 3rd ventricle. 6-Pineal recess. 7-Aqueduct. 8-Superior medullary vellum. 9-Fastigium. 10-Inferior medullary vellum. 11-Foramen of Magendie. 12-Obex

3.7 Aqueduct of Sylvius

On high-resolution bSSFP imaging, the lumen of the aqueduct should be clearly visible, and the diameter should be roughly equal for most of its length (i.e. with no funnelling). On flow-sensitive T2 pulse sequences, the flow-void should be very obvious and blend into lower-intensity flow-voids of the 3rd and 4th ventricle. The extent and intensity of flow-voids in these structures is highly dependent on the parameters of pulse sequence used (e.g. TE, ETL, slice thickness) and therefore, the sequence parameters should be locked and not changed between patients in order to reliably assess changes of hydrodynamics amongst individual patients. If you rely on a specialist (i.e. a neuroradiologist) to interpret images of your patients for you, beware that there is a room for inter-rater variability. This subjective assessment of flow-voids could in theory be solved by relying more on flow curves of phase contrast

CSF flow study, however, the ROI for these curves is usually drawn manually by a technologist and this process can be burdened with inter-operator bias as well.

3.8   Fourth Ventricle

The fourth ventricle has a somewhat complex three-dimensional shape, however, it can be sufficiently conceptualised as an elongated CSF-filled space with five nooks or recesses. In the sagittal plane, the central dorsal recess is the **fastigium**, a triangular structure pointing towards the cerebellum. Cranially from fastigium, the fourth ventricle narrows towards the aqueduct and caudally from fastigium it narrows towards **obex** and **foramen of Magendie**. Then the two lateral recesses continue as **foramina of Luschka**. The **choroid plexus** can be found inside the fourth ventricle and continues out via the outflow foramina. On Sagittal imaging, both the superior and inferior medullary velum should be inwardly convex. If not, consider the possibility of increased pressure in the 4th ventricle. An enlarged cisterna magna might be a normal finding, occasionally it can accompany an important pathology.

3.9   Subarachnoid Spaces

SA spaces are located between arachnoid and pia mater and contain blood vessels, delicate connective tissue and in the case of basal cisterns also cranial nerves. The width of SA spaces increases with age due to parenchymal volume loss, but can vary considerably also amongst individuals of similar age. Barely perceptible SA spaces in elderly individuals might mean a life-threatening hydrocephalus, but can be physiological in a teenager or young adult. Therefore, assessment of SA spaces should be done with care in correlation with age and clinical history of the patient. Depending on sequence parameters, exceptionally thin SA spaces can also cause incomplete fluid suppression on FLAIR sequences and should not be mistaken for pathological contents of the SA space which could otherwise mean SA haemorrhage or meningitis.

4   Imaging Features of Hydrocephalus

The following text breaks down imaging signs and features of hydrocephalus at each level of the ventricular system. Many, if not all, of these features could be included under the umbrella term of "big ventricles", however, knowledge of the below-mentioned should help to a) better distinguishing subtle hydrocephalus from age-related volume loss, b) detect the level of obstruction and c) differentiate ongoing ventricular hypertension from old changes after decompression (spontaneous or surgical). For the same reason, the individual signs and features are discussed in the appropriate anatomical context.

4.1 Lateral Ventricles

Not all parts of the ventricular system have the same compliance and as the pressure in the ventricles increases, the most compliant parts will dilate first. In the case of lateral ventricles, this "soft part" is the temporal horns (Fig. 6) [7]. Measurements vary, but **temporal horn width** above 3 mm (measured on axial slice, AC-PC line) is suggestive of hydrocephalus. A potential pitfall is mesiotemporal atrophy as seen e.g. In AD or FTLD. However, in cases where atrophy is the main driving factor for enlargement of temporal horns, collateral sulcus will be widened, as opposed to ventricular hypertension, where the collateral sulcus will be effaced. A similar mechanism can lead to **blunting of the occipital horns**, which are usually sharp or even imperceptible.

Another widely used measure of lateral ventricular dilation is the **Evans' index** (measurement method can be seen in Fig. 5). Normal Evans' index is below 0.3, but a portion of "successful ageing brains" (see chapter "Differential diagnosis of neurodegenerative disorders") will have Evans' index above that as well. The index is also dependent on the selection of the slice (interpreter-dependent) and tilt of the axial plane in which you measure (technologist-dependent). Therefore, Evans' index is not a precise measurement, is difficult to accurately reproduce and should not be used to monitor lateral ventricular width during follow-ups—in those cases a simple measurement of bifrontal ventricular width (along with assessment of temporal horns) will be sufficient.

Long-standing hydrocephalus will lead to thinning or even formation of **defects in the septum pellucidum,** detection of which can be important for further neurosurgical management.

Periventricular T2-hyperintensity (Fig. 7), if accompanying other signs of hydrocephalus, is highly suggestive of interstitial periventricular oedema, which is caused either by stagnation of interstitial fluid in the periventricular brain parenchyma or back-leak of CSF fluid [8]. In some cases, it can be difficult to distinguish from glial changes or ependymitis granularis, which despite its name is an inconsequential finding [9].

4.2 Foramen of Monro

The two most important things you should look for are the presence of a) **flow-voids** through the foramen and b) **obstructive lesions** in the area.

Intensity of flow-voids through foramina of Monro can vary amongst individuals but as long as your flow-sensitive T2 sequence is set up right, they will be detectable

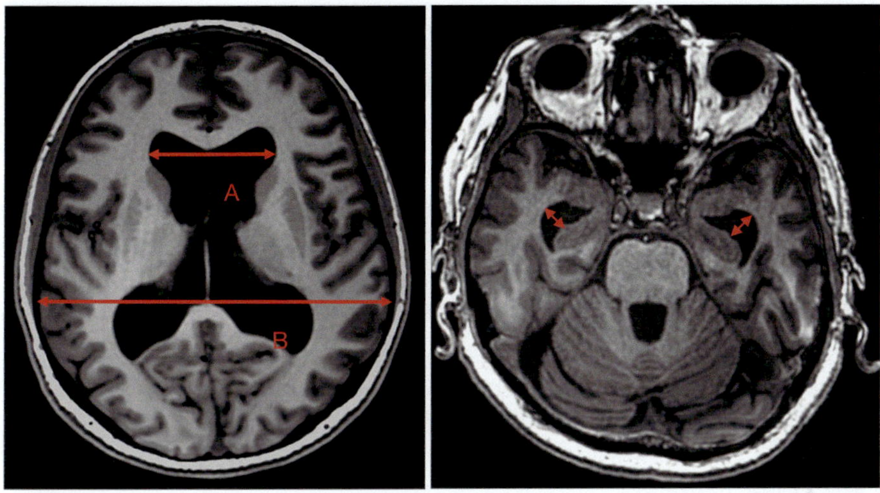

Fig. 5 Evans index and temporal horn width. Image on the left shows measurement of Evans index (A/B). Values above 0.3 can be considered abnormal, but occasionally are seen in elderly without any other neurological disorder ("successfully aging brain"). Image on the right shows measurement method of temporal horn width

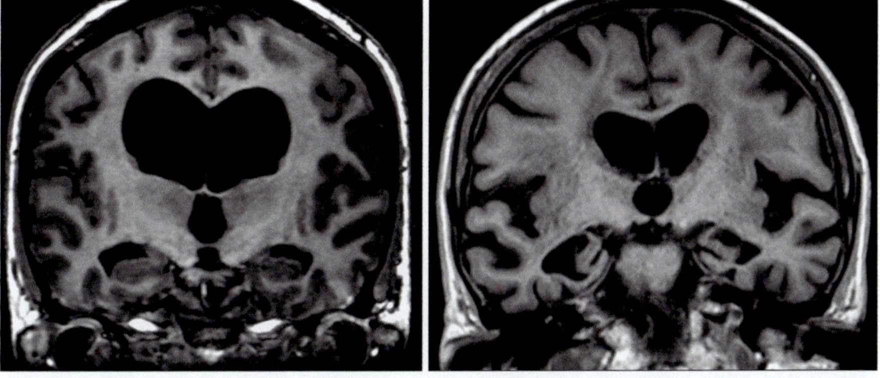

Fig. 6 Distended temporal horns. Enlarged temporal horns can be seen in the setting of increased intraventricular pressure as well as in cases of mesiotemporal atrophy. Assessment of collateral sulci (and surrounding sulci) can help differentiate the cause as in cases of increased intraventricular pressure, collateral sulci remain closed. In cases of mesiotemporal atrophy, collateral sulci are widened. (see chapter on differential diagnosis of neurodegenerative disorders)

in all or almost all healthy individuals. Windowing might help to increase their conspicuity.

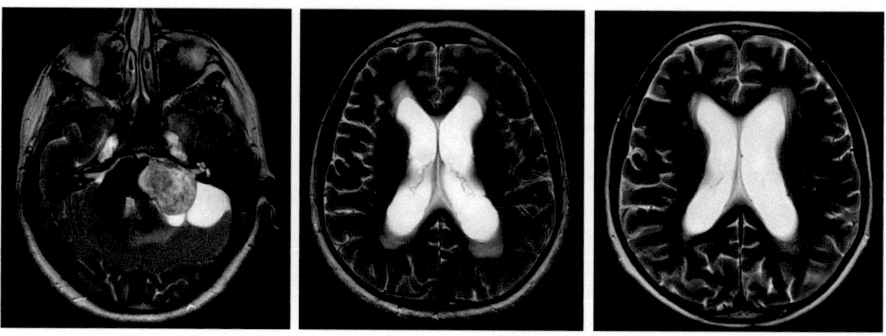

Fig. 7 Interstitial oedema. Patient with large vestibular schwannoma (left) presenting with dilated supratentorial ventricles and periventricular interstitial oedema (centre). After surgical resection of schwannoma, the interstitial oedema starts to resolve (right)

4.3 Third Ventricle

The third ventricle is considered **dilated if its width is above 10 mm** (measured on axial slices). However, an exceedingly narrow, **"slit-like" third ventricle** can also be a sign of pathology and can occur in the case of stenosis of the foramen of Monro or in idiopathic intracranial hypotension (which can be a result of long-standing intracranial *hyper*tension e.g. after ruptured meningocele).

Assessment of the **third ventricular recesses** (Fig. 8) can be extremely helpful, as these will be dilated and blunted in case of obstruction downstream. In addition to the recesses, the **floor** of the third ventricle and **lamina terminalis** can bulge outward as well. Normal anatomy of the third ventricle and distention of its recesses and floor are noted in Fig. 4.

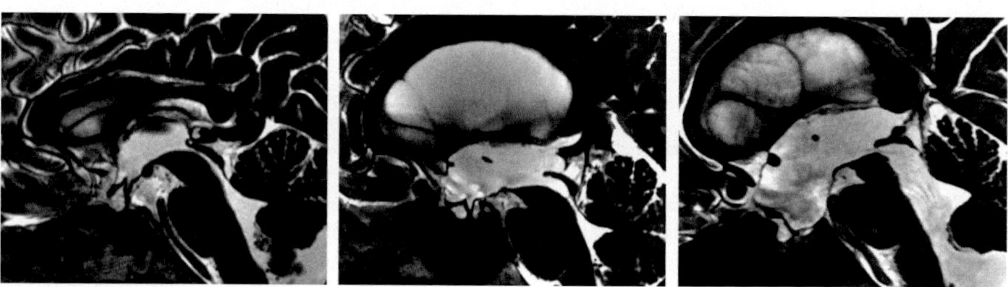

Fig. 8 Dilation of 3rd ventricle. In a healthy individual (left), the recesses of the 3rd ventricle are slim and sharp and lamina terminalis and the floor of the third ventricle slightly concave. In case of increasing intraventricular pressure (in the centre—notice the aqueductal web), these structures start to bulge out. On the right is a patient with advanced, long-standing hydrocephalus, with even more severe features of ventricular distention and remodelation of bony sella turcica

4.4 Aqueduct of Sylvius

Funnelling of the aqueduct (Fig. 9) is a sign of possible obstruction, usually at its vertex. The funnel can be oriented both ways (tapering up or down).

Absence of flow-void is on 3D T2 flow-sensitive acquisition (1) a strong predictor of obstruction, but an unusually prominent flow-void can also be a sign of pathological CSF hydrodynamics, typically in case of iNPH or LOVA [10].

Occasionally, aqueductal flow-void can be missing even if the obstruction is upstream (foramen of Monro) or downstream (outflow foramina of the 4th ventricle), so be sure to thoroughly examine the whole ventricular system.

The proportions of the aqueduct (its length and narrow diameter) mean that **debris** (e.g. ruptured dermoid cyst) or **blood clots** (intraventricular haemorrhage) (Fig. 10) can get stuck here and cause obstruction. Certain debris (e.g. fat) and even blood products can have T2 signal intensity close to CSF, so if unsure of the contents of the aqueduct, examine MPR of acquired 3D T1 sequence. T2 SPACE/CUBE sequences and DWI sequences (or even more importantly their b0 images) often have some degree of fat suppression, which can be useful if compared to axial 2D T2 FSE/TSE sequences.

One of the more common causes of aqueductal stenosis is a thin **obstructing web**, which can be congenital or acquired. The web might be imperceptible on conventional imaging and the only clue might be distention of the third ventricular recesses or absence of flow-void through the aqueduct. In order to visualise a thin web, high-resolution bSSFP sequences might be necessary.

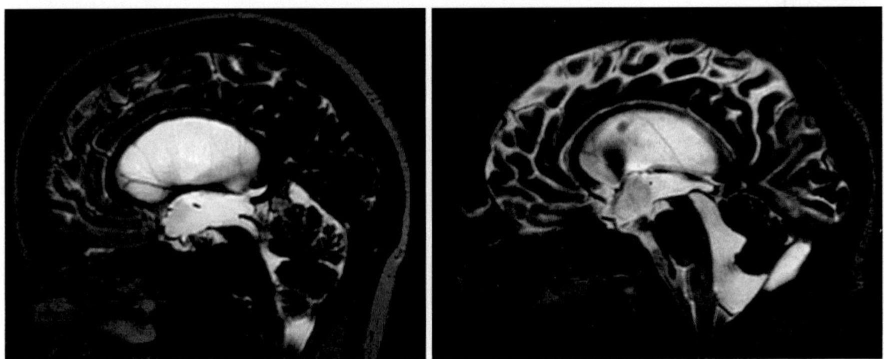

Fig. 9 Aqueductal funnelling. Two cases of aqueductal obstructions, with funnelling in downstream direction (left) and upstream direction (right)

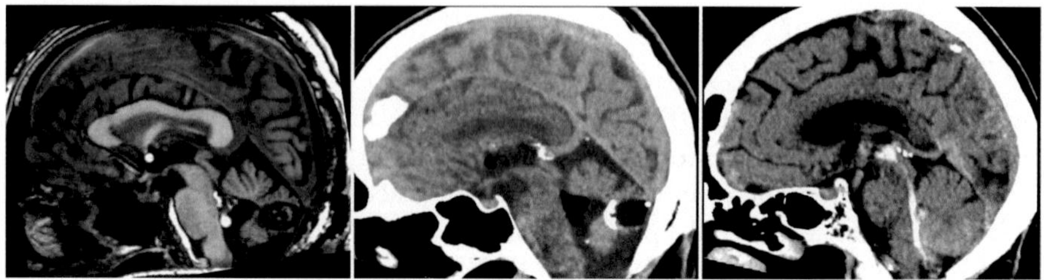

Fig. 10 Pathological contents of the aqueduct. T1w image on the left and CT image in the centre show ruptured cerebellar dermoid cyst, with propagation of its lipid contents (hyperintense on T1w, hypodense on CT) through the aqueduct into the third ventricle. Notice how the oily droplet sits independently in the 3rd ventricle. Patient presented with severe headaches to which the passage of dermoid contents via aqueduct might have contributed. Headaches subsided before imaging studies. Image on the right shows different patients with IVH and blood clot extending from 3rd ventricle through aqueduct to 4th ventricle

4.5 Fourth Ventricle

Distension of the 4th ventricle will manifest as loss of the concave shape of its roof and blunting of fastigium. In severe cases, the floor of the 4th ventricle can bulge out as well and push the brain stem forward (Fig. 11). If not sure whether the brainstem is compressed by the mass effect, inspect the prepontine cistern and cerebellopontine angles. The prepontine cistern should not be effaced and the facial and vestibulocochlear nerves should be clearly visible on T2 imaging—if they appear impinged between the skull and the brainstem, suspect significant compression of the brain stem. Flow-voids of the 4th ventricle are best assessed on axial slices, where they can be nicely followed from the aqueduct to the outflow foramina.

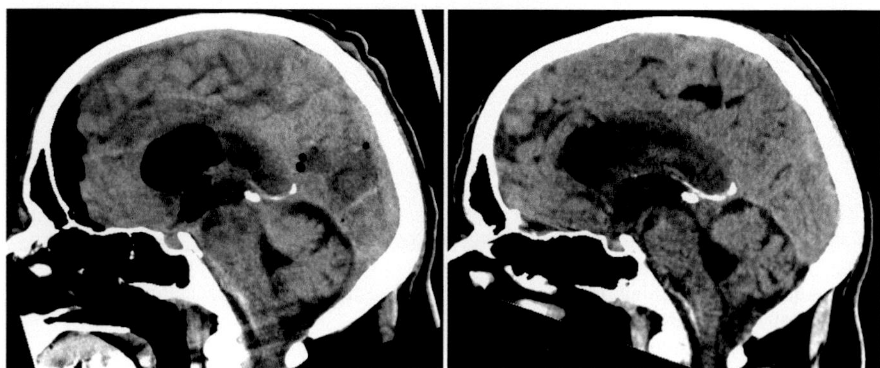

Fig. 11 Distention of the 4th ventricle. Postoperative CT 1 day (left) and 5 days (right) after surgery shows dilation of the 4th ventricle between the studies. Concave contours of the ventricular roof are lost, fastigium is blunted and brainstem bows slighty forward (image on the right). Notice the blood in front of the brain stem, which likely played a part in development of hydrocephalus

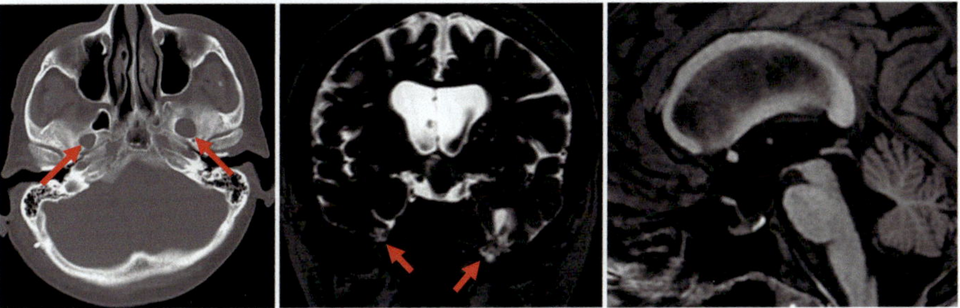

Fig. 12 Features of Long-standing hydrocephalus. CT image on the left shows dilated foramen ovale on both sides (arrows). Heavily T2 weighted image in the centre shows protrusion of meninges and brain parenchyma (i.e. encephalomeningocele) through the dilated foramina (arrowheads), and overlying temporal lobe has substantial atrophy and gliosis. This patient suffered from intractable epilepsy. T1w image on the right shows bulged floor of the 3rd ventricle, partially empty sella and remodelation of bony sella turcica, all signs of long-standing hydrocephalus

4.6 Features of Hydrocephalus Outside the Ventricles

Depending on duration and degree of hydrocephalus, signs of elevated intracranial pressure might manifest outside of ventricles as well. These include empty sella with or without remodelling of the bony sella turcica and encephalomeningoceles. Any imaging study with newly detected hydrocephalus should be interrogated for signs of these conditions, as occasionally empty sella secondary to hydrocephalus can lead to hypopituitarism [11] and encephalomeningoceles can lead to intractable epilepsy [12] (Fig. 12).

5 Imaging Differential Diagnosis of Causes of Hydrocephalus

5.1 Introduction and Classification

At any point along its path, CSF flow can be obstructed by blood clots, tumours, inflammatory adhesions, septations or cysts. These will be amongst the most common causes of hydrocephalus in adults. In addition to this, other causes, often of idiopathic origin, can occur at certain levels. The most notable of these causes are summarised in the following text.

There are many different classifications of hydrocephalus, but this section will be keeping to the common clinical division to communicating and non-communicating, more closely laid out in Table 2. Since the majority of clinical classifications are derived from morphological features of hydrocephalus, imaging findings play a major role in the workup and management of hydrocephalus.

Table 2 Diagram showing the commonly used clinical classification of hydrocephalus. We will follow this classification in this chapter

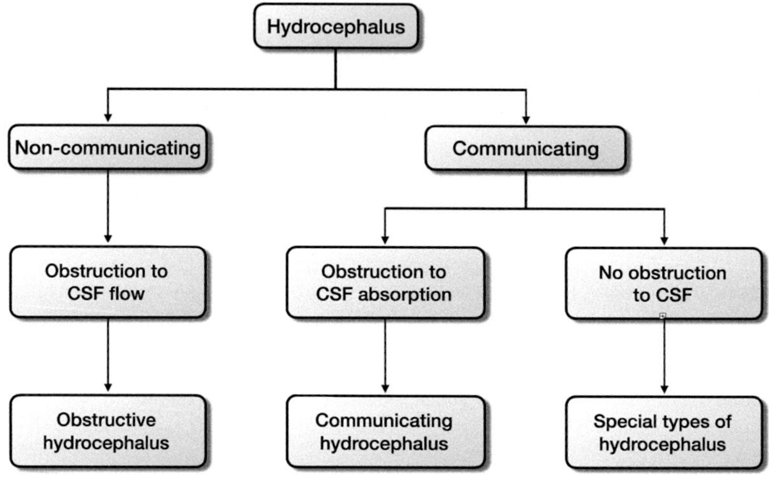

5.2 Non-Communicating Hydrocephalus

Obstruction Inside the Lateral Ventricles

Just like any other part of the ventricular system, lateral ventricles can be obstructed by a clot, tumours, septations or cysts of various origin. If these are found inside the lateral ventricles, it leads to signs of hydrocephalus that are limited only to a portion of the ventricle (Fig. 13). Alternatively, lateral ventricles can be compressed by an extra-ventricular lesion such as EDH or SDH; however, these usually cause obstruction at the foramen of Monro. If an obstructing lesion is not immediately obvious, try to look for a transitional zone between dilated and non-dilated ventricle, as this might be the location of an obstructing web.

Obstruction of the Foramen of Monro

The most typical lesion of foramina of Monro leading to hydrocephalus is the colloid cyst. They typically manifest as round lesions between the roof of the third ventricle and foramina of Monro, hyperdense on CT and of variable signal on MRI. While the vast majority of these are asymptomatic, in time they may grow and occasionally cause life-threatening acute hydrocephalus (Fig. 14) [13].

If there are signs of dilated lateral ventricles, the remainder of the ventricular system is slim and there is no obvious obstruction, consider the possibility of **idiopathic stenosis of foramina of Monro** [14]. In this entity of unknown origin, there is no detectable cause of obstruction beyond stenotic foramina of Monro, with no

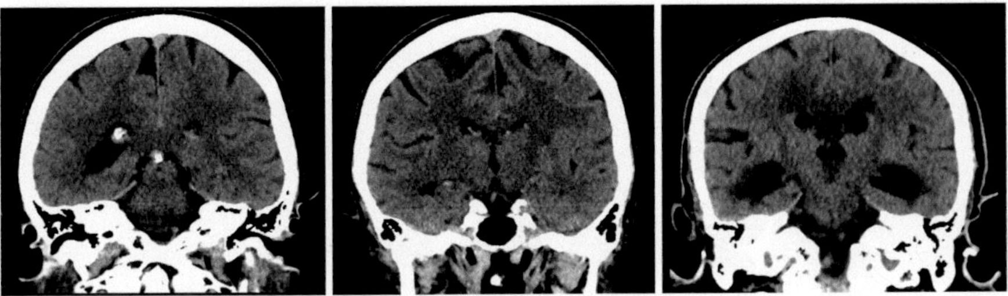

Fig. 13 Obstruction inside lateral ventricles. Patient with simple choroid plexus cyst in the antrum of right lateral ventricle (left and centre image) with mild compensatory dilation of its temporal horn. In the absence of periventricular interstitial oedema and clinical symptoms, this finding doesn't require further management. On the right, a patient with marked dilation of temporal horns with relative preservation of frontal horn width, pointing to the location of obstruction, which was inflammatory adhesions in the antra due to ventriculitis. Notice the periventricular interstitial oedema, most likely a combination of inflammatory changes and decompensated hydrocephalus

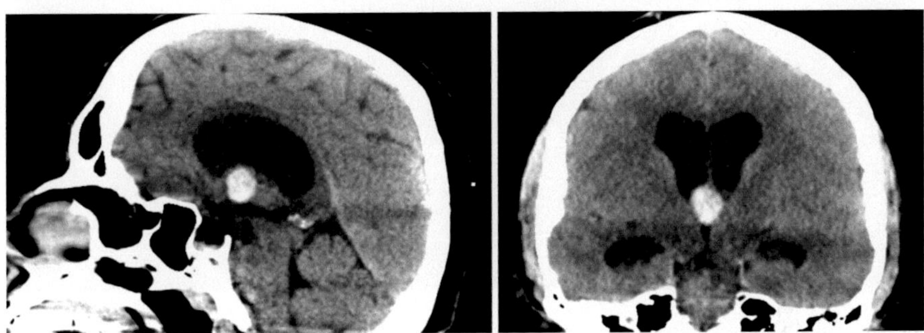

Fig. 14 Colloid cyst. Hyperdense oval lesion of the roof of the third ventricle, protruding into foramina Monroi and causing obstructive hydrocephalus (notice the temporal horns). Typical findings for colloid cyst

discernible flow-voids. One of the hallmarks of this disorder is the striking contrast between dilated lateral ventricles and narrow, slit-like third ventricle (Fig. 15) [15].

Obstruction of the 3rd Ventricle

Third ventricle is a favourite location for several tumours, including craniopharyngioma, germinoma or rosette-forming glioneuronal tumour (Fig. 16) [16]. In the case of the latter two, CSF seeding is a common occurrence and can help to narrow down the differential. Third ventricle can be also compressed by lesions within the parenchyma, such as gliomas or metastases.

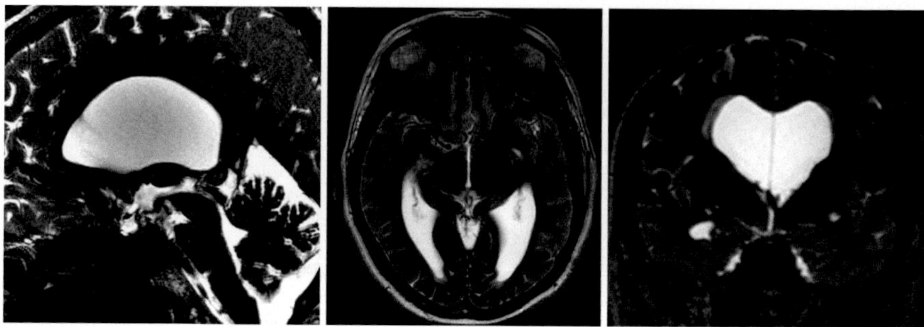

Fig. 15 Idiopathic stenosis of foramina of Monro. Dilated lateral ventricles, slit-like third ventricle and absence of flow-voids through foramina of Monro are highly suggestive of bilateral Idiopathic stenosis of foramina of Monro. In these cases, look for defects in septum pellucidum as it can impact further management

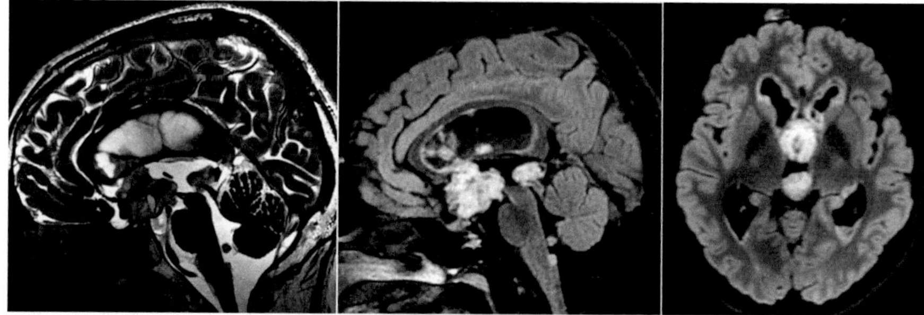

Fig. 16 Third ventricle tumour causing hydrocephalus. Tumour of the third ventricle in a young adult, filling most of its ventral volume, with extensive CSF seeding including but not limited to all ventricles, entry into the aqueduct and obex. The ventricles are enlarged given the young age, a sign of developing hydrocephalus, at least partially due to sub-occlusion of the aqueduct. Histology confirmed Rosette-forming glioneuronal tumour. Similar behaviour with "double midline" presentation and CSF seeding can be seen with germinoma

Aqueductal Obstruction

The aqueduct can be compressed from the outside, e.g. by mesencephalic gliomas, or from the inside, e.g. by cysts or webs. Sometimes the intra-aqueductal lesion is not well demarcated on conventional imaging, and thin-slice imaging might be needed. This is true especially for aqueductal webs, but sometimes also for thin-walled cysts with signal characteristics identical to CSF. If an adult presents with an aqueductal web, features of long-standing hydrocephalus and no relevant neurological history, the term Late-onset idiopathic aqueductal stenosis (LIAS) is used [17] (Fig. 17).

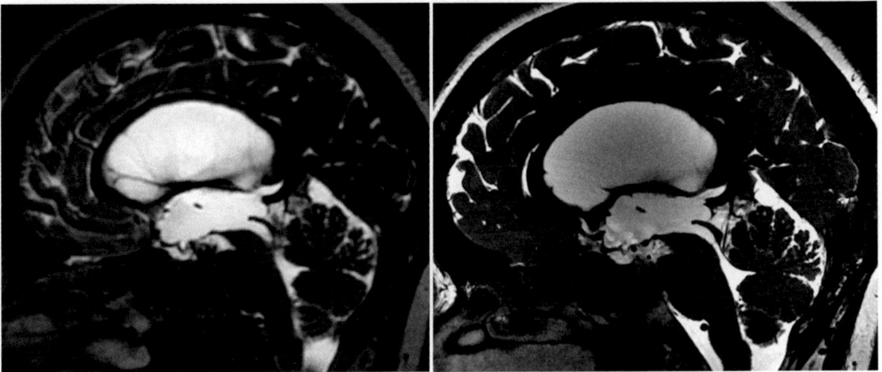

Fig. 17 Aqueductal web. Sagittal 3D T2 imaging on the left shows bowing of the corpus callosum as a sign of dilated lateral ventricles, distended third ventricle, lack of flow-voids through aqueduct and normal-sized 4th ventricle. SSFP imaging on the right elucidates thin aqueductal web as the causative pathology

Obstruction of the 4th Ventricle

The most common fourth ventricular tumours causing obstruction in the adult population include ependymomas, subependymomas or choroid plexus tumours [18]. Metastases are a common occurrence in the posterior fossa too and can cause compression of the ventricle, just like large vestibular schwannomas (see Fig. 7) or gliomas.

Similarly to the third ventricle, both inflow (aqueduct) and outflow (foramina of Magendie and Luschae) from the fourth ventricle can be obstructed at the same time, and this relatively uncommon condition is called **trapped 4th ventricle** [19]. This usually occurs in a post-surgery setting with ventriculoperitoneal shunt or third ventriculostomy draining the more proximal parts of the ventricular system (Fig. 18).

Obstruction of Foramina Magendie and Luschka

The outflow foramina of the 4th ventricle are usually plugged by a tumour of the fourth ventricle or by blood after intraventricular propagation of intra-axial haemorrhage. Bleeding, meningitis or surgery can also lead to scarring in the area which will impede the flow of CSF into the subarachnoid space.

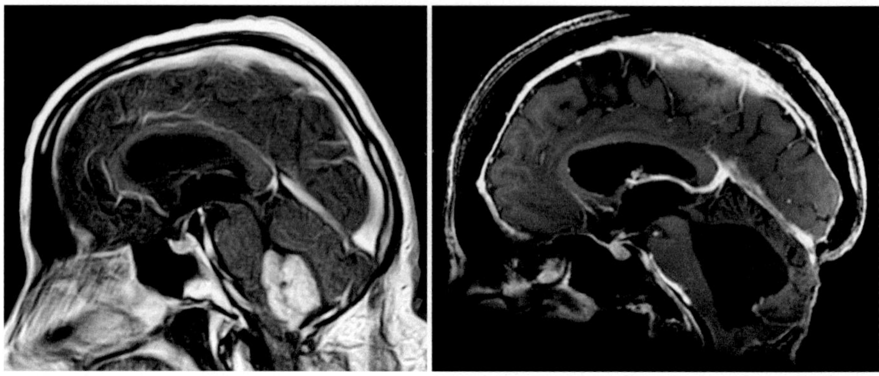

Fig. 18 Obstruction of the 4th ventricle. Post-contrast T1w image on the left shows vividly enhancing mass within the 4th ventricle, protruding into foramina of Magendie and Luschka, exerting mass effect on posterior fossa structures. Biopsy confirmed ependymoma. On the right a markedly dilated 4th ventricle in disproportion to other parts of the ventricular system in a patient who underwent surgical treatment for abscess of the posterior fossa and insertion of ventriculoperitoneal shunt (not shown). A thin web can be seen spanning the aqueduct. These findings should prompt further evaluation for the possibility of trapped 4th ventricle

5.3 Communicating Hydrocephalus

Post-Meningitis and Post-Haemorrhage Hydrocephalus

Inflammation of the leptomeninges leads to release of various cytokines (including TGF-β), which trigger fibrogenic response within the CSF spaces [20] and subsequent impairment of CSF flow through ventricular system, SA spaces, VRS and/or glymphatic system. This can happen as a result of CNS infection or sterile inflammation following SA or intraventricular haemorrhage (see Figs. 19 and 20) and at various time points after the initial insult [19]. In these cases, patient history (or prior imaging) is the most important clue for diagnosis.

Hydrocephalus Due to Meningeal Infiltration

Hydrocephalus can also result from infiltration of leptomeninges by a tumour, usually lymphoma. If detectable on MR, leptomeningeal lymphoma will typically manifest as diffuse leptomeningeal enhancement, with possible involvement of cranial nerves, spinal cord and its nerve roots [21]. A certain proportion of CNS lymphomas are radiologically occult [22] and hydrocephalus might be the only clue to diagnosis. In even rarer cases, hydrocephalus can be caused by non-neoplastic infiltration of the meninges, seen for example in Erdheim-Chester disease [23].

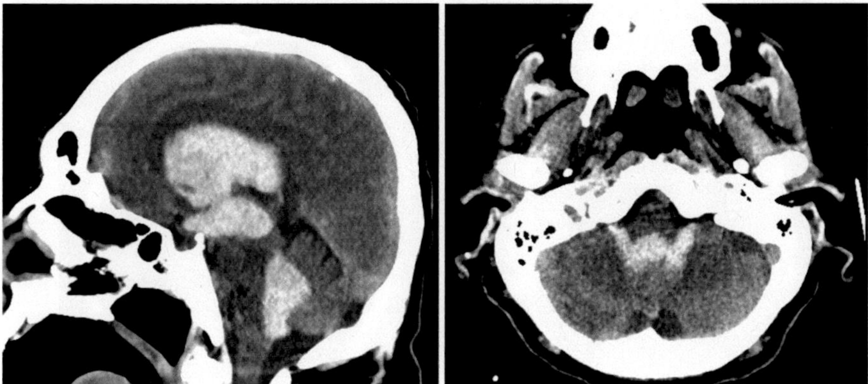

Fig. 19 Intraventricular haemorrhage causing hydrocephalus. Extensive intraventricular haemorrhage essentially forming a cast of the ventricular system, including foramina of Magendie and Luschka (left). Notice the sulcal effacement, a sign of life-threatening hydrocephalus

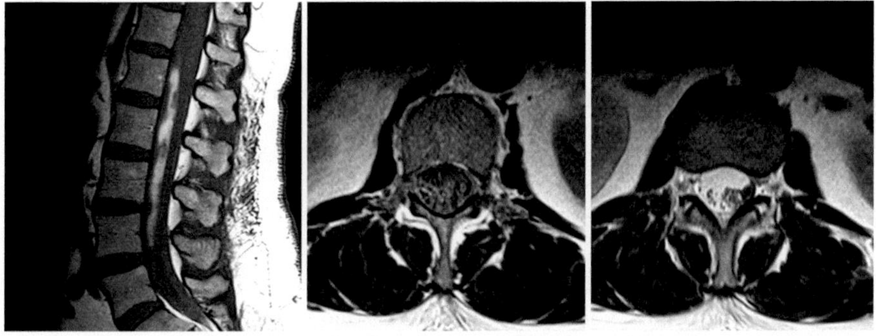

Fig. 20 Spinal cord arachnoiditis. Sagittal T1w scans (left) showing hyperintense blood anterior to spinal cord. On axial T2w, the hypointense blood can be seen surrounding the fibres of cauda equina, localising the blood into subarachnoid space. On axial T2w slices three months later (right), some of the fibres of cauda equina clump together as a result of sterile inflammatory process (arachnoiditis) with subsequent fibrogenesis. While not as nicely visible there, similar processes occur intracranially as a result of SAH, IVH or meningitis and can cause obstruction at various levels, including ventricular foramina and perivascular spaces

5.4   Special Types of Hydrocephalus

Overproduction Hydrocephalus

A rare cause of hydrocephalus is seen in the setting of choroid plexus papilloma, carcinoma or hyperplasia [24], where it is thought that these entities cause hydrocephalus by overproduction of CSF. Unfortunately, in certain cases, hydrocephalus does not

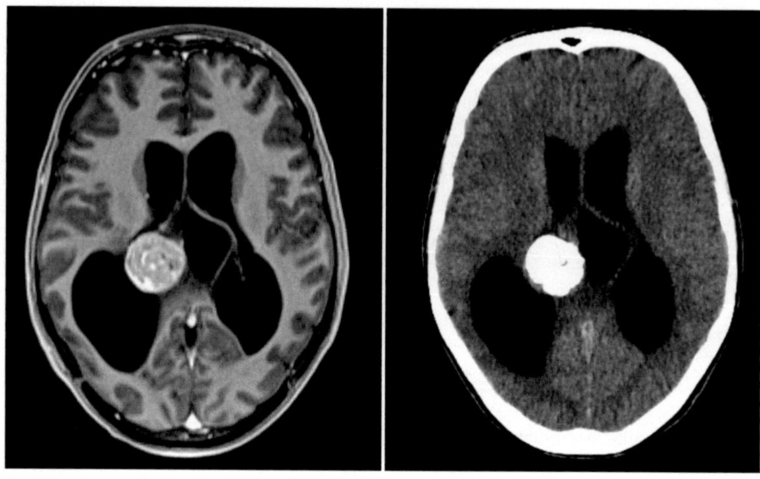

Fig. 21 Choroid plexus papilloma in young adult. Lobulated, enhancing mass with calcifications and closely related to the choroid plexus. Notice enlarged ventricles, most likely due to combination of overproduction and obstructions created by tumour-related septations

resolve even after complete surgical resection, implying additional mechanisms might be at play (Fig. 21).

Long-Standing Overt Ventriculomegaly in Adults

LOVA is a relatively new entity [25] with two major subdivisions: LOVA with and without patent aqueduct. Closed aqueduct LOVA and LIAS are considered the same entity by some authors, especially since the imaging findings and subsequent management are similar. Therefore, the following text focuses on open-aqueduct LOVA, which poses a bigger diagnostic dilemma and is a major differential diagnosis of iNPH.

The clinical tetrad of LOVA includes a) macrocephaly, b) long-term ventriculomegaly, c) clinical symptoms of increased intracranial pressure and d) absence of secondary cause of aqueductal obstruction. Evidence of long-term triventriculomegaly includes partial empty sella, remodelation of sella turcica or meningoceles (see Fig. 12).

Differentiating open-aqueduct LOVA from iNPH can be challenging since there is significant overlap in imaging findings. Features like younger age, macrocephaly,[3] bulging of the third ventricle and presence of enlarged cisterna magna have been found to associate more closely with LOVA than iNPH [26]. An enlarged cisterna magna is accompanied by movement of the whole cerebellum into a more cranial

---

[3] Defined as head circumference above 98th percentile adjusted for sex [27]. For males, this is 53.8 cm and for females 52.9 cm.

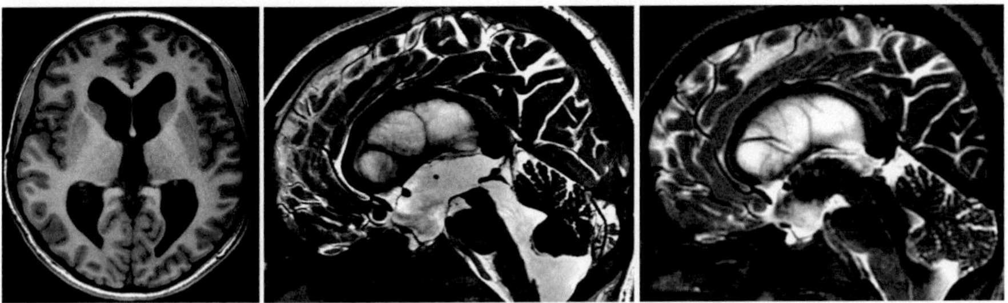

Fig. 22 Open-aqueduct LOVA. MRI of a 42-year-old female with chronic headaches and visual disturbances, with bulging of the 3rd ventricle and maintained flow through the ventricular system. Cisterna magna is spacious and inferior follia of cerebellum are effaced. Remodelation of bony sella turcica and partially empty sella point to a long-standing hydrocephalus. In the setting of macrocephaly and otherwise uneventful history, these findings are highly suggestive of open-aqueduct LOVA

position and effacement of inferior folia, which is a relatively characteristic finding (Fig. 22).

Idiopathic Normal Pressure Hydrocephalus

Imaging features of iNPH have been discussed in more detail in previous chapters. What follows is a table comparing the major imaging features of iNPH, LOVA and LIAS—the common differential when assessing adults with newly found hydrocephalus (Table 3).

Table 3 Features of open-aqueduct LOVA, iNPH and LIAS

	OA-LOVA	iNPH	LIAS
Callosal angle	Sharp	Sharp	Normal
DESH score	Low	High	Low
Empty sella	Common	Common	Common
Remodelling of sella	Minority of cases	Rare	Rare
Third ventricle bulging	Common	Uncommon	Common
Enlarged cisterna magna	Very common	Common	Rare

Adapted from Palandri et al. [16]. OA-LOVA: open-aqueduct long-standing overt ventriculomegaly in adults. iNPH: Idiopathic Normal Pressure Hydrocephalus. LIAS: Late-onset idiopathic aqueductal stenosis

6 Key Points

- A standardised MRI protocol with focus on high-resolution (e.g. CISS, FIESTA-C) and sagittal flow-sensitive sequences (e.g. 3D T2 SPACE, CUBE) is necessary to increase the diagnostic accuracy of hydrocephalus.
- Hydrocephalus is more than just enlarged ventricles and knowledge of relevant ventricular anatomy and individual features of hydrocephalus helps to increase sensitivity to hydrocephalus and its causes.
- Long-standing hydrocephalus can occasionally lead to complications like hypopituitarism or epilepsy; therefore, it is important to actively look for these complications.
- Many classifications of hydrocephalus exist, the most clinically relevant classifications usually rely on morphology of the hydrocephalus and therefore put a great emphasis on imaging findings.
- Open-aqueduct LOVA can look similar to iNPH, including the sharp callosal angle. Younger age, macrocephaly, bulging of the third ventricle and enlarged cisterna magna might help differentiate.

Funding This chapter was supported by the Ministry of Health of the Czech Republic institutional grant no. NU23-04–00551.

References

1. Ucar M, Guryildirim M, Tokgoz N, Kilic K, Borcek A, Oner Y, Akkan K, Tali T. Evaluation of aqueductal patency in patients with hydrocephalus: three-dimensional high-sampling-efficiency technique (SPACE) versus two-dimensional turbo spin echo at 3 Tesla. Korean J Radiology: Official J Korean Radiol Soc. 2014;15(6):827–35. https://doi.org/10.3348/kjr.2014.15.6.827.
2. Stratchko L, Filatova I, Agarwal A, Kanekar S. The ventricular system of the brain: anatomy and normal variations. Semin Ultrasound CT MR. 2016;37(2):72–83. https://doi.org/10.1053/j.sult.2016.01.004.
3. Born CM, Meisenzahl EM, Frodl T, Pfluger T, Reiser M, Möller HJ, Leinsinger GL. The septum pellucidum and its variants. An MRI study: an MRI study. European Archives of Psychiatry and Clinical Neurosci 2004;254(5):295–302. https://doi.org/10.1007/s00406-004-0496-z
4. Donauer E, Moringlane JR, Ostertag CB. Cavum vergae cyst as a cause of hydrocephalus, ?Almost Forgotten??: successful stereotactic treatment. Acta Neurochir. 1986;83(1–2):12–9. https://doi.org/10.1007/bf01420502.
5. Funaki T, Makino Y, Arakawa Y, Hojo M, Kunieda T, Takagi Y, Takahashi JC, Miyamoto S. Arachnoid cyst of the velum interpositum originating from tela choroidea. Surg Neurol Int. 2012;3(1):120. https://doi.org/10.4103/2152-7806.102334.
6. Damle NR, Ikuta T, John M, Peters BD, DeRosse P, Malhotra AK, Szeszko PR. Relationship among interthalamic adhesion size, thalamic anatomy and neuropsychological functions in healthy volunteers. Brain Struct Funct. 2017;222(5):2183–92. https://doi.org/10.1007/s00429-016-1334-6.

7. Missori P, Paolini S, Peschillo S, Mancarella C, Scafa AK, Rastelli E, Martini S, Fattapposta F, Currà A. Temporal horn enlargements predict secondary hydrocephalus diagnosis earlier than Evans' index. Tomography: A J Imaging Res 2022;8(3):1429–1436. https://doi.org/10.3390/tomography8030115

8. Kim H, Jeong E-J, Park D-H, Czosnyka Z, Yoon BC, Kim K, Czosnyka M, Kim D-J. Finite element analysis of periventricular lucency in hydrocephalus: extravasation or transependymal CSF absorption? J Neurosurg. 2016;124(2):334–41. https://doi.org/10.3171/2014.11.JNS14138.

9. Sze G, De Armond SJ, Brant-Zawadzki M, Davis RL, Norman D, Newton TH. Foci of MRI signal (pseudo lesions) anterior to the frontal horns: histologic correlations of a normal finding. AJR Am J Roentgenol. 1986;147(2):331–7. https://doi.org/10.2214/ajr.147.2.331.

10. Krauss JK, Regel JP, Vach W, Jüngling FD, Droste DW, Wakhloo AK. Flow void of cerebrospinal fluid in idiopathic normal pressure hydrocephalus of the elderly: can it predict outcome after shunting? Neurosurgery 1997;40(1). 67–73; discussion 73–4. https://doi.org/10.1097/00006123-199701000-00015

11. Krejčí T, Krejčí O, Mrůzek M, Röschlová I, Lipina R. Non-communicating hydrocephalus with a primary empty sella presenting with growth hormone deficiency and delayed puberty successfully treated by endoscopic third ventriculocisternostomy. Acta Neurochir. 2021;163(2):511–4. https://doi.org/10.1007/s00701-020-04481-9.

12. Pettersson DR, Hagen KS, Sathe NC, Clark BD, Spencer DC. MR imaging features of middle cranial Fossa encephaloceles and their associations with epilepsy. AJNR Am J Neuroradiol. 2020;41(11):2068–74. https://doi.org/10.3174/ajnr.A6798.

13. Tenny S, Thorell W. Colloid brain cyst. In StatPearls [Internet]. StatPearls Publishing; 2022.

14. Raz E, Fatterpekar G, Davis AJ, Huang PP, Loh JP. Mystery case: idiopathic bilateral stenosis of the foramina of Monro. Neurology. 2012;79(18):e166–7. https://doi.org/10.1212/WNL.0b013e318271f792.

15. Gomez-Ruiz N, Polidura MC, Crespo Rodriguez AM, Arrazola García J. Idiopathic stenosis of foramina of Monro in an asymptomatic adult patient: a rare entity radiologists should be aware of. BJR Case Reports. 2020;6(2):20190102. https://doi.org/10.1259/bjrcr.20190102.

16. Elwatidy SM, Albakr AA, Al Towim AA, Malik SH. Tumors of the lateral and third ventricle: surgical management and outcome analysis in 42 cases. Neurosciences (Riyadh, Saudi Arabia) 2017;22(4):274–281. https://doi.org/10.17712/nsj.2017.4.20170149

17. Fukuhara T, Luciano MG. Clinical features of late-onset idiopathic aqueductal stenosis. Surgical Neurol. 2001;55(3):132–136. discussion 136–7. https://doi.org/10.1016/s0090-3019(01)00359-7

18. Sufianov R, Pitskhelauri D, Bykanov A. Fourth ventricle tumors: a review of series treated with microsurgical technique. Front Surgery 2022;9:915253. https://doi.org/10.3389/fsurg.2022.915253

19. Panagopoulos D, Karydakis P, Themistocleous M. The entity of the trapped fourth ventricle: a review of its history, pathophysiology, and treatment options. Brain Circulation. 2021;7(3):147–58. https://doi.org/10.4103/bc.bc_30_21.

20. Kuo L-T, Huang AP-H. The pathogenesis of hydrocephalus following aneurysmal subarachnoid hemorrhage. Int J Mol Sci. 2021;22(9):5050. https://doi.org/10.3390/ijms22095050.

21. Haldorsen IS, Espeland A, Larsson E-M. Central nervous system lymphoma: characteristic findings on traditional and advanced imaging. AJNR Am J Neuroradiol. 2011;32(6):984–92. https://doi.org/10.3174/ajnr.A2171.

22. Boshrabadi AP, Naiem A, Ghazi Mirsaeid SS, Yarandi KK, Amirjamshidi A. Hydrocephalus as the sole presentation of primary diffuse large B-cell lymphoma of the brain: report of a case and review of literature. Surg Neurol Int. 2017;8(1):165. https://doi.org/10.4103/sni.sni_446_16.

23. De Macêdo LP, Ferreira USM, Ferreira YDO, de Carvalho Júnior EV, Faquini IV, Almeida NS, Azevedo-Filho HRC. Erdheim-Chester disease with intracranial involvement causing hydrocephalus: case report. Interdisciplinary Neurosurgery: Adv Techniques and Case Managem. 2020;21(100722): 100722. https://doi.org/10.1016/j.inat.2020.100722.

24. Fujimura M, Onuma T, Kameyama M, Motohashi O, Kon H, Yamamoto K, Ishii K, Tominaga T. Hydrocephalus due to cerebrospinal fluid overproduction by bilateral choroid plexus papillomas. Child's Nervous Syst: ChNS: Official J Int Soc Pediatric Neurosurgery. 2004;20(7):485–8. https://doi.org/10.1007/s00381-003-0889-8.
25. Kiefer M, Eymann R, Steudel WI. LOVA hydrocephalus—a new entity of chronic hydrocephalus. Nervenarzt. 2002;73(10):972–81. https://doi.org/10.1007/s00115-002-1389-x.
26. Palandri G, Carretta A, La Corte E, Giannini G, Martinoni M, Mantovani P, Albini-Riccioli L, Tonon C, Mazzatenta D, Elder BD, Conti A. Open-aqueduct LOVA, LIAS, iNPH: a comparative clinical-radiological study exploring the "grey zone" between different forms of chronic adulthood hydrocephalus. Acta Neurochir. 2022;164(7):1777–88. https://doi.org/10.1007/s00701-022-05215-9.
27. Oi S, Shimoda M, Shibata M, Honda Y, Togo K, Shinoda M, Tsugane R, Sato O. Pathophysiology of long-standing overt ventriculomegaly in adults. J Neurosurg. 2000;92(6):933–40. https://doi.org/10.3171/jns.2000.92.6.0933.

Imaging Differential Diagnosis of Neurodegenerative Disorders

Vojtěch Sedlák, Petr Skalický, Adéla Bubeníková, Helen Whitley, and Ondřej Bradáč

Abstract Imaging methods are a major tool in diagnosis of neurodegenerative disorders, as they can detect morphological changes specific for individual conditions. MRI is the dominant imaging modality, but since major disease-specific morphological changes often occur only later in disease course, when the diagnosis is clinically obvious, standardised protocol and image interpretation are necessary to detect and correctly interpret often subtle signs of neurodegenerative disorders in their earlier stages. This chapter provides the basis for setup of an optimal MRI protocol and correct interpretation and presents the most important imaging features of neurodegenerative disorders that are often on the differential along with iNPH.

Keywords Differential diagnosis · Imaging · Cerebrospinal fluid flow · Magnetic resonance imaging · Normal pressure hydrocephalus

Abbreviations

AD	Alzheimer's disease
ADC	Apparent diffusion coefficient
AIE	Autoimmune encephalitis
bSSFP	Balanced steady-state free precession
BRAVO	Brain volume imaging
CISS	Constructive interference in the steady state

V. Sedlák
Department of Radiology, Military University Hospital, Prague, Czech Republic

P. Skalický · A. Bubeníková · O. Bradáč (✉)
Department of Neurosurgery, Second Faculty of Medicine, Charles University and Motol University Hospital, Prague, Czech Republic
e-mail: ondrej.bradac2@fnmotol.cz

A. Bubeníková · H. Whitley · O. Bradáč
Department of Neurosurgery and Neurooncology, First Faculty of Medicine, Charles University and Military University Hospital, Prague, Czech Republic

© The Author(s), under exclusive license to Springer Nature Switzerland AG 2023
O. Bradac (ed.), *Normal Pressure Hydrocephalus*,
https://doi.org/10.1007/978-3-031-36522-5_18

CJD	Creutzfeldt-jakob disease
CSF	Cerebrospinal fluid
CT	Computed tomography
DWI	Diffusion weighted imaging
DAT	Dopamine active transporter
EPI	Echoplanar imaging
ERICA	Entorhinal cortical atrophy
FDG	Fluorodeoxyglucose
FIESTA	Fast imaging employing steady-state acquisition
FIESTA-C	Fast imaging employing steady-state acquisition-constructive interference
FLAIR	Fluid attenuated inversion recovery
FSE	Fast spin echo
GM	Grey matter
HD	Huntington's disease
iNPH	Idiopathic normal pressure hydrocephalus
LBD	Lewy body dementia
MPR	Multiplanar reconstruction
MPRAGE	Magnetisation prepared rapid gradient echo
MRI	Magnetic resonance imaging
MSA	Multiple system atrophy
MTA	Medial temporal lobe atrophy
MUSE	Multi-shot echoplanar imaging
PAC	Spicture archive and communication system
PC	Phase contrast
PD	Parkinson's disease
PET	Positron emission tomography
PROPELLER	Periodically rotated overlapping parallel lines with enhanced reconstruction
PSP	Progressive supranuclear palsy
RESOLVE	Readout segmentation of long variable echo-trains
SNR	Signal-to-noise ratio
SPACE	Sampling perfection with application optimised contrasts using different flip angle evolution
SSFP	Steady-state free precession
SWI	Susceptibility weighted imaging
TSE	Turbo spin echo
VD	Vascular dementia
WMH	White matter hyperintensities

1 Introduction

In this chapter, we will discuss the imaging appearances of neurodegenerative disorders that may share clinical features of iNPH. The focus will be mostly on MRI, but nuclear medicine and CT findings will be mentioned whenever they might be helpful. The following text is not an exhaustive list of signs and findings, instead it is meant to provide a guide to most high-yield imaging features that can lead you towards the correct diagnosis. The chapter starts with setting up an optimal MRI protocol and a MRI reading checklist to increase diagnostic accuracy. Then, the chapter continues by discussing imaging features of individual neurodegenerative disorders and where appropriate contrasts them with iNPH imaging findings.

2 Recommended MRI Protocol

As patients with neurodegenerative disorders often present on a spectrum with regards to clinical and morphological brain changes, a standardised MRI protocol and systematic approach are needed to make sure that you extract the most information from acquired scans and correctly interpret the findings. This is even more important as many clinically ambiguous cases will also have ambiguous findings on MRI and so rather than being a confirmatory test, MRI will contribute to diagnosis by effectively increasing or decreasing the likelihood of clinically suggested diagnosis.

As with any other indication for brain MRI, the optimal diagnostic protocol for investigation of neurodegenerative disorders is a matter of dispute amongst radiologists. However, Table 1 summarises a protocol that the majority of neuroradiologists would find sufficient or even satisfactory for diagnosing iNPH and other neurodegenerative disorders.

Table 1 Recommended MR protocol for investigation of adult-onset hydrocephalus

Pulse sequence	Estimated time [3T]
Mandatory sequences	
2D Ax DWI	< 1 min
3D T1 (MPRAGE OR BRAVO)	3–4 min
2D Ax T2 (FSE or PROPELLER)	2 min
2D Ax T2 FLAIR	2 min
3D Sag T2	2 min
3D Ax SWI (or T2* GRE)	4 (2) min
Optional sequences	
3D Sag SSFP (CISS, FIESTA…)	3 min
CSF flow study	4 min
3D ASL perfusion	4 min

When it comes to the neurodegenerative MRI protocol, pulse sequences can be grouped into 2. The first group is the standard "always on" or "mandatory" sequences that should always be included under any circumstance. These will provide you with the majority of information and usually will clue you into the right diagnosis. However, in certain cases, the "optional" sequences can yield some valuable information you would not be able to obtain otherwise.

2.1 Standard Sequences

When interpreting the neurodegenerative brain MRI, the main workhorse sequence is your **3D T1 weighted**. Make sure you allocate enough time to acquire a high SNR isotropic data, with good resolution (1 mm is ideal) and tissue contrast. This usually means IR-prepped, spoiled GRE sequences (i.e. MPRAGE, BRAVO, etc.) (Fig. 1). The acquisition plane is mostly a matter of preference, but make sure to order MPR reconstructions in all neurodegenerative brain MRI studies and better yet, all brain studies, to get a feel for normal, so you are confident when evaluating the abnormal. Axial and sagittal MPR planes can be reconstructed in the usual manner (axials in identical plane to 2D sequences, sagittals precisely parallel to the sagittal plane). However, coronal MPRs should be reconstructed in two planes: perpendicular to a) the AC-PC line and b) the long axis of the hippocampi. Reconstructing your coronals parallel to the brain stem instead of perpendicular to the hippocampal long axis is also acceptable as these two planes are closely aligned in most subjects. If your institution uses a PACS viewer capable of working with volumetric data and real-time MPR, that is even better and you can skip the in-console MPR reconstructions.

Axial T2 sequences will not play such a dominant role in diagnosis of dementias as in some other brain MRI applications. T2 scans will be helpful in consulting FLAIR findings due to their better resolution and SNR. Some studies also suggest higher sensitivity of T2 scans to glial changes of thalamus and posterior fossa structures

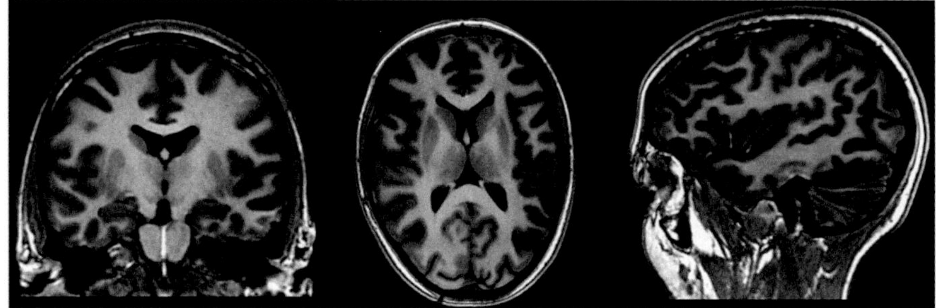

Fig. 1 An example of a good quality 3D T1 BRAVO sequence, in 1 mm isotropic resolution. Acquisition time was 4 min on a 3 T scanner. Any further increase in time acquisition and image quality will have a dubious impact on diagnostic accuracy

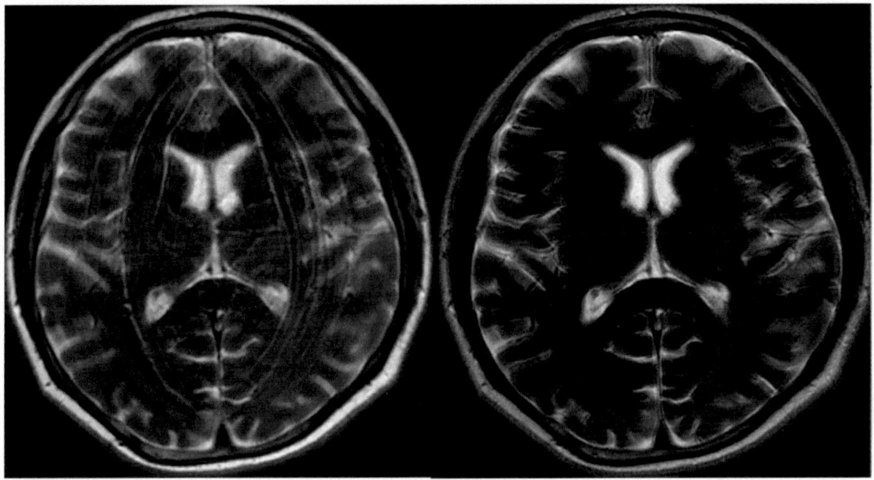

Fig. 2 Reduction of motion artifacts with a PROPELLER sequence. A healthy volunteer was asked to intermittently move their head during both, T2 FSE and PROPELLER acquisitions. There is noticeable reduction of motion artifacts with PROPELLER compared to standard FSE sequence

(1). The standard in brain imaging is to use T2 FSE/TSE sequences with Cartesian readout. However, a thing to consider in suspected iNPH/neurodegenerative disease patients is to use T2 acquisition with **radial read-out**, for instance PROPELLER, BLADE, or MultiVane due to their intrinsic **motion-correction** (Fig. 2) (2). This is because a s large proportion of patients with suspected neurodegenerative disorders will have notable motion artefacts on the majority of used sequences. In case you decide to implement these pulse sequence designs, keep in mind that susceptibility and flow-related artefacts will be reduced, compared to classic Cartesian FSE/TSE. All major vendors provide T2 sequences with radial read-out as standard options preinstalled on their scanners.

T2 FLAIR sequences are best for assessing the amount and distribution of glial changes in the brain, which are common in iNPH and many other neurodegenerative disorders. They are also important for detecting cortical defects due to multi-infarct dementias, which might be missed on regular T2, especially if small, as CSF and gliosis have a similar signal intensity on plain T2 imaging. PROPELLER/BLADE versions of T2 FLAIR are available as well and worth considering.

DWI output of modern MR scanners to PACS consists of three volumes: a **DWI image** (also called trace image), an **ADC map** and a **b0 image**. A potential pitfall when interpreting primary DWI images (i.e. trace images) is the so-called **T2 shine through** artefact (arguably a misnomer[1]) where the apparent hyperintensity of the

---

[1] Since diffusion trace images are formed from T2 images by modulating the signal by water diffusivity in a given voxel, all signal in diffusion trace images is the residual T2 signal "shining through".

DWI image is not due to true diffusion restriction but due to high T2 values of underlying pathology as DWI sequences are essentially modified, diffusion-sensitised T2 sequences. Therefore, any suspected pathology on DWI images should be correlated with ADC maps, which contain diffusion information free of T2 effects. Occasionally, ADC maps show pathology even in cases where DWI images look normal. This is called "**T2-washout**" and is seen, for example, in some cases of diffuse glioma [1].

The third output from DWI sequence (along with DWI images and ADC maps) is the b0 image, which is a non-diffusion weighted T2 SE-EPI image, potentially useful when the MRI protocol did not contain any SWI/T2* sequences, as SE-EPI images contain some amount of T2* weighting.

DWI is due to its fast readout resilient to motion artefacts; however, the same mechanism causes DWI sequences to be anatomically distorted, most notably around paranasal sinuses and skull base. The main role of DWI will be to rule out recent ischemia especially in patients with signs of vascular dementia, and in this scenario, these artefacts usually do not cause issues. When CJD is on the differential, however, adding multi-shot EPI DWI (RESOLVE, MUSE) to your protocol is advisable, as the above-mentioned artefacts could make the physiological cortex appear unusually hyperintense mimicking pathology, or do the opposite—obscure pathological changes. The above-mentioned multi-shot EPI techniques reduce anatomical distortion at the expense of increased imaging time.

Over recent years, **susceptibility weighted imaging** has made its way into standard brain MRI protocols in many institutions. In the case of neurodegenerative disorders, SWI comes in handy when evaluating for presence of hypertensive encephalopathy, superficial siderosis or cerebral amyloid angiopathy. Faster alternative to SWI is a conventional 2D T2* GRE sequence; however, this comes at a cost of spatial resolution and inability to reliably differentiate calcium deposits from microbleeds [2].

2.2 *Optional Sequences*

As iNPH is a disease with compromised CSF flow dynamics, quantifying the flow of CSF would seem promising. To do so *a phase contrast CSF flow study* sequence is set up, with a slice perpendicular to the long axis of the aqueduct, with low velocity encoding, lower than is usually done for MRI venography. However, in recent years, scientific literature has become split on the actual utility of assessing the CSF flow through aqueduct using phase contrast imaging. One should be very careful when employing such technique and do so only after gaining enough experience by testing the PC sequence on many patients, preferably also a non-neurodegenerative cohort, as the absolute values of CSF flow through the aqueduct seem to be scanner-dependent [3].

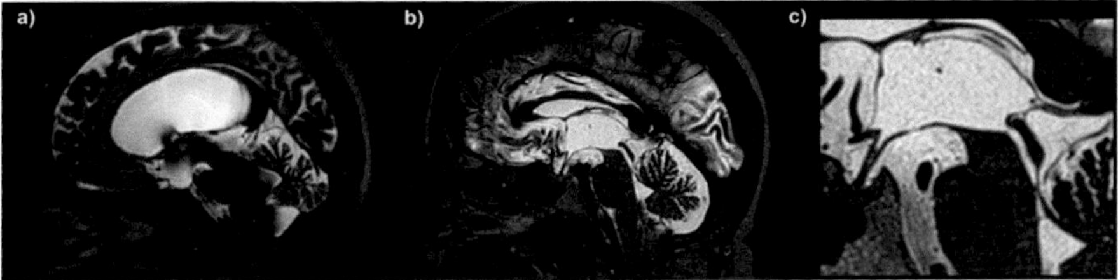

Fig. 3 High-resolution and flow-sensitive 3D sequences. a) Flow-sensitive 3D T2 CUBE sequence demonstrating vast flow-voids through the aqueduct and neighbouring ventricles due to hyperdynamic CSF flow in this patient with suspected iNPH. b) Patient with missing flow-voids through the aqueduct on this flow-sensitive sequence due to its closure. Notice the presence of flow-voids in prepontine cistern created by pulsations of the basilar artery, acting as an internal control. c) High-resolution bSSFP image of the same patient as in "b)", depicting an obstruction at the caudal end of the aqueduct. Also notice less prominent flow-voids in the prepontine cistern on this flow-insensitive, but high-res sequence

What seems to be a more reasonable option is to perform **single 3D T2 flow-sensitive acquisition** (CUBE, SPACE) in the sagittal plane through the median structures of the brain (Fig. 3). This should provide enough information on morphology of the aqueduct, ventricles and all the ventricular foramina and also provide a clear answer as to whether flow through these structures is present (comparable to PC CSF flow study, [4]). Furthermore, presuming the same sequence parameters will be used for each examination, it is also possible to subjectively quantify the flow through the aqueduct based on the extent and intensity of flow-voids[2] in the aqueduct and adjacent ventricles. Depending on sequence parameters, hyperdynamic CSF flow (often seen in the case of iNPH) will usually cause flow-voids to fill most of the third and fourth ventricles. On the other hand, complete absence of flow-void through the aqueduct strongly suggests aqueductal obstruction (6), e.g. due to a web. Modern scanners come with an option called flow-compensation which decreases the conspicuity of flow-voids, so make sure that this option is turned off to increase your sensitivity to flow.

If the cause of obstruction is not clear, adding a high-resolution **bSSFP sequence** (i.e. FIESTA-C, CISS) in sagittal orientation is helpful, as certain small structures, such as aqueductal web or cyst wall might need resolution approaching 0.5 mm isotropic in order to reliably visualise them.

Visualising cerebral metabolism was not a feasible option for non-contrast MRI for a long time. In recent years, however, all major MRI vendors started shipping their own version of **arterial spin labelling** pulse sequence, providing an option to assess blood flow through individual parts of the brain, which in many studies seems to be correlating nicely with FDG-PET [5]. However, as this is not yet a widespread

---

[2] A phenomenon of flow-related signal loss in MRI, due to time-of-flight and spin-phase effects. While disliked by some authors, the term "flow-voids" is in wide-spread clinical use, and for the sake of conciseness, we will use the term in this book as well.

clinical practice, one should exercise caution when interpreting these and become an experienced ASL-reader before relying on them too heavily.

3 Nuclear Medicine Imaging

Nuclear medicine is an important adjunct in the diagnosis of neurodegenerative disorders and can assess alterations of regional metabolism and perfusion which are present in many neurodegenerative disorders. It is also possible to use specific radiotracers to assess for integrity of dopaminergic pathways in suspected Parkinson's disease (so-called DaT scan) or to evaluate amyloid load in the brain (Amyloid PET using tracers like Pittsburg substance B or Flutemetamol).

4 Computed Tomography

CT should not be used routinely for diagnosis of neurodegenerative disorders, except in cases where MRI is contraindicated (e.g. claustrophobia, incompatible pacemaker). Therefore, the majority of CT scans with findings suggestive of neurodegenerative disease are done for other reasons, for example, as part of the workup for altered mental state, trauma or stroke. However, if CT is used, modern scanners with their volumetric acquisitions can nicely depict volume changes present in many neurodegenerative disorders, and if your PACS system contains thin slices (1 mm or less), there is also a possibility of reconstructing those in any plane you wish. A major advantage CT has over MRI is its relatively minimal sensitivity to motion, as the majority of patients (even iNPH patients) can stay still for the few seconds during which the brain CT is acquired.

5 Systematic Approach to Neurodegenerative MRI Reading

To ensure you extract the most information from the scan and do not overlook the subtle findings that can be the only clue to the correct diagnosis, a systematic approach is needed. This is even more important when evaluating neurodegenerative disease on MRI as in this setting, hard signs are few and far between.

There is no single universally best systematic approach to reading any scan, and so rather than going to great lengths about the approach itself, we offer a diagnostic checklist in Table 2, and we recommend that you create a systematic reading routine of your own based on this. The checklist is not comprehensive, instead it focuses on findings important for neurodegenerative MRI assessment and therefore should be used as an adjunct to your current, more general approach.

Table 2 Diagnostic checklist for neurodegenerative MR reading

T1 Axial	T2/FLAIR
– General brain morphology	– Degree and distribution of WMH
– Atrophy? Focal/general	– Signs of hydrocephalus/periventricular edema
– Hydrocephalus? Ventricular width and shape	– Flow void through aqueduct
– Obvious malacia	– Sulci width and contents (i.e. blood in CAA)
– Basal ganglia signal intensity	
– Shape of mesencephalon	**SWI/T2***
– Width of cerebellar peduncles	– Amount and distribution of blooming artefacts
	– Superficial cortical siderosis?
T1 Sagittal	– SWI hypointensity in precentral or other gyri
– Antero-posterior gradient of sulcal widening	
– Callosal bowing	**DWI**
– Shape and thickness of corpus callosum	– Signs of recent ischemia
– Width of pars marginalis of cingulate sulcus	– DWI hyperintensity of cortex, thalamus, and basal ganglia
– Shape and size of ventricles	– ADC map abnormality
– Aqueductal width	
– Shape and size of brainstem structures	**High-res sagittal SSFP through midline** (FIESTA, CISS)
– Mammillary bodies	– Patency of aqueduct
– Temporal lobes, hippocampi, amygdalae	– Foramina of Monro, Magendie, and Luschka
– Silvian fissure width	– Shape of the third ventricle
– Cerebellar atrophy	– Distention of supraoptic, infundibular, pineal, and suprapineal recesses
T1 Coronal, perpendicular to AC-PC line	**Flow-sensitive sagittal T2 sequence through midline** (SPACE, CUBE)
– Sulcal crowding at vertex	– Presence of flow-voids in aqueduct and other foramina
– Callosal angle	
T1 Coronal, perpendicular to long axis of hippocampi	
– Mesiotemporal lobe—hippocampus, amygdala, parahippocampal gyrus	
– Width of temporal horns, choroidal fissure	
– MTA score, ERICA score	

6   Normal Ageing Brain

It is hard to diagnose any neurodegenerative disorder without having an idea of what a normal ageing brain looks like. The following text therefore discusses the main changes that occur as a person ages [6, 7] (Fig. 4, Table 3).

Volume changes mostly involve white matter, with relative preservation of grey matter volume. An exception to this is the volume of the caudate nucleus which slowly decreases with age. These changes cause symmetric enlargement of the ventricles, the subarachnoid and perivascular spaces with age. The cerebellum can also lose a bit of volume, especially from the posterior vermis.

White matter T2 hyperintensities (Fig. 5) (WMHs) are almost ubiquitous after the age of 65. As a rough rule of thumb, one small WMH per decade of age is acceptable and probably should not be interpreted as pathology. Also normal are thin hyperintensities lining the ventricles, especially in the area of frontal horns (frontal horn "caps") and splenium of the corpus callosum. The transition point where "age-appropriate" WMHs become a possibly significant pathology is extremely fuzzy,

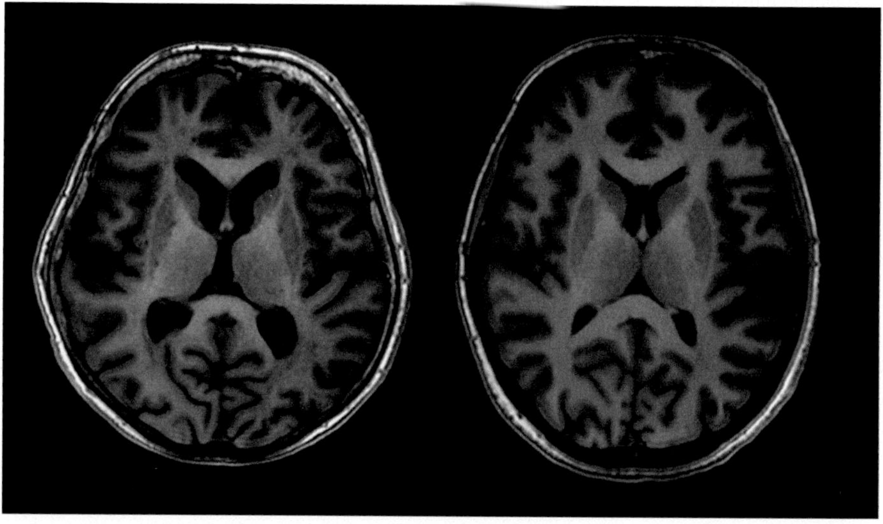

Fig. 4 Ageing brain. Brain of clinically healthy 79-year-old individual showing generalised atrophy, involving mostly gray matter with Evans' ratio 0.3. Brain of a 40-year-old patient for comparison on the right

Table 3 Normal findings in a "successfuly ageing brain"	
	Mild generalised volume loss, especially in the WM
	Small and sparce WMH, about 1 per decade of age
	Calcifications in globus pallidus
	T2 linear hypointensities in visual, sensory and motor cortices

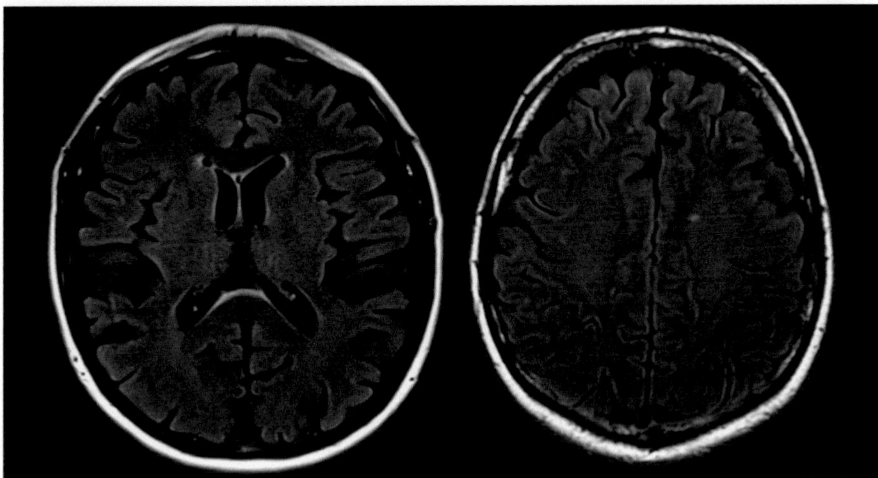

Fig. 5 White matter T2 hyperintensities. With age, linear periventricular T2/FLAIR hyperintensities can develop, which are especially notable around splenium of corpus callosum (image on the left). Image on the right shows a 62-year-old patient with few WMH in centrum semiovale. One small WMH per decade is acceptable. No more WMHs were found elsewhere, and so this finding can be considered appropriate for age

and there is large overlap between "normal" brain and brain that is possibly affected by small vessel disease, for example. In a normal brain however, WMHs will not enhance and will not show diffusion restriction on DWI. If these are present, think of a recent ischemic lesion first.

SWI/T2* hypointensities in the globus pallidus are caused by calcium deposition and are normal in patients above 40 years of age. Sometimes they can be quite striking even in otherwise healthy elderly individuals and should not be mistaken for Fahr disease [8]. They can also be nicely seen on CT as hyperdense calcium-density clusters in the globus pallidus.

On DWI, ADC values of otherwise normal appearing white matter will slowly increase with age. Also, after the age of 50, DWI signal intensity in motor, sensory or visual cortices might differ from surrounding grey matter, but this is only due to age-related iron deposition in the cortex of these areas, which influences the T2 component of DWI signal, causing it to be more hypointense then cortex elsewhere [9]. This phenomenon is sometimes referred to as **"T2 black lines"** and can be also appreciated on SWI and to a lesser extent on regular T2 FSE images. It is important not to mistake this finding for pathology, like superficial cortical siderosis (e.g. as seen in cerebral amyloid angiopathy) or amyotrophic lateral sclerosis (where damage to upper motor neurons manifests as decreasing signal on the SWI/T2* weighted sequence) (Fig. 6, Table 3).

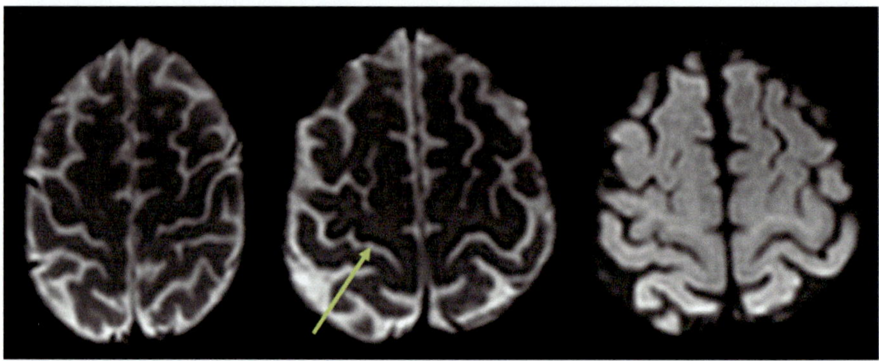

Fig. 6 "T2 black lines". B0 image taken from a DWI sequence (middle image) shows linear hypointensity along the cortex of precentral gyrus in an elderly patient (arrow). Contrast this with younger patient (on the left) in whom the "T2 black lines" are less prominent. These T2 signal changes can cause the affected cortex to appear unusually hypointense on trace DWI images (right) compared to neighbouring white matter. This is due to iron deposition and is a normal finding seen with ageing. B0 images of DWI sequences are especially susceptible to these phenomena, but it can be also seen on SWI or regular T2 FSE

7 Pathology

7.1 Alzheimer's Disease

AD is strikingly common in populations above 60–70 years old, and therefore, it is important to acknowledge this high pre-test probability even before looking at the scan and actively search for its signs in any elderly individual. Despite the imaging features of developed AD being fairly specific, these patients often come for their first scan before the diagnosis is obvious both clinically and radiologically. Therefore, the role of MRI imaging is usually to a) detect signs favouring diagnosis of AD and b) rule out other possible causes of dementia (like small vessel disease, post-ischemic changes or iNPH), with the latter arguably being more important for the further management of the patient. PET/CT, either with FDG or amyloid agents as a radiotracer, tends to show specific abnormalities earlier in the disease course.

On MRI, the hallmark finding of AD is volume loss with mesiotemporal and parietal predominance.

Mesial temporal atrophy involves most notably the hippocampi and parahippocampal gyri, with subsequent widening of surrounding CSF spaces—temporal horns of lateral ventricles, choroidal fissures and collateral sulci. These changes are striking even relatively early in the disease course and are important to look for in any elderly patient. In an attempt to diminish subjectivity in assessment, several visual scoring systems have been developed, with the **MTA score** and **ERICA score** being the most commonly used. They can be seen employed in both research and clinical settings alike and their imaging features are listed in Tables 4 and 5.

Table 4 MTA score

Assessing plane: parallel to long axis of brain stem, level of anterior pons	
MTA = 0	No or minimal amount of CSF around hippocampus
MTA = 1	Slight widening of choroid fissure
MTA = 2	Mild enlargement of temporal horn, mild loss of hipocampal volume
MTA = 3	Markedly widened temporal horn and choroid fissure, moderate hipocampal atrophy
MTA = 4	Gross loss of hippocampal volume and structure
Cut-offs	MTA ≥ 1 for patients 70 years or younger
	MTA ≥ 1.75 for patients above 70

Table 5 ERICA score

Assessing plane: parallel to long axis of brain stem, at the level of mammilary bodies	
ERICA = 0	Normal finding
ERICA = 1	Widening of collateral sulcus
ERICA = 2	Lifting of parahippocampal sulcus off of tentorium ("tentorial cleft sign")
ERICA = 3	Gross loss of volume of entorhinal cortex and parahippocampal gyrus
Cut-offs	ERICA ≥ 2

The **MTA score** was developed in the late 1990s [10] and relies on the **volume changes of the hippocampi themselves** (Fig. 7, Table 4). As hippocampi shrink, the surrounding CSF spaces (choroid fissure, temporal horns of lateral ventricles and collateral sulcus) dilate. Dilation of these spaces is then assessed on MRI and an MTA score between 0 and 4 is given for each side. Most concise studies average the results for both hippocampi and/or give transitional (i.e. 1.5) scores for a single hippocampus, and therefore, final results like 1.75 or 2.5 are often seen. Cut-off values for diagnosis of AD vary with age, and different authors propose slightly different values for different groups—with an impact on sensitivity and specificity.

One of the more practical cut-offs is the one proposed by Vanhoenacker et al. [11]. They determined that the MTA score is suggestive of AD if ≥ **1 for patients 70 years old or younger** and MTA ≥ **1.75 for patients above 70 years old**. The diagnostic accuracy of these cut-offs was 0.77 and 0.74, respectively. Of note is the high 90% sensitivity in the above 70 cohort.

Although the MTA score focuses on hippocampi themselves, there is strong evidence showing that **entorhinal atrophy precedes hippocampal atrophy** in the AD pathogenic process [12, 13], and the volume of the entorhinal cortex is relatively maintained in normal ageing. Also, increased size of ventricles with relative preservation of hippocampal volume (which can happen for example in iNPH) can bias the results of MTA scoring.

Realisation that the **entorhinal cortex is one of the first structures affected by AD** led to the development of the **ERICA score** (Fig. 8, Table 5) [14]. The ERICA score is calculated on coronal sections parallel to the long axis of the brainstem at

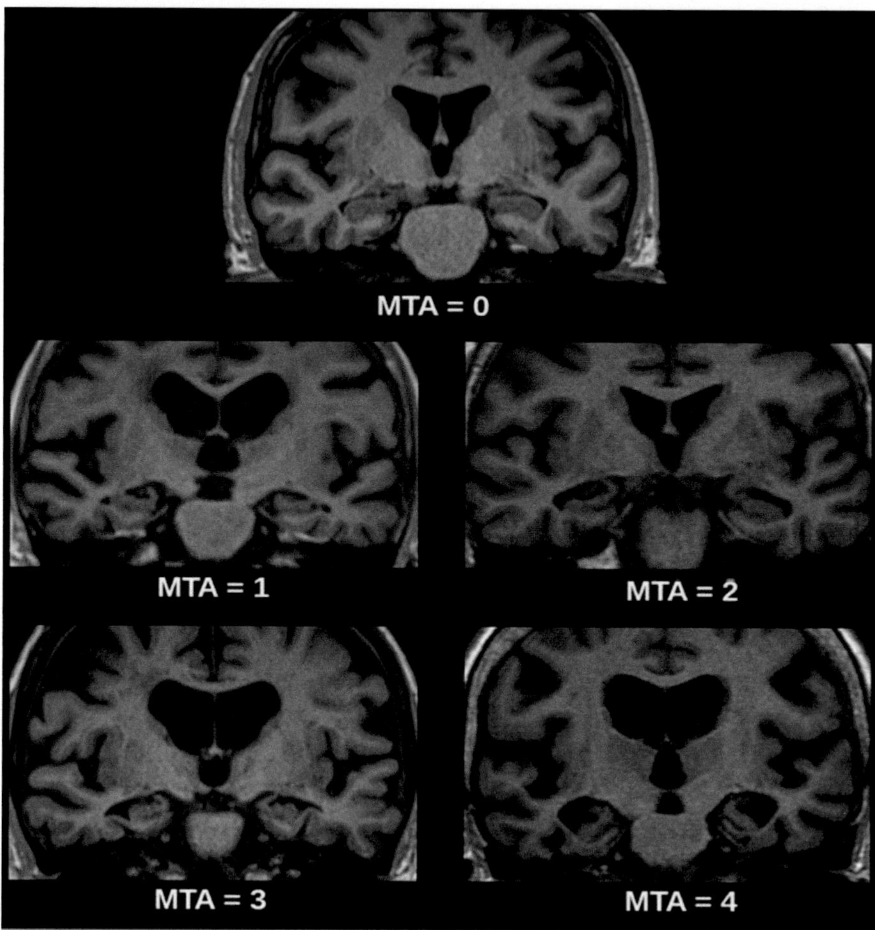

Fig. 7 MTA score. MTA = 0 is found in normal ageing and shows minimal or no CSF around the hippocampi. In MTA = 1, choroid fissures start to dilate. In MTA = 2, temporal horns of lateral ventricles distend as well. In MTA = 3, hippocampal atrophy becomes obvious. In MTA = 4, hippocampus undergoes marked atrophy and structure loss

the level of mammillary bodies, with possible values between 0 and 3. An ERICA **score of 2 or 3** was highly suggestive of AD, with sensitivity of 83%, specificity 98% and diagnostic accuracy of 91% in the initial study on 120 patients (60 AD and 60 non-AD). The diagnostic accuracy of MTA score in the same study was 74%.

The question then arises: what scoring system to use? Both are valuable as their knowledge shines some light on the volume changes happening in different stages of AD. According to some studies [15], the MTA score can be slightly more sensitive (90% sensitivity in patients above 70, when using a cut-off MTA score of 1.75), while ERICA is more specific to AD. Therefore, one would argue that in order to

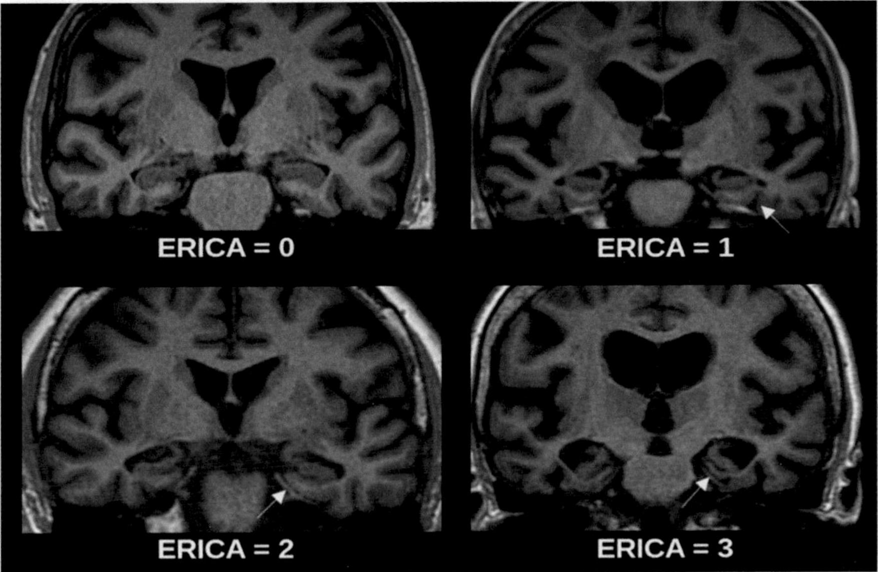

Fig. 8 Entorhinal cortical atrophy (ERICA) score. ERICA score 0 implies no entorhinal atrophy. In ERICA = 1, widening of collateral sulcus can be seen. Main finding of ERICA 2 is elevation of parahippocampal gyrus off tentorium. In ERICA 3, gross atrophy and structure loss of entorhinal cortex can be seen

rule out AD, MTA is more useful, and ERICA will perform better when confirming the diagnosis.

Another location of disproportionate atrophy is the precuneus, which can be nicely assessed in the sagittal plane. The most consistent feature of **precuneal atrophy** is widening of pars marginalis of cingulate sulcus and parieto-occipital fissure, but widening of sulci within the cuneus itself may also be present. As is the case with hippocampal and entorhinal atrophy, a visual rating scale for parietal atrophy has been developed for parietal atrophy to enhance diagnostic accuracy—the posterior atrophy score [16] (Fig. 8).

Importantly, **parietal atrophy is not a prominent feature of FTLD**, one of the main diagnostic considerations during AD workup. In FTLD, temporopolar atrophy may mimic the mesial temporal atrophy in AD, confounding the MTA and ERICA scores. However, in FTLD, parietal atrophy is not dominant, and the relatively normal volume of precuneus is in contrast to the atrophy of frontal and/or temporal lobes. This can be nicely seen on parasagittal sections (Fig. 9).

In AD, volume changes in parietal and temporal regions will be preceded by regional hypoperfusion on PWI and decreased uptake of glucose on FDG-PET. PET using amyloid or tau agents shows abnormal uptake even earlier and can help differentiate Alzhemier's patients from LATE patients. Amyloid PET might also be useful in determining patients who would benefit from amyloid-targeted therapy.

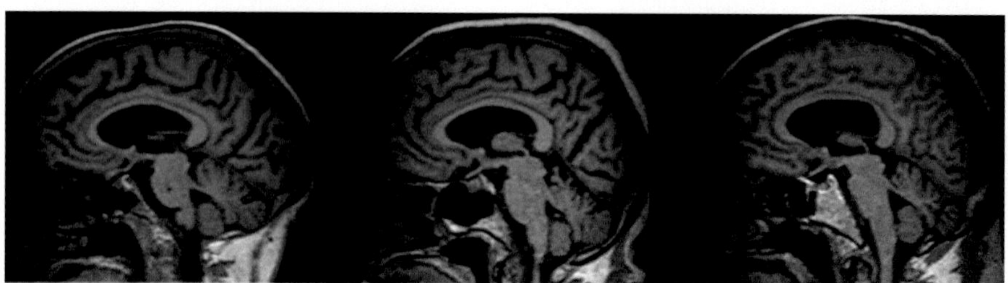

Fig. 9 FTLD vs. AD vs. iNPH: As both can present with temporal and even mesial temporal atrophy, distinguishing AD and FTLD can be challenging. Parasagittal T1 sections can be extremely useful in this setting. AD (centre image) will present with atrophy more pronounced in the parietal lobe, while the atrophy in FTLD (left) will preferentially involve the frontal lobes. For comparison, sagittal view of a patient with earlier signs of iNPH (right) is shown. In this case, instead of atrophy, the dominant feature is the crowding of sulci, most pronounced around pars marginalis of cingulate gyrus (the cingulate gyrus sign). Also note the bulging of the isthmus of corpus callosum—this is a sagittal view correlate to narrow callosal angle

7.2 Limbic-Predominant Age-Related TDP-43 Encephalopathy

LATE is a common, most likely underdiagnosed entity, with up to 25% of patients above 80 having LATE-associated neuropathological changes at autopsy [17]. It has imaging findings very similar to AD, making it **virtually impossible to distinguish** these two on conventional MR and CT scans. Making the matter worse is the fact that AD and LATE often coexist.

Most patients with LATE will therefore manifest on imaging **with temporoparietal volume loss**, especially in mesial temporal and precuneal regions, just like AD patients. Occasionally, signs favouring LATE can be seen. For instance, 1) Hippocampal T2 hyperintensity (due to non-epileptogenic sclerosis), 2) more rostrocaudal involvement of the amygdala and hippocampus (LATE tends to affect amygdalas more profoundly than AD) and 3) somewhat asymmetric involvement of mesial temporal lobes.

However, arguably the most suggestive imaging feature of LATE is negative amyloid PET, in a patient with suspected AD.

7.3 Posterior Cortical Atrophy

The most important finding that should raise suspicion of PCA is parietal and especially **precuneal atrophy** in a patient between 50 and 65 years old, in the correct clinical setting. Milder atrophy can also be seen in the occipital lobes (25% of PCA patients develop visual hallucinations) or temporal lobes. Importantly though, mesial temporal lobes initially appear normal, and atrophy will be absent or dubious at best.

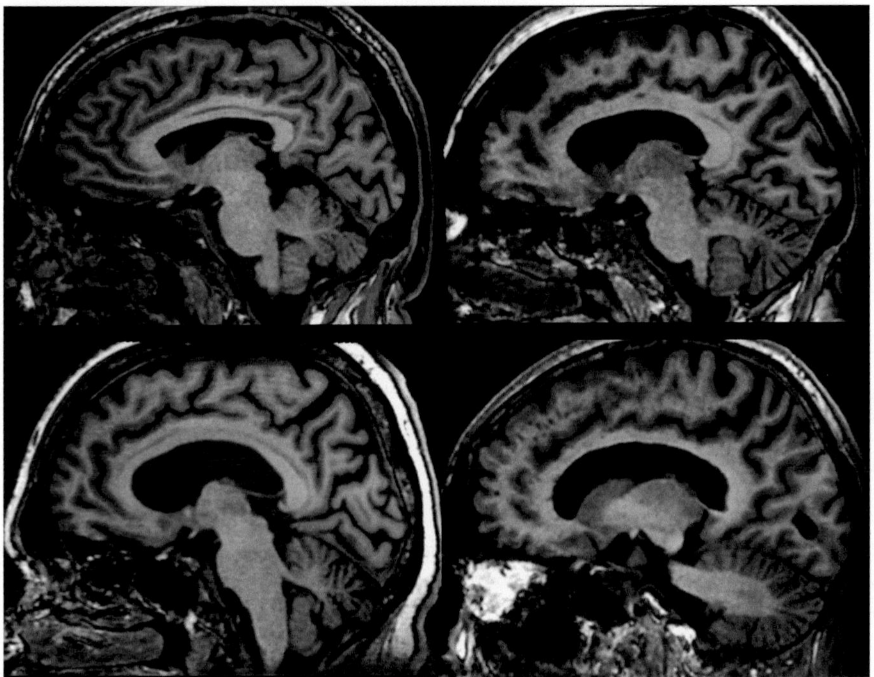

Fig. 10 Parasagittal T1 images showing progressing amounts of precuneal atrophy. On top left patient with no precuneal atrophy and thin pars marginalis of the cingulate sulcus, that is no wider than the surrounding sulci (Koedam 0). Top right image showing increased width of pars marginalis, but no obvious gyral atrophy (Koedam 1). Bottom left image shows mild gyral atrophy (Koedam 2), and image on the bottom right shows forming knife-like gyri in the precuneus (Koedam 3)

Similarly to mesiotemporal atrophy, several semiquantitative grading systems for parietal atrophy exist, the most commonly used being the **posterior cortical atrophy score** by Koedam et al. [16] (Fig. 10).

7.4 Vascular Disorders Causing Dementia

Vascular dementia encompasses all the causes of cognitive dysfunction which result from vascular brain damage. In the context of dementia of the elderly, virtually all cases of vascular dementia are acquired, usually as a result of atherosclerosis, arteriolosclerosis, thromboembolic disease or cerebral amyloid angiopathy. It is the second most common cause of dementia, and the prevalence increases sharply after 55–60 years of age. Some authors [18] classify VD based on the exact aetiology, which is helpful in terms of what imaging findings one should expect in the context of VD.

Table 6 Complications of cerebral amyloid angiopathy

Intracranial haemorrhage
– Microhaemorrhage in lobar and cerebellar distribution
– Macrohaemorrhage in the same distribution as above
– Subarachnoid haemorrhage, usually at the convexities
Cognitive impairment due to
– Ischemic leukoencephalopathy
– Microinfarcts and lacunes
– Lobar microhaemorrhages
– Subarachnoid haemorrhage (Amyloid spells)
Inflammatory complications:
– Inflammatory cerebral amyloid angiopathy
– Cerebral amyloidoma

Small vessel disease will manifest as large, confluent areas of gliosis in the cerebral white matter and basal ganglia. Some authors suggest that at least 25% of white matter should be affected by small vessel disease-related gliosis (leukoaraiosis) in order to qualify for VD [19].

Leukoaraiosis can be combined with foci of lobar haemorrhage on SWI/T2* sequences, which in a normotensive elderly patient is highly suggestive of **cerebral amyloid angiopathy**. CAA results from the deposition of amyloid protein in the walls of small- to medium-sized cortical, subcortical and leptomeningeal arteries. CAA can cause both ischemic and hemorrhagic complications, which are shown in Table 6. Importantly, all of these manifestations will have predilection for the more superficial regions (lobar, cortico-subcortical, and in case of SAH even the brain surface) as these are preferential areas of amyloid deposition.

The main imaging feature of CAA is the presence of the above-**mentioned SWI/ T2* blooming hypointensities** (Fig. 11) in the periphery of cerebrum and cerebellum, which is in contrast to hypertensive encephalopathy, whose microhemorrhages are distributed mostly in the basal ganglia, brainstem and sometimes in the cerebellum also. In addition, CAA can present with **superficial cortical siderosis** (Fig. 11)—deposits of hemosiderin along the brain surface due to recurrent subarachnoid haemorrhage. In rarer cases, these signs can be accompanied by subcortical white matter vasogenic edema, which in a patient with established or suspected CAA is suggestive of *Inflammatory cerebral amyloid angiopathy*. Importantly, CAA often coexists with AD.

Post-stroke dementia will manifest as regions of encephalomalacia and/or gliosis with size and location corresponding with the features of the patient's dementia. In these cases, it is essential to consult DWI and ADC maps to rule out possible recent ischemia. Also, in case of multiple smaller infarctions in multiple vascular territories, consider the possibility of recent embolic shower, as this might have a major impact on further management.

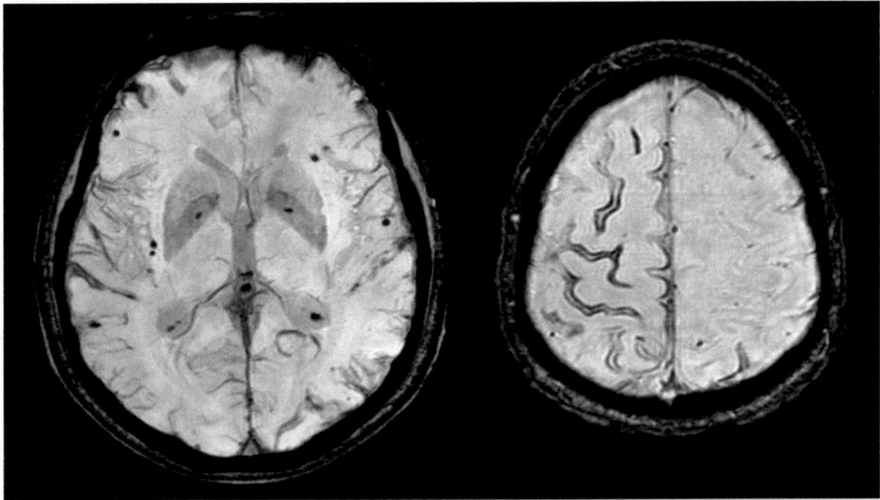

Fig. 11 Cerebral amyloid angiopathy on SWI. SWI showing peripheral blooming hypointensities (on the left) and superficial cortical siderosis (on the right). In normotensive elderly patient, these findings are highly suggestive of CAA

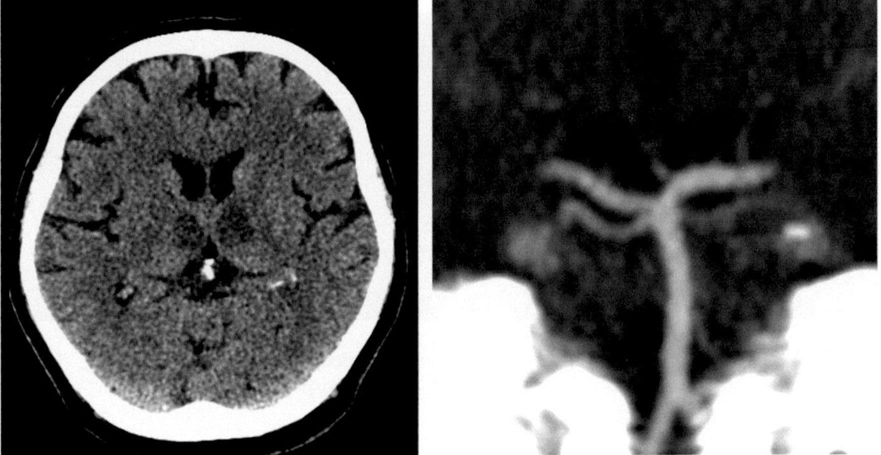

Fig. 12 Artery of percheron territory infarct. Image on the left showing symmetrical subacute infarctions in ventromedial thalami. CT angiogram (right) shows a stub of percheron artery arising from the P1 segment of the left posterior cerebral artery. Patient presented with confusion and dizziness, subsequent neurological evaluations uncovered a combination of anterograde and retrograde amnesia. Imaging and clinical findings classic for the infarction of the artery of percheron

Combination of small ischemic regions on DWI/ADC and foci of haemorrhage on SWI/T2* indicates the possibility of **vasculitis** (both primary CNS or systemic) or **disseminated intravascular coagulopathy,** which can take a more chronic course with possible acute exacerbation. Imaging of vasculitis is especially of note, since at the time of writing this book, excellent results are being reported when employing **vessel wall imaging** sequences in diagnosing vasculitis and other vascular disorders of the CNS [20].

Thalamic dementia is usually a result of bilateral thalamic disorders, i.e. due to small vessel disease, stroke (either sequential or as an occlusion of artery of Percheron) [21] or metabolic disorders (Wernicke-Korsakoff, osmotic demyelination syndrome). Beware that FLAIR sequences are relatively insensitive to glial changes in the posterior fossa and thalamus, and these structures should be always thoroughly interrogated on T2WI as well, and otherwise up to 50% lesions might be missed, according to some studies [22] (Fig. 13).

Vascular dementias can also occur in the younger populations (i.e. < 50), and in such cases, inherited causes like CADASIL, CARASIL, Fabry disease and others should be considered.

Glial changes can be semiquantitatively rated using Fazekas score (Table 7) [23], which rates separately periventricular and deep white matter (Fig. 13, Table 7).

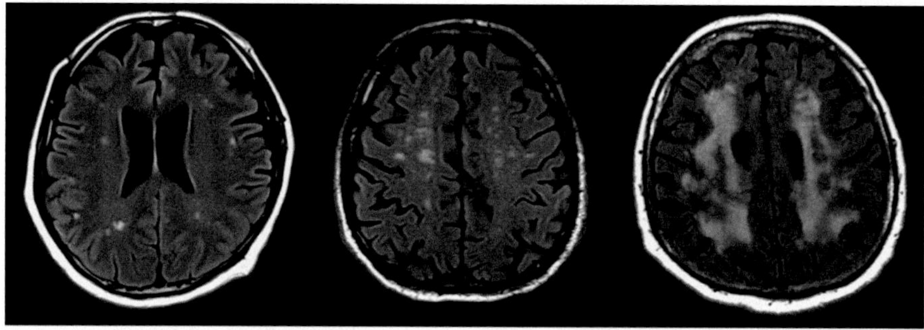

Fig. 13 White matter hyperintensities. Glial changes of deep white matter of varying degrees. These could be rated (from left to right) Fazekas 1, 2 and 3, respectively

Table 7 Fazekas score

Grade	Periventricular WM	Deep WM
0	Absent	Absent
1	Frontal horn caps, pencil-thin lining	Punctate foci
2	Smooth halo	Beginning confluence
3	Irregular signal extending to deep WM	Large confluent WMH areas

Table 8 Causes of vascular dementia and their main imaging features

Small vessel disease	Confluent WMH in deep WM and periventricular distribution
CAA	SWI/T2* blooming lesions in lobar distribution
Post-stroke dementia	Malacia and gliosis in the area of former stroke
Chronic DIC	Diffuse foci of bleeding and ischemia
Vasculitis	Diffuse foci of bleeding and ischemia, vessel wall thickening
Thalamic dementia	Bilateral thalamic gliosis and/or malacia

7.5 Parkinson Disease and Lewy Body Dementia

A challenging diagnosis to make on conventional MRI, to say the least, the main role of MRI in the diagnosis of PD and LBD is to rule out other possible causes of parkinsonian clinical presentation, i.e. PSP, CBD or MSA. Although rare, these are seen in regular clinical practice and often have fairly specific imaging features.

Imaging features of PD, LBD and its variants are often fairly unremarkable, showing only mild generalised atrophy, which may be more noticeable in frontotemporal regions; however, mesial temporal lobes will be spared of major atrophy unlike in AD. Currently a promising imaging sign is under investigation—the "absent swallow tail sign" (Fig. 14) on SWI images. Some preliminary studies show up to 90% diagnostic accuracy for PD and LBD [24], but certain other studies failed to reproduce the results, struggling to find any meaningful association between the sign and PD or LBD [25, 26]. Further investigation is therefore needed before this sign enters regular clinical practice, and even then, it will be most likely confined only to 7 T and some 3 T MR systems. An alternative to this approach might be quantitative susceptibility mapping [27].

PWI can be also helpful, showing frontotemporal, and especially occipital hypoperfusion, which can be easily remembered due to the notorious association of LBD with visual hallucinations. The above-mentioned perfusion changes form the so-called cingulate island sign, where relatively normal perfusion values of the posterior cingulate on sagittal reconstructions contrast with hypoperfusion of occipital and frontal lobes.

However, the most established imaging method for evaluating Parkinson's disease is the nuclear medicine dopamine transporter (DaT) scan, which shows dramatically decreased uptake in the striatum (Fig. 14).

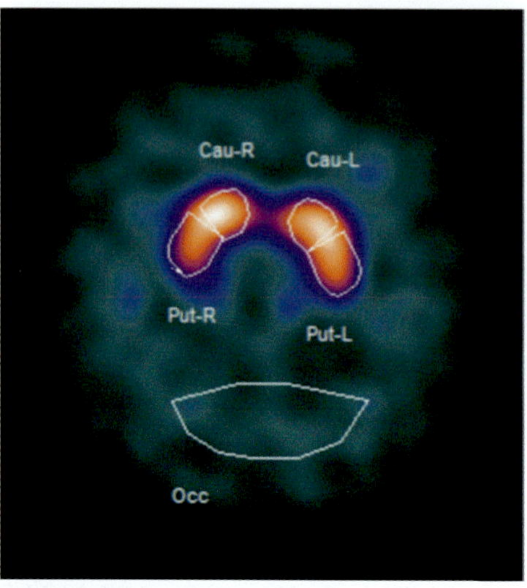

Fig. 14 Normal DaT scan. DaT scan showing normal uptake in striatum. This comma-shaped pattern is lost in patients with Parkinson's disease and instead is replaced by period-shaped uptake

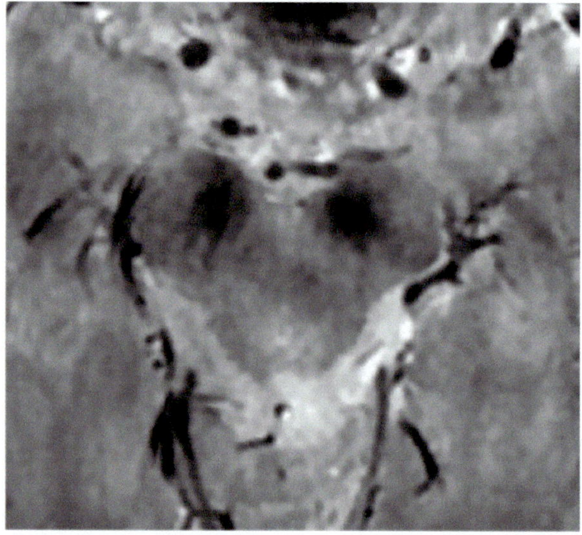

Fig. 15 Swallow tail sign. In a healthy individual on SWI images, the posterior third of otherwise hypointense substantia nigra is split into two, reminiscing the tail of a swallow. In PD, the hyperintense part of the posterior third of substantia nigra (which houses nigrosome-1) will undergo iron deposition and will turn isointense with the rest of the substantia nigra, effectively losing the appearance of the swallow's tail. In this image of a healthy individual, you can see normal swallow tail appearance of substantia nigra, especially on the right. Asymmetricity of findings is common and can possibly be one of the reasons behind the bad reproducibility of studies investigating swallow tail sign

7.6 *Frontotemporal Lobar Degeneration*

Frontotemporal dementia is the most common cause of early onset (<65 years) dementia, with several distinct gene mutations associated with individual clinical subtypes. The more specific findings of individual FTLD subtypes are noted in Table 9.

The key to imaging diagnosis of FTLD is in the name—expect **atrophy in frontal and/or temporal lobes**, symmetric or asymmetric based on the subtype. In some less common subtypes, parietal, fronto-opercular, caudate or even generalised atrophy may occur as well. Expect T2/FLAIR hyperintensity in the areas of severe volume loss as a sign of gliosis [28].

Unlike in AD, the **parietal lobe will usually be relatively spared** of atrophy, which is a helpful clue to differentiate these two entities (Figs. 16 or 9).

Nuclear medicine may be helpful in distinguishing FTLD from other causes of dementia. FDG-PET and HMPAO-SPECT will show hypometabolism and hypoperfusion, respectively, before the involved areas will undergo eventual atrophy. Amyloid PET will assess the possibility of AD.

FTLD is also associated with other neurodegenerative disorders, most importantly **PSP, CBD** and **ALS**. These can occur in the same individual suffering from FTLD or can be an important clue in a family history. Checking for specific imaging findings of these disorders is a must in any patient with suspected FTLD. The main findings of **ALS** are T2 hyperintensity along the corticospinal tracts (better seen on FLAIR), and hypointensity of the precentral gyri on SWI maybe even T2* sequences. PSP and CBD are discussed separately in this text later on.

Table 9 Patterns of atrophy in frontotemporal lobar degeneration

Behavioural variant FTLD	Bilateral frontal lobes
Semantic variant of PPA	Left temporal lobe
Non-fluent variant of PPA	Left frontal operculum and insula
Logopenic variant of PPA	Left temporal lobe, parietal lobe
FTLD-FUS	Bilateral caudate nuclei
FTLD-TDP due to GRN mutation	Right frontal, temporal and parietal lobes
FTLD-TDP due to C9orf72 mutation	Generalised atrophy, possibly sparing occipital lobes
FTLD-tau due to MAPT mutation	Bilateral temporal lobes

Adapted from [28]

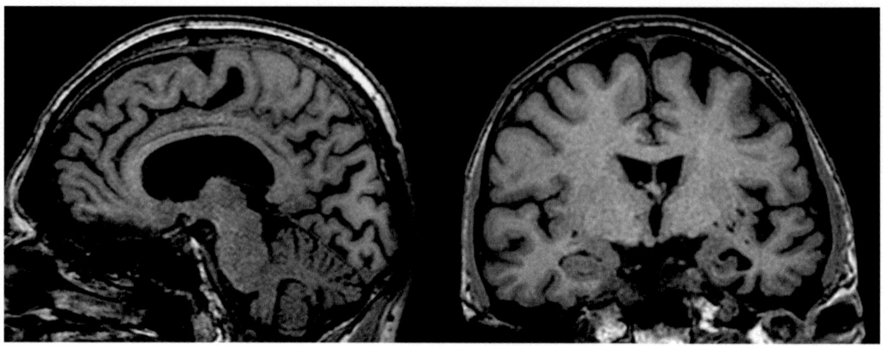

Fig. 16 FTLD. T1w image on the left showing frontal atrophy contrasting with relative preservation of volume in precuneus and around pars marginalis gyrus cinguli. Findings suggestive of behavioural variant of FTLD. On the right a coronal T1w image of a patient with semantic variant of primary progressive aphasia, showing striking asymmetric atrophy of the left temporal lobe

7.7 Progressive Supranuclear Palsy

Diagnosing patients with PSP can be challenging, and therefore, the patients will often go on to develop classical MRI findings before the diagnosis of PSP is made. In the literature, there are many (subjective) signs, the most notorious being the **hummingbird sign**. Contrary to the popular belief, it does not refer to brain stem taking on the shape of the hummingbird on sagittal sections (as with a little bit of fantasy every brainstem looks so), but instead it refers to the concavity of the upper aspect of the midbrain, which should usually be flat or convex [29]. This concavity ("forehead" of the hummingbird) is a sign of advanced midbrain atrophy, which is a hallmark finding in PSP. Still, calling a hummingbird sign should be done with great care as it is a subjective marker, and its presence should mainly raise a suspicion for midbrain atrophy and prompt a search for some other signs of neurodegenerative disease.

There are two major indexes that can be used when diagnosing PSP on imaging. The first and arguably more useful is the **midbrain-to-pons area ratio** [30, 31], which can be easily measured on the majority of PACS viewers and all workstations, simply by drawing out the outlines of pons and midbrain and dividing the areas of the former with the later. Normal values are around 0.25, with values around and **under 0.12** strongly suggestive of PSP in the correct clinical setting. Also important to note is that midbrain atrophy can be the result of other pathologies (i.e. cerebral peduncle atrophy due ischemic stroke in the motor areas) and many patients with iNPH have midbrain-to-pons area ratio between 0.15 and 0.20 (Fig. 17).

Another, more recent (and more complicated) approach is the MRI parkinsonism index (comes in 2 iterations, the more recent was introduced in 2018), which claims to improve diagnostic accuracy in distinguishing PSP patients from PD patients and healthy controls (accuracy of 99.5% and 100%, respectively) [32] (Fig. 17).

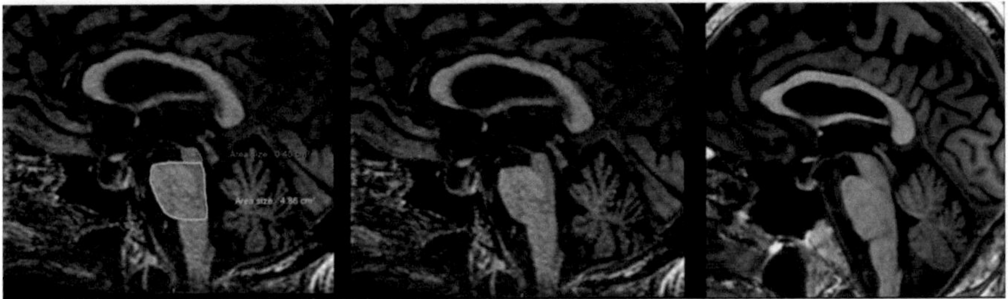

Fig. 17 Midbrain-to-pons area ratio. Patient with profound atrophy of mesencephalon (middle). Measurement method of midbrain and pons area is shown on the left—contours of midbrain and pons are delineated using freehand ROI tool—majority of modern PACS viewers should then be able to calculate the area of the drawn ROI. Normal appearing mesencephalon for comparison on the right

7.8 Multiple System Atrophy

According to the 2008 consensus paper [33], MSA is divided into two major subtypes: MSA-C with predominance of cerebellar symptoms and MSA-P with predominance of parkinsonian symptoms. Being familiar with this division is useful, as the pathology on imaging is in the expected locations for the respective variant.

MSA-C will present with **T2 hyperintensities in middle cerebellar peduncles** and in pons, where the hyperintensities form the so-called **hot cross bun sign**. However, keep in mind that the hot cross bun sign refers exclusively to T2 hyperintense cross on the background of darker pons, as with a little bit of fantasy the inverse (dark cross on less dark pons) can be seen even in normal individuals.

MSA-P signs are usually more subtle, usually consisting of T2 hyperintensities on the putamen/external capsule interface (suggestive of diagnosis on 1.5 T, but possibly a normal finding on 3 T) or T2* hypointensity of the putamen itself (due to high iron deposition) [34].

A DaT scan may be helpful in ruling out PD (Fig. 18).

7.9 Corticobasal Degeneration

The hallmark of CBD is **asymmetric cortical atrophy**, more severe on the side contralateral to the clinical symptoms. The most affected location tends to be the **superior parietal lobule,** and the atrophy then wanes with distance from this location (Fig. 19). This pattern of atrophy will usually be accompanied by T2/FLAIR hyperintensity of the affected gyri, secondary expansion of the adjacent lateral ventricle and atrophy of corpus callosum, especially its body. Involvement of basal ganglia manifests as atrophy, T2 hyperintensity or both [35].

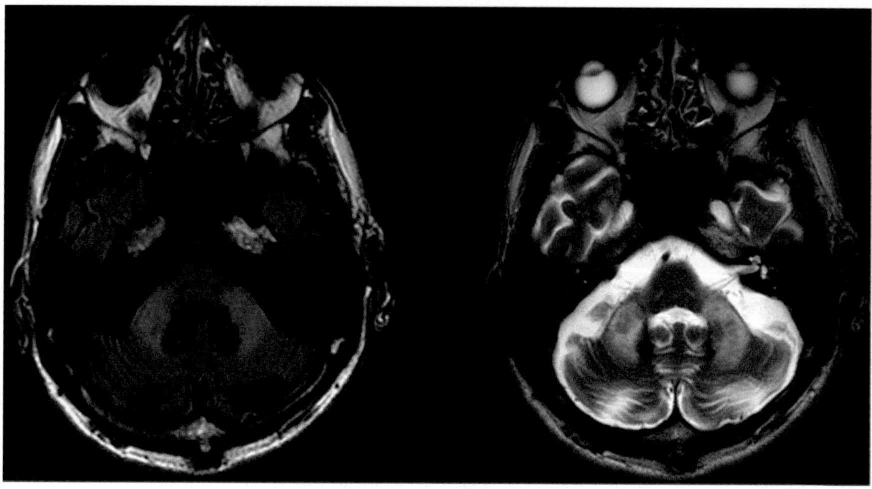

Fig. 18 T2 hyperintensity in MCP, consistent with the diagnosis of MSA-C

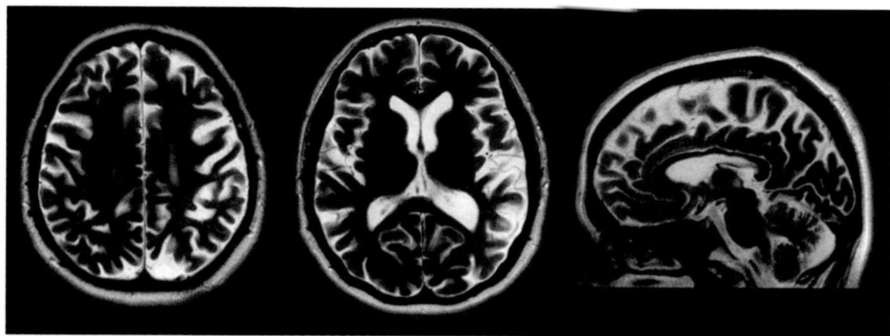

Fig. 19 Corticobasal degeneration. Asymmetric parietal atrophy, which less severely also involves surrounding areas of frontal and temporal lobes. Atrophy of corpus callosum can also be appreciated on sagittal T2 (on the right)

7.10 Autoimmune Encephalitis

AIE, also known by its former name as limbic encephalitis, consists of two major entities with regards to its aetiology, epidemiology and prognosis—paraneoplastic and non-neoplastic AIE.

Paraneoplastic AIE (Fig. 20) is a complication of an underlying tumour, and therefore, its epidemiology and age of onset will correlate with those of the causative tumour. The more common tumours causing AIE include small cell lung cancer, lymphomas or ovarian tumours. In these cases, neurological symptoms precede tumour detection on average by 6–12 months [36]. Therefore, suspected AIE should

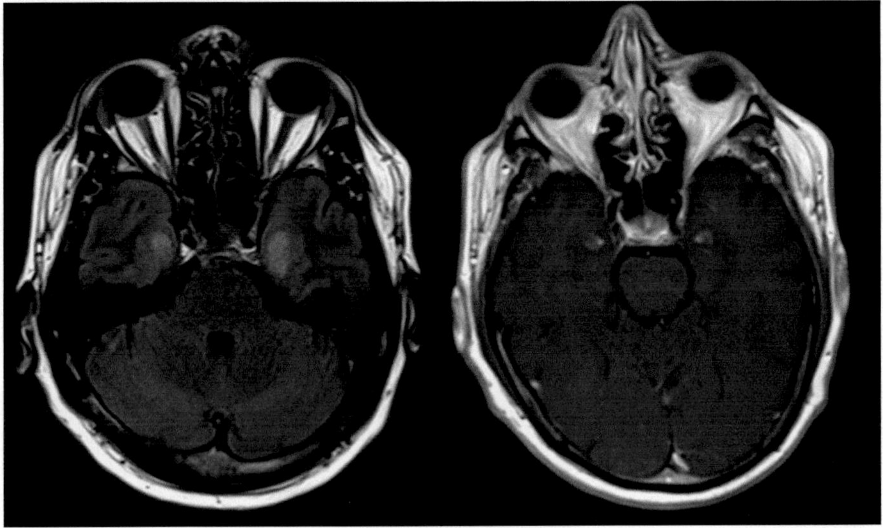

Fig. 20 Autoimmune encephalitis. T2/FLAIR hyperintensity in medial temporal lobes, accompanied by patchy enhancement post-gadolinium. These findings are suggestive of AIE and should prompt search for possible underlying malignancy

prompt immediate oncological screening, since tumour removal can stop or even reverse the disease progression.

Non-neoplastic limbic encephalitis is usually seen in younger female patients, often in the context of other autoimmune disorders.

Imaging features of AIE are varied, and 40% of patients may have normal imaging findings [37]. In the case of positive MRI findings, the most common include **T2/ FLAIR hyperintensities in mesial temporal lobe, thalamus and insula. Patchy enhancement** of involved areas can be seen. In case of diffusion restriction or signs of haemorrhage of the involved areas, think of HSV encephalitis instead, but the disease course is usually vastly different.

AIE can be accompanied by **autoimmune myelopathy** as well, which presents with **longitudinally extensive, tract-specific, and symmetric T2 hyperintensites** in the spinal cord (Fig. 21). AI myelopathy can occur also on its own, without AIE [38].

7.11   HIV Encephalopathy

HIV encephalopathy is a term used for a spectrum of imaging findings of HIV-associated dementias [39]. The main imaging findings are diffuse, asymmetric cerebral atrophy, out of proportion considering the age of the patient, and symmetric, confluent periventricular T2/FLAIR hyperintensities of the white matter. In the

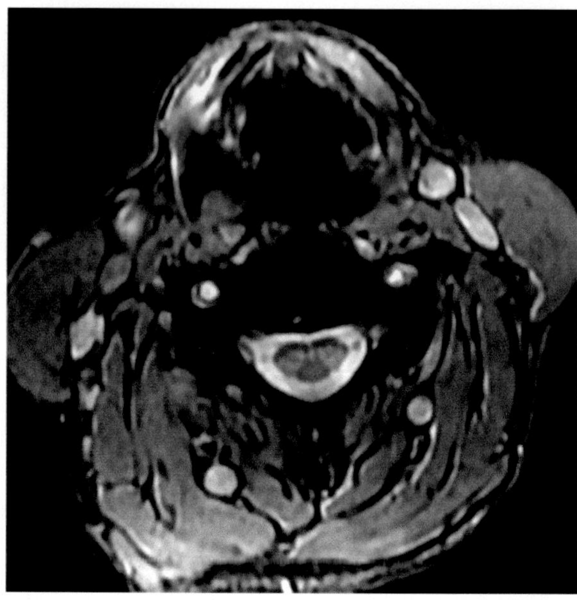

Fig. 21 Paraneoplastic myelitis. T2* section at the level of cervical spine shows symmetric T2 hyperintensity contained to lateral collumns—corticospinal tracts. These changes were present along the whole length of the imaged segment. Longitudinally extensive, tract-specific myelopathy is highly suspicious for paraneoplastic myelitis

setting of progressive disease, both clinically and radiologically, consider the possibility of progressive multifocal leukoencephalopathy or immune reconstitution inflammatory syndrome.

7.12   Creutzfeld-Jakob Disease

CJD is a rapidly progressive neurodegenerative disorder, with life expectancy less than a year after the symptom onset. There are several types with possibly different imaging findings [40]. The most common MR findings include DWI hyperintensity of the cortex, striatum and thalamus, where the famous hockey stick sign can be seen. Of note is the fact that ADC values vary based on the disease stage and that the perceived DWI hyperintensity is a combination of T2 and ADC abnormalities in the image.

7.13   Other Less Common Causes of Cognitive Decline

What follows is the "notable mentions" section where we will briefly discuss entities which might present with dementia symptoms, but will usually be off the table in differential diagnosis by the time the possibility of iNPH is raised—either because of the disease course, patients age or known comorbidities. However, they might still be worth considering especially when a patient's precise medical history is unknown.

Chronic Subdural hematomas usually present in the setting of trauma, however, up to 15% of patients (especially elderly) will have no definite history of a traumatic event. Majority of patients will have altered mental state, and in up to 50% of cases, pupillary abnormalities might be seen [41]. Diagnosis is usually made on CT, which nicely depicts crescentic extra-axial fluid collection, with densities correlating with age of the bleeding. Signs of acute-on-chronic SDH include hyperdense gravity-dependent sediment in otherwise hypodense SDH or septated SDH with areas of acute, hyperdense blood. Watch out for swirly appearance of the SDH contents of various densities, which is concerning of hyperacute bleed.

Brain tumours can have varying presentations from focal signs to neuropsychiatric symptoms or seizures. The most common brain tumours include meningiomas, gliomas and metastases.

Post-radiation necrosis is seen in the context of radiotherapy due to intracranial tumours and can present months, years or even decades after the cessation of radiotherapy. Imaging is variable based on the stage of the process and may include large confluent white matter T2/FLAIR hyperintensities due to leukoencephalopathy or vasogenic edema, areas of blooming on T2*/SWI due to microangiopathy of radiation-induced vascular malformations or even tumoriform enhancement on post-gadolinium T1WI.

Abscesses will manifest as single (69% of patients) or multiple lesions, usually in a supratentorial location (90%). The main imaging findings include peripheral enhancement, usually smoother than in case of necrotic tumours, low ADC values of liquefied centre and dual rim sign (Fig. 22). Beware that only 12% of patients have the classic clinical triad (fever, headache and focal neurologic signs) and normal white blood cell count can be found in up to one third of patients [42].

Demyelinating disorders will usually present in a younger population than iNPH, but occasionally can be seen in the elderly as well. Somewhere between 3 and 12% of MS patients are diagnosed after the age of 50 [43] but only less than 1% are

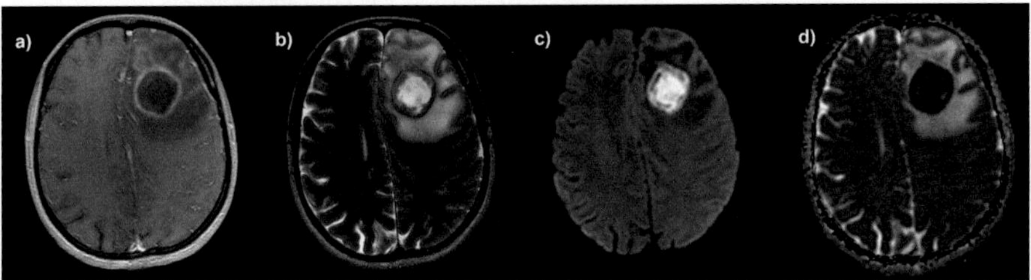

Fig. 22 Cerebral abscess. Centrally necrotic lesion with ring enhancement on post-contrast T1w (a) dual ring sign on T2w (b) and with diffusion restriction on DWI/ADC [1, 2]

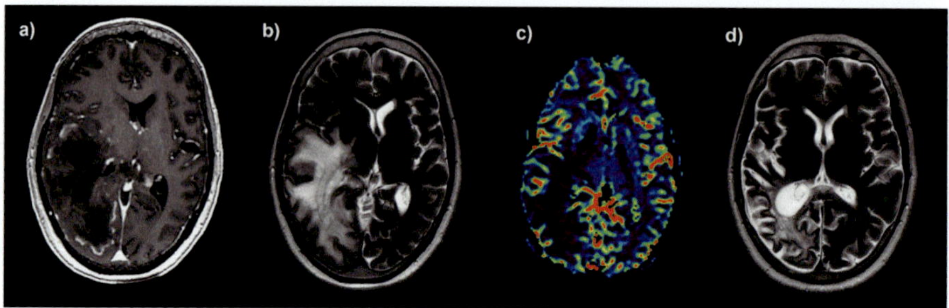

Fig. 23 Tumefactive demyelinating lesion. A 57-year-old female patient presenting with decreased psychomotor speed and hemineglect. Initial MR (a–c) shows T2 hyperintense lesion located mostly in parietal and occipital lobes, with discontinuous peripheral enhancement and decreased rCBV on PWI. On a follow up scan 7 months later, atrophy and gliosis is evident in the former distribution of TDL

diagnosed after the age of 60 [44]. Acute disseminated encephalimyelitis can also occur after the age of 65 [45].

Caudate atrophy is a hallmark of **Huntington's disease**, but recognising this feature is not easy using plain visual assessment alone. Morphometry might be of help, but if your institution lacks the appropriate software built-in into your PACS, there are two proposed measurements that can make the diagnosis of caudate atrophy less subjective (Table 10). However, when applying these measurements, two things are important to keep in mind. First is the fact that caudate atrophy is not specific to Huntington's disease [46]. And second, perhaps more important, is the fact that studies establishing these measurements have been done on populations significantly younger than what is usual with other neurodegenerative populations [47] and since ventricles enlarge with age due to parenchymal volume loss, caudate heads move farther apart, and these volume changes might confound these measurements (for more information see section on normal ageing brain).

Table 10 Measurements used in diagnosis of Huntington's disease

	FH/CC ratio	CC/IT ratio
Measurement plane	Axial plane parallel to AC-PC line, level of caudate heads	
Normal values	2.2–2.6	0.09–0.12
Suggestive of HD	< 1.8	> 0.16

FH/CC ratio Frontal horn width to intercaudate distance ratio. *CC/IT* Intercaudate distance to inner table ratio

8 Key Points

- Early in the disease course, the imaging features of many neurodegenerative disorders are subtle. To detect and correctly interpret those, a dedicated, standardised protocol is necessary.
- Structured MRI reading and reporting is recommended to increase the reliability in detecting soft signs of neurodegenerative disorders. Active search for individual signs is needed.
- Familiarity with normal age-related changes of the brain is important.
- Useful scoring systems exist, especially for mesiotemporal and parietal atrophy, with established correlations with the appropriate pathological entities.

The most common neurodegenerative disorders include Alzheimer's disease, vascular dementia, frontotemporal lobar degeneration, Lewy body dementia and iNPH. Deeper knowledge of morphological changes occurring in these disorders is the most high-yield.

Acknowledgements This chapter was supported by the Ministry of Health of the Czech Republic institutional grant no. NU23-04-00551.

References

1. Casey S. "T2 washout": an explanation for normal diffusion-weighted images despite abnormal apparent diffusion coefficient maps. AJNR Am J Neuroradiol. 2001;22(8):1450–1.
2. Azad R, Mittal P, Malhotra A, Gangrade S. Detection and differentiation of focal intracranial calcifications and chronic microbleeds using MRI. J Clin Diagnostic Research: JCDR, 2017;11(5);TC19–TC23. https://doi.org/10.7860/JCDR/2017/24076.9846
3. Bradley WG. CSF Flow in the brain in the context of normal pressure hydrocephalus. Am J Neuroradiol. 2015;36(5):831–838 (online). Available at: http://www.ajnr.org/content/36/5/831. Accessed 12 July 2020.
4. Ucar M, Guryildirim M, Tokgoz N, Kilic K, Borcek A, Oner Y, Akkan K, Tali T. Evaluation of aqueductal patency in patients with hydrocephalus: three-dimensional high-sampling-efficiency technique (SPACE) versus two-dimensional turbo spin echo at 3 Tesla. Korean J Radiol Official J Korean Radiol Soc. 2014;15(6):827–35. https://doi.org/10.3348/kjr.2014.15.6.827.
5. Musiek ES, Chen Y, Korczykowski M, Saboury B, Martinez PM, Reddin JS, Alavi A, Kimberg DY, Wolk DA, Julin P, Newberg AB, Arnold SE, Detre JA. Direct comparison of FDG-PET and ASL-MRI in Alzheimer's Disease. Alzheimer's Dementia: J Alzheimer's Assoc. 2012;8(1):51–59 (online). Available at: https://www.ncbi.nlm.nih.gov/pmc/articles/PMC3264701/.
6. Mora F. Successful brain aging: plasticity, environmental enrichment, and lifestyle. Dialogues Clin Neurosci. 2013;15(1):45–52 (online). Available at: https://www.ncbi.nlm.nih.gov/pmc/articles/PMC3622468/.
7. Osborn AG, Salzman KL, Jhaveri MD. Diagnostic imaging. Brain. Salt Lake City, Utah: Amirsys; Philadelphia, Pa. 2016.
8. Mufaddel AA, Al-Hassani GA. Familial idiopathic basal ganglia calcification (Fahr's disease). Neurosciences (Riyadh, Saudi Arabia). 2014;19(3):171–7.

9. Korogi Y, Hirai T, Komohara Y, Okuda T, Ikushima I, Kitajima M, Shigematu Y, Sugahara T, Takahashi M, T2 Shortening in the visual cortex: effect of aging and cerebrovascular disease. n.d. (online). Available at: https://www.ncbi.nlm.nih.gov/pmc/articles/PMC8338507/pdf/9127035.pdf. Accessed 12 Apr 2022.

10. Wahlund L-O, Julin P, Lindqvist J, Scheltens P. Visual assessment of medial temporal lobe atrophy in demented and healthy control subjects: correlation with volumetry. Psychiatry Res Neuroimaging. 1999;90(3):193–9.

11. Vanhoenacker A-S, Sneyers B, De Keyzer F, Heye S, Demaerel P. Evaluation and clinical correlation of practical cut-offs for visual rating scales of atrophy: normal aging versus mild cognitive impairment and Alzheimer's disease. Acta Neurologica Belgica 2017;117(3):661–669.

12. Braak H, Braak E. Neuropathological stageing of Alzheimer-related changes. Acta Neuropathologica. 1991;82(4):239–59.

13. Du AT, Schuff N, Kramer JH, Ganzer S, Zhu XP, Jagust WJ, Miller BL, Reed BR, Mungas D, Yaffe K, Chui HC, Weiner MW. Higher atrophy rate of entorhinal cortex than hippocampus in AD. Neurology. 2004;62(3):422–427.

14. Enkirch SJ, Traschütz A, Müller A, Widmann CN, Gielen GH, Heneka MT, Jurcoane A, Schild HH, Hattingen E. The Erica score: an MR imaging–based visual scoring system for the assessment of entorhinal cortex atrophy in Alzheimer disease. Radiology. 2018;288(1):226–333.

15. Vanhoenacker A-S, Sneyers B, De Keyzer F, Heye S, Demaerel P. Evaluation and clinical correlation of practical cut-offs for visual rating scales of atrophy: normal aging versus mild cognitive impairment and Alzheimer's disease. Acta Neurologica Belgica. 2017;117(3).661–669.

16. Koedam ELGE, Lehmann M, van der Flier WM, Scheltens P, Pijnenburg YAL, Fox N, Barkhof F, Wattjes MP. Visual assessment of posterior atrophy development of a MRI rating scale. Eur Radiol. 2011;21(12):2618–2625.

17. Nelson PT, Dickson DW, Trojanowski JQ, Jack CR, Boyle PA, Arfanakis K, Rademakers R, Alafuzoff I, Attems J, Brayne C, Coyle-Gilchrist ITS, Chui HC, Fardo DW, Flanagan ME, Halliday G, Hokkanen SRK, Hunter S, Jicha GA, Katsumata Y, Kawas CH. Limbic-predominant age-related TDP-43 encephalopathy (LATE): consensus working group report. Brain. 2019;142(6):1503–27.

18. Iemolo F, Duro G, Rizzo C, Castiglia L, Hachinski V, Caruso C. Pathophysiology of vascular dementia. Immun Ageing 2009;6(1) online. Available at: https://immunityageing.biomedcentral.com/articles/10.1186/1742-4933-6-13.

19. Prins ND, Scheltens P. White matter hyperintensities, cognitive impairment and dementia: an update. Nat Rev Neurol. 2015;11(3):157–165.

20. Ferlini L, Ligot N, Rana A, Jodaitis L, Sadeghi N, Destrebecq V, Naeije G. Sensitivity and specificity of vessel wall MRI sequences to diagnose central nervous system angiitis. Front Stroke 2022;1.https://doi.org/10.3389/fstro.2022.973517

21. Porta-Etessam J, Martínez-Salio A, Berbel A, Benito-León J, García-Muñoz A, Kesler P, Mateo S. Thalamic dementia due to infarct of the left thalamus and genum of the right internal capsule. Revista De Neurologia. 2001;33(11):1043–1046 (online). Available at: https://pubmed.ncbi.nlm.nih.gov/11785031/. Accessed 12 Apr 2022.

22. Bastos Leite AJ, van Straaten ECW, Scheltens P, Lycklama G, Barkhof F. Thalamic lesions in vascular dementia. Stroke. 2004;35(2):415–9.

23. Fazekas F, Chawluk JB, Alavi A, Hurtig HI, Zimmerman RA. MR signal abnormalities at 1.5 T in Alzheimer's dementia and normal aging. AJR A J Roentgenol. 1987;149(2):351–356. https://doi.org/10.2214/ajr.149.2.351.

24. Schwarz ST, Afzal M, Morgan PS, Bajaj N, Gowland PA, Auer DP. The 'Swallow Tail' appearance of the healthy Nigrosome—a new accurate test of Parkinson's disease: a case-control and retrospective cross-sectional MRI study at 3T. PLoS ONE. 2014;9(4):e93814.

25. Kim DS, Tung GA, Akbar U, Friedman JH. The evaluation of the swallow tail sign in patients with parkinsonism and gait disorders. J Neurol Sci. 2021;428:117581 (online). Available at: https://pubmed.ncbi.nlm.nih.gov/34333378/. Accessed 12 Apr 2022.

26. Prasuhn J, Neumann A, Strautz R, Dreischmeier S, Lemmer F, Hanssen H, Heldmann M, Schramm P, Brüggemann N. Clinical MR imaging in Parkinson's disease: how useful is the swallow tail sign? Brain Behavior. 2021;11(7).

27. Langkammer C, Pirpamer L, Seiler S, Deistung A, Schweser F, Franthal S, Homayoon N, Katschnig-Winter P, Koegl-Wallner M, Pendl T, Stoegerer EM, Wenzel K, Fazekas F, Ropele S, Reichenbach JR, Schmidt R, Schwingenschuh P. Quantitative susceptibility mapping in Parkinson's disease. PLOS ONE. 2016;11(9):e0162460.

28. Meeter LH, Kaat LD, Rohrer JD, van Swieten JC. Imaging and fluid biomarkers in frontotemporal dementia. Nat Rev Neurol. 2017;13(7):406–19.

29. Pandey S. Hummingbird sign in progressive supranuclear palsy disease. J Res Med Sci The Official J Isfahan Univ Med Sci. 2012;17(2):197–8.

30. Cui S-S, Ling H-W, Du J-J, Lin Y-Q, Pan J, Zhou H-Y, Wang G, Wang Y, Xiao Q, Liu J, Tan Y-Y, Chen S-D. Midbrain/pons area ratio and clinical features predict the prognosis of progressive Supranuclear palsy. BMC Neurol. 2020;20(1):114. https://doi.org/10.1186/s12883-020-016 92-6.

31. Massey LA, Jäger HR, Paviour DC, O'Sullivan SS, Ling H, Williams DR, Kallis C, Holton J, Revesz T, Burn DJ, Yousry T, Lees AJ, Fox NC, Micallef C. The midbrain to pons ratio: a simple and specific MRI sign of progressive supranuclear palsy. Neurology. 2013;80(20):1856–61. https://doi.org/10.1212/WNL.0b013e318292a2d2.

32. Morelli M, Arabia G, Salsone M, Novellino F, Giofrè L, Paletta R, Messina D, Nicoletti G, Condino F, Gallo O, Lanza P, Quattrone A. Accuracy of magnetic resonance parkinsonism index for differentiation of progressive supranuclear palsy from probable or possible Parkinson disease. Mov Disord. 2011;26(3):527–33.

33. Gilman S, Wenning GK, Low PA, Brooks DJ, Mathias CJ, Trojanowski JQ, Wood NW, Colosimo C, Durr A, Fowler CJ, Kaufmann H, Klockgether T, Lees A, Poewe W, Quinn N, Revesz T, Robertson D, Sandroni P, Seppi K, Vidailhet M. Second consensus statement on the diagnosis of multiple system atrophy. Neurology. 2008;71(9):670–6.

34. Lee J-Y, Yun JY, Shin C-W, Kim H-J, Jeon BS. Putaminal abnormality on 3-T magnetic resonance imaging in early parkinsonism-predominant multiple system atrophy. J Neurol. 2010;257(12):2065–2070 (online). Available at: https://pubmed.ncbi.nlm.nih.gov/20652301/. Accessed 12 Apr 2022.

35. Tokumaru AM, O'uchi T, Kuru Y, Maki T, Murayama, S, Horichi Y. Corticobasal degeneration: MR with histopathologic comparison. Am J Neuroradiol. 1996;17(10):1849–1852 (online). Available at: http://www.ajnr.org/cgi/content/abstract/17/10/1849. Accessed 12 Apr 2022.

36. Graus F, Keime-Guibert F, Reñe R, Benyahia B, Ribalta T, Ascaso C, Escaramis G, Delattre JY. Anti-Hu-associated paraneoplastic encephalomyelitis: analysis of 200 patients. Brain: A J Neurol. 2001;124(Pt 6):1138–1148 (online). Available at: https://www.ncbi.nlm.nih.gov/pub med/11353730. Accessed 26 Apr 2020.

37. Oyanguren B, Sánchez V, González FJ, de Felipe A, Esteban L, López-Sendón JL, Garcia-Barragán N, Martínez-San Millán J, Masjuán J, Corral I. Limbic encephalitis: a clinical-radiological comparison between herpetic and autoimmune etiologies. Eur J Neurol. 2013;20(12):1566–70.

38. Flanagan EP, McKeon A, Lennon VA, Kearns J, Weinshenker BG, Krecke KN, Matiello M, Keegan BM, Mokri B, Aksamit AJ, Pittock SJ. Paraneoplastic isolated myelopathy: clinical course and neuroimaging clues. Neurology. 2011;76(24):2089–2095 (online). Available at: https://pubmed.ncbi.nlm.nih.gov/21670438/. Accessed 12 Apr 2022.

39. Antinori A, Arendt G, Becker JT, Brew BJ, Byrd DA, Cherner M, Clifford DB, Cinque P, Epstein LG, Goodkin K, Gisslen M, Grant I, Heaton RK, Joseph J, Marder K, Marra CM, McArthur JC, Nunn M, Price RW, Pulliam L, Robertson KR, Sacktor N, Valcour V, Wojna VE. Updated research nosology for HIV-associated neurocognitive disorders. Neurology. 2007;69(18):1789–1799. https://doi.org/10.1212/01.WNL.0000287431.88658.8b

40. Fragoso DC, da Gonçalves Filho ALM, Pacheco FT, Barros BR, Aguiar Littig I, Nunes RH, Maia Júnior ACM, da Rocha AJ. Imaging of Creutzfeldt-Jakob disease: imaging patterns and their differential diagnosis. RadioGraphics. 2017;37(1):234–257.

41. Jallo, J., & Loftus, C. M. (Eds.). (2009). *Neurotrauma and critical care of the brain* (1st ed.). Thieme Medical.
42. Radoi M, Ciubotaru V, Tataranu L, Tataranu L, Bagdasar-Arseni Brain abscesses: clinical experience and outcome of 52 consecutive cases. n.d. (online). Available at: https://www.rev istachirurgia.ro/pdfs/2013-2-215.pdf. Accessed 12 Apr 2022.
43. Awad A, Stüve O. Multiple sclerosis in the elderly patient. Drugs Aging. 2010;27(4):283–94.
44. White AD, Swingler RJ, Compston DAS. Features of multiple sclerosis in older patients in south wales. Gerontology. 1990;36(3):159–64.
45. Ceronie B, Cockerell OC. Acute disseminated encephalomyelitis in an older adult following prostate resection. ENeurologicalSci. 2019;14:40–2. https://doi.org/10.1016/j.ensci.2018.11.006.
46. Josephs KA, Whitwell JL, Parisi JE, Petersen RC, Boeve BF, Jack CR Jr, Dickson DW. Caudate atrophy on MRI is a characteristic feature of FTLD-FUS: caudate atrophy in FTLD-FUS. Eur J Neurol The Official J Eur Federation Neurol Soc. 2010;17(7):969–75. https://doi.org/10.1111/j.1468-1331.2010.02975.x.
47. Ho VB, Chuang HS, Rovira MJ, Koo B. Juvenile Huntington disease: CT and MR features. AJNR Am J Neuroradiol. 1995;16(7):1405–12.
48. Tamhane AA, Arfanakis K. Motion correction in periodically-rotated overlapping parallel lines with enhanced reconstruction (PROPELLER) and turboprop MRI: Motion CORRECTION in PROPELLER- and Turboprop-MRI. Magn Reson Med. 2009;62(1):174–82. https://doi.org/10.1002/mrm.22004.

Application of Machine Learning Methods in NPH

Arnošt Mládek, Václav Gerla, Awista Zazay, and Ondřej Bradáč

Abstract Machine learning (ML) is the adaptation of data models using statistical techniques. In the healthcare domain, the most common application of machine learning is predictive medicine, i.e., determining the probability of whether specific treatments will be effective for a patient based on various attributes and treatment context. The vast majority of applications for machine learning and precision medicine also require data, which the systems then learn using supervision. Artificial neural network (ANN) technologies have been successfully used in medical research for several decades. They are commonly used to classify data to determine the likelihood of a patient developing a particular disease. The complex tool of deep learning (ML) with the ability to self-learn from incremental data is increasingly applied, e.g., in radiomics or image data analysis, where it is used to detect clinically relevant image patterns beyond what the human eye can perceive.

Keywords Machine learning · Neural network · Artificial intelligence · Deep learning · Classification algorithms

Abbreviations

AD	Alzheimer's disease
AdaBoost	Adaptive Boosting
ANN	Artificial neural network

A. Mládek (✉) · A. Zazay · O. Bradáč
Department of Neurosurgery and Neurooncology, 1st Medical Faculty, Charles University and Military University Hospital, Prague, Czech Republic
e-mail: arnost.mladek@lf1.cuni.cz

A. Mládek · V. Gerla
Department of Cognitive Systems and Neurosciences, Czech Institute of Informatics, Robotics and Cybernetics, Czech Technical University, Prague, Czech Republic

O. Bradáč
Department of Neurosurgery, 2nd Medical Faculty, Charles University and Motol University Hospital, Prague, Czech Republic

© The Author(s), under exclusive license to Springer Nature Switzerland AG 2023
O. Bradac (ed.), *Normal Pressure Hydrocephalus*,
https://doi.org/10.1007/978-3-031-36522-5_19

AUC	Area under the curve
BP	Backpropagation
CSF	Cerebrospinal fluid
CV	Cross-validation
CWT	Continuous wavelet transform
DET	Determinism
DL	Deep learning
DT	Decision trees
ECG	Electrocardiogram
ELD	External lumbar drainage
En	Entropy
FT	Fourier transform
GaussNB	Gaussian Naïve Bayes
GBDT	Gradient Boosting Decision Tree
GradientBoost	Gradient Boosting
HMM	Hidden Markov Models
HO	Hyperparameter optimization
ICP	Intracranial pressure
KNN	K-nearest neighbors
LAM	Laminarity
LIT	Lumbar infusion test
LogReg	Logistic regression
LOOCV	Leave-One-Out Cross-Validation
LR	Logistic regression
ML	Machine learning
NB	Naïve Bayes
NPH	Normal pressure hydrocephalus
PSD	Power spectral density
RF	Random forest
RL	Reinforcement learning
RQA	Recurrence quantification analysis
ROC	Receiver operating characteristic
S3VM	Semi-supervised support vector machines
SFS	Sequential Forward Selection
SVM	Support vector machines
TT	Trapping time
XGBoost	EXtreme Gradient Boosting

1   Introduction

Current computer-assisted neurosurgery research is based mainly on statistical analysis combined with practice guidelines and evidence-based research. However, these approaches have various limitations such as the unsuitability to analyze nonlinear parameters, impracticality for analyzing large datasets, and the possibility of human bias [1]. Machine learning (ML) involves algorithms learning patterns in huge and complex datasets generating useful predictive outputs at the required accuracy level. The use of ML in neurosurgery has the potential to bring substantial improvements in prediction and diagnosis. The application of ML algorithms to new large datasets can also reveal novel trends and relationships that may have beneficial implications for clinical practice in medicine [2].

2   Types of Learning Problems

The four main types of learning problems can be defined in ML: supervised, unsupervised, reinforcement, and semi-supervised learning.

- Supervised learning trains algorithms with datasets that contain pre-labeled outcomes for each case in order to solve prediction and classification problems. Supervised learning algorithms include logistic regression (LR), naïve Bayes (NB) approaches, K-nearest neighbors (KNN), support vector machines (SVM), decision trees (DT), artificial neural networks (ANN), Hidden Markov Models (HMM) [3, 4], and others.
- Unsupervised learning uses unlabeled datasets and allows the algorithm to extract features and patterns. A typical representative of unsupervised learning is cluster analysis. Clustering is a learning exploratory technique that allows identifying structure in the input data without prior knowledge of their distribution. The main idea is to classify the objects based on a similarity measure where similar objects are assigned to the same class [5].
- Reinforcement learning (RL) is learning by making and correcting mistakes that optimize decision making based on stages [6]. The RL framework consists of an agent that takes actions in a given environment. Those actions have an associated immediate reward. The goal of the learning process is to maximize the long-term reward, which is a function that depends on the sum of all the rewards that are collected over time.
- Semi-supervised learning allows the use of non-labeled data in conjunction with a small amount of labeled data aimed at improving the predictive performance [7, 8]. This approach is usually used as an extension of various supervised or unsupervised methods, e.g., semi-supervised Support Vector Machine (S3VM) [9] or semi-supervised clustering algorithms [10].

2.1 Feature Extraction End Selection

ML methods are not usually applied directly to the clinical datasets, and descriptive features are extracted from processed signals, or images [11–14]. ML methods then operate on these derived features. Basic types of features used in clinical practice are statistical parameters (e.g., minimum and maximum values, mean values, standard deviation, etc.) and clinical characteristics (e.g., age, weight, and medication). More complex features include power spectral density (PSD), morphological features [15], entropy- or fractal-based features, and others.

In some cases, ML algorithms can automatically derive features from input data and work with them, e.g., deep learning (DL) protocols. However, these approaches generally require extensive datasets to calculate the final prediction or classification model. Therefore, it is often not feasible to use these advanced algorithms in clinical practice.

A false assumption is that a large number of features would improve the discrimination capabilities of a ML algorithm. In fact, by reducing the feature space vector dimensional (feature selection), the ML provides more compact and easily interpretable results. Thereby, the performance of the ML is improved and the speed of the system increased [16].

2.2 Overview of ML Models

In the following text, we briefly outline basic principles of three selected ML approaches that are often used in prediction and classification tasks.

Support Vector Machine

The essence of SVM can be described by four basic concepts [17]: 1) the separating hyperplane that represents a straight line in a high-dimensional space that separates objects as points into two classes, 2) the maximum-margin hyperplane that adopts the maximal distance from any one of the given points, 3) the soft margin which allows some data points to push their way through the margin of the separating hyperplane without affecting the final result, and 4) the kernel function that projects data from a low-dimensional space to that of a higher dimension where the data will become linearly separable (Fig. 1).

SVM has been successfully used to predict risk of cerebrospinal fluid shunt failure in children [18], early recurrence of glioblastoma [19], detection of normal pressure hydrocephalus (NPH) during a presymptomatic stage [20], motor outcomes, speech, tremor, rigidity, bradykinesia, and akinesia [21].

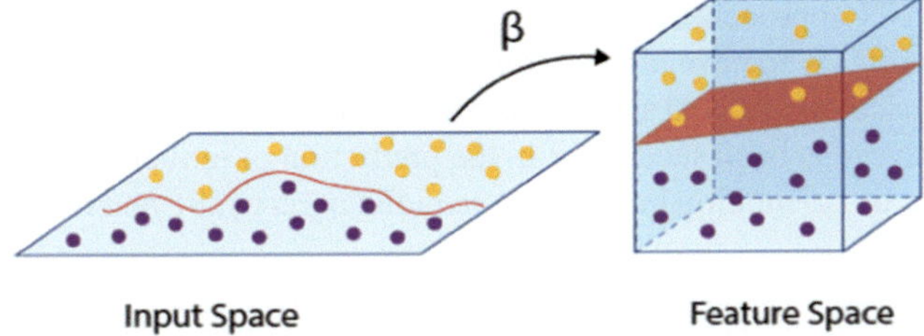

Fig. 1 The nonlinear classification by SVM. Illustration of the concept of treating the objects to be classified as points in input space (left) and finding a hyperplane that linearly separates them in higher dimensional space (right). The transformation β is referred to as the kernel function

Artificial Neural Networks

The basic building block of the artificial neural network (ANN) is the artificial neuron, which is a digital construct that tries to simulate the basic behavior of a biological neuron. An artificial neuron works in such a way that information propagates from the inputs through the input weights and activation function to the output. ANNs work with artificial neurons arranged in several layers (Fig. 2). The architecture of the most advanced ANN (e.g., DL networks) can contain up to tens to hundreds of such layers.

The main advantage of ANNs over conventional methods lies in their ability to solve highly complex problems. However, ANNs are often criticized for their poor interpretability, since it is difficult for humans to take the symbolic meaning behind the learned ANN models.

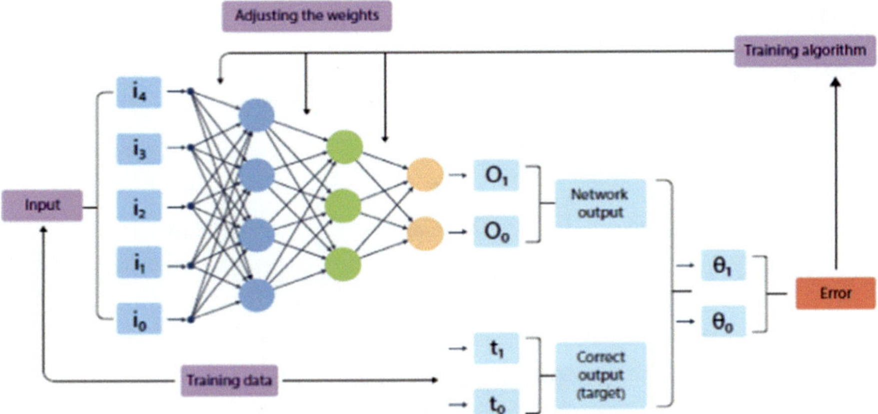

Fig. 2 Schematic representation of ANN learning procedure. This approach is referred to as back-propagation (BP) or backward propagation of errors. A BP algorithm is designed to test for errors working back from the output to the input nodes

Various ANN approaches have been successfully used in neurosurgery, such as predicting patients who have lumbar spinal canal stenosis [22], idiopathic NPH [23], pediatric ventriculoperitoneal shunt infections in children [24], and brain tumors [25, 26]. ANNs have also been successful in the prediction of intracranial pressure (ICP) trends [27], beam orientation in stereotactic radiosurgery [28], and for brain ventricle parcellation [29].

Decision Trees

Decision trees (DTs) are widely used classifiers because of their intelligible nature that resembles human thinking [30]. DTs are constructed via algorithms that identify ways to split input data based on different conditions. DT performance is highly competitive through the use of ensembles (a combination of multiple decision trees). A top-ranked algorithm is eXtreme Gradient Boosting (XGBoost) (Fig. 3). In XGBoost, the DTs are consecutively built and the algorithm tries to learn from wrongly classified observations by adding a higher weight on them in the subsequently built trees [31].

DTs approaches were used in predicting intraoperative and perioperative complications [32], surgical decision making in vestibular schwannoma cases [33], and in the area of spinopelvic chordoma surgery [34].

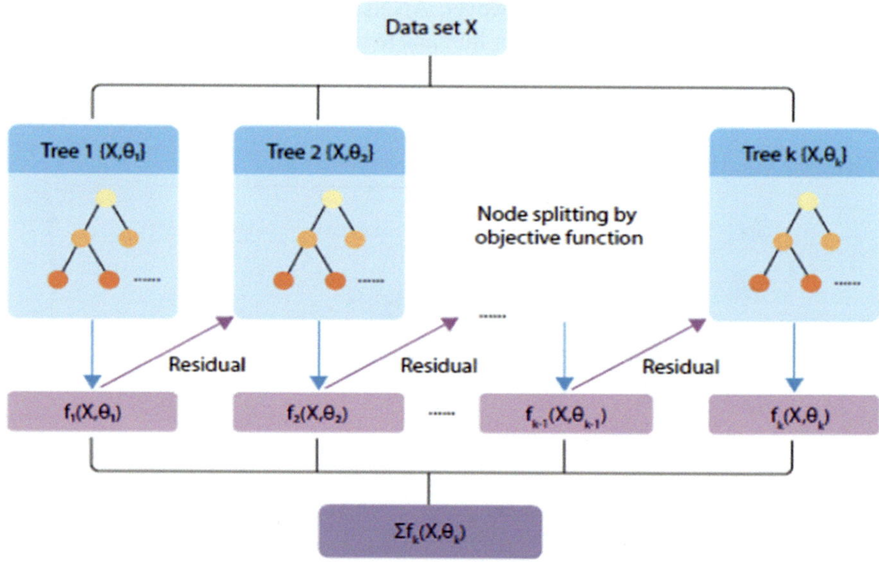

Fig. 3 Schematic representation of eXtreme Gradient Boosting (XGBoost) algorithm

2.3   Model Assessment

For ML applications, performance measurement is an essential task [35]. The performance and reliability of ML algorithms can be measured and optimized by using the following widely known diagnostic tests: confusion matrix, accuracy, precision, sensitivity, specificity, and F1 score. These metrics offer to optimize deployed prediction and classification models.

In neurosurgery (or medicine in general), it is advisable to use the receiver operating characteristic (ROC) curve [36], which is defined as a plot of sensitivity as the y coordinate versus 1-specificity as the x coordinate across different ML method settings.

2.4   Limitations

Neurosurgical-based research has inherent limits because of several biases limiting the adoption of ML in clinical research. The data are mostly based on subjective impressions of surgeons. Bias could arise from the fact that surgeons who are more exposed to neurosurgical ML can value it more positively than those who do not routinely make use of it [37].

ML methods themselves also have their limits. They can often lead to so-called under- and over-fitting (Fig. 4) [38]. Under-fitting is a scenario where a classification model is too simple compared to the problem being solved. Over-fitting is the opposite of under-fitting, occurring when the model is overtrained or too complex. The key problem also arises from the structure of the processed data. A learning algorithm is trained on a set of training data, but then it is applied to make predictions on new data points, which leaves the door open to the possibility of various errors [38]. This phenomenon is more noticeable on smaller datasets where model performance cannot be sufficiently verified. Various issues could also appear on imbalanced datasets where the target class has an uneven distribution of observations (e.g., healthy versus diseased classes have disproportionately different numbers of observations).

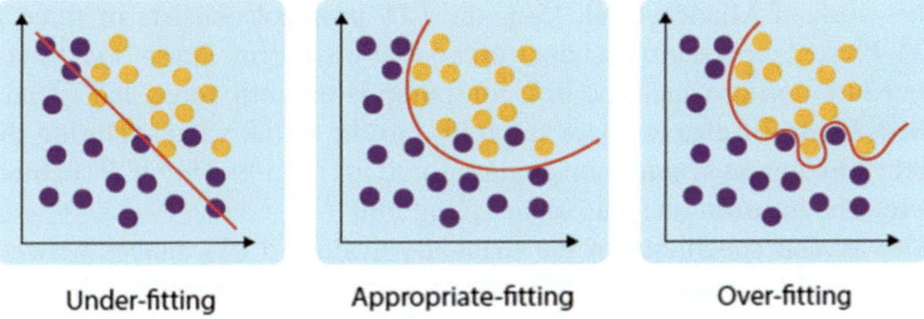

Fig. 4 Training data points plotted to show under-fitting, appropriate fitting, and over-fitting. The red line corresponds to the separating hyperplane of the trained classifier

The number of published ML studies in the field of neurological surgery is skyrocketing as the application of ML algorithms to new, large datasets can reveal novel trends and relationships that may have beneficial implications for clinical practice in medicine [1, 2, 35, 37, 39–41]. ML techniques can provide high-value predictions without human intervention which may assist in making better decisions in real time. They provide the convenience of setting many clinical features as inputs and have the ability to analyze the data as a whole [1, 2]. The use of ML applications to provide clinical decision support in neurological surgery is highly heterogeneous. The densest cluster of research papers focuses on various topics in spinal surgery, such as the preoperative evaluation, planning, and outcome prediction. The three most widely applied algorithms are neural networks, logistic regression, and support vector machines; neural network models frequently outperform other algorithms on supervised learning tasks [2]. The following ML applications in the field of neurological surgery have been published: prediction of surgical satisfaction in patients with spinal canal stenosis [39], beam orientation in stereotactic radiosurgery [28], automated navigation system for deep brain stimulator placement [3, 4], brain tumor classification segmentation [25, 26, 42], and decision support in critical care [43]. Please note that the listing is far from being complete. For a detailed overview of ML applications in neurosurgery and in medicine in general, please consult the following large-scale reviews [1, 2, 35, 37, 39–41, 44–48].

3 Lumbar Infusion Test-based Data

The purpose of the lumbar infusion test (LIT) is to assess the adequacy of CSF compliance via the infusion of a fluid challenge (Fig. 5). A common measure determining whether patients are likely to be responsive to shunting is the resistance to CSF outflow Rout (mmHg ml^{-1}.min) [49] which is calculated as the pressure difference divided by the infusion rate [50]. There are various Rout cut-off points as there is no threshold that is widely accepted. The Rout of 12 mmHg ml^{-1}.min is considered to be close to the sought-after value [51] and was used in our study [52] to label the patients as LIT positive (Rout > 12 mmHg ml^{-1}.min) or negative (Rout < 12 mmHg ml^{-1}.min).

In the work of Mládek et al. [52], the LIT protocol consists of three phases (Table 1). Phase I represents the unperturbed ICP waveform. Phase II is the standard LIT procedure during which the infusion pump is on until a new ICP steady state is reached. Phase III characterizes the return to the initial values. During the LIT, the patient's ECG was synchronously monitored for time-locking ICP segmentation procedure. The infusion rate was set at 1.5 ml min^{-1}.

Sensitivity and specificity of the manually evaluated LIT ranges between 56–100% and 50–90%, respectively [53, 54]. Nonetheless, it provides a helpful diagnostic tool to reveal the reduced cerebrospinal fluid (CSF) compliance indicative of NPH [55–58]. The temporary external lumbar drainage (ELD) is superior to the LIT

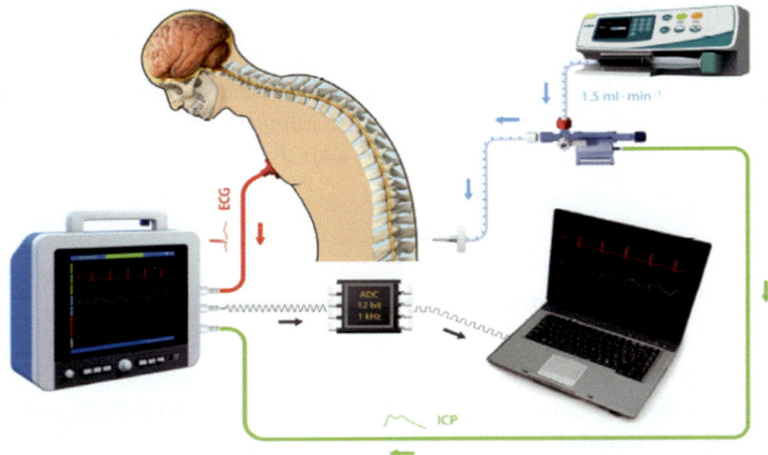

Fig. 5 Illustration of the LIT setup. Saline is administered by an infusion pump at a constant rate of 1.5 ml.min^{-1} into the subarachnoid space (blue arrows). The needle is connected via a fluid-filled tubing system and a three-way stop cock to a disposable pressure transducer. The transducer is electrically connected to a bedside monitor (green line), which displays ICP (*green*) and electrocardiogram (ECG) (*red*) onto a monitor and simultaneously relays the analog data through ADC to a computer (*gray analog and digital signal*)

Table 1 Description of the LIT phases I–III. The mean phase lengths are in minutes

Phase	Infussion pump	Length (min)	ICP trend	Motive
1.	Off	2	Steady	Equilibration of the ICP waveform, offset level
2.	On	20	Increase	Main phase, testing of CSF absorptive capacity
3.	Off	5	Decrease	Testing of the recovery rate

in terms of positive predictive value (80–100%), sensitivity (50–100%), and specificity (60–100%) [55]. ELD yields the highest accuracy of shunt-responsiveness prediction and is usually recommended for NPH diagnosis [59].

Currently, there is limited literature providing insight into ICP/CSF factors that predispose individuals toward shunt responsiveness. Knowledge of new predictive markers could contribute to NPH management. Therefore, we developed ML algorithms to predict which patients are more likely to experience clinical improvements after surgery. In our study [52], we analyzed ICP waveforms recorded throughout the LIT and extracted numerous signal features, rather than reducing the LIT outcome to one number, Rout, which is usually done. We then developed ML algorithms with the ability to reveal complex relations between the ICP signal features and the ELD outcome to predict which patient is more likely to respond to CSF drainage.

3.1 Design of the Study

The study group included 96 subjects that met selection criteria. Subjects were classified as NPH (46) and non-NPH (50) according to the ELD outcome. Both groups consisted of possible NPH patients, with the NPH group having positive ELD (ELD+).

3.2 Data Processing and Feature Extractions

The calculated ICP features can be clustered into seven groups: temporal dynamics based (F01–F11), integral based (F12–F13), nonlinear based (F14–F21), continuous wavelet transform based (CWT, F22–F28), recurrence quantification analysis based (RQA, F29–F40), heart rate based (HR, F41–F42), and ECG locking based (F43–F48). For illustration of selected ICP features, see Fig. 6.

Temporal-dynamics-based features (F01–F11) describe the ICP waveform evolution in time. F01 corresponds to the Q0.99–Q0.01 quantile difference, which is basically the ICP elevation throughout the infusion phase (phase II) of the LIT. Utilization of quantiles instead of averages prevents artificial spikes that may bias the results. Integral-based features (F12–F13) represent the area under the curve (AUC, mmHg min) of a time normalized ICP and differ in the input signal only. Nonlinear-based features (F14–F21) are routinely employed in signal processing to

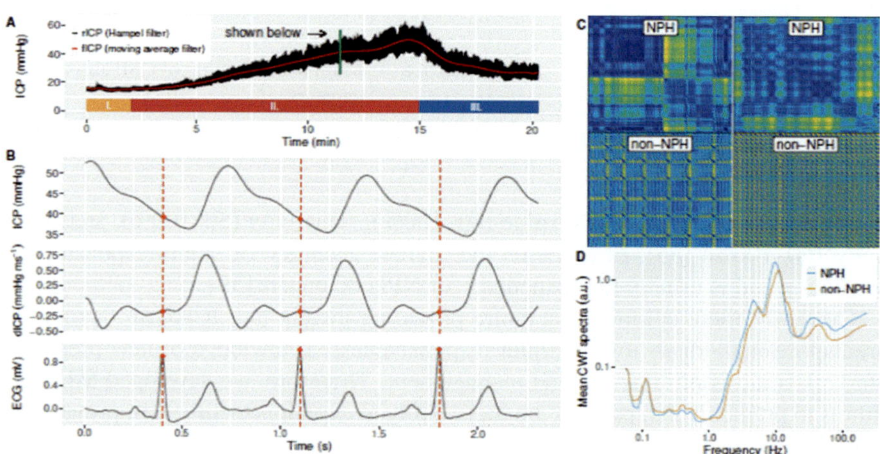

Fig. 6 A. Illustration of the LIT recording, with colored boxes indicating the three phases. B. Detail of the ICP inset. Top: ICP, middle: ICP time derivative (dICP), and bottom: ECG. C. Example of ICP recurrent maps calculated from two NPH (top row) and two non-NPH (bottom row) patients. D. Illustration of mean continuous wavelet transform (CWT) spectra for NPH (*blue*) and non-NPH (*orange*) patients

extract complex spatial and temporal patterns. An ICP signal reflecting the intricate CSF dynamics is inherently non-stationary and nonlinear with a frequency spectrum that is not consistent over time [60]. It is therefore reasonable to exploit nonlinear analysis techniques to characterize ICP from this perspective. There are three types of nonlinear ICP features used in the present study: a modified Shannon entropy (En; F14, F15, F20), a logarithmic energy entropy (LogEn; F16, F21), and Higuchi fractal dimension (HFD; F17-F19). Shannon entropy [61] is characterized by the degree of uncertainty associated with the occurrence of the result and provides a measure of signal disorder. Logarithmic energy entropy is a function of signal energy instead of probabilities. Higuchi's algorithm [62] represents an efficient and noise insensitive method for calculating the discrete time series fractal dimension which quantifies the signal's complexity and self-similarity. CWT-based features (F22–F28) were calculated using the CW transform; a method of time–frequency analysis, which builds on the classical short-time Fourier transform (FT). The wavelet transform $W\psi$ of a continuous signal f is defined as:

$$\left[W_\psi f\right](a, b) = \int_{-\infty}^{+\infty} f(t)\psi_{a,b}^*(t)\mathrm{d}t = \int_{-\infty}^{+\infty} f(t)\frac{1}{\sqrt{a}}\psi^*\left(\frac{t-b}{a}\right)\mathrm{d}t$$

where ψ^* is the complex conjugate of the mother wavelet, $\psi_{a,b}{}^*$ is the complex conjugate of the transform kernel, a represents the dilatation, and b is the time shift. RQA-based features (F29–F40) originate in the recurrence quantification analysis (RQA), a type of nonlinear data analysis which identifies the number and duration of recurrences. Natural processes can have a distinct recurrent behavior such as periodicity and irregular cyclicity. Moreover, the recurrence of states, in the meaning that states become arbitrarily close after some time, is a fundamental property of deterministic dynamical systems and is typical for nonlinear or chaotic systems. In the RQA technique, the ICP waveform is represented in the form of a recurrent plot defined as

$$R_{ij} = \Theta\bigl(\varepsilon - \left\|x_i - x_j\right\|\bigr), \quad i, j = 1, 2, \ldots, N$$

where N is the number of the considered states, theta is the phase space trajectory, ε is the threshold distance, ||...|| is the norm, and $\Theta()$ the Heaviside function. The binary R_{ij} matrix serves as an alternative 2D view of the ICP waveform from which global features can be calculated: determinism (DET), trapping time (TT), entropy (En), and laminarity (LAM). DET refers to the percentage of recurrence points which form diagonal lines and is defined as:

$$\mathrm{DET} = \sum_{l=l_{min}}^{N} lP(l) \cdot \left(\sum_{l=1}^{N} = lP(l)\right)^{-1}$$

where P(l) is the histogram of the lengths l of the diagonal lines. LAM refers to the percentage of recurrent points that form vertical lines which can be calculated as follows:

$$\text{LAM} = \sum_{v=v_{\min}}^{N} v P(v) \cdot \left(\sum_{v=1}^{N} v P(v) | \right)^{-1}$$

where P(v) is the histogram of the lengths v of the vertical lines. TT represents the length of the vertical recurrence plot lines:

$$\text{TT} = \sum_{v=v_{\min}}^{N} v P(v) \cdot \left(\sum_{v=v_{\min}}^{N} P(v) | \right)^{-1}$$

The Shannon entropy of the probability distribution of the diagonal line lengths p(l) is defined as:

$$E_n = - \sum_{l=l_{\min}}^{N} -p(l) \ln p(l).$$

Dimension (dim) and delay time (tau) parameters for the phase space construction were set based on the dataset estimates to 3 and 8, respectively.

ECG R-wave positions were used to calculate both the heart rate mean (F41) and median (F42). In the ECG locking-based features (F43–F48), ECG R-waves were used to segment the ICP into one cardiac cycle intervals.

3.3 ML Models and Parameters

In the study [52], the performance of the following eight ML models implemented in the Scikit-Learn Python library [63] was put to test: Random Forest (RF), Logistic Regression (LogReg), Gaussian Naïve Bayes (GaussNB) [46], Support Vector Model (SVM), Adaptive Boosting (AdaBoost), Extra-trees (ExtraTrees), Gradient Boosting (GradientBoost), and eXtreme Gradient Boosting (XGBoost).

By default, the recommended ML model parameter values were used. Also, the suitability of parameter settings with respect to the solved task were checked and selected parameters were adjusted accordingly (Table 2). The hyperparameter optimization (HO) of ML models was not used. Even though the HO procedure might further improve the nominal accuracy of the classification, it can be at the expense of the actual model performance due to over-fitting. In addition, HO in combination with two nested cross-validations (CVs) could be extremely computationally demanding.

Table 2 Parameter values of used ML approaches

ML model	Class in scikit-learn library	Parameters setting
RF	sklearn.ensemble.RandomForestClassifier	*
LogReg	sklearn.linear_model.LogisticRegression	*
GaussNB	sklearn.naive_bayes.GaussianNB	var_smoothing = 1e-11
SVM	sklearn.svm.SVC	dual = false
AdaBoost	sklearn.ensemble.AdaBoostClassifier	learning_rate = 0.2
ExtraTrees	sklearn.ensemble.ExtraTreesClassifier	max_depth = 6
GradientBoost	sklearn.ensemble.GradientBoostingClassifier	learning_rate = 0.2
		max_depth = 6
XGBoost	xgboost.sklearn.XGBoost	learning_rate = 0.2
		max_depth = 6

For all remaining unlisted parameters, recommended values were used
*The algorithm uses the recommended values of all parameters.

3.4 Cross-Validation Scenario

In the study [52], two nested cross-validations were utilized. An inner-stratified fivefold CV was used in a Sequential Forward Selection (SFS) algorithm. In SFS, the features were sequentially added according to its highest contribution to the chosen criterion; the classification mean accuracy over all CV cycles was applied in this case.

An outer Leave-One-Out Cross-Validation (LOOCV) was applied to make predictions on data not used to train the model. In LOOCV, each patient was chosen once to be the test set and all remaining patients were used as a train set. The model was trained N times, where N is the number of patients, and was validated on a single patient. The result characteristics such as accuracy, sensitivity, specificity, and AUC were averaged over all LOOCV cycles. This approach is a computationally demanding procedure to perform, but it results in a reliable and unbiased estimate of the ML model performance.

3.5 Study Results and Implications

Table 3 compares accuracies, AUCs, sensitivities, and specificities for all ML algorithms developed. From these algorithms, the XGBoost classifier showed the best discrimination potential with 80.2% accuracy, 0.887 AUC, 86.0% sensitivity, and 73.9% specificity when all 48 features are considered. The manual Rout-based classification displays significantly lower concordance with ELD outcomes with accuracy, sensitivity, and specificity of 62.5%, 62.0%, and 63.0%, respectively. Because of its superior discrimination and balanced accuracy, the XGBoost classifier was selected for calibration and further testing. Figure 7 shows the detailed performance of the XGBoost classifier. In terms of AUC (0.891), accuracy (82.3%), and sensitivity (86.1%), the highest predictive potential was obtained for eight features (Fig. 7A–B). Figure 7D shows the XGBoost model ROC curve when 1, 8, or all 48 features are considered. The feature importance (Fig. 7E) indicates the most seminal predictors for NPH/non-NPH discrimination, with relative importance ranking based on usage frequency in the model. The calibration curve (Fig. 7F) indicates strong concordance between the estimated and observed probabilities.

The principal feature with the highest feature importance (FI) is F01 (Fig. 7), the ICP elevation in phase II, which is the unscaled Rout value. F01 is higher in NPH patients ($p = 1.4e^{-5}$, FI = 62), in line with the original principle of the LIT. The remaining features, F02–F48, are difficult to interpret as they lack a clear clinical correlate, and a physiological explanation is rather speculative. Despite often being unexplainable, features F02–F48 enhance our XGBoost model to increase the prediction accuracy by approximately 20% compared to the actual Rout-based manual evaluation. This finding illustrates the greatest asset of the ML algorithms: the ability to explore complex multidimensional feature space and reveal clinically exploitable information hidden within, otherwise unreachable via common statistical techniques. Clearly, ML-based evaluation of the LIT cannot, at least for now, replace ELD completely. Still, an in-depth LIT ICP analysis may reveal a subset of patients that could be indicated for permanent CSF drainage.

The benefit of our ML model is illustrated in Fig. 8. While patients P1–P2 show an easy-to-recognize ICP elevation typical for non-NPH and NPH diagnosis, P3–P4 represent the gray-zone patients. Unlike the Rout-based assessment which failed for P3–P4, our ML model correctly predicted the ELD outcome in all patients P1–P4.

Table 3 Comparison of the AUCs, accuracies, sensitivities, and specificities of tested ML models

Model	AUC	Accuracy (%)	Sensitivity (%)	Specificity (%)
Rout	NA	62.5	62.0	63.0
RF	0.707	68.5	72.0	63.0
LogReg	0.711	70.8	80.0	60.9
GaussNB	0.688	71.6	84.0	52.2
SVM	0.728	71.9	86.0	56.5
AdaBoost	0.707	75.0	84.0	65.2
ExtraTrees	0.817	76.0	82.0	69.6
GradientBoost	0.895	79.2	86.0	71.7
XGBoost	0.887/0.891 (8)	80.2/82.3 (8)	86.0/86.1 (8)	73.9/78.3 (7)

In XGBoost X/Y (Z): X refers to the performance obtained for all 48 features, Y represents the highest performance obtained for optimal number of features, Z is the optimal feature number. NA: not available

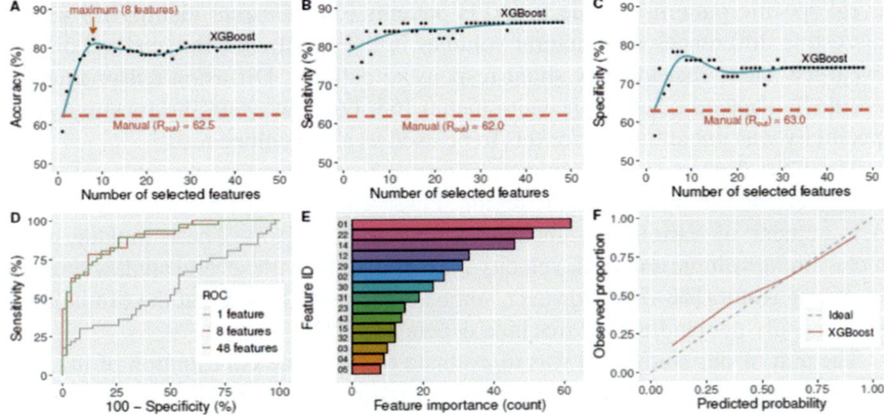

Fig. 7 XGBoost model performance. A, B, and C: dashed red lines symbolize the performance of Rout-based manual classification. D: ROC curves for 1, 8, and 48 features. E: Ranking the calculated features according to their importance in the model. F: Calibration curve of the XGBoost model. The dashed gray line denotes ideal calibration, which represents a perfect agreement between probabilities predicted by the model and actual outcome probabilities observed in the underlying data. Specifically, the predictions of a model whose calibration curve is closer to the dashed line are better estimates of the actual probability of NPH/non-NPH status

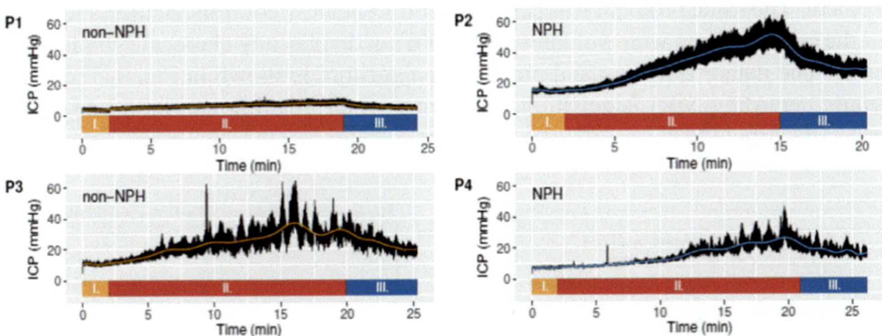

Fig. 8 ICP measured during LIT of four selected patients P1–P4; non-NPH (orange: P1 and P3) and NPH (blue: P2 and P4). While P1–P2 are representatives of patients where the manual Rout-based classification correctly discriminates between NPH and non-NPH, P3–P4 illustrate those gray zone patients in which Rout-based classification fails. Specifically, Rout of P3 and P4 is 13.8 and 7.3 mmHg ml^{-1}.min, respectively, therefore assigning them to the opposite class. All P1–P4 patients were classified according to ELD using our XGBoost ML model

4   Phase-Contrast MRI-Based Data

Our recent study [64] demonstrates that the DESH score lacks sufficient sensitivity and specificity to be applied as a stand-alone diagnostic or prognostic marker for iNPH. Our group has also tested the hypothesis that structural volume analysis can reveal specific patterns unique to iNPH patients [64]. Despite identifying several interesting differences in structural volumes in iNPH patients, this method did not reveal any signs that identify shunt-responsive patients. Diffusion tensor imaging repeatedly showed changes in white matter [65, 66], but again the sensitivity and specificity was not sufficient for this to be used as a standalone test.

The CSF flow void phenomenon observed in the cerebral aqueduct of iNPH patients has led to interest in this region. Phase-contrast MRI allows for a detailed measurement of various parameters of CSF motion [67]. These include aqueductal stroke volume and peak velocity measurements, with several studies showing promising results [68–70]. However, some authors have stated that the examination is technically demanding and machine dependent [71].

The aim of our study [72] was to evaluate the possible contribution of machine learning algorithms in enhancing results of MRI flowmetry in NPH diagnostics. In contrast to the previous published studies, we have looked at the method from a wider perspective of all the available flowmetry features.

4.1 Design of the Study

The final study group included 30 iNPH patients who completed the study MRI protocol. The same protocol was performed on 15 healthy controls. Subjects selected for the control group were volunteers who did not display any classical symptoms of iNPH. The data acquisition and processing algorithm is shown in Fig. 9. Technical details regarding MRI acquisitions and image interpretation can be found in the respective article [72].

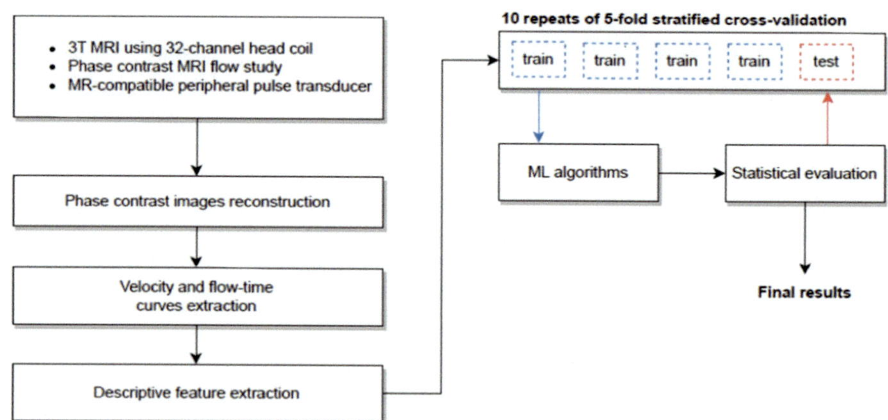

Fig. 9 Diagram summarizing methodology of the study

4.2 Feature Extraction

For each patient, seven CSF flowmetry vectors have been obtained directly from the MRI: aqueduct area, peak positive velocity, peak negative velocity, average velocity, positive flow rate, negative flow rate, and average flow rate. Each vector is composed of 32 points evenly distributed along one cardiac cycle. To calculate CSF flow features, 32 points of each vector were interpolated by a cubic spline. The features of a given vector were calculated using the piece-wise smooth interpolating function, and these features characterize the spline behavior. Altogether, the phase-contrast MRI test provided 87 basic features.

4.3 Machine Learning Details

A set of 87 selected complex features were calculated for each patient (85 + age and sex). The whole patient dataset was divided into training and testing parts by the k-fold (k = 5) cross-validation (CV). We improve k-fold CV by using stratified re-sampling, which ensures that the relative class frequencies (iNPH and control) are sufficiently preserved in each fold according to the original class frequencies in the full dataset. Stratified k-fold CV is useful for small and/or imbalanced datasets (30 iNPH and 15 control patients in our case) [73]. Another improvement was the repetition of the k-fold stratified CV process N times (N = 10), enabling an estimate of the mean and standard deviation in a performance.

The following eight different state-of-the-art ML models were deployed using the aforementioned robust CV design: Multilayer perceptron (MLP), Gaussian Naive Bayes (GaussNB), Gradient Boosting Decision Tree (GBDT), Logistic Regression (LogReg), Extra Trees (ExtraTrees), Random Forest (RF), XGBoost (XGB), and Adaptive Boosting (AdaBoost). The listed algorithms are implemented and described in the Scikit-Learn Python library63 and were run in Python 3.8.

Due to better repeatability of the proposed solution, default settings of all algorithms were used. Accuracy, sensitivity, specificity, receiver operating characteristic (ROC), and area under the ROC curve (AUC) were used to compare performance of all ML methods.

4.4 Study Results and Implications

Within the scope of phase-contrast MRI, all major parameters were inspected: peak positive and negative velocity, peak amplitude, average velocity, aqueductal area, and positive, negative, and average flow. Using the t-test for a direct comparison, significant differences were found with p-values of less than 0.05 in 47 of the 85 tested features. Many of the parameters are not easy to interpret. The most distinctive parameters with a p-value of less than 0.005 were peak negative velocity, peak amplitude, and negative flow.

Table 4 compares accuracies, sensitivities, specificities, and AUCs for all ML algorithms developed. From these algorithms, the AdaBoost classifier showed the highest specificity and best discrimination potential overall with $80.4 \pm 2.9\%$ accuracy, $72.0 \pm 5.6\%$ sensitivity, $84.7 \pm 3.8\%$ specificity, and 0.812 ± 0.047 AUC. The highest sensitivity was $85.7 \pm 5.6\%$ reached by the GaussNB model, and the best AUC was 0.854 ± 0.028 by ExtraTrees classifier. The final ROCs and calibration curves for all ML models are presented in Fig. 10.

Table 4 Mean value and standard deviation of the accuracy, sensitivity, specificity, and AUC computed over 10 CV repetitions

Model	Accuracy	Sensitivity (%)	Specificity (%)	AUC
Multilayer perceptron	72.0 ± 3.4	54.7 ± 5.6	80.7 ± 5.5	0.750 ± 0.048
Gaussian Naïve Bayes	73.8 ± 2.4	85.7 ± 5.6	73.3 ± 2.4	0.770 ± 0.009
Gradient boosting decision tree	73.8 ± 4.3	64.0 ± 3.7	78.7 ± 6.5	0.747 ± 0.064
Logistic regression	76.9 ± 4.0	65.3 ± 5.6	82.7 ± 4.9	0.808 ± 0.029
Extra trees	77.3 ± 1.9	73.3 ± 4.7	79.3 ± 4.9	0.854 ± 0.028
Random forest	78.2 ± 4.0	74.7 ± 5.6	80.0 ± 4.1	0.813 ± 0.027
XGBoost	79.6 ± 1.9	72.0 ± 5.6	83.3 ± 2.4	0.840 ± 0.037
Adaptove boosting	80.4 ± 2.9	72.0 ± 5.6	84.7 ± 3.8	0.812 ± 0.047

Individual models are sorted according to the resulting accuracy (from lowest to highest)

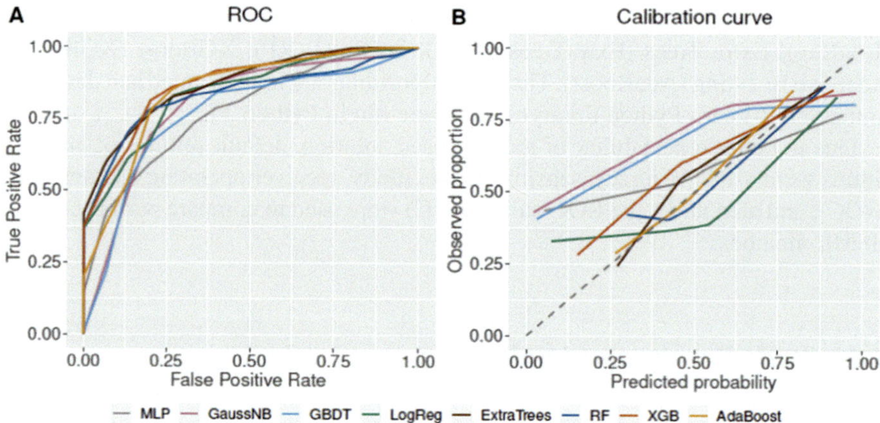

Fig. 10 ROC (left) and calibration curves (right) for all individual ML models. The dashed diagonal line represents the performance of an ideal model, where the predicted outcome would correspond perfectly with the actual outcome

The importance of a feature by AdaBoost was computed as the normalized total reduction of the criterion brought by that feature (the higher, the more important the feature). It is also known as the Gini importance [63]. Feature importance differs a lot from the significance counted with the chi-square test. No "major" feature regardless of importance had any importance for the AdaBoost classifier, and the most significant parameters played only a minor role in its computations.

Since MRI has become more broadly available, many scientists have had great hopes in phase-contrast MRI, which seemed to promise the long anticipated biomarker for selecting shunt-responsive iNPH patients [74]. Unfortunately, it has become clear that phase-contrast MRI is not easy to interpret as its results vary according to the MRI machine used [71]. This led to the fact that not many authors really tested this method, and the literature on this topic is scarce. The current articles focus on one or a few parameters of phase-contrast MRI. The most studied parameters are peak mean velocity and aqueductal stroke volume. The results are rather controversial. There is a study by Tawfik et al. [69] which shows great results for both parameters with a diagnostic accuracy of 92.5–93.3% for peak mean velocity and 100% for aqueductal stroke volume. However, these results were not supported by other authors. On the contrary, aqueductal stroke volume was identified as a poor predictor of shunt responsiveness by Blitz et al. [75]. This unfavorable result was also supported by other authors [76].

In the study Vlasak et al. [72], we have looked at all of the available parameters of phase-contrast MRI examination. The flow curve is defined by seven vectors: aqueduct area, peak positive velocity, peak negative velocity, average velocity, positive flow rate, negative flow rate, and average flow rate. We have identified the three most distinct parameters with a p-value less than 0.005 with direct comparison using a t-test: peak negative velocity, peak amplitude, and negative flow. These findings may be related to the increased ICP pulsatility in iNPH patients observed from invasive ICP monitoring [77], while the altered negative flow and higher peak amplitude observed on phase-contrast MRI in normal conditions could represent increased ICP pulsatility observed in overnight ICP monitoring [78]. The results of ICP monitoring on shunt response prediction in the literature vary [78–80], but the role of altered wave characteristics observed in our study with regards to prediction of shunt response has yet to be clarified.

As stated above, machine learning approaches have already been successfully utilized in medical research. To our knowledge, no machine learning approach has been applied to enhance the results of CSF flowmetry. We have considered this method beneficial, because some of the flowmetry features are difficult to interpret as they lack a clear clinical correlation, and their physiological explanation is rather speculative and under further investigation. Also, the importance of individual features does not necessarily correlate with the p-values. Using this method, we achieved a sensitivity of up to 85% and specificity of 84%. The best accuracy was 80%. The highest-performing ML algorithm was the Adaptive Boosting. This model showed a good calibration and discrimination on the testing data with 80.4% accuracy, 72.0% sensitivity, 84.7% specificity, and 0.812 AUC. Unfortunately, with the wide variety of published results of phase-contrast MRI, it is not easy to make a direct comparison. Nonetheless, contrary to some papers [75, 76], our results show the benefit of using the phase-contrast MRI method in distinguishing iNPH group from healthy controls. However, we cannot confirm the results of Tawfik et al. [69].

The developed ML models were optimized for highly accurate prediction rather than explanation. Thus, model parameters cannot be simply deployed for the purpose of explaining the effect of individual features on the differentiation of iNPH and healthy patients. Some of the frequently used ML models (especially ensemble-based algorithms) allow the use of the optimization of hyperparameters. This could further improve the performance of the ML models. This approach could be used in the future if the dataset were enlarged. Further external validations of data from multiple neurosurgical centers would be necessary before applying these approaches in clinical practice.

5 Synopsis of Other ML Studies Dealing With NPH

5.1 MRI/CT-Based ML Studies

In 2014, Virhammar et al. [81] applied logistic regression models on various MR imaging features with shunt outcome as a dependent variable. It was found that a small callosal angle, wide temporal horns, and occurrence of disproportionately enlarged subarachnoid space hydrocephalus were common in patients with iNPH and were significant predictors of a positive shunt outcome.

A new method for automatically segmenting and labeling the ventricular system of NPH patients was suggested by Ellingsen et al. [11]. Their technique named RUDOLPH integrated a two segmentation approach: a patch-based tissue classification method (S3DL, subject specific sparse dictionary learning) with a registration-based multi-atlas labeling method (MALP-EM, multi-atlas label propagation with expectation–maximization). This combination was shown to provide a robust segmentation and labeling of the lateral, third, and fourth ventricles of the brain. In comparison with other segmentation techniques, it demonstrated substantial improvements in labeling the enlarged ventricles, indicating that the proposed strategy may be a viable option for the diagnosis of NPH.

Benedetto et al. [23] described a novel, quantitative approach to assessing CT images of suspected NPH patients. Their SILVER index represented a reliable method to easily evaluate DESH; however, prospective clinical studies were required to elucidate its effective role in the clinical assessment of the patients. A similar investigation has been conducted by Gunter et al. [13] from the Mayo Clinic. They created an automated classifier for imaging characteristics of DESH. MRI data were parcellated for CSF and overlaid with a database of > 100 sulcal regions. The CSF volume in each region was then summed up and normalized. AUC values calculated for each region individually then determined the ML model feature selection. The selected regions were used to train the SVM classification model. In line with that, Shao et al. [29] proposed a modified a deep neural network-based method to perform accurate ventricular parcellation, even with grossly enlarged ventricles, from MRI. The proposed technique yields robust segmentation of the ventricular system and provides more accurate results in cases of dilated ventricles.

A similar approach employing deep learning classification with a 3D convolutional ladder network was used by Irie et al. [82] in order to differentiate patients with NPH and Alzheimer's disease (AD). The authors acknowledge that building and training of a convolutional neural network without over-fitting was limited by the small number of samples. To address this problem, a residual extraction phase followed by a neural network classification was introduced. The group of Irie has shown that the deep learning approach supplemented with the residual extraction algorithm has the potential to discriminate between NPH, HC, and AD.

Rau et al. [20] developed a SVM-based classifier of MR brain images for automatic detection of NPH patterns during a presymptomatic stage. The following anatomical regions appeared to be seminal to recognize NPH pattern: the fourth ventricle, gray matter and CSF volumes of caudate, the left basal forebrain, and the right parietal operculum. Wu et al. [83] conducted a fine segmentation-based volumetric analysis of MRI data and demonstrated its potential to reliably differentiate CSF drainage responders from other patients with iNPH like as well as to predict neurological outcome after shunting. A linear support vector machine was embraced into the recursive feature elimination. The authors applied a class-weighting procedure to address the disproportion in the size of responders and non-responders groups. It was also shown that the classification accuracy significantly changes with the selected segmentation granularity.

5.2 ICP-Based ML Studies

In 2006, Schmidt et al. [84] introduced a mathematical model in which ICP was estimated using hemodynamic parameters (TCD characteristics) derived from arterial blood pressure and cerebral blood flow. The proposed model uses fuzzy pattern classification to identify clusters of the sample space; in each cluster a local ICP estimator was defined. The calculated ICP is considered as a weighted sum of local ICP estimations.

Calisto et al. [15, 16] developed and implemented an automatic system, which extracts 20 morphological parameters and features of one ICP pulse wave (e.g., mean, absolute minima and maxima, leading edge slope, subpeak amplitude, etc.) and provides with respective trends and statistics. The extracted parameters were shown to correlate with diagnosis, e.g., NPH pathology. A similar study using WEKA classification software was conducted by Galeano et al. [85].

In 2016, Nucci et al. [86] developed and trained an artificial neural network aiming to assess the clinical status based on various morphological pulse pressure waveform patterns and compared it to well-known characteristics like outflow resistance, elastance index, etc. The developed morphology based classification model estimates the global ICP and its ability to reflect or predict perturbation in CSF dynamics.

5.3 Other Studies

The following articles go beyond graphical (MRI/CT) or temporal (ICP, ABP) data and build.

ML models on different inputs. Muscas et al. [87] developed a prognostic ML classifier based on a random forest model allowing accurate subject-based risk stratification identifying low-risk patients with subarachnoid hemorrhage for shunt dependency. All patients were described by 32 features including patient-related (age, gender, ASA, Karnofsky score), disease-related (Hunt-Hess score, GCS, clinical vasospasm), radiological (Fisher, BNI, ICH or IVH, etc.), and treatment-related (aneurysm treatment, treatment timing, treatment complications, etc.).

Sotoudch et al. [88] proposed a ML predictive model for treatment response after shunting NPH patients using radionomics and clinical features. The random forest model provided the best performance in treatment prediction when only clinical data (iNPHGS and Modified Rankin Scale) were considered (AUC = 0.71). The prediction potential of the SVM model was significantly enhanced when radiomics features were taken into account (AUC = 0.8). Augmentation of the model with age and sex did not raise the prediction performance though.

Jeong et al. [89] applied deep learning algorithms for vision-based gait analysis to estimate temporal-spatial gait parameters. In the study, gait performance was investigated before and after cerebrospinal fluid tap test in NPH patients. The quantitative gait data were simultaneously collected from the vision-based gait analysis system using deep learning algorithms for monocular videos and the GAITRite gait analysis system. It was shown the variability of the stride length and time, both measured by the gait analysis algorithm, were correlated with FAB scores.

6 Key Points

- Machine learning is the use and development of computer systems that are able to learn and adapt without following explicit instructions.
- There are four types of ML: supervised, unsupervised, reinforcement, and semi-supervised.
- Among the frequently used ML models are support vector machines (SVM), artificial neural networks (ANN), and decision trees.
- ML model can be under- or over-fitted, either of which leads to inferior results when tested on new data.

7 Funding and Acknowledgements

This chapter was supported by the Ministry of Health of the Czech Republic institutional grant no. NU23-04–00551.

Research outcomes reported in the present chapter were supported by the Charles University Grant Agency (GAUK, 1068120).

References

1. Celtikci E. A systematic review on machine learning in neurosurgery: the future of decision-making in patient care. Turk Neurosurg. 2018;28:167–73. https://doi.org/10.5137/1019-5149. JTN.20059-17.1.
2. Buchlak QD, Esmaili N, Leveque J-C, Farrokhi F, Bennett C, Piccardi M, Sethi RK. Machine learning applications to clinical decision support in neurosurgery: an artificial intelligence augmented systematic review. Neurosurg Rev. 2020;43:1235–53. https://doi.org/10.1007/s10 143-019-01163-8.
3. Taghva A. An automated navigation system for deep brain stimulator placement using hidden Markov models. Neurosurgery 2010;66:108–117. discussion 117. https://doi.org/10.1227/01. NEU.0000365369.48392.E8.
4. Taghva A. Hidden semi-Markov models in the computerized decoding of microelectrode recording data for deep brain stimulator placement. World Neurosurgery. 2011;75:758-763.e4. https://doi.org/10.1016/j.wneu.2010.11.008.
5. Serra A, Fratello M, Cattelani L, Liampa I, Melagraki G, Kohonen P, Nymark P, Federico A, Kinaret PAS, Jagiello K, Ha MK, Choi J-S, Sanabria N, Gulumian M, Puzyn T, Yoon T-H, Sarimveis H, Grafstr¨om R, Afantitis A, Greco D. Transcriptomics in toxicogenomics, Part III: data modelling for risk assessment. Nanomaterials 2020;10:708. https://doi.org/10.3390/nan o10040708.
6. Martın-Guerrero JD, Lamata L. Reinforcement learning and physics. Appl Sci 2021;11. https://doi.org/10.3390/app11188589.
7. Kostopoulos G, Karlos S, Kotsiantis S, Ragos O, Tiwari S, Trivedi M, Kohle ML. Semi-supervised regression: a recent review. J Intell Fuzzy Syst. 2018;35:1483–500. https://doi.org/10.3233/JIFS-169689.
8. Zoli M, Staartjes VE, Guaraldi F, Friso F, Rustici A, Asioli S, Sollini G, Pasquini E, Regli L, Serra C, Mazzatenta D. Machine learning–based prediction of outcomes of the endoscopic endonasal approach in Cushing disease: is the future coming? Neurosurgical Focus FOC. 2020;48:E5. https://doi.org/10.3171/2020.3.FOCUS2060.
9. Ding S, Zhu Z, Zhang X. An overview on semi-supervised support vector machine. Neural Comput Appl. 2015;28:969–78.
10. Bair, E. Semi-supervised clustering methods. Wiley interdisciplinary reviews. Computat. Stat. 2013;5:349–361. https://doi.org/10.1002/wics.1270.
11. Ellingsen LM, Roy S, Carass A, Blitz AM, Pham DL, Prince JL. Segmentation and labeling of the ventricular system in normal pressure hydrocephalus using patch-based tissue classification and multi-atlas labeling. Proc SPIE–the Int Soc Opt Eng. 2016;9784:97840G. https://doi.org/10.1117/12.2216511.
12. Cherukuri V, Ssenyonga P, Warf BC, Kulkarni AV, Monga V, Schiff SJ. Learning based segmentation of CT brain images: application to postoperative hydro-cephalic Scans. IEEE Trans Biomed Eng. 2018;65:1871–1884. https://doi.org/10.1109/TBME.2017.2783305.
13. Gunter NB, Schwarz CG, Graff-Radford J, Gunter JL, Jones DT, Graff- Radford NR, Petersen RC, Knopman DS, Jack CR. Automated detection of imaging features of disproportionately

enlarged subarachnoid space hydrocephalus using machine learn-ing methods. NeuroImage: Clin. 2019;21:101605. https://doi.org/10.1016/j.nicl.2018.11.015.

14. Duan W, Zhang J, Zhang L, Lin Z, Chen Y, Hao X, Wang Y, Zhang H. Evaluation of an artificial intelligent hydrocephalus diagnosis model based on transfer learning. Med. 2020;99:e21229. https://doi.org/10.1097/MD.0000000000021229.

15. Calisto A, Galeano M, Serrano S, Calisto A, Azzerboni B. A new approach for inves- tigating intracranial pressure signal: filtering and morphological features extraction from continuous recording. IEEE Trans Bio-Med Eng. 2013;60:830–837. https://doi.org/10.1109/TBME.2012. 2191550.

16. Calisto A, Bramanti A, Galeano M, Angileri F, Campobello G, Serrano S, Azzerboni B. A preliminary study for investigating idiopatic normal pressure hydrocephalus by means of statistical parameters classification of intracranial pressure recordings. *Annual International Conference of the IEEE Engineering in Medicine and Biology Society*. 2009;2629–2632. https://doi.org/10.1109/IEMBS.2009.5335371.

17. Noble WS. What is a support vector machine? Nat Biotechnol. 2006;24:1565–1567. https://doi.org/10.1038/nbt1206-1565.

18. Hale AT, Riva-Cambrin J, Wellons J. C, Jackson EM, Kestle JRW, Naftel RP, Hankinson TC, Shannon CN. Hydrocephalus clinical research network, machine learning predicts risk of cerebrospinal fluid shunt failure in children: a study from the hydrocephalus clinical research network. Child's Nerv Syst: Official Journal of the International Society for Pediatric Neurosurgery 2021;37:1485–1494. https://doi.org/10.1007/s00381-021-05061-7.

19. Akbari H, Macyszyn L, Da X, Bllello M, Wolf RL, Martinez-Lage M, Biros G, Alonso-Basanta M, O'Rourke DM, Davatzikos C. Imaging surrogates of infiltration obtained via multiparametric imaging pattern analysis predict subsequent location of recurrence of glioblastoma. Neurosurg. 2016.

20. Rau A, Kim S, Yang S, Reisert M, Kellner E, Duman IE, Stieltjes B, Hohenhaus M, Beck J, Urbach H, Egger K. SVM-based normal pressure hydrocephalus detection. Clin Neuroradiol. 2021;31:1029–1035. https://doi.org/10.1007/s00062-020-00993-0.

21. Watts J, Khojandi A, Shylo O, Ramdhani RA. Machine learning's application in deep brain stimulation for parkinson's disease: a review. Brain Sci. 2020;10. https://doi.org/10.3390/brainsci10110809.

22. Azimi P, Benzel EC, Shahzadi S, Azhari S, Mohammadi HR. Use of artificial neural networks to predict surgical satisfaction in patients with lumbar spinal canal stenosis: clinical article. J Neurosurg: Spine. 2014;20:300–305. https://doi.org/10.3171/2013.12.SPINE13674.

23. Benedetto N, Gambacciani C, Aquila F, Di Carlo DT, Morganti R, Perrini P. A new quantitative method to assess disproportionately enlarged subarachnoid space (DESH) in patients with possible idiopathic normal pressure hydrocephalus: the SILVER index. Clin Neurol Neurosurg. 2017;158:27–32. https://doi.org/10.1016/j.clineuro.2017.04.015.

24. Habibi Z, Ertiaei A, Nikdad MS, Mirmohseni AS, Afarideh M, Heidari V, Saberi H, Rezaei AS, Nejat F. Predicting ventriculoperitoneal shunt infection in children with hydrocephalus using artificial neural network. Child's Nerv Syst: Official Journal of the International Society for Pediatric Neurosurgery. 2016;32:2143–2151. https://doi.org/10.1007/s00381-016-3248-2.

25. Jones TL, Byrnes TJ, Yang G, Howe FA, Bell BA, Barrick TR. Brain tumor classification using the diffusion tensor image segmentation (D-SEG) technique. Neuroophthalmol. 2015;17:466–476. https://doi.org/10.1093/neuonc/nou159.

26. Havaei M, Davy A, Warde-Farley D, Biard A, Courville A, Bengio Y, Pal C, Jodoin P-M, Larochelle H. Brain tumor segmentation with deep neural networks. Med Image Anal. 2017;35:18–31. https://doi.org/10.1016/j.media.2016.05.004.

27. Swiercz M, Mariak Z, Krejza J, Lewko J, Szydlik P. Intracranial pressure processing with artificial neural networks: prediction of ICP trends. Acta Neurochir. 2000;142:401–6. https://doi.org/10.1007/s007010050449.

28. Skrobala A, Malicki J. Beam orientation in stereotactic radiosurgery using an artificial neural network. Radiotherapy and Oncol: J Europ Soc Therapeutic Radiol Oncol. 2014;111:296–300. https://doi.org/10.1016/j.radonc.2014.03.010.

29. Shao M, Han S, Carass A, Li X, Blitz AM, Shin J, Prince JL, Ellingsen LM. Brain ventricle parcellation using a deep neural network: application to patients with ventriculomegaly. NeuroImage Clinical 2019;23:101871. https://doi.org/10.1016/j.nicl.2019.101871

30. Jena M, Dehuri S. Decision tree for classification and regression: a state-of-the art review. Informatica 2020;44. https://doi.org/10.31449/inf.v44i4.3023.

31. Abualdenien J, Borrmann A. Ensemble-learning approach for the classification of levels of geometry (LOG) of building elements. Adv Eng Inform 2022;51:101497. https://doi.org/10.1016/j.aei.2021.101497.

32. Cãnete-Sifuentes L, Monroy R, Medina-Pérez MA. A review and experimental comparison of multivariate decision trees. IEEE Access 2021;9:110451–110479. https://doi.org/10.1109/ACCESS.2021.3102239.

33. Gadot R, Anand A, Lovin B, Sweeney A, Patel A. Predicting surgical decision-making in vestibular schwannoma using tree-based machine learning. Neurosurg Focus. 2022;52:E8. https://doi.org/10.3171/2022.1.FOCUS21708.

34. Karhade AV, Thio Q, Ogink P, Kim J, Lozano-Calderon S, Raskin K, Schwab JH. Development of machine learning algorithms for prediction of 5-year spinal chordoma survival. World Neurosurgery. 2018;119:e842–7. https://doi.org/10.1016/j.wneu.2018.07.276.

35. Segato A, Marzullo A, Calimeri F, De Momi E. Artificial intelligence for brain diseases: a systematic review. APL Bioeng. 2020;4:041503. https://doi.org/10.1063/5.0011697.

36. Japkowicz N, Shah M (Eds). In: Evaluating learning algorithms: a classification perspective. Cambridge University Press; 2011.

37. Staartjes VE, Stumpo V, Kernbach JM, Klukowska AM, Gadjradj PS, Schr̈oder ML, Veeravagu A, Stienen MN, van Niftrik CHB, Serra C, Regli L. Machine learning in neurosurgery: a global survey. Acta Neurochirurgica 2020;162:3081–3091. https://doi.org/10.1007/s00701-020-04532-1.

38. Dietterich T. Overfitting and undercomputing in machine learning. ACM Comput Surv. 1995;27:326–7. https://doi.org/10.1145/212094.212114.

39. Azimi P, Mohammadi HR, Benzel EC, Shahzadi S, Azhari S, Montazeri A. Artificial neural networks in neurosurgery. J Neurol Neurosurg Psychiatry. 2015;86:251–6. https://doi.org/10.1136/jnnp-2014-307807.

40. Senders JT, Staples PC, Karhade AV, Zaki MM, Gormley WB, Broekman MLD, Smith TR, Arnaout O. Machine learning and neurosurgical outcome prediction: a systematic review. World Neurosurgery. 2018;109:476-486.e1. https://doi.org/10.1016/j.wneu.2017.09.149.

41. Senders JT, Zaki MM, Karhade AV, Chang B, Gormley WB, Broekman ML, Smith TR, Arnaout O. An introduction and overview of machine learning in neurosurgical care. Acta Neurochir. 2018;160:29–38. https://doi.org/10.1007/s00701-017-3385-8.

42. Juan-Albarracín J, Fuster-Garcia E, Manjón JV, Robles M, Aparici F, Martí-Bonmatí L, García-Gómez JM. Automated glioblastoma segmentation based on a multiparametric structured unsupervised classification. PloS One 2015;10:e0125143. https://doi.org/10.1371/journal.pone.0125143.

43. Johnson AEW, Ghassemi MM, Nemati S, Niehaus KE, Clifton DA, Clifford GD. Machine learning and decision support in critical care. In: Proceedings of the IEEE. Institute of Electrical and Electronics Engineers 2016. p. 104, 444–466. https://doi.org/10.1109/JPROC.2015.2501978. 19

44. Deo RC. Machine learning in medicine. Circulation. 2015;132:1920–30. https://doi.org/10.1161/CIRCULATIONAHA.115.001593.

45. Obermeyer Z, Emanuel EJ. Predicting the future—big data, machine learning, and clinical medicine. N Engl J Med. 2016;375:1216–9. https://doi.org/10.1056/NEJMp1606181.

46. Ghahramani Z. Probabilistic machine learning and artificial intelligence. Nature. 2015;521:452–9. https://doi.org/10.1038/nature14541.

47. Jordan MI, Mitchell TM. In: Machine Learning: Trends, perspectives, and prospects. Science (New York, N.Y.) 2015;349:255–260. https://doi.org/10.1126/science.aaa8415.

48. Pahwa B, Bali O, Goyal S, Kedia S. Applications of machine learning in pediatric hydrocephalus: a systematic review. Neurol India. 2021;69:S380–9. https://doi.org/10.4103/0028-3886.332287.

49. Meier U. The importance of the intrathecal infusion test in the diagnostics of normal pressure hydrocephalus. Biomedizinische Technik Biomed Eng. 2001;46:191–9.

50. Borgesen SE, Gjerris F. Relationships between intracranial pressure, ventricular size, and resistance to CSF outflow. J Neurosurg. 1987;67:535–9. https://doi.org/10.3171/jns.1987.67.4.0535.

51. Kim D-J, Kim H, Kim Y-T, Yoon BC, Czosnyka Z, Park K-W, Czosnyka M. Thresholds of resistance to CSF outflow in predicting shunt responsiveness. Neurol Res. 2015;37:332–40. https://doi.org/10.1179/1743132814Y.0000000454.

52. Mládek A, Gerla V, Skalický P, Vlasák A, Zazay A, Lhotská L, Beneš V, Beneš V, Bradáč O. Prediction of shunt responsiveness in suspected patients with normal pressure hydrocephalus using the lumbar infusion test: a machine learning approach. Neurosurgery 2022;90:407–418. https://doi.org/10.1227/NEU.0000000000001838.

53. Hebb AO, Cusimano MD. Idiopathic normal pressure hydrocephalus: a systematic review of diagnosis and outcome. Neurosurgery 2001;49:1166–1184. discussion 1184–1186. https://doi.org/10.1097/00006123-200111000-00028.

54. Skalický P, Mládek A, Vlasák A, De Lacy P, Beneš V, Bradáč O. Normal pressure hydrocephalus-an overview of pathophysiological mechanisms and diagnostic procedures. Neurosurgical Rev. 2020;43:1451–1464. https://doi.org/10.1007/s10143-019-01201-5.

55. Marmarou A, Bergsneider M, Klinge P, Relkin N, Black PM. The value of supplemental prognostic tests for the preoperative assessment of idiopathic normal-pressure hydrocephalus. Neurosurgery 2005;57:S17–28. discussion ii–v. https://doi.org/10.1227/01.neu.0000168184.01002.60.

56. Ryding E, Kahlon B, Reinstrup P. Improved lumbar infusion test analysis for normal pressure hydrocephalus diagnosis. Brain and Behav. 2018;8:e01125. https://doi.org/10.1002/brb3.1125

57. Kahlon B, Sundbärg G, Rehncrona S. Comparison between the lumbar infusion and SF tap tests to predict outcome after shunt surgery in suspected normal pressure hydrocephalus. J Neurol Neurosurgery and Psychiatry 2002;73:721–726. https://doi.org/10.1136/jnnp.73.6.721.

58. Kahlon B, Sundarg G, Rehncrona S. Lumbar infusion test in normal pressure hydrocephalus. Acta Neurol Scand. 2005;111:379–84. https://doi.org/10.1111/j.1600-0404.2005.00417.x.

59. Walchenbach R, Geiger E, Thomeer R, Vanneste J. The value of temporary external lumbar CSF drainage in predicting the outcome of shunting on normal pressure hydrocephalus. J Neurol Neurosurg Psychiatry. 2002;72:503–6. https://doi.org/10.1136/jnnp.72.4.503.

60. Dai H, Jia X, Pahren L, Lee J, Foreman B. Intracranial pressure monitoring signals after traumatic brain injury: a narrative overview and conceptual data science framework. Front Neurol. 2020;11:959. https://doi.org/10.3389/fneur.2020.00959.

61. Shannon CE. A mathematical theory of communication. The Bell Syst Techn J. 1948;27:379–423. https://doi.org/10.1002/j.1538-7305.1948.tb01338.x,ConferenceName:TheBellSystemTechnicalJournal.

62. Higuchi T. Approach to an irregular time series on the basis of the fractal theory. Physica D. 1988;31:277–83. https://doi.org/10.1016/0167-2789(88)90081-4.

63. Pedregosa F, Varoquaux G, Gramfort A, Michel V, Thirion B, Grisel O, Blondel M, Prettenhofer P, Weiss R, Dubourg V, Vanderplas J, Passos A, Cournapeau D, Brucher M, Perrot M, Duchesnay E. Scikit-learn: machine learning in python. The J Mach Learn Res. 2011;12:2825–30.

64. Vlasak A, Skalicky P, Mladek A, Vrana J, Benes V, Bradac O. Structural volumetry in NPH diagnostics and treatment-future or dead end? Neurosurg Rev. 2021;44:503–14. https://doi.org/10.1007/s10143-020-01245-y.

65. Keong NC, Pena A, Price SJ, Czosnyka M, Czosnyka Z, DeVito EE, Housden CR, Sahakian BJ, Pickard JD. Diffusion tensor imaging profiles reveal specific neural tract distortion in normal pressure hydrocephalus. PloS One 2017;12:e0181624. https://doi.org/10.1371/journal.pone.0181624.

66. Hoza D, Vlasak A, Horınek D, Sames M, Alfieri A. DTI-MRI biomarkers in the search for normal pressure hydrocephalus aetiology: a review. Neurosurgical Rev. 2015;38:239–244. discussion 244. https://doi.org/10.1007/s10143-014-0584-0.

67. Sakhare AR, Barisano G, Pa J. Assessing test-retest reliability of phase contrast MRI for measuring cerebrospinal fluid and cerebral blood flow dynamics. Magn Reson Med. 2019;82:658–70. https://doi.org/10.1002/mrm.27752.

68. Algin O, Hakyemez B, Parlak M. The efficiency of PC-MRI in diagnosis of normal pressure hydrocephalus and prediction of shunt response. Acad Radiol. 2010;17:181–7. https://doi.org/10.1016/j.acra.2009.08.011.

69. Tawfik AM, Elsorogy L, Abdelghaffar R, Naby AA, Elmenshawi I. Phase-contrast MRI CSF flow measurements for the diagnosis of normal-pressure hydrocephalus: observer agreement of velocity versus volume parameters. AJR Am J Roentgenol. 2017;208:838–43. https://doi.org/10.2214/AJR.16.16995.

70. Witthiwej T, Sathira-ankul P, Chawalparit O, Chotinaiwattarakul W, Tisavipat N, Charnchaowanish P. MRI study of intracranial hydrodynamics and ventriculoperitoneal shunt responsiveness in patient with normal pressure hydrocephalus. J Med Assoc Thailand = Chotmaihet Thangphaet 2012;95:1556–1562.

71. Bradley WG. Magnetic resonance imaging of normal pressure hydrocephalus. Semin Ultrasound CT MR. 2016;37:120–8. https://doi.org/10.1053/j.sult.2016.01.005.

72. Vlasak A, Gerla V, Skalicky P, Mladek A, Sedlak V, Vrana J, Whitley H, Lhotska L, Benes V, Benes V, Bradac O. Boosting phase-contrast MRI performance in idiopathic normal pressure hydrocephalus diagnostics by means of machine learning approach. Neurosurg Focus. 2022;52:E6. https://doi.org/10.3171/2022.1.FOCUS21733.

73. Ojala M, Garriga GC. Permutation tests for studying classifier performance. In: 2009 Ninth IEEE international conference on data mining. 2009. p. 908–913. ISSN:–8486. https://doi.org/10.1109/ICDM.2009.108.

74. Bradley WG, Scalzo D, Queralt J, Nitz WN, Atkinson DJ, Wong P. Normal pressure hydrocephalus: evaluation with cerebrospinal fluid flow measurements at MR imaging. Radiology. 1996;198:523–9. https://doi.org/10.1148/radiology.198.2.8596861.

75. Blitz AM, Shin J, Balédent O, Pagé G, Bonham LW, Herzka DA.; Moghekar, A. R.; Rigamonti, D. Does phase-contrast imaging through the cerebral aqueduct predict the outcome of lumbar CSF drainage or shunt surgery in patients with suspected adult hydrocephalus? AJNR Amer J Neuroradiol. 2018;39:2224–2230. https://doi.org/10.3174/ajnr.A5857.

76. Shanks J, Markenroth Bloch K, Laurell K, Cesarini KG, Fahlstr̈om M, Larsson E-M, Virhammar J. Aqueductal CSF stroke volume is increased in patients with idiopathic normal pressure hydrocephalus and decreases after shunt surgery. AJNR American J Neuroradiol. 2019;40:453–459. https://doi.org/10.3174/ajnr.A5972

77. Eide PK, Sorteberg W. Diagnostic intracranial pressure monitoring and surgical management in idiopathic normal pressure hydrocephalus: a 6-year review of 214 patients. Neurosurgery. 2010;66:80–91. https://doi.org/10.1227/01.NEU.0000363408.69856.B8.

78. Eide PK, Sorteberg W. Outcome of surgery for idiopathic normal pressure hydrocephalus: role of preoperative static and pulsatile intracranial pressure. World Neurosurgery. 2016;86:186-193.e1. https://doi.org/10.1016/j.wneu.2015.09.067.

79. Nabbanja E, Czosnyka M, Keong NC, Garnett M, Pickard JD, Lalou DA, Czosnyka Z. Is there a link between ICP-derived infusion test parameters and outcome after shunting in normal pressure hydrocephalus? Acta Neurochir Suppl. 2018;126:229–32. https://doi.org/10.1007/978-3-319-65798-1_46.

80. Qvarlander S, Lundkvist B, Koskinen L-OD, Malm J, Eklund A. Pulsatility in CSF dynamics: pathophysiology of idiopathic normal pressure hydrocephalus. J Neurol Neurosurg Psychiatry. 2013;84:735–41. https://doi.org/10.1136/jnnp-2012-302924.

81. Virhammar J, Laurell K, Cesarini KG, Larsson E-M. Preoperative prognostic value of MRI findings in 108 patients with idiopathic normal pressure hydrocephalus. AJNR Am J Neuroradiol. 2014;35:2311–8. https://doi.org/10.3174/ajnr.A4046.

82. Irie R, Otsuka Y, Hagiwara A, Kamagata K, Kamiya K, Suzuki M, Wada A, Maekawa T, Fujita S, Kato S, Nakajima M, Miyajima M, Motoi Y, Abe O, Aoki S. A novel deep learning approach with a 3D convolutional ladder network for differential diagnosis of idiopathic normal pressure hydrocephalus and Alzheimer's disease. Magnetic Resonance in Med Sci: MRMS: an Official J

Japan Soc Magnet Resonance in Med. 2020;19:351–8. https://doi.org/10.2463/mrms.mp.2019-0106.

83. Wu D, Moghekar A, Shi W, Blitz AM, Mori S. Systematic volumetric analysis predicts response to CSF drainage and outcome to shunt surgery in idiopathic normal pressure hydrocephalus. Eur Radiol. 2021;31:4972–80. https://doi.org/10.1007/s00330-020-07531-z.

84. Schmidt B, Bocklisch SF, Pässler M, Czosnyka M, Schwarze JJ, Klingelh¨ofer J. Fuzzy pattern classification of hemodynamic data can be used to determine noninvasive intracranial pressure. Acta Neurochirurgica. Supplement 2005;95:345–349. https://doi.org/10.1007/3-211-32318-x_71.

85. Galeano M, Calisto A, Bramanti A, Angileri F, Campobello G, Serrano S, Azzerboni B. Classi-fication of morphological features extracted from intracranial pressure recordings in the diag-nosis of normal pressure hydrocephalus (NPH). In: Annual International Conference of the IEEE Engineering in Medicine and Biology Society. 2011. p. 2768–2771.

86. Nucci CG, De Bonis P, Mangiola A, Santini P, Sciandrone M, Risi A, Anile C. Intracra-nial pressure wave morphological classification: automated analysis and clinical validation. Acta Neurochirurgica. 2016;158:581–588. discussion 588. https://doi.org/10.1007/s00701-015-2672-5.

87. Muscas G, Matteuzzi T, Becattini E, Orlandini S, Battista F, Laiso A, Nappini S, Limbucci N, Renieri L, Carangelo BR, Mangiafico S, Della Puppa A. Development of machine learning models to prognosticate chronic shunt-dependent hydrocephalus after aneurysmal subarach-noid hemorrhage. Acta Neurochir. 2020;162:3093–105. https://doi.org/10.1007/s00701-020-04484-6.

88. Sotoudeh H, Sadaatpour Z, Rezaei A, Shafaat O, Sotoudeh E, Tabatabaie M, Singhal A, Tanwar M. The role of machine learning and radiomics for treatment response prediction in idio-pathic normal pressure hydrocephalus. Cureus. 2021;13: e18497. https://doi.org/10.7759/cureus.18497.

89. Jeong S, Yu H, Park J, Kang K. Quantitative gait analysis of idiopathic normal pressure hydro-cephalus using deep learning algorithms on monocular videos. Sci Rep. 2021;11:12368. https://doi.org/10.1038/s41598-021-90524-9.

Treatment and Outcome

Shunt Technology for the Treatment of Hydrocephalus

Christoph Miethke

Abstract Improvement in medical device technology depends on financial aspects, knowledge, creativity, commitment, cooperation and resources. In the best case, concrete tasks come from the clinicians, which are then worked on by technicians in constant dialogue with the clinicians. The completion of such development projects means that a new product is available for clinical use. The decisive milestone in this regard is usually an approval of a medical device. Especially in the field of technology for the treatment of normal pressure hydrocephalus (NPH), the competence to develop proposals for innovations with regard to significant patient benefits lies with technicians, since the understanding of technical possibilities and physical laws of hydraulic systems does not belong to the core competences of neurosurgeons and can only be part of them in exceptional cases. Exactly here seems to be a central challenge regarding the further improvement of shunt systems for the treatment of NPH. This chapter describes shunt technology for the treatment of hydrocephalus, introduces different types of shunt systems available for clinical usage and outlines the future directions of shunt devices development.

Keywords Shunt · Shunt technology · Valves · Hydrocephalus · Normal pressure hydrocephalus · Ventriculoperitoneal shunt · Ventriculoatrial shunt · Lumboperitoneal shunt

Abbreviations

AGV	Gravitational valve
ASD	Anti-siphon device
BMI	Body mass index
CSF	Cerebrospinal fluid
DP	Differential pressure

C. Miethke (✉)
Christoph Miethke GmbH, Potsdam, Germany
e-mail: christoph.miethke@miethke.com

© The Author(s), under exclusive license to Springer Nature Switzerland AG 2023
O. Bradac (ed.), *Normal Pressure Hydrocephalus*,
https://doi.org/10.1007/978-3-031-36522-5_20

DPV   Differential pressure valve
DSV   Dual switch valve
FRD   Flow reduction devices
GCA   Gravity compensating device
ICP   Intracranial pressure
IVP   Intraventricular pressure
LP   Lumboperitoneal
LPV   Low pressure valve
MPV   Medium pressure valve
NPH   Normal pressure hydrocephalus
OSV   Orbis-Sigma-Valve
REM   Rapid eye movement
SA   Shunt assistant
SAR   Subarachnoid space
SCD   Siphon-control device
SG   Siphon-guard
SpR   Space of the spinal canal
VA   Ventriculoatrial
VP   Ventriculoperitoneal

1   Introduction

Although the introduction of shunts was an historical breakthrough in the treatment of hydrocephalus more than 60 years ago, the basic physics is still a matter of controversy. This is reflected by a high number of completely different valve constructions and by the limited clinical evidence for implanted valve types. A conclusion of a clinical study such as "subdural effusions occurred in 71% of patients with a low pressure valve (LPV) shunt and in 34% with an medium pressure valve (MPV) shunt...." [1] is counteracted by a statement by Drake who published the findings that "two new valve designs did not significantly affect shunt failure rates" [2]. However, one of the valve types investigated in Drake's study is said to significantly reduce "the risk of mechanical complications" referring to another study [3].

One explanation for these conflicting statements can be found in the fact that the clinical outcome does not only depend on the valve type but on the disease aetiology, patient's age, shunt type (lumboperitoneal, LP; ventriculoperitoneal, VP; ventriculoatrial, VA), duration of follow-up and surgical aspects. Another explanation is that a clinical study which includes all types of available hardware has never been performed. In addition to these aspects of shunt-based treatment, there is the fact that the evidence for the effectiveness of shunts for the treatment of normal pressure hydrocephalus (NPH) has not been shown until now [4]. At the conference "Hydrocephalus 2022" in Gothenburg Marc Luciano reported a prospective randomised study to be performed which investigates the effectiveness of shunting in a placebo-controlled group of patients diagnosed for NPH. Again at the same conference, the outcome of 12 patients with a new shunt from the ventricles into the sinus after 6 months was reported to have shown lower complication rates than generally reported in the literature [5].

Considering these diverse aspects, the question arises: what is scientifically known about the shunt treatment of hydrocephalus? Is the choice of which valve to be implanted based on a clear understanding of technical features or on the relationship to a company or its representatives or based on the surgical education? "I implant the shunt I was trained on!" How deeply is the fact ongoingly reflected that the surgery takes 30 min to an hour, but the shunt establishes hydraulic conditions for years?

The approach in this chapter is to present some technical facts and the important differences of the available valve systems. There are significant differences leading systematically to different pressure conditions which in the author's opinion is the background for long lasting clinical problems, and severe complaints of many patients which could, at least partially, have been avoided based on careful technical reflection of the used hardware. It is not the author's objective to know everything about hydrocephalus, shunts and shunt technology; however, what is presented is the author's interpretation of the requirements and different proposals for treatment, in order to open discussion about what we understand and what we do not know. The reader's critical interest is highly appreciated.

2 A Manufacturer's Opinion on Shunt Technology

Modern medicine is dominated by technical achievements which have introduced new options for diagnosis and treatment. While the development of drugs is already in early stages [6] based on clinical research, the development of medical devices is focused on solutions proposed by engineers understanding the open tasks, technology and physics.

The situation can be compared to the discussion about the importance of digitalization. There is a group of digital freaks diving deeply into their digital world. On the other hand, there are the experts who have outstanding knowledge on a certain topic (lawyers, physicians, artists....), however these experts have no idea at all about digital technology and only limited understanding for the new opportunities based on digital approaches. Only the lively discussion between these two groups can accelerate digital innovations. Similarly, neither the physicians nor the engineers alone can accelerate digital innovations. Consequently, it should be an important task for leaders in the medical device industry to pay close attention to the ongoing discussion about successes, evidence and the discussion about open questions and unresolved problems during scientific conferences in their field. It should be a question of responsibility to present the scientific basis for their products at these conferences or in scientific journals. Up until now, the priority of technology has too often only focused on selling products. Too often, industry engagement is reduced to marketing presentations. In addition to the considerations of clinical findings, scientific, physical and technical arguments should be responsibly presented by scientists from the industry.

At the conference "Hydrocephalus 2022" in Gothenburg, there was a session about technical advances in treatment and diagnostics [7]. Whereas the first speaker claimed that neurosurgeons have been accepting and using findings and improvements over the past decades, and the second speaker complained about the lack of progress and innovations over the past decades. These two contradictory statements surprisingly did not lead to excited discussions. However, the discussion should be led by people with competence in the field of technical solutions for the treatment of hydrocephalus and people who present new concepts and ideas but even more important, who present improved products for clinical use.

In the history of valve development, there have been numerous projects which failed completely. One can find two different types of failed projects. The first type is represented by people who investigated only principles without including thoughts about product development. They clearly undervalue the difficulties to develop functioning products based on ideas which actually can be implanted and clinically used. A typical example is the proposal for an adjustable anti-siphon device (ASD) [8]. These innovations describe basically an idea, but not at all the real solution. Such proposals are far away from clinical use. In the vast majority of cases, these innovations are discussed during conferences academically, called to be promising proposals and are soon after forgotten [9]. Whether or not, these new thoughts were promising but deeply unrealistic or not at all feasible is an open question. One problem is always the funding of the development. In these cases, obviously nobody has been willing to invest the money needed to develop a product. Sometimes not even the inventor really trusts the value of their own invention. It is easy to talk about opinions. It is challenging to invest and risk private money.

Another type of failed innovation actually is not innovative at all. Well-known principles are presented in a different technical design. No additional new advantage for the treatment is introduced but only another competitive product. An example in the field of shunts for the treatment of hydrocephalus is the so-called diamond valve [10], which is a silicone slit valve without any improvement for the hydraulic management of shunts in contrast to existing solutions (in this case flow reducing devices). In this group the motivation for the development is simply based on financial interest. Another example is the so-called Beverly valve which was presented by a French company announcing a new solution; however, the basic principle was a kind of ASD which works systematically depending on the undefined subcutaneous pressure, consequently without predictable characteristics [11]. This is well known as a significant weak point of ASDs [12] and consequently the decisive knock-out criteria.

All over the world, the requirements for the approval of new products are becoming increasingly difficult and elaborated. The general approach is to ensure that only safe and reliable products are available for clinical use, and consequently, the best technology is offered to the patients. Within the scientific community, the effort to achieve approval is generally completely undervalued. Nowadays, it is not difficult to invent new solutions. The approval, however, is the long-distance run and the decisive obstacle. There is no international acceptance regarding the approval of medical devices. One has to claim for the approval country by country. The international acceptance would facilitate the situation without serious risks.

Many of the innovative medical devices are not based on ideas of physicians but technicians. It is reasonable that companies have to invest the money to develop new products promising improvement at the end for the patients in terms of treatment or diagnosis. All over the world, the only chance to establish new products for clinical use is if a company invests the money needed for development and approval. The approval contains clinical data which confirm the theory. However, these data should be collected financially and scientifically independent of the influence of a company. It should be of public interest to investigate new products if the concept is based on convincing scientific arguments. These arguments should be presented at scientific conferences based on scientific rules and facts. Unfortunately, the independent clinical research is often based on financial marketing interest of medical device companies and not on clinical evidence. Therefore, the benefit of these investigations is simply focusing on the company's interest and not on the scientific value [13].

3   Function of Shunts

The introduction of shunts for treatment of hydrocephalus was an historical breakthrough for paediatric hydrocephalus. Soon after, the importance of shunts was also seen for adult hydrocephalus of different aetiologies. However the reliable lowering of the intracranial pressure is a life-saving solution for newborns, patients with NPH do not have a problem with overpressure. Nevertheless, for all patients who undergo shunt surgery, the principle is the same. A shunt establishes an artificial hydraulic connection between a compartment physiologically filled with cerebrospinal fluid (CSF) and another compartment within the body by the implantation of a device. In any case, the goal of this intervention is to interfere with the pressure or the pressure dynamics within the CSF system. The characteristic of the artificial connection defines the resulting pressure dynamics within the CSF system. Consequently, the characteristic of a valve defines the function of a shunt, but additionally as well the dimension (length, inner diameter) and the location of the entrance to the CSF system and the location of the exit (where the CSF is drained to).

The CSF formed in the lateral ventricles is transported further within the CSF system by means of the ependyma lining the ventricular walls. However, the CSF flow is mainly due to the ventricular CSF production and the arterial pulse wave, which propagates into the CSF space [14]. From the inner ventricular system, the CSF finally reaches the subarachnoid space via the foramina Luschke and the foramen Magendie. The outflow from the subarachnoid space occurs mainly via the granulations arachnoideae, which are also called Pacchioni's granulations. These are structures reminiscent of cauliflowers in appearance, which protrude into the central venous vessel and through which the CSF is released into the venous blood. In adults, the CSF system has a volume of 120 to 150 ml. Approximately, 23 ml per hour is used as a reference value for the average CSF production in adults. The CSF volume in the two side ventricles is around 20–30 ml in healthy adults, the III. and IV. ventricles contain about 5 ml each, 25 ml fills the subarachnoid space with the cisterns and another 75 ml fills the spinal section of the cerebrospinal fluid system [15].

The volume distribution in the compartments of the CSF system, which are connected by narrow channels, suggests that they are of great importance for dynamic intracranial pressure processes, especially when considering the locally different levels of compliance. The pressure in the CSF system is kept within narrow limits by the balance between CSF production and CSF resorption. CSF production is relatively constant, independent of blood pressure, while absorption into the venous blood depends on the venous pressure. The range of physiological intracranial pressure is below 13 cmH_2O. The scientific literature has repeatedly debated the limits of physiological intracranial pressure, particularly with regard to its position dependence [16–19]. For the lying position, a mean intracranial pressure of about 13 cmH_2O (13 mbar) above the ambient pressure is assumed to be the typical mean value, although there are sometimes significant deviations [20]. For ethical reasons, historical measurements on healthy volunteers are unimaginable today. However, the values determined at the time still appear plausible today [21]. The historical measurements on healthy volunteers did not include measurements in a standing position [20]. It is generally assumed that the normal intracranial pressure is due to spinal compliance. This means that pressure increases in the spinal canal due to changes in position lead to a rapid uptake of CSF and consequently to a significant drop in intraventricular pressure, at least temporarily. Whether this is always the case as a physiological phenomenon, whether the pressure initially falls and then remains low, or whether the spinal canal is continuously filled by CSF production and the intraventricular pressure increases again until physiological absorption finally resumes, remains to be seen. Considering the volume of the different compartments and the related compliance as well as the dimensional individual variation of the connecting foramina, it becomes obvious that the posture-dependent dynamic change of the pressure within the different compartments might be very different from human to human (Fig. 1).

A shunt inserted into one or several compartments of the CSF system and connected to another compartment within the body affects both the dynamic pressure as well as the absolute pressure within the system. The change depends on the location of the CSF extraction and into which compartment the CSF is diverted.

Nowadays, as a first choice, the CSF is drained into the abdominal cavity. In addition, the derivation into the venous system, into the pleural space, or the subgaleal region [22] is clinically performed. The main reason for the preference of shunting into the abdomen is the risk for the patient in case of an infection. An infection of the peritoneum is less dangerous than the infection within the blood system and it leads to a lower mortality [23]. Long-term follow-up revealed the fact of severe complications due to thrombosis [24]. If shunted into the venous system, the first choice is the atrium of the right heart. There are only limited papers about the superiority of atrial shunts in comparison with abdominal shunts [25]. A second option is the

Fig. 1 Graphic representation of the volume distribution of the CSF (S: lateral ventricle, III.: third ventricle, IV.: fourth ventricle, SAR: subarachnoid space, SpR: space of the spinal canal). The ratio of the areas of the squares corresponds to the ratios of the designated volumes

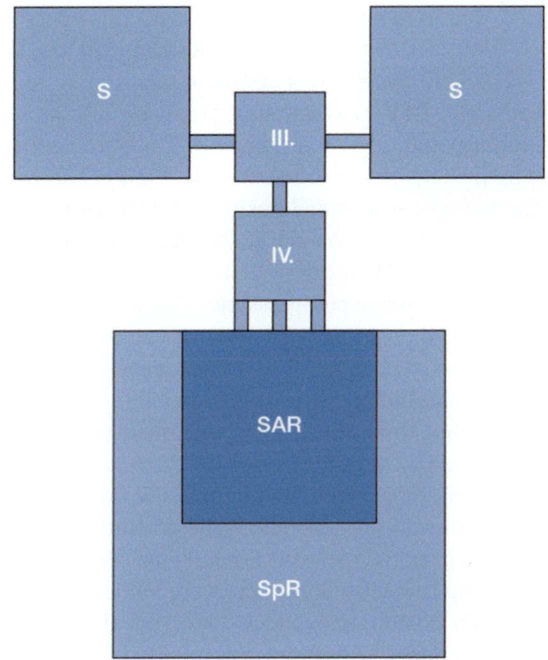

drainage into the sinus. There are several different proposals, generally it is seen to be more physiological [26–28]. Although these approaches produce repeatedly excited discussion during scientific conferences [29, 30], they have never been successfully introduced into clinical practice.

If technically the same shunt is implanted, the resulting pressure within the CSF system will be significantly different. Vice versa, a shunt being sufficient for a drainage into the abdomen is likely not necessarily sufficient for a drainage into another compartment. Very often, the valve within a shunt system is seen as a single component establishing an intracranial pressure (ICP) within the shunt system. It is the truth however, that the physics of the whole shunt defines the outcome and has to be understood for the choice of the valve.

The most often implanted shunt is the VP shunt. Normally, the tip of the ventricular catheter is placed within one of the side ventricles. Whether the ventricular catheter is placed parietally, occipitally or frontally has no impact on the result of the shunt. In any case, an artificial connection from the side ventricle to the abdominal cavity is created. If there is no stenosis between the different compartments of the CSF system (communicating hydrocephalus), the physical situation is even the same for a LP shunt or a connection between the III. ventricle or the IV. ventricle and the abdomen. This is not particularly true for an LP shunt when there is a stenosis restricting outflow between the spinal canal and the cranial ventricular system. The implantation of an LP shunt is definitely dangerous in the case of an aqueduct stenosis, since in this case, due to the considerable pressure difference between the spinal canal and the III. ventricles or the side ventricles can lead to a herniation of the cerebellum [31].

The CSF system is a complex physical system which is affected by breathing, heart rate, CSF production, CSF absorption as well as physical activity (running, jumping) and, above all, posture. The complexity can be illustrated and discussed with the help of simplified models. Figure 2 shows a box which is filled with a fluid (for example water) and positioned differently. The walls of the box are not elastic. Due to the gravity on earth, a hydrostatic pressure that depends on the position of the box is established.

The fluid is not compressible. The walls are stiff. There is no volume shift due to the changed position of the box. However, the hydrostatic pressure is changing with the positional change. This is true regardless of the absolute pressure within the box. The differential pressure at the lowest point within the vertical box is much higher than within the horizontally positioned box. This means that the highest pressure within the box is at the bottom of the box in the vertical position.

Exactly this is true for the pressure within the CSF system. The pressure at the different locations depends on the posture. In the lying position, the pressure within the ventricles and the spine is nearly the same, whereas a human in an upright position shows significantly higher pressure values if a steady state is achieved. This might lead to a posture-dependent flow from the ventricles into the spine depending on the compliance within these compartments and the hydraulic resistance within the connecting channels. Due to the low volumes within the different compartments of the CSF system, the steady state of posture depending on pressure changes should nearly immediately be established after postural changes. The principle is shown in Fig. 3. The model differs from Fig. 2 in so far as now there are two elastic windows within the walls of the box. The elastic deformation of the box depends on the pressure acting on the window.

In the vertical position, the deformation of the elastic parts of the walls is the lowest if the box is horizontally positioned. The pressure difference within the box is the lowest (dp2). The volume shift remains minimal. It becomes significant in the fully upright position of the box. Whereas the model of Fig. 3 demonstrates the principles within the CSF system, Fig. 4 is closer to the pressure changes within

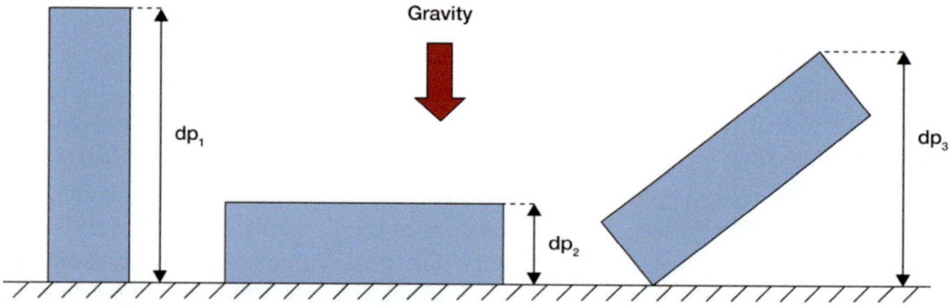

Fig. 2 Modelling hydrostatic pressure depending on the position of a box with stiff walls

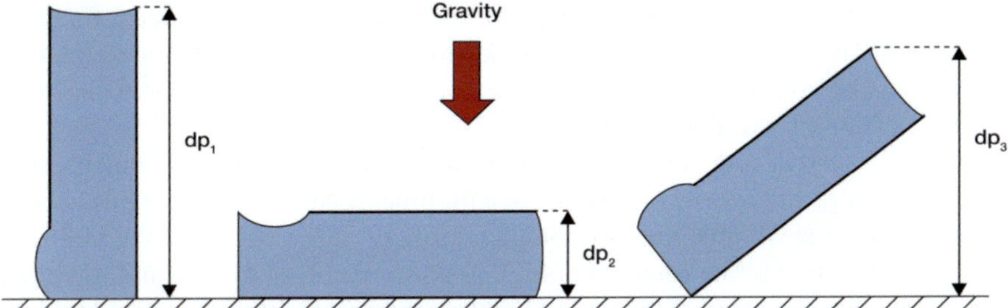

Fig. 3 Modelling hydrostatic pressure depending on the position with elastic walls of the box

the abdominal cavity. Both models help to understand and discuss the functioning of a shunt. The volumes of the compartment of the CSF system are very low. The consequence is that a shunt easily allows the drainage of the whole volume several times per hour. This means that without a valve, a shunt would introduce an artificial compartment to the CSF system dramatically defining the resulting pressures.

The compliance of the box in Fig. 3 is significantly lower than within those shown in Fig. 4. One side of the box is completely elastic, which leads to a significant volume shift if the position is changed from horizontal to the vertical position. The higher pressure in the lower part as well as the lower pressure in the upper part of the box is the reason why the bigger part of the fluid volume is now moving into the lower part of the box.

The purpose of a shunt is to withdraw fluid from the CSF system and thereby consequently lower the CSF pressure. A small withdrawal of CSF leads to significant changes of this pressure. A withdrawal of even a minimal amount of fluid would not be possible from the box with stiff walls (Fig. 2). The box with a compliance (Fig. 3) would allow a limited withdrawal of fluid with only moderate pressure changes. However, such an amount of fluid drained into the box with a large elastic sidewall (Fig. 4) would not change the pressure situation due to the enormous compliance of the system. Whereas the pressure within the abdominal cavity is posture-dependent, the pressure of the atrium of the right heart is less affected by postural changes. CSF

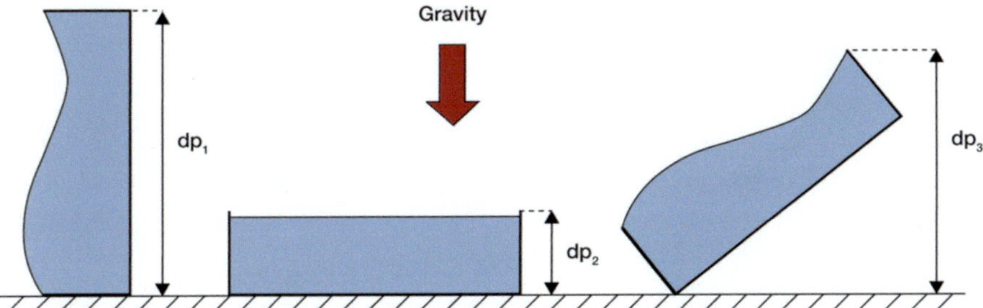

Fig. 4 Modelling hydrostatic pressure depending on the position within a box with flexible walls

can be drained into either the abdomen or the atrium of the right heart in a sufficiently controlled manner. However, the posture-dependent changes in relation to the CSF system must be considered. This is true for both the location of withdrawal of CSF and the location of introduction of CSF.

The CSF system is a sensitively balanced hydraulic circulation, which establishes physiological pressure situations for a lifetime. A shunt influences this balance dramatically. In newborns, the physiological growth of the skull and the brain can be horribly disturbed. The problem of high pressure is solved by implanting a shunt with a DPV, but the price of this is too low pressures in the upright position. Overdrainage in shunted toddlers can happen for different reasons. Possibly the most important one is posture related over-drainage in the upright position even for a couple of minutes. In this situation, the components of the skull are in contact too early. Due to this contact, the bone components grow together earlier than what is physiologically normal with the consequence that the intracranial volume available for the physiological growth of the brain is too small (Fig. 5).

Thickening of the skull is well documented as one possible consequence of overshunting in early childhood. The mechanisms of bone growing described in the literature [32, 33] are complex. However, the background and mechanism leading to thickening of the skull in some patients is still not understood. The following thesis may stimulate alternative explanations and scientific investigations on the subject.

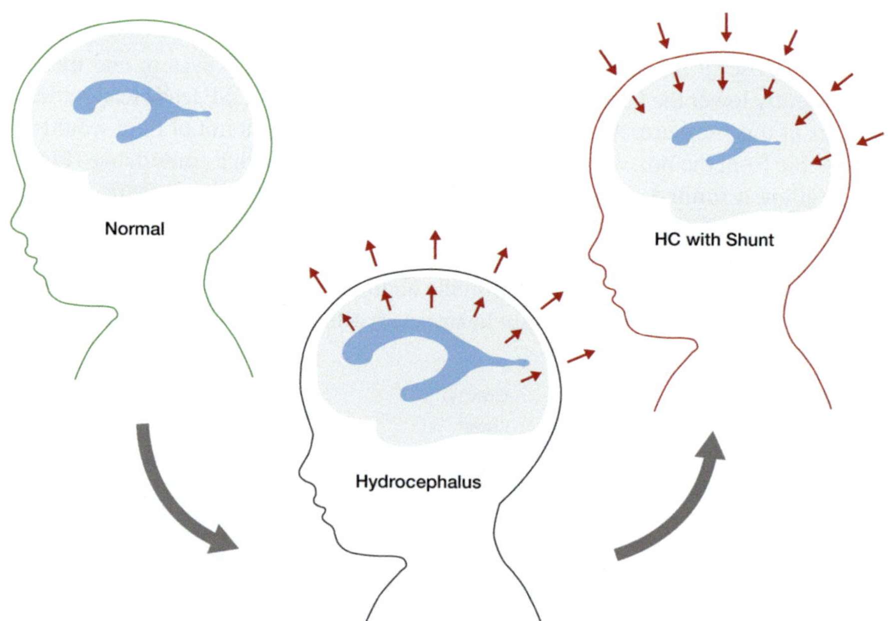

Fig. 5 Development of hydrocephalus: before shunting abnormal growth, after over-shunting, skull becomes smaller than normal. The intracranial volume is too small for the growing brain

Physiologically there is no tension within the skull, because the parts of the bone are not connected. Due to the shrinking of the head circumference after shunting, the bone components are in contact earlier than physiologically intended and start to grow together. This early closure of the skull changes the normal mechanical situation completely. Normally, there is no tension at all within the bone components of the skull. Based on the growth of the brain requiring more intracranial space, the bone starts thickening to lower the tension within its structure. The opposite reaction is known in artificial hip joints, where the metallic stem within the femur lowers the stress within the cortical bone with the consequence of osteolysis [34]. While in artificial hip joints, the cortical bone begins to thin due to stress relaxation, and in shunted newborns, the bone starts thickening to lower artificial tension. More intracranial space is needed for the growing brain, and the thickening of the skull leads to the opposite result; the intracranial space is lowered by the bone growing partially into the cranium. As a long-term consequence, the intracranial space becomes filled with brain tissue at the expense of the CSF-filled intracranial components. Slit-like ventricles are going to be established with a long-term consequence of the development of a slit-ventricle syndrome which occurs many years after the responsible shunt has been implanted [35–41]. The shunt establishing a non-physiological pressure for many years is often seen as the best shunt, because it worked for many years without serious complaints. However, this shunt is the reason for severe problems for shunted adolescents and young adults (Fig. 6).

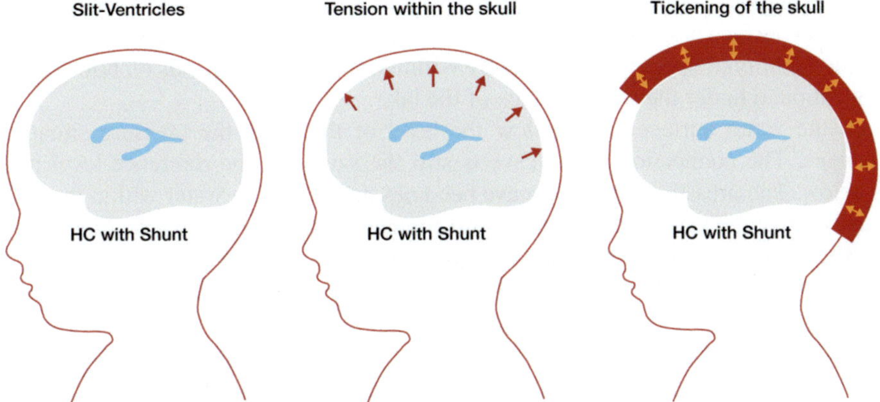

Fig. 6 Dilemma of over-drainage in shunted newborns: early closure of the skull leads consequently to thickening of the skull

4 Hydrostatic Pressure and the Siphon Effect

The problem of over-drainage has been recognised ever since the first shunts were implanted successfully for the treatment of hydrocephalus. Since these early days, over-drainage was and partially still is seen as a complication which is acceptable in comparison with the outstanding importance of the pioneering success of shunts. The explanation of this kind of complication is widely seen in the so-called siphon effect.

The siphon effect describes a specific hydraulic system. To understand the siphon effect, it is necessary to understand hydrostatic pressure. The principle of the hydrostatic pressure explains and describes why the water level of a lake is flat regardless of the shape of the lake. At the surface of the lake, the pressure is everywhere the same. Based on this aspect, the pressure within the lake in the same depth is everywhere the same. The hydrostatic pressure depends only on the depth, the density of the fluid (in case of the lake water) and the gravity. The gravity index is constant as well as the density of the water. Water is not compressible. Accordingly, the hydrostatic pressure within a lake depends only on the depth. Figure 7 shows vessels of different shapes. The pressure within the vessels is in all cases the same, only depending on the depth. The deeper the point of interest, the higher the pressure is.

Just as hydrostatic pressure increases with a deeper point of interest, the opposite is true as well. At a less deep point of interest, the hydrostatic pressure is lower. If the pressure at the surface is the atmospheric pressure, the hydrostatic pressure can even be below it, consequently negative. Figure 8 shows a picture of a lake. Under the water surface is an opening connected to a cave. The cave is filled with water and has no additional opening. The pressure within the cave just depends on how deep it is positioned under the water surface of the lake.

If the water surface sinks below the level of the cave, the pressure situation changes. The connection to the cave is still the same but the reference level now is below. The pressure within the cave becomes negative. The water within the cave cannot leave the cave because there is no connection to the atmospheric pressure.

The understanding of the hydrostatic pressure facilitates the understanding of the siphon effect. Although it is obvious that the surface of a lake defines the reference

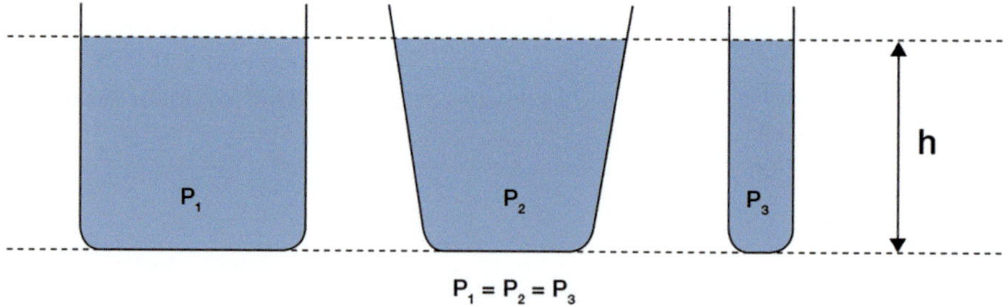

Fig. 7 Hydrostatic pressure depending on the depth only

a

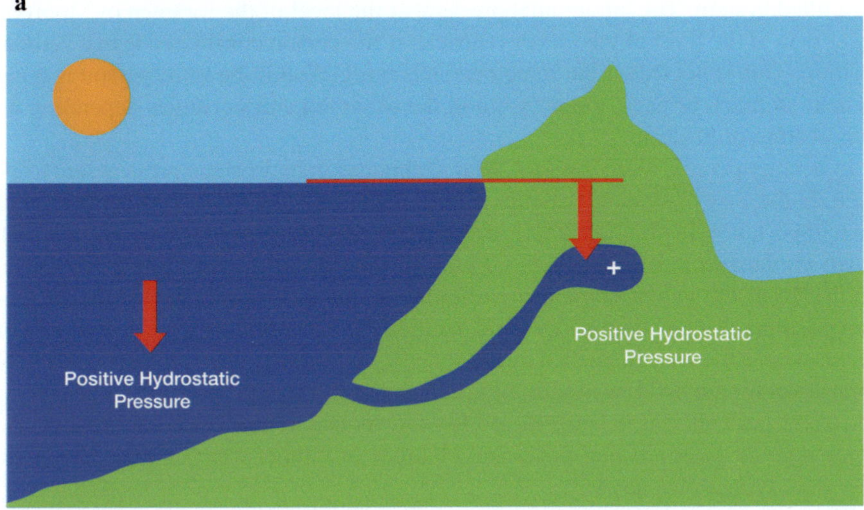

b

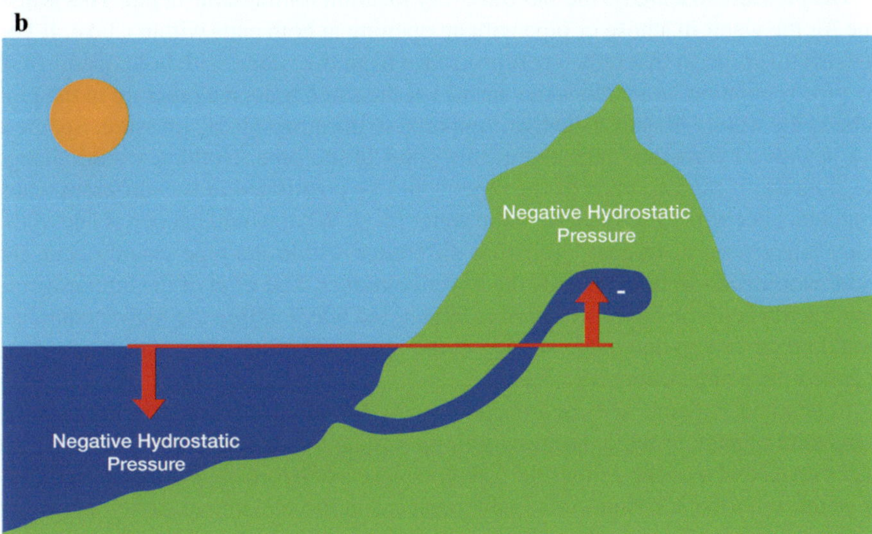

Fig. 8 **a** Water filled cave under the water surface of the ocean. **b** Water filled cave above the water surface of the ocean

level regarding the hydrostatic pressure within a lake, it is more challenging to determine the reference level within a shunted patient. However, the physical principle to analyse the situation is the same. The physiological intraventricular pressure is known to be between − 5 cm of water (vertical) and 18 cm of water (supine). Above or below theses values, the intraventricular pressure is pathological [20]. To interpret these values, it is necessary to know the location of the values. Within a physiological ventricular system filled with CSF, there is a hydrostatic pressure gradient like in any fluid filled system. The intracranial pressure at the level of the foramen of Monro is lower than at the level of the fourth ventricle, if the person considered is in a vertical position. This is not true if the same person is lying. And if the same person is lying on their stomach or back, the pressure in the observed areas changes depending on their posture or position.

In healthy people, these position-related changes in hydrostatic pressure are irrelevant. In the case of shunted patients, on the other hand, the same consideration is of great importance. In principle, this is true regardless of the type of shunt (VA, VP, LP). When implantation of shunts was introduced into the treatment of hydrocephalus, the design of the valves contained within these shunts simply reflected the recumbent position of the patient under consideration. The first shunts were developed for infants whose life was threatened by hydrocephalus and who were almost exclusively lying down for the first few months of life. Against this background, the vertical position of the patients was not considered further. As late as the 1990s, most paediatric neurosurgeons believed that positional changes in infants were unimportant since they were lying down anyway.

The pressure in a lake is the same at every location for the same depth. This is also true for the water in a hose or pipe with an opening at both ends within a lake. If you now lift this pipe so that only a part protrudes from the water, with both openings of the pipe remaining under the water surface at the same time, the pressure in the pipe outside the water becomes negative compared to the atmospheric pressure. So, there is a negative hydrostatic pressure at this point in the pipe. Nothing would change the situation if the two ends of the pipe would be positioned in two different water containers but with exactly at the same water level. What would happen if one of the water tanks were lowered? A pressure difference within the pipe would occur, the water would start to flow towards the lower container. The level of the higher would sink, the level of the lower would rise. In fact, the water within the higher container would be moved up due to the suction at the other end of the pipe. This mechanism is called the siphon effect (Fig. 9).

In shunted patients with hydrocephalus, by far more important is the postural dependent change in the pressure within the implanted drainage system. While the water surface of the lake defines the reference level for hydrostatic pressure in a body of water, with the VP shunt this is the pressure in the abdominal cavity. However, the pressure conditions in the abdomen are not as static as in a lake. The reference point and the associated pressure in the abdominal cavity depend crucially on the

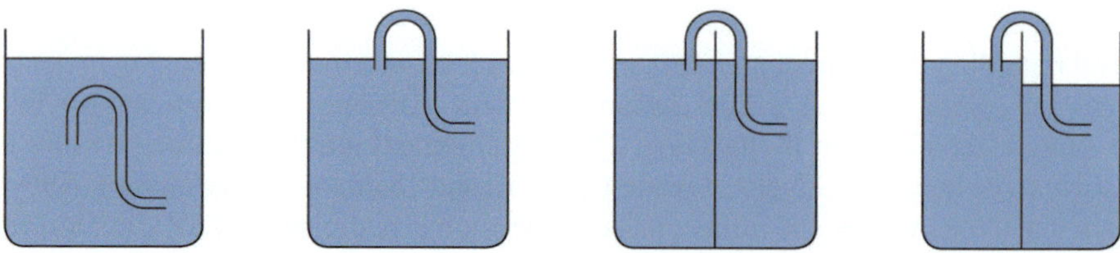

Fig. 9 Siphon effect and the negative hydrostatic pressure in a pipe connecting two water containers

position. In the horizontal position of the patient, the zero level (reference level) corresponds to the highest point of the skin. Lying on the back, this corresponds to the surface of the stomach, lying on the stomach corresponds to the level of the surface of the back. This assessment is based on the assumption that although the pressure situation in the peritoneum can be temporarily increased by muscle tension, it cannot be reduced; on average, however, the pressure situation in the abdomen corresponds to a container filled with water up to the highest skin surface. In the upright position, the reference point migrates to the upper part of the abdomen. Vertically, the reference point (zero level: the peritoneal pressure is equal to the atmospheric pressure) varies more depending on individual anatomic structures and personal circumstances such as body mass index (BMI) or physical condition. However, it seems reasonable to use the lowest point of the sternum as a reference point when standing.

Based on direct measurement there are no data reported in the literature about the intra- abdominal pressure. However, measurements in the bladder have been shown to represent the intra-abdominal pressure convincingly under certain circumstances. It is important that the bladder is filled with some urine but without leading to an elastic tension within the bladder tissue [42–44].

It is possible to measure the intra-abdominal pressure in shunted patients indirectly by using a telemetric transducer. As the intraventricular pressure (IVP) is based on the intra-abdominal pressure in shunted patients, the measurement of the IVP allows the calculation of the reference level within the abdominal cavity. For sure, this is true only for a correctly working valve and the knowledge of its performance characteristic. The measured value of the IVP as a steady state in the lying or standing position represents the abdominal pressure, if the opening pressure of the valve is subtracted. Concretely, if a telemetric sensor [45] is used, which is positioned within a reservoir, the measured value allows to calculate the abdominal pressure. As an example, if the pressure for the standing position is measured with a frontally implanted telemetric pressure transducer with − 5 cm of water and a valve is implanted with an opening pressure of 25 cm of water, the reference level can be calculated by subtracting the opening pressure from the measured value. The zero level in this case would be approximately 30 cm vertically below the reservoir. Though this value is not exact, such measurements, however, could be very valuable to learn more about the range of values in vivo and possibly to learn about complications. Such an investigation could significantly improve the general understanding of the functioning of shunts and shed light on the importance and physical principle of the abdominal pressure in shunt success.

In any shunt, the siphoning occurs depending on the posture. However, the siphoning is not the reason for any kind of over-drainage or other complication. Rather, the systematic reason for over-drainage lies in the hydrostatic pressure within the shunt system that arises due to its position. Figure 10 demonstrates the difference for the case with or without a siphoning effect and the same hydrostatic pressure acting on the system. The control of the flow regulating the filling of the water level in both containers is based on exactly the same physical principle, the hydrostatic pressure. In this way, the term "Siphon effect" is confusing.

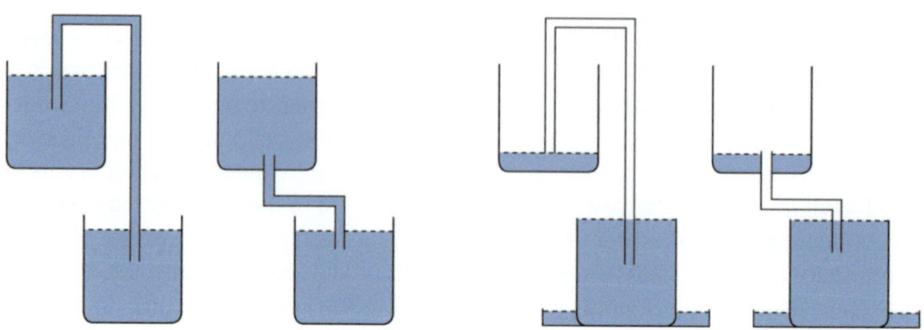

Fig. 10 Comparison of the hydrostatic pressure with and without siphoning: both upper containers empty to the same filling level

The situation is similar when comparing VP shunts with LP shunts. The hydrostatic pressure is relevant wherever there is a hydraulic connection between different compartments. In VP shunts, it is always the connection of the CSF system with the abdomen. It does not matter how the connection is made, whether it is along the spinal canal and then along a tube, or directly from the ventricle along a tube into the abdomen, it makes no difference. The only decisive question is whether there is an open connection between the different compartments. In case of aqueductal stenosis, there might still be a connection; however, the flow is limited throughout the stenosis. Clinically this difference has an outstanding importance.

In Japan, it has become more and more popular to implant a LP shunt in patients with NPH [46, 47]. The lumboperitoneal derivation was viewed critically, mainly because of the risk of cerebellar herniation, especially in hydrocephalus with aqueductal stenosis. Due to the successful implantation of VP shunts, LP shunts were only used in exceptional cases. The background to the renaissance of LP shunts in Japan was obviously a question of finding alternatives to the VP shunt to avoid access to the CSF system in the head area with impairment of the brain.

To discuss the key differences in shunts, it is helpful to consider their operating principle without a valve. Understanding what would happen without a valve informs what the valve should do. While a valve was definitely necessary in the first VA shunts to prevent backflow of blood into the ventricles, a valve did not have the same importance in VP shunts, especially in patients with NPH. The strategy of implanting an adjustable valve with an initial high setting of up to 20 cm of water was simply based on the fear of over-drainage in the upright position of the patient. Reflux of fluids from the abdomen into the ventricular system of the brain is not as dangerous as reflux of blood. However, an artificial hydraulic connection between the ventricular CSF system without an integral valve physically interacts with the valve. The valveless shunt defines flow through the shunt more than most implanted valves. This is especially true for adjustable or non- adjustable DPVs.

As demonstrated in the model in Fig. 10, there is no difference between the hydraulic system between LP and VP shunts statically. However, the flow along the two systems is entirely different. Interestingly, this difference is especially important when the patient is in a vertical position. In the horizontal position, the differential pressure between the ventricular system and the abdomen is not dangerous. Shunted without a valve the resulting IVP can be above and hardly below the atmospheric pressure. Figure 11 shows the ventricular system in principle. The area represents the volumes of the different compartments.

Most of the CSF volume is located in the spinal canal. Only small volumes are found in the third and fourth ventricles. The two lateral ventricles each contain about one-third of the spinal volume. The compartments are connected to the spinal canal. The side ventricles via the short foramen of Monro to the third ventricle, the third ventricle via the aqueduct to the fourth ventricle. In each of the ventricles, the withdrawal of fluid leads to a corresponding change of pressure in the other compartments depending on the compliance. High compliance means that limited withdrawal hardly changes the pressure within the chamber of withdrawal. Withdrawal of fluid from a compartment with low compliance changes the pressure immediately and consequently in the connected compartments. The range and the time shift depend on the dimension of the connecting canal and the volume of withdrawal.

The comparison of the flow through an LP shunt and a VP shunt does not show significant differences in the horizontal position. Even without a valve such a shunt allows only a limited outflow due to the pressure difference between the two connected compartments. The CSF mainly produced from the choroid plexus in the two side ventricles passes along the third and the fourth ventricle, flowing into the spinal canal from where it is drained into the abdomen in case a LP shunt is implanted. If a VP shunt is implanted, the CSF is going to be drained directly from the place

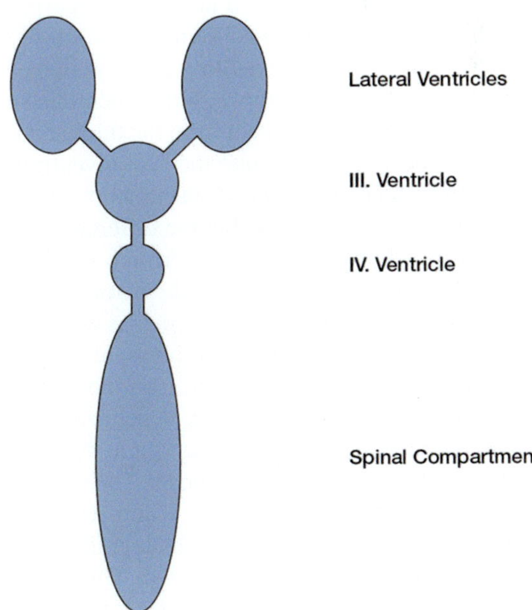

Fig. 11 Scheme of the ventricular CSF system

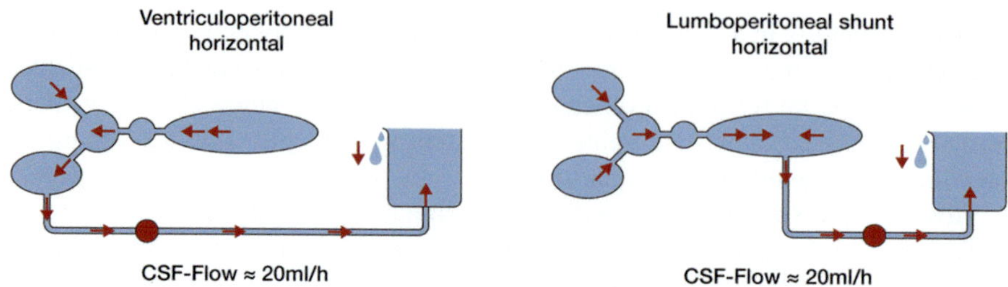

Fig. 12 Comparison of LP shunt and VP shunt for the horizontal position

of its origin along the shunt into the abdomen. For the lying position, it is hardly possible to imagine that there is a significant difference between the two different drainage methods. The volume of CSF being produced is going to be drained along the shunt in both cases without a significant decrease of the pressure within the CSF system below the atmospheric pressure because there is no driving force, no hydrostatic pressure artificially established within the system. Based on this consideration, a patient with NPH could clearly take a benefit from a valveless shunt (Fig. 12).

The situation is markedly different when the patient is in a vertical position. Here, too, drainage and pressure response depend on the compliance of the affected compartment. In contrast to the horizontal position, the possible drainage volume can be much higher depending on the hydrostatic pressure as a measure of the patient's body size. The key difference between the LP shunt and the VP shunt in the upright position is the dynamic change following a change in the patient's posture. The static end result is again the same. If no valve is incorporated in the shunt and the drainage in both cases has reached a constant flow (corresponding to CSF production of about 20 ml per hour), then the resulting pressure in the ventricular system is the same for both methods. However, the way in which this situation is established is different. In VP drainage, CSF is drawn from the third and fourth ventricles, the subarachnoid space and the spinal canal into the lateral ventricle where the ventricular catheter is placed. From there, it is drained via the shunt into the abdominal cavity. The resistance between and compliance within the different compartments, as well as the stiffness of the surrounding brain tissue, determine whether, when, and how quickly the lateral ventricles collapse, a hygroma or hematoma develops and negative pressure builds up, leading to clinical limitations such as dizziness, headache or nausea.

As stated, the static resulting pressure condition for LP shunts is the same as soon as a steady state is achieved, and the production rate is equal to the drainage along the shunt. But the posture-dependent change reveals more risk depending on the individual structure of the whole system. Most dangerous is the case of a complete or partial aqueduct stenosis. The withdrawal of fluid from the spinal canal immediately causes the pressure within this compartment to decrease. Hereby a pressure gradient is established which pulls the upper part of the brain downwards. An upper brain herniation is created. This mechanism is the background for the fact that the LP shunt was not popular for decades especially in patients with NPH. Nowadays, patients with an aqueduct stenosis are treated endoscopically. With open foramina and an open aqueduct, the LP shunt does not introduce from a physical point of view more risk than the VP shunt. Against this background, the Japanese approach to choose the LP shunt more often again is understandable. However, for the LP shunt as well as for the VP shunt, the problem of the posture-dependent hydrostatic pressure has to be solved by a valve integrated into the shunt system. Without the compensation of the hydrostatic pressure, non-physiological low values can lead to severe complications like bleeding, slit ventricles, shift of the midline of the brain or other clinical complications (Fig. 13).

In summary, it should be emphasised that it is not the siphon effect but the systematically occurring hydrostatic pressure within the peritoneal drainage and to a lesser extent within the atrial drainage which is the real problem or the central task for the valves to be integrated into the shunt system. The high number of parameters such as individual circumstances and anatomical structures could explain the very different clinical outcomes after shunt with different valve types. Consideration of a valveless shunt clearly demonstrates the physical principle of the shunt and helps to define the requirements for the integrated valves. The fact that patients with NPH usually do not have aqueductal stenosis is what allows successful implantation of LP shunts in this patient group. However, hydrostatic pressure in the vertical position must be considered. In addition, complications and their explanation should take into account the reflection of the flow direction from the site of CSF production, essentially the choroid plexus in the lateral ventricles, to the abdominal cavity, as well as the different compliance and volumes in the different compartments (Fig. 14).

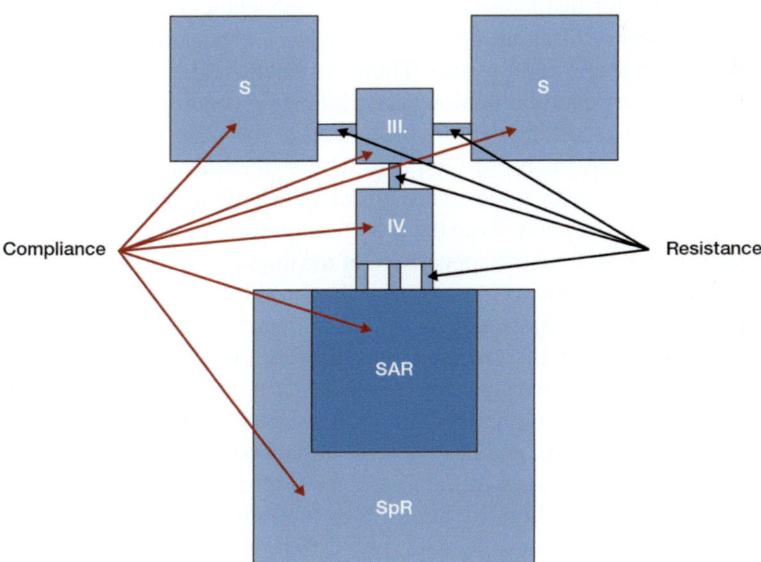

Fig. 13 Volume, resistance and compliance within the CSF system

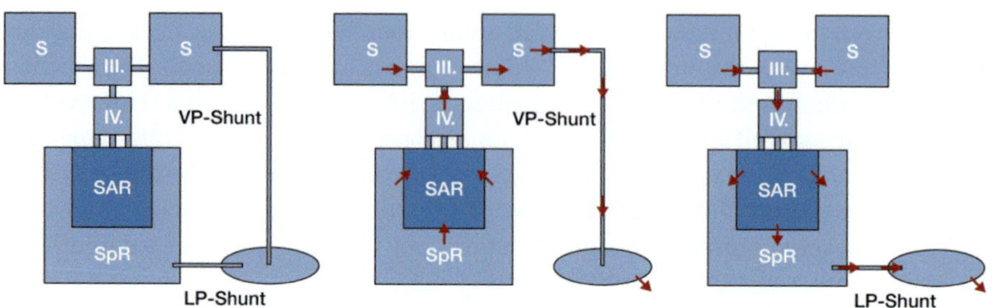

Fig. 14 Comparison of LP shunt and VP shunt for the horizontal position

5 Valve Designs

Basically, valves can be distinguished by the technical design, the physical principle implemented and the post-operative intervention option for optimising therapy or treating complications. In addition, there is the drainage type, which can entail specific functional and space requirements that have a lasting effect on the success of the treatment. As a result, a large number of different solutions are offered for the treatment of hydrocephalus, which can also lead to very different clinical results in terms of their range of functions. In general, it can be said that the treatment of NPH by implantation of a valve-guided drainage system has established itself as a very successful therapy.

Another aspect for distinguishing valves is the technical design. But here, too, there are always very different opinions and views, especially with regard to the material used, the shape and the size. These parameters address first and foremost the surgical boundary conditions, alongside the healing conditions after implantation and the expectation regarding the safe placement of the valve and the least possible impairment of the patient by the implant. The evaluation of such parameters in medical technology is also subjected to objective criteria and personal inclinations or preferences of the surgeon. Even the presentation form of the packaging can play a role. In essence, it is about the appearance of the implant against the background of the marketing aspects of the respective manufacturer. However, shape, material and size of the implant have objectively an impact on the clinical success of the shunt.

As for the shape, both the thickness and the width or area of the top view vary considerably. Since the valve is placed retroauricularly in the vast majority of cases, the thickness of the device is most important. A flat design prevents the implant from being visible under the skin and has the least impact on the patient's daily life. The larger the implant in plan view or the longer the implant, the more important is the deformation property to primarily conform to the radius of curvature of the skull without functional limitations. To date, two different views have been realised: a metallic, flat housing that does not allow deformation and a less flat but soft housing made of silicone that elastically adapts to the patient's individual conditions. There is no evidence of superiority of one approach over the other. The risk of skin perforation at the implant is low, although such complications can occur with both solutions. In addition to these aspects, there is a technical fact behind the two approaches that is not obvious at first glance and whose relevance can hardly be proven clinically. Metal housings have the advantage over plastic housings in that they can reliably protect the actual mechanism of the flap with a low wall thickness. Comparable protection by a silicone wall requires a significantly greater wall thickness. This means that compared to metal housings, a larger proportion of the valve volume can be used for the essential, desired function. In principle, there may be an opportunity here to increase the functional reliability of valves.

Consequently, this aspect has been realised with the so-called *DUALSWITCH VALVE* (DSV) [48]. The valve was designed especially for the treatment of patients with NPH. It should be placed in the chest region, which allows a larger housing. Within the larger housing, a more reliable and robust valve mechanism could be established to guarantee a stable function of the valve. The physical principle behind the concept is the definition of pressure: $p = F/A$. Pressure is defined as force over area. Using this equation, the opening force of a valve can be calculated. The force of a spring to guarantee the required opening pressure depends on the area of the valve seat. The smaller the valve seat, the lower the spring force for a constant opening pressure must be. Conversely, the larger the area of the valve seat is, the bigger the spring force establishing the same opening performance. However, the disturbing force due to particles within the CSF or changed viscosity remain at the same level regardless of the area of the valve seat. In other words, the larger the area of the valve seat, the more reliable the valve mechanism becomes. The evidence of this principle has been reported in different papers [49–53]. Whenever the functional reliability of a valve is challenged, the best guarantee for a reliable function is given for the DSV, within a spring force is realised which is more than 200 times stronger than in any other valve available.

Due to early complications following the successful introduction of shunts for the treatment of paediatric hydrocephalus, a standard for testing the function of valves was developed and adopted, but without specifying requirements for valve function. Accuracy, correct, precise opening and closing characteristics and how to measure them in case of dispute have been well described without defining what a valve should do (ASTM 0647). The only consensus in science about the requirements for shunts so far is that they must provide a hydraulic connection between the CSF system and the drainage compartment (abdominal cavity, atrium of the right heart) and promise a complication-free course with good clinical results. What this means remains an open question. With this in mind, it is clear that the physical, hydraulic performance of valves is far more interesting than the technical design in terms of material, shape and size. Since adjustable valves were introduced as early as the late 1980s, the principles can be generally considered as adjustable or non-adjustable valves [54]. The adjustability of the valves naturally opens up useful treatment options: in cases of over- or under-drainage, non-invasive adjustment of the operating performance of the implanted device may avoid revisions. To date, there is no class 1 evidence from a prospective, randomised multicentre trial of the superiority of adjustable versus non-adjustable valves [55–57].

Figure 15 gives an overview of the available valve technology. Logically, adjustability is useful for any type of proposed solution; however, the technology for adjustment has only been developed for one type of differential pressure valves (DPVs) as well as for gravity valves. All adjustable DPVs feature a ball-in-cone valve mechanism. The other two pressure valves, silicone diaphragm valves and silicone slit valves, are only available as non-adjustable solutions.

There are basically two different groups of valves: the DPVs and the group of devices that take into account the hydrostatic pressure generated by the position. While the silicone slot valves are hardly available nowadays and are rarely implanted in Europe, the United States or Japan, the silicone diaphragm valves are still widely used. Independent tests of various simple DPVs showed a surprising range of values, without being able to prove which valve was the correct one [58]. Some valves functioned like a valveless tube, while others did not seem to open at all. The most technically precise valve designs are the ball-in-cone valves. These valves usually contain a stainless steel (or titanium) spring that presses a sapphire or ruby ball against a valve seat, which is also made of metal or ruby (sapphire). Sapphire balls guarantee the best possible roundness and surface quality to produce an optimum opening and closing mechanism on the valve seat. Ball-cone valves differ essentially in the design of the spring and the diameter of the valve seat. The larger the diameter, the stronger the spring force to determine the opening pressure and the more reliably the valve works.

DPVs do not address hydrostatic pressure at all. From a technical point of view, they are simply designed only for the lying position of the patient. It is known that the risk of over-drainage increases if the opening pressure of the valve is low and vice versa: a high setting decreases the risk of complications due to over-drainage. On the other hand, low settings promise a superior clinical outcome in contrast to high settings. The so-called Holter-valve has often been used. This valve consisted of a silicone tube with a closed end and slits in its wall. The stiffness of the material and the

	Fixed	Adjustable
Differential Pressure Valves		
→ Silicon Slit Valves	✓	✗
→ Membran Valves	✓	✗
→ Ball Cone Valves	✓	✓
Devices Incorporating Vertical Hydrostatic Pressure		
→ Anti Siphon Valves	✓	✗
→ Flow Regulated Valves	✓	✗
→ Gravitational Valves	✓	✓

Fig. 15 Table of available valve designs

texture of the slit defines the opening characteristic. Modern DPVs are always ball-in-cone designs with a precise functioning. The graph in Fig. 16 represents the typical characteristic of these old designs and reveals the limited accuracy. For ball-in-cone valves, the variation is by far lower, the valves are by far more reliable regarding their tolerances. These valves act technically great, precise and reliable. With regards to hydrostatic pressure, whether a valve works precisely is questionable if the physics of VP shunts are ignored and non-physiological values within hydrocephalus patients are systematically established. Many patients, however, seem to become adapted to this situation without serious complaints and the human body seemingly is able to get used to this kind of non-natural condition. However, it is impossible to predict who will suffer severely from this situation with the consequence of a subdural bleeding and, especially in patients with NPH, a clinical condition which is worse than before surgery. In particular for this group of patients, the clinical outcome and the complication rate have been doubted [59, 60]. One explanation for this is the poor technical characteristic of simple DPVs (Fig. 17).

Be that as it may, DPVs are still regularly used today, for example, in patients with post-haemorrhagic hydrocephalus. Whether a valveless shunt, i.e. just a tube, would provide the same clinical success is an open question. Some published work

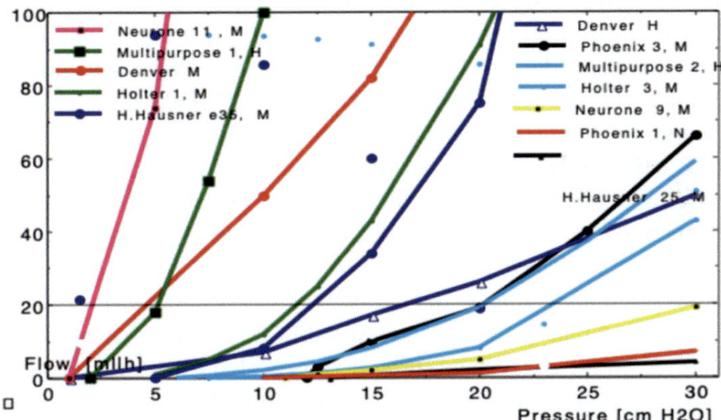

Fig. 16 Pressure flow characteristic of different DP valves [61]

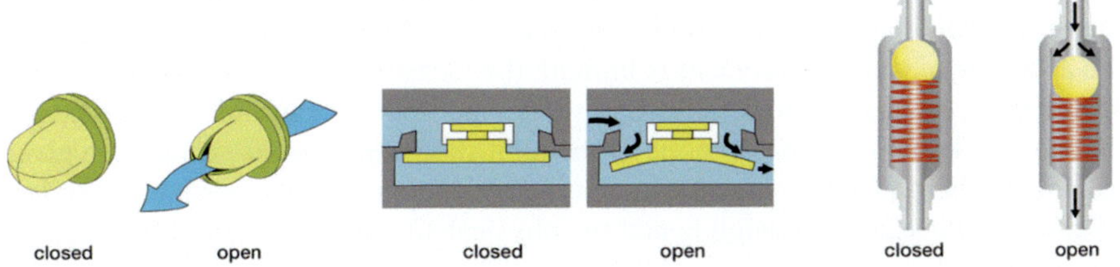

Fig. 17 Three types of DPVs (silicone-slit valve, membrane valve, ball-in-cone valve)

supports this, as does consideration of the physics of shunts, particularly DPVs with a low-pressure setting [62]. The only advantage of these valves will be the reflux protection, which is possibly not mandatory for VP shunts.

The importance of the counterbalance of the hydrostatic pressure within VP shunts has been impressively reported in early studies with the first gravitational devices. The systematic comparison of the data demonstrated for the group with larger ventricles (limited decrease of the ventricular size after shunting), smaller enlargement of the subdural space and significantly lower number of subdural effusions (hygromas, hematomas) which required surgical treatment, than for the group of DPVs [49, 63].

The possibility of adjusting the operating characteristics of implanted shunts non-invasively was introduced in the late 80s of the twentieth century. This technology was developed to avoid revisions in case of under-drainage and especially in case of over-drainage. In the 90s, these devices became very popular. In Japan, the use of a "programmable" valve was defined as the golden standard for the treatment of hydrocephalus, although adjustable valves have exactly the same problems and disadvantages as non-adjustable DPVs. It is clear to everyone that if you move a bucket of water from the vertical to the horizontal position, the situation changes completely.

The fact that this is also the case with implantable drains for the treatment of hydrocephalus still does not correspond to the general neurosurgical understanding. One can draw very different conclusions from this for the requirement of the function of hydrocephalus valves; however, one cannot seriously believe that one and the same valve function is the best conceivable solution for all body positions. In standing position, the hydrostatic pressure sucking in the ventricle occurs in the shunt system, which cannot be compensated by a DPV. In the supine position, low but positive pressures relative to the atmosphere are clinically targetable, especially for NPH. Thus, with up righting, adjustable valves would have to be set to a high opening pressure or, with recumbency, to a rather low value, if not the lowest possible value.

There is an ongoing scientific debate about the useful setting of DPVs in NPH [64–68]. On the one hand, it is recommended to add an anti-siphon system to the adjustable valve, on the other hand, it is recommended to choose the optimal valve setting taking into account the patient's height and BMI. A statement such as "The relationship between ICP and opening pressure valves is linear but not predicted by simple hydrodynamics" [69] could be interpreted as questioning the reliability of the physics. However, a valve, like all other medical devices, in principle follows clearly understood rules and is based on engineering evidence. Now, if clinically measured values appear to contradict physical laws, the explanation can only be that the accuracy of the measurement is limited, the measured values do not represent a steady state, or the measured value represents superimposed physiological processes that are not known or seen. In none of the published papers is an explanation given as to what alternative physical phenomena might explain why the posture-dependent hydrostatic pressure is negligible and the physical situation for control by shunts is the same for the upright position of the patient and the horizontal. It seems confusing that the vertical position of patients is not considered to be of comparable importance

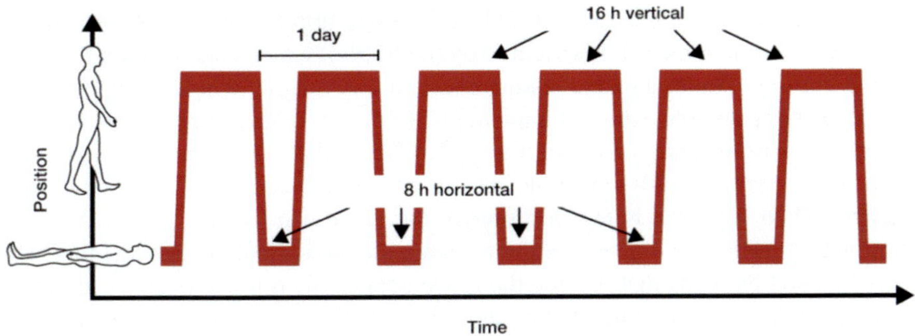

Fig. 18 In average humans are in upright position on third of the day

to the supine position, even though patients with NPH spend many more hours per day standing upright than lying down (Fig. 18).

The strategy of initially starting with a very high setting and carefully acclimatising the brain structure to the pressures defined by the shunt may reduce the risk of severe complications due to over-drainage. However, the conditions are far from physiological and represent only a compromise rather than an optimal approach. This strategy delays the onset of adequate drainage and, particularly in patients with NPH, counteracts the intended approach of lowering ICP during deep sleep to prevent the occurrence of B waves. All available adjustable DPVs offer a maximum valve adjustment up to 20 cm of water column. There is one exception that offers adjustment up to 40 cm of water column. While 20 cm of water can compensate for the hydrostatic pressure in the upright position of the patient, the less the taller the patient is, the adjustment up to 40 cm of water in the lying position is more likely to lead to a quasi-occlusion of the shunt. During the night, such a shunt acts as if there were no shunt and consequently no treatment. To overcome problems due to over-drainage, a kind of trouble shooting adjustment has been introduced. It is called virtual off what as well means the adjustment to 40 cm of water. Such an adjustment interrupts the treatment for the time of this high adjustment to overcome the critical clinical condition due to over-drainage.

In addition to inadequate operation, unwanted adjustment due to magnetic fields in daily life plays an important role for adjustable valves. For this reason, valves have been invented and are available for clinical use that are equipped with a braking mechanism that prevents uncontrolled adjustment even during MRI examinations. Valves that do not have such a safety mechanism should no longer be used. In addition, adjustable valves should be magnetically readable, making X-ray control unnecessary for the vast majority of cases.

In order to make unintentional adjustment of the valves impossible, two different technical principles have been implemented. The first is a simple mechanical brake, normally active, which can be deactivated by a discreet pressure from the outside on the body of the device (*proGAV*®). This eliminates the friction that normally prevents the movement of the adjustment rotor and allows the rotation of the rotor by magnetic fields applied from the outside [70, 71]. If the force applied on the device is taken away, the position of the rotor is secured by the friction which acts between the rotor and the housing. An unintended readjustment by any magnetic field is impossible.

The second principle, which is implemented differently in different valve designs, uses magnetism to create a kind of brake [72–75]. In two cases, the rotor inside the device can be rotated only when the rotor is moved upward from the outside by a magnet. When the rotor is moved upward, the valve can be moved to a different position by turning the magnet. Without such a magnetic field, the rotor is mechanically blocked by walls that impede the movement of the rotor. Therefore, although not impossible, it is very unlikely that the valve position will change unintentionally (Certas plus). In this design, the spring force acting on the valve ball depends on the rotation of the rotor. When the rotor is turned, the force is directly adjusted to the new position of the rotor. In this case, the spring acts parallel to the valve axis. The situation is similar with the second design. Also in the second design (Strata), the rotor is moved upward by an external magnetic field and rotated by the rotation of the external field (the magnet). When the adjustment tool is removed, a spring in the valve pushes the rotor against the bottom of the housing where it is trapped in that position Each position corresponds to a different pressure level because the bottom of the housing is of variable thickness. Depending on the thickness, the spring is pressed slightly more or less against the valve ball. The adjustment is therefore perpendicular to the valve axis. The changed setting is detected when the rotor reaches its final position. There are reports in the literature of unintentional adjustments with both types of valves, although this should be technically very unlikely [76, 77].

Another design uses the attractive forces of magnets to provide a reliable locking mechanism for the rotor. Again, the adjustment works as a function of the rotation of the rotor. However, the rotor is locked by two attracting magnets until a special external magnet opens this locking mechanism (Polaris). Neither magnetic fields of daily life nor an MRI examination can unintentionally adjust the valve [73]. The adjustment is achieved by changing the length of the spring acting on the valve ball. The change is possible when the locking mechanism is opened by a specific magnetic field applied to the valve from outside and this magnetic field is turned to the desired position.

In summary, the differences of the available adjustable valves in terms of ease of use, shape, technical solutions and material are far from being as important as the safety against accidental adjustment and, more importantly, the limited hydraulic performance. In principle, these valves act like non-adjustable DPVs, always as a compromise between the vertical and the horizontal position of the patient. Against this background, soon after the successful introduction of shunts for the treatment of hydrocephalus, the first proposals have been made to optimise cerebrospinal fluid drainage for the standing body position.

The second group of valve designs (Fig. 15) contains the different proposals to improve the clinical perspective of the valves of the first group, the adjustable or non-adjustable DPVs. Three different principles are used clinically today. Very often, these valves are all referred to as anti-siphon devices. This is very confusing and partly the result of limited reflection on the differences that sometimes not everyone wants to highlight. The anti-siphon device (ASD) is a brand name for a valve principle. The term ASD does not describe a group of devices or a classification.

This group of valves or valve components is defined by the fact that their designs consider a vertical hydrostatic pressure within the shunt system. The technology behind them offers three different principles. The first one introduced is the ASD. Similar to this device is the so-called siphon-control-device (SCD). The second type is a system to keep a constant flow throughout a shunt regardless of the active differential pressure acting on the device. Two products are clinically used today: the Orbis-Sigma-Valve (OSV), which is not intended to be used together with an additional valve, and the so-called siphon-guard, which is always used in addition to a DPV. The last type of this group uses the gravity of metallic balls in the upright position of the patient to increase the overall working pressure reasonably (gravity compensating device [GCA], *SHUNTASSISTANT*® [SA]). Such a device is used additionally to a DPV (like the ASD, SCD). Both additionally used types are as well available integrated in one housing.

If two valves are installed in series, the opening characteristics of both devices must be added together. For each device, the decisive factor is which absolute pressure is present at the outlet and which at the inlet. If the difference between these values is greater than the opening pressure of the valve, the valve opens and allows the discharge until the difference has dropped to the opening or closing pressure of the device. The various valves together transmit the atmospheric pressure (zero level) to the ventricles. Within the ventricles, the pressure depends on the location of the measurement. Above zero level, the pressure becomes negative, below positive (Fig. 19).

The addition of the opening pressures of the various valves applies to all devices, where the devices are positioned within the shunt system, and retroauricular or thoracic has no influence on the function of the devices. The only exceptions are

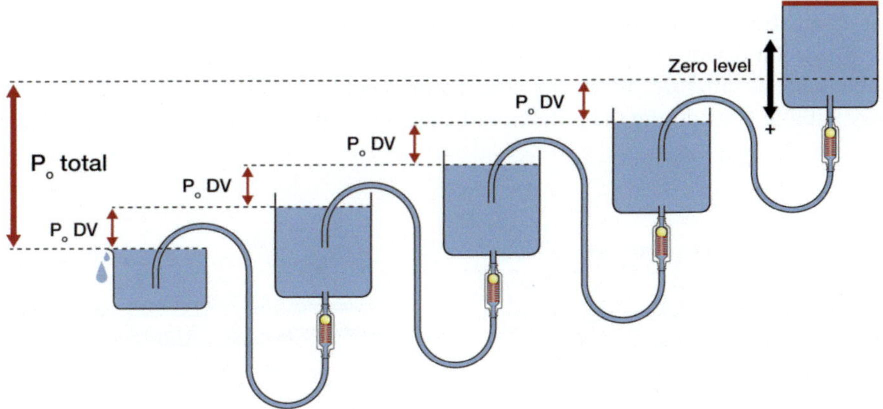

Fig. 19 Differential pressure valve in series: the individual opening pressures must be added together

the ASD and the SCD. Function depends on the position of the implantation. Too high a positioning increases the opening pressure, too low a positioning weakens the intended compensation of the hydrostatic pressure. Such devices should be implanted retroauricularly without exception.

The ASD was the first device proposed to limit the risk of over-drainage. Its principle separates the proximal pressure acting within the device from the distal pressure. Hereby the proximal pressure defines the opening of the device nearly independent of the negative distal pressure. If the device is closed, the proximal pressure is acting on an area which is many times larger than the area where the distal pressure is acting on. If there is a hanging water column creating a distinct negative pressure at the outlet of the ASD, it has an only slight impact on the opening performance of the device. The water column creates a suction within the ASD, which creates a closing force between the valve seat and the closing membrane. However, this suction force is by far smaller than the proximal force which is established by the ventricular pressure. If the ICP increases regardless of whether or not the patient is standing, the proximal force becomes stronger than the distal closing force. The device opens (Fig. 20).

The ASD/SCD concept is therefore a very elegant solution to eliminate the influence of the distal water column and to avoid the risk of over-drainage in the upright position of the patient. Figure 21 shows an example of the calculation of the principle of operation. The units are omitted here to make the relationship between the forces clear. In the upright position of an adult patient, the proximal pressure is about 10 cm of water and the distal negative pressure could be 40 cm of water. Since the proximal area is about 20 times larger than the distal area, the proximal force is five times stronger than the distal suction force. If there is no suction force because the patient is lying down, then there is no force opposing the opening pressure and consequently the opening pressure becomes lower. The diaphragm is more easily moved away from the valve closure at the centre by the proximal ventricular pressure. Conversely, the greater the distal negative pressure, the higher the opening pressure. That is, the larger a patient is, the higher the opening pressure in the upright position.

The main disadvantage of this device is the strict dependence of its function on subcutaneous pressure. While the device works very well and reliably in the laboratory without considering the influence of subcutaneous pressure, it seems impossible

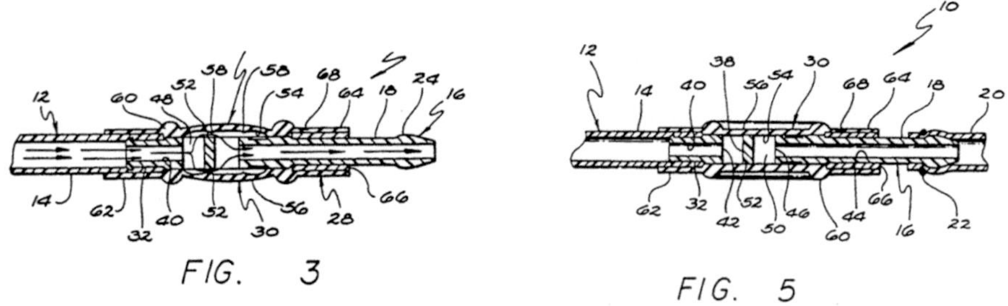

Fig. 20 Schematic drawing of the ASD taken from the patent (left open, right closed)

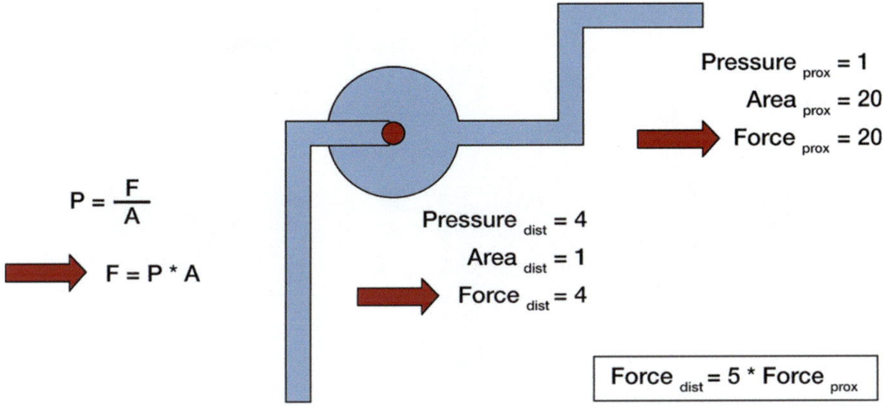

Fig. 21 Proximal force within the ASD/SCD defines the opening characteristics

to predict the opening characteristics of this device after implantation. Simulation of fluctuating subcutaneous pressures also highlights the enormous importance of this drawback in the laboratory for a possible drainage outcome or specifically for increased ventricular pressures. In addition to the proximal and distal forces, there is a third force acting on the membrane. This force acts from the outside of the implant on the entire membrane surface, so that it increases the opening pressure depending on the magnitude of the force or pressure. In fact, however, this force is neither known nor can it be calculated systematically. What is the pressure exerted by the skin that curves over the implant? If there is a scar over the implant or if the patient is lying on the device (during the night?), the opening properties are significantly increased. This may worsen over time as the tissue over the implant changes due to natural processes. This is the reason why the ASD/ SCD is viewed critically and has not been able to establish itself clinically [78, 79] (Fig. 22).

The second type of valves that take into account the vertical hydrostatic pressure in a VP shunt is the flow reducer technology. It is important to mention that the flow reducers do not regulate the flow. This would require an engineering solution to measure the actual flow and regulate it according to specific requirements. The term flow control is a marketing term. What is correct is that these devices limit or reduce flow. The idea behind flow reducing valves is to limit the flow to physiological ranges, regardless of the differential pressure applied to the device. Figure 23 shows the principle of the OSV [80].

If CSF below a flow of about 20 ml per hour is to be drained via the device, the valve has no significant resistance (phase I). To allow a flow of more than 20 ml per hour, the resistance increases (phase II). If the differential pressure rises above 40 cm of water, the valve opens without further resistance, so that the pressure across the valve does not become significantly higher than 40 cm of water (phase III) (Fig. 24).

The major problem with this approach is the technical difficulty of reasonably setting the flow within the required range. Small particles, which are often present in CSF, significantly affect the possible flow. In vivo, the valve may operate quite

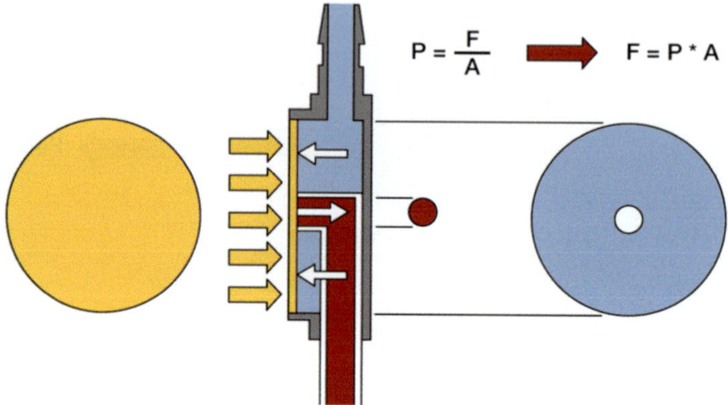

Fig. 22 Principle of the ASD/SCD: the greatest influence on the device comes from the subcutaneous pressure

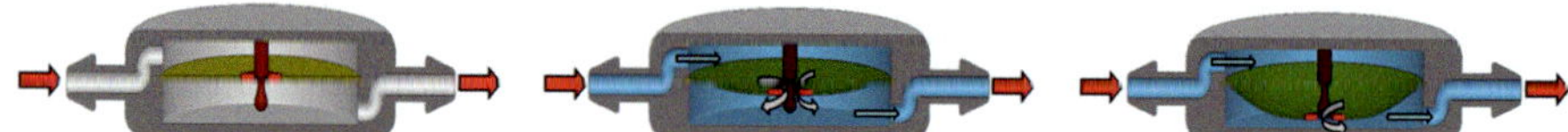

Fig. 23 Principle of the OSV: Stage I (left) low resistance, stage II (centre) limited flow by narrowing the outlet area, stage III (right) high pressure area with low resistance increase with increasing flow

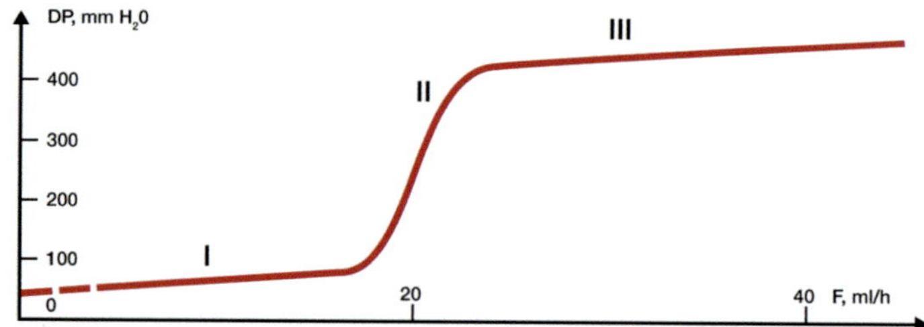

Fig. 24 Flow pressure characteristic of the OSV

differently from the ideal curve, and even in in vitro studies, the measured values do not always correspond to the expected values [81]. Another important obstacle of this device is the fact that it limits the flow regardless of the reason for increased flow rates. It is known that especially patients with NPH benefit from low ICP. However, high CSF rates might as well occur due to high CSF production, e.g. during the deep sleep in the night (Rapid eye movement, REM) [82].

Clinical results support this criticism. Three different valve types, a DPV, a DPV in combination with an SCD and a DPV in combination with an OSV, were comparatively investigated in a prospective randomised study in paediatric hydrocephalus. The results for all investigated variants were in principle comparable. Interestingly, the results revealed significant differences with respect to the different valve designs of the participating centres, each of which included more than 25 patients in the study. The centre in which the inventor of the OSV was the neurosurgeon in charge found much better survival rates for the OSVs than the other centres (Fig. 25). This aspect could be explained by the fact that in the field of hydrocephalus therapy, decisions are often made less on the basis of facts and evidence and more on personal judgement and experience. Indisputable evidence is scarce. Unfortunately, the results of the study support the widely held belief that the surgeon's experience regarding implantation technique is more important than the design of the valve, even though implantation takes only 30 to 60 min, and the valve determines the clinical outcome for months and years thereafter.

A similar type of flow reduction is the so-called siphon-guard (SG). Unlike the OSV, the SG has two parallel internal paths. The main central pathway contains a ball mechanism that is closed when the flow (the differential pressure acting on the device) increases significantly above physiological levels. If this occurs, the CSF is diverted through a spiral narrowed channel that creates significantly higher resistance, reducing the flow through the valve. However, safe switching between these two states appears to be critical. Laboratory studies have shown that there is a systematic risk that the central occlusion of the mid-channel remains permanently activated [83, 84]. This may increase the risk of under-drainage or hypertension. Both designs, the OSV and the SG, reduce the risk of over-drainage, but also increase the risk of under-drainage because they cannot distinguish whether or not high flow is caused by hydrostatic pressure or for other reasons.

As already mentioned, the SG is not an ASD because its operating principle is completely different and consequently its performance is also different. Sometimes, it is also called a gravitational valve, which is also wrong. The SG (like the OSV) does not act in a posture- dependent manner. The weight of the ball in the device to close the passage in the vertical position is not comparable to the weight of metal balls used in gravity valves. Therefore, there is no recommendation from the manufacturer to implant this device parallel to the body axis. Because of the different hydraulic and physical performance, it is necessary to carefully differentiate between the three types of valves taking into account the vertical hydrostatic pressure.

The third type of these devices is the group of posture-dependent gravity valves. While adjustable solutions have not been proposed and clinically established for the other two principles (ASD, SCD or flow reduction devices (FRD)), an adjustable valve is also available for gravitational technology (Fig. 15). It is surprising that the adjustability of valves is generally well accepted and their clinical potential is highly valued, but the fact that this is especially true for the upright position, as humans spend more time in an upright than in a supine position during the day, has hardly been addressed since the introduction of valves. Although the adjustment of the DPVs is also effective in the vertical position, the adjustment is not equally useful for both postures. Raising the opening pressure when standing leads to unwanted and harmful pressures when lying down; conversely, lowering the pressure significantly increases the risk of over-drainage.

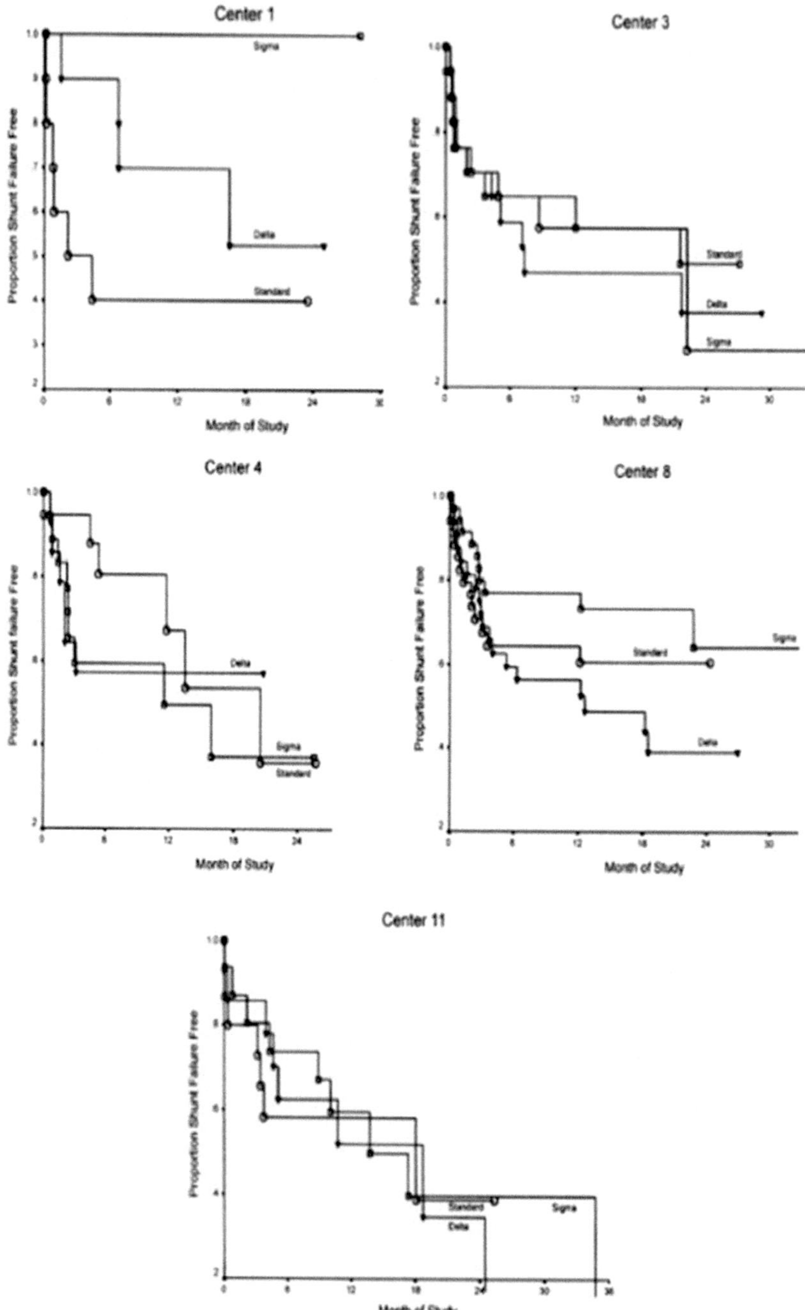

Fig. 25 Kaplan–Meier curves for the shunt failure in the paediatric population examined in different participating centres of a randomised trial

The general principle of gravitational valves uses the gravity of metallic balls to create a posture-dependent opening pressure of the devices. The specific weight of metal is widely different. On the one hand stainless steel balls are used, on the other hand tantalum balls. The benefit of tantalum is its high specific weight. With a density of 17 kg per litre, it is more than two times heavier than stainless steel. This means that bodies of small volumes can create comparatively high gravitational forces. Instead of using several balls out of stainless steel to create the required opening force, with tantalum balls only one ball is needed. One ball reduces the friction within the ball and the wall of the housing, which increases the overall precision of the device. However, such differences are of limited importance for the clinical outcome.

The first gravitational valve was introduced for LP drainages. It was recognised that for this type of drainage, the hydrostatic pressure compensation is important; however, this principle has never been considered to be important for VP shunts as well. The first gravitational valve for VP shunts was the DSV. This valve had two chambers in parallel. The first valve chamber integrated a DPV adjusted to the lying position, and the second chamber contained a valve adjusted to the standing position. The respective chamber is activated by a tantalum ball which opens and closes the low-pressure path depending on the posture. Here again, the specific weight of tantalum allows to establish a reliable switching function. The valve was designed to be implanted in the chest region. The background is that the two valves within the DSV have a large membrane to increase its working reliability. The larger the area is where the pressure is acting, the more reliable the valve becomes. Secondly, the chest is a good indicator for the position of the patient. For gravitational devices, it is important to be implanted in parallel to the body axis. A drawback of the DSV is that it offers only two different valve characteristics. In an inclined position, it may switch to the low-pressure stage too early and thus allow over-drainage. Clinical reports about results after implanting the DSV, however, could demonstrate the importance of the gravitational principle (Fig. 26).

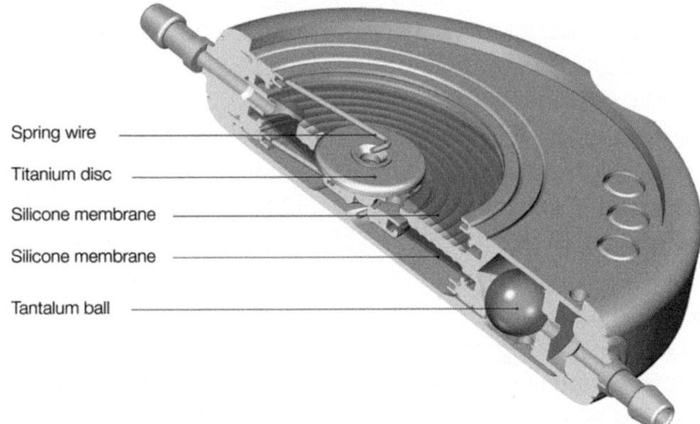

Fig. 26 Principle of the DSV switching between two valve chambers depending on posture

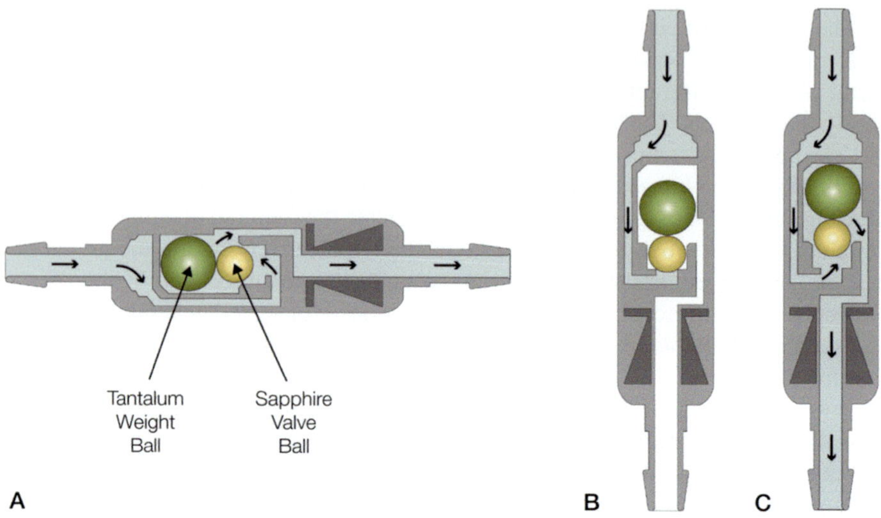

Fig. 27 Principle of a gravitational valve with a tantalum ball acting vertically directly against the hydrostatic pressure

The other gravitational principle being integrated in hydrocephalus valves uses the weight of a metallic ball directly acting against a valve seat. The gravity of the ball counteracts against the hydrostatic pressure while the patient is upright. The opening pressure of such valves is defined by the closing area of the valve seat and the weight of the ball. In some gravitational valves, different opening characteristics of the valve are established by choosing one, two, three or even for balls. In other devices, the opening pressure is realised by different sizes of the valve seat. The smaller the valve seat, the higher the opening pressure becomes with the same gravitational force acting on the seat (Fig. 27).

There are gravitational valves of different manufacturers available. They can be distinguished by the material used, the shape and the size. Important is the implantation under reflection of the gravitational force in parallel to the body axis. This precise and reliable positioning of the horizontal-vertical valve, which was proposed by Hakim already in the 1970s, was a challenge and possibly the reason that it never became very popular. The fear of subdural effusions was too great, and a VP shunt was almost preferred, especially in NPH patients. The DSV is the second device available for implantation in a LP shunt [85], but despite the good results with this valve, the LP shunt is still not very popular today. Figure 28 gives an overview about available gravitational valves.

Gravity valves have the potential to systematically equalise hydrostatic pressure. The most important study to demonstrate the strength of this technology is the so-called SVASONA study, which investigated the influence of a gravity valve in a prospective randomised trial with NPH patients [87]. An adjustable valve was implanted with or without a gravitational unit. Up to now, only four class one studies

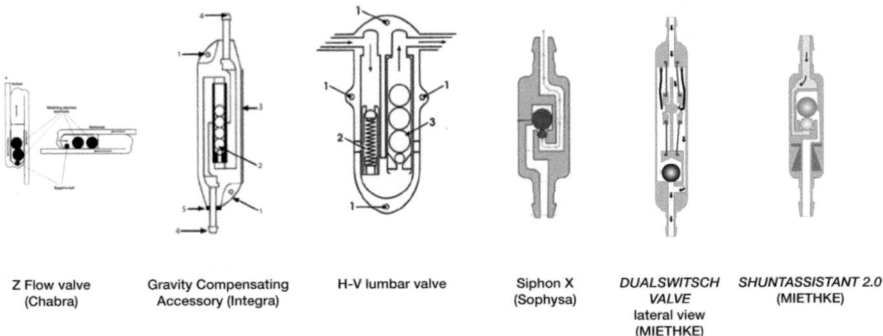

Fig. 28 Available gravitational valves at the market developed by different manufacturers (the size of the drawing does not represent the actual size) [86]

have ever been performed in the field of shunt therapy. Class one study means that it was prospective, randomised, controlled and performed as a multicentre study. The first was the Drake study, performed and published in 1998 in which a DPV with or without a SCD and an OSV has been investigated in a paediatric population. The results did not show any evidence for any valve type. The second study was published by Boon et al. who compared the results after implanting a medium pressure (MPV) or low pressure (LPV) DPV in patients with NPH. The authors concluded: "Outcome was better for patients who had an LPV shunt than for those with an MPV shunt, although most differences were not statistically significant. The authors advise that patients with NPH be treated with an LPV shunt". They found a significantly higher rate of subdural effusions in the LPV group (71%) compared with the MPV group (34%), with no significant clinical impact on patient outcome. The third prospective, randomised, controlled, multicentre study was published in 1999 by Pollack, who compared an adjustable DPV with a conventional, non-adjustable DPV. The goal of the study was not to prove the superiority of one valve design, but to show that the results for both groups were comparable and that adjustable valves could be used safely in the treatment of hydrocephalus, which the authors successfully demonstrated. The SVASONA study was published in 2013 and brought clear evidence for the beneficial impact of the gravitational unit to the complication rate due to over-drainage in patients with NPH (Fig. 29).

The investigators could enrol 145 patients with idiopathic NPH, 137 of whom could be analysed after reaching the endpoint of the study. They found highly significantly different results. Six months after surgery, 29 patients of the group without a gravitational unit and 5 patients with a gravitational unit had developed a subdural effusion. The consequence of the results was the premature discontinuation of the patient recruitment. As a conclusion the authors stated: "Implanting a gravitational rather than another type of valve will avoid one additional over- drainage complication in about every third patient undergoing VP shunting for idiopathic NPH".

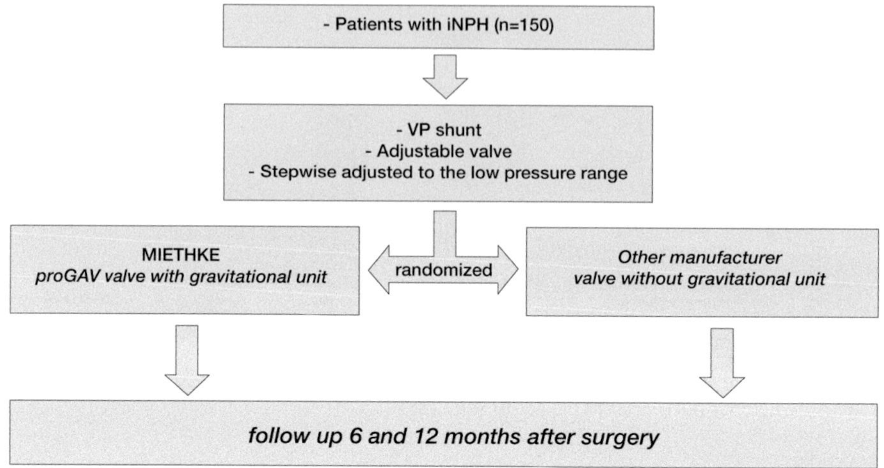

Fig. 29 Scheme of the SVASONA study to investigate the impact of gravitational device on the outcome of NPH patients [87]

There are some limitations to this study. For example, it focuses only on a single valve. Flow- reducing devices and ASD/SCD were not considered. It is possible that the complication rate would be similar for these devices. However, this would need to be shown in another study. Another limitation is the design, which requires consistent lowering of the valve setting. This requirement is based on the hypothesis that lowering the ICP allows for a better clinical outcome for NPH patients. Whether comparable clinical outcomes might result with DPVs that are not lowered has not been investigated. However, even without being able to answer all the questions, the results of the study provide very impressive support for the theoretical expectations that arise from the physical study of VP shunts. From a technical point of view, it is very clear that gravity compensation must have an effect on the pressure situation in the drained compartment. If this pressure is kept close to the atmospheric level, i.e. if the sucking influence of a hanging water column is compensated, the risk of subdural effusion decreases.

Adjustability of the gravitational unit is often equated with DP adjustment along with a non-adjustable gravitational unit, since DP unit adjustment increases or decreases the opening power for both body positions. However, independent adjustment of shunt power in the vertical position is useful in many cases even without increasing DP unit pressure. For example, a clinical problem in the treatment of NPH is disease progression. After insertion of a shunt, deterioration of the clinical condition is sometimes observed after initial satisfactory improvement. In these cases, lowering the valve setting is the only perspective, although lowering the opening pressure increases the risk of subdural effusions. If the DPV is already set to the lowest possible setting, the only option is controlled over-drainage in the vertical position [88–90]. With an adjustable DPV, such a manoeuvre is impossible (Fig. 30).

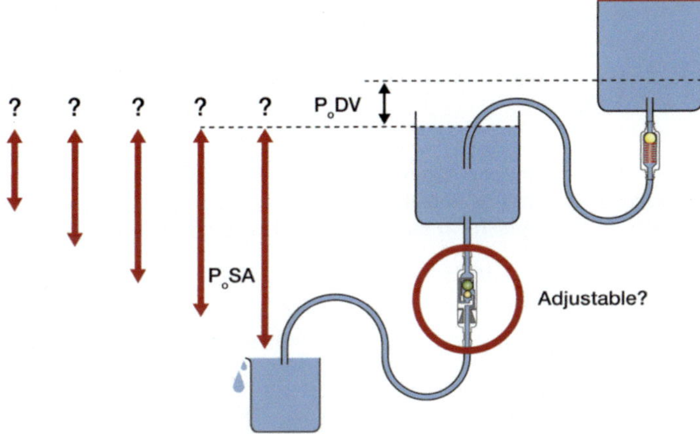

Fig. 30 Adjustment of the gravitational unit of a VP shunt

A similar aspect can be observed in the lumbar puncture test, which is performed to diagnose NPH. In this test, a certain amount of CSF (30–50 ml) is collected without knowing the pressure response. However, clinical improvement shortly after the puncture or even a day later is a strong indicator that the shunt is responding. Withdrawal of such a volume of fluid from the ventricular system can easily create a significant negative pressure. Often the patient initially shows marked clinical improvement, but after some time, the old condition returns. The former ICP value is reached again.

For these reasons, the adjustment of the gravity valve could be more important than the adjustment of the DPV. The principle is based on the adjustment of a spring force acting against the gravity of a tantalum ball in the upright position. Figure 31 shows the principle of this design schematically. When set to zero, such a device provides a non-invasive option equivalent to an invasive lumbar puncture. A very low setting can be made for a few minutes or even longer and then readjusted to values that can counteract hydrostatic pressure. Adjustment of gravity-dependent vertical opening pressure thus opens up new opportunities for the diagnosis and treatment of NPH, especially in re-worsening conditions of the NPH patient. However, there is currently no clinical evidence to support this perspective.

The opening pressure of the adjustable gravitational valve (*M.blue*®) depends on the posture and the adjustment. At the highest setting, the increase of pressure starts with the first movement from the horizontal in the vertical position. With the adjustment of the spring acting against the gravity of the tantalum ball, the gravitational counterbalance starts delayed. As lower, the adjusted opening pressure is as later the gravitational force influences the operating characteristic of the device (Fig. 32).

The introduction of gravity valve (AGV) adjustment has provided an additional means of non-invasively interfering with the hydraulic properties of an implanted shunt. However, the question arises whether or not both adjustment options are

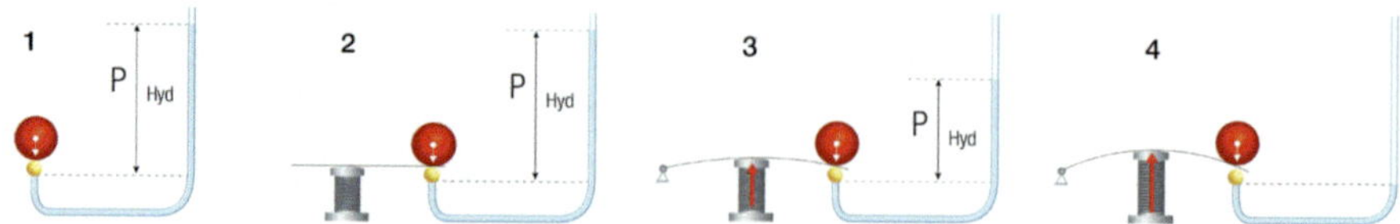

Fig. 31 Principle of the adjustment of a gravitational force: 1 – hydrostatic principle; 2 – adjustable spring between tantalum ball and valve ball; 3 – adjustment is partially lowering the gravitational force of the tantalum ball; 4 – gravity of the tantalum ball is deactivated, the ball is moved up and does not create a flow resistance

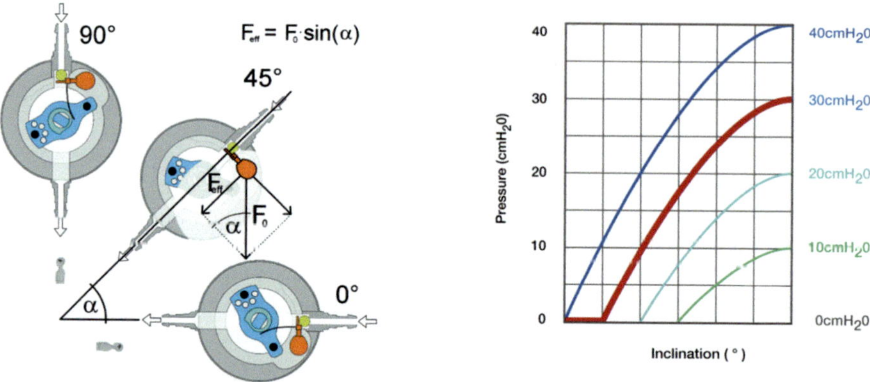

Fig. 32 Design of the adjustable gravitational valve and performance characteristic depending on posture and adjustment

clinically necessary or valuable for a good clinical outcome. Particularly in NPH, a low DPV setting is likely to be beneficial for outcome. A reasonable setting to optimise treatment could be made with the AGV. Since it is open whether both units are needed and the AGV may promise more therapeutic options, it is reasonable to develop an AGV with a non-adjustable DP unit. Such a unit is implemented in the *M.blue*®. This valve consists of the spring adjustment unit to define the action of the tantalum weight and a fixed pressure DPV integrated in the distal outlet part of the titanium housing. The DP unit is available with various fixed pressures. Of course, like all other gravitational valves, it is important that this device is implanted parallel to the body axis (Fig. 33).

6   The Adjustment of Flow

Although the shunt treatment is a very successful neurosurgical intervention there are still many open questions and unsolved problems. This is the background for the fact that again and again new ideas are proposed and there is no agreed evidence

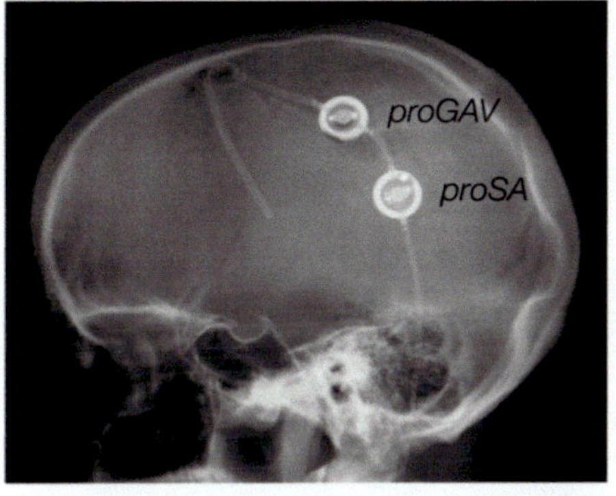

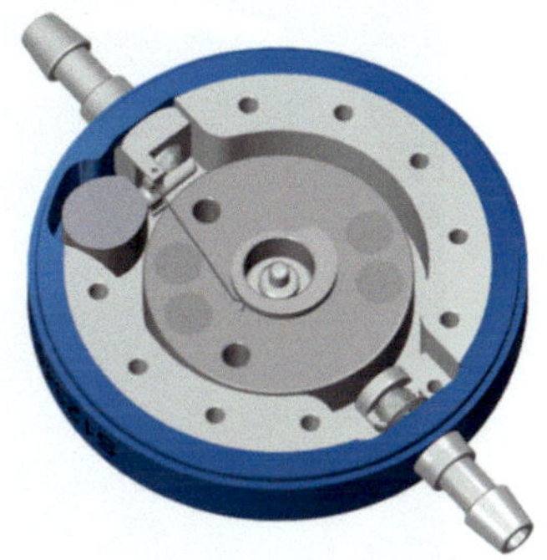

Fig. 33 Are two adjustment unit needed? X-ray of an implanted AGV together with an adjustable DP valve (left), Schematic description of an *M.blue*® with a fixed pressure DP valve at the distal outlet of the device (right)

about basic technical and functional aspects of shunting. The failure rate in paediatric hydrocephalus due to shunt blockage is high and the problem is unsolved, methods to check shunt independency are not available and the question of how to treat slit-ventricle syndrome successfully is not answered. The first mentioned problem refers to the small housing required and consequently small space available for reliable valve technology for newborns and young children. Larger devices (like the DSV) improve the reliability of the valve mechanism; however, they are too large to be implanted in this patient group.

The second and third problem could be addressed by developing an adjustable flow reduction device that could be implanted in conjunction with an AGV. Adjustment of flow alone cannot offer and promise a reasonable perspective, since it is and will be completely unknown what setting could guarantee physiologic pressure (ICP) values. However, together with reasonable pressure control, it could add significant value to treatment in some patients. In particular, in patients with slit ventricle syndrome or in over-drained neonates, a flow-reducing device combined with an adjustable gravitational valve could support an improvement in the clinical outlook of affected patients. Usually, patients with slit ventricle syndrome are very difficult to treat. The valve setting is either too low or too high. Or it works for some time, then it fails. For patients, this is often a nightmare (Fig. 34).

Adjustment of flow could significantly affect ICP with respect to changes due to dynamic pressure amplitudes. The crying child could actively pump the ventricles empty. Patients with slit ventricles have pathologically low compliance. Low outflowing fluid volumes correspond with high pressure changes within the ventricles. However, shunts easily allow flow up to a hundred times greater than the production rate. When a valve opens because the differential pressure rises significantly above its opening pressure, the total resistance of a shunt is independent of the compliance of the ventricles. Due to pressure changes caused by movement (change of position, running, jumping), the fluid is drained by this movement.

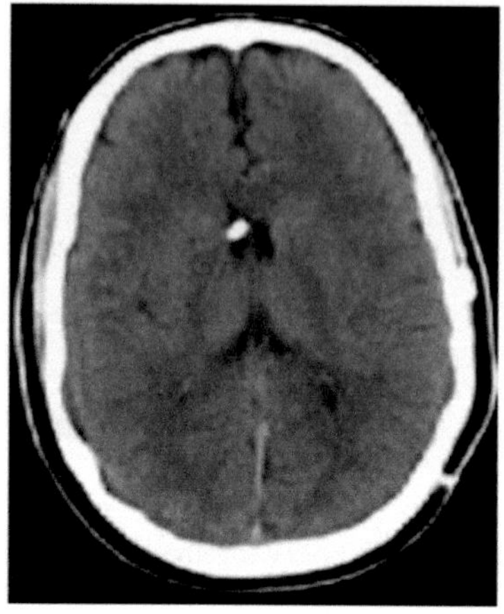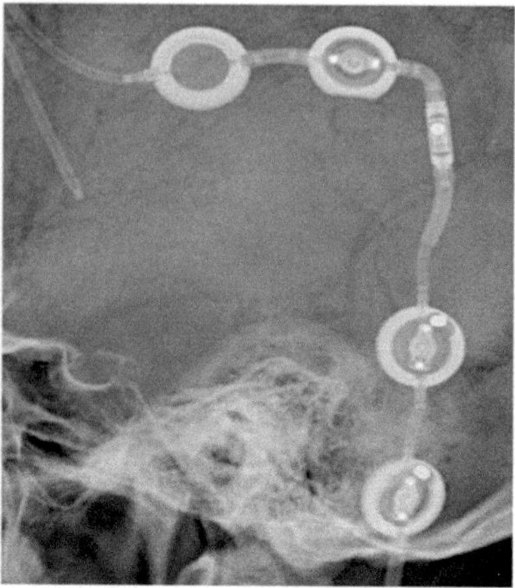

Fig. 34 CT scan of a patient with slit ventricles (left); X-ray of a shunted patient with a serious of gravitational valves (right) with on opening pressure of 102 cm of water in the upright and 2 cm of water in the horizontal position of the patient

The hydrostatic pressure in both vessels in Fig. 35 (left) is the same. However, when the same amount of liquid is drained, the pressure behaviour in the two chambers is completely different. The thin vessel with a small surface area drains quickly, resulting in a rapid pressure drop, while the pressure in the other vessel remains almost unchanged. This model demonstrates the need for reduced drainage in compartments with low compliance. Pressure regulation within the ventricles of patients with low compliance is a challenge for shunt systems. Even very small flow rates can significantly alter the ICP in a negative manner. Even the installation of multiple gravity valves cannot reliably prevent this (Fig. 35, right). Simply setting the opening pressure much higher than physically reasonable avoids drainage in the upright position and thus the influence of dynamic pressure changes due to patient movement. Introducing an additional flow setting could allow for more reasonable vertical valve opening characteristics if the volume of fluid drained remains low during pressure peaks. Flow adjustment dampens fluid outflow and reduces the influence of short-term pressure fluctuations. The set means pressure is easier to control.

Figure 36 explains the effect of flow reducing. The resistance depends on the length of the pathway with reduced inner diameter. The resistance of a tube is highly dependent on its diameter. In the case of a round catheter, the outflow resistance depends on the radius to the fourth power. This means that the smaller the radius, the greater the outflow resistance and the longer a pressure-driven outflow of liquids takes. According to the Hagen–Poiseuille law, the flow can be calculated as follows:

$$\dot{V} = \frac{dV}{dt} = \frac{\pi \cdot r^4}{8 \cdot \eta} \frac{\Delta p}{l}$$

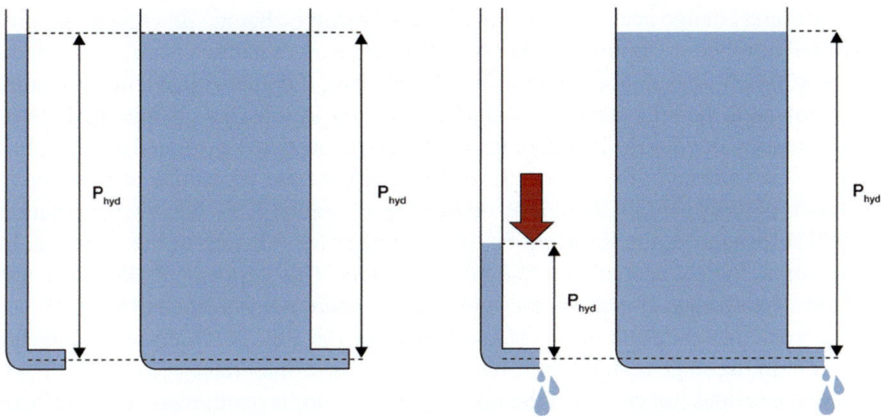

Fig. 35 Model to illustrate the effect of varying compliance on drainage outcome

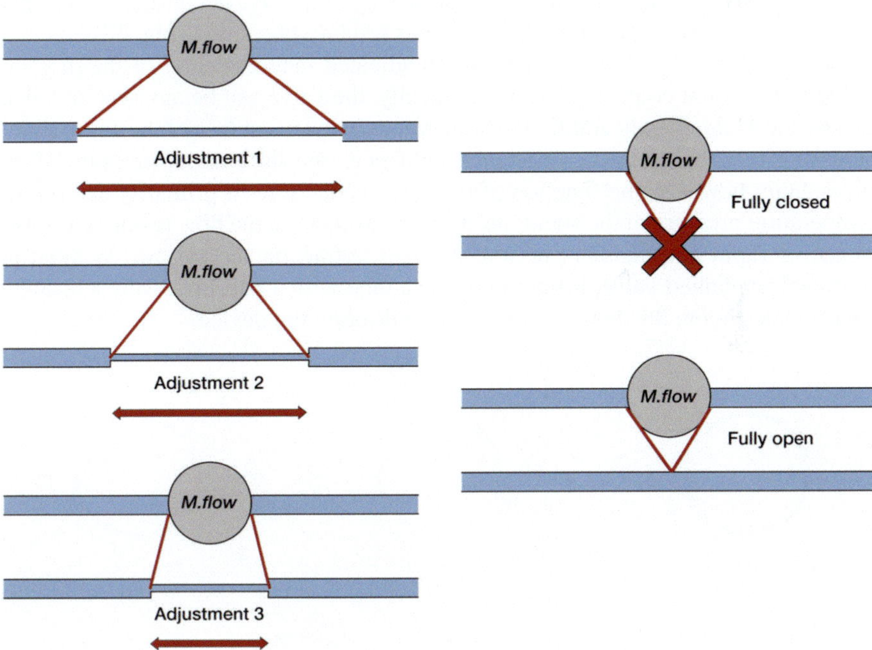

Fig. 36 Illustration of the principle of operation of the *M.flow*® Left: Resistance setting; Right: Device fully off (top) and fully on (bottom)

$\dot{V}$: volume change according to the time; dV: volume change; dt: change in time; π: natural number; r: radius; Δp: pressure difference; η: dynamic viscosity; l: length.

The *M.flow*® does not contain a valve mechanism. It contains just a narrow canal which connects the inlet and the outlet of the implant. A rotor covers this small canal and its position defines the length of the narrowed pathway to be drained through. For the lowest resistance of the device, the opening of the rotor is positioned right above the outlet. In this position, there is no additional resistance at all. Next to the position of highest resistance, the rotor can be turned further for full stop of the drainage. In this position, the device closes the shunt completely. This adjustment allows the test of shunt dependency. If needed, the shunt can be opened again immediately.

The mode of operation of the *M.flow*® is shown in Fig. 36. A drainage catheter has a certain drainage resistance. If the *M.flow*® is now integrated into this catheter, the resistance does not change if the opening in the rotor is positioned directly above the outlet. If the rotor is now twisted, the resistance depends on the final position of the opening in the rotor above the channel. The longer the outflowing channel, the higher the resistance and the lower the flow through the valve at constant differential pressure. In the closed position, the outflow is reliably prevented (Fig. 37).

Thus the *M.flow*® allows the flow to be adjusted independently of the pressure setting of the shunt control valve. Theoretically, the valve can be any type of valve, because the *M.flow*® only additionally intervenes in the resistance of the entire shunt. Increasing or decreasing the resistance influences the differential pressure of the entire shunt; however, the function of the valve is decisive. It primarily determines the operating pressure of the shunt; the *M.flow*® influences the flow result as a consequence of rapid and sudden pressure changes acting on the system. Without an additional implanted valve, it functions like a tube with a non-invasively adjustable inner lumen. Figure 38 shows a cross section through the device.

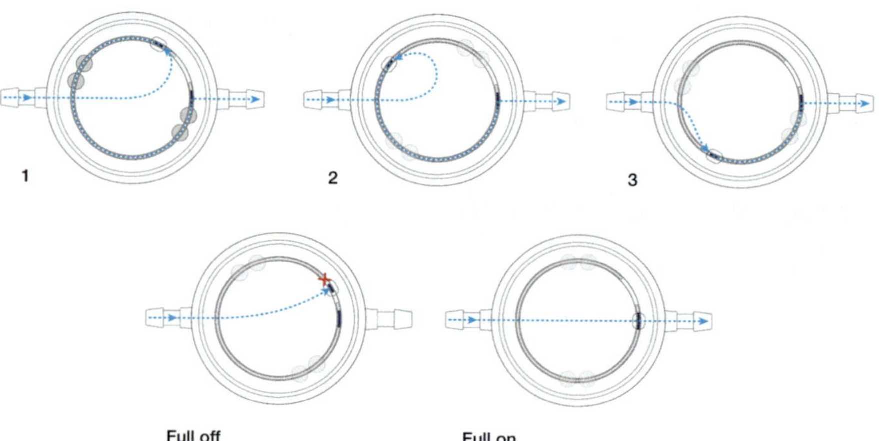

Fig. 37 Adjustments the device design for different rotor positions

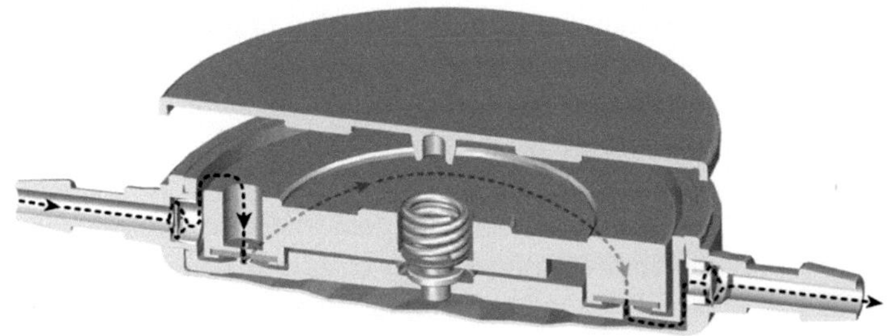

Fig. 38 Cross section of the *M.flow*® for adjusting the flow through a shunt

7 The Fairy Tale of Smart Shunts

More than 40 years ago, Rekate proposed a closed-loop system to control ICP [91]. Since then, numerous similar approaches have been published; none of these ideas have been available for clinical use though. In the first view, this sounds surprising. Reviewing the different proposals reveals a couple of understandable reasons.

First, the authors do not differentiate by patient group or aetiology. However, shunt failure is completely different in paediatric hydrocephalus, post-haemorrhagic hydrocephalus or NPH. In many of these articles, the introduction mentions that there have been no realistic improvements in recent decades and that "Current technology remains relatively rudimentary with advances coming along every few years as companies battle to retain market share." In addition, the motivation for their own activities is generally described by the continued poor results after shunting. However, the statement like "It is generally estimated that 40% of shunts fail within 2 years and 98% have failed within 10 years" ignores successes in improved treatment and progress in understanding of shunts at least of the years after 2000. It is not true, neither for the paediatric population nor for the adult population, that 98% of shunts fail within 10 year or 40% within 2 years [92, 93]. On the one hand, the authors mention that the deep understanding of the pathophysiology of CSF circulation is a prerequisite for the development of an intelligent shunt, on the other hand, they do not differentiate between the significance of a shunt failure and the clinical course and treatment success up to this point, they also do not differentiate between the reasons for the revision of a shunt and especially not between the different patient collectives. A non-responder in the NPH group is a completely different case than a neonate with shunt blockage and post-haemorrhagic hydrocephalus. However, both cases fail and negatively affect the survival rate. However, the failure rate in infants is not a matter of not understanding CSF physiology, which may be the reason for failure in the NPH patient, among others, but a consequence of limited space for the implant to establish reliable valve function. On the other hand, the reason for failure in NPH could also be, e.g. a wrong indication or the implantation could be too late, since it is known (one of the clinical achievements of recent years) that clinical success depends on the timing of implantation of a shunt: the later it is implanted, the worse the clinical status at the time of implantation, the worse and more disappointing the outcome. In any case, one cannot generalise from shunt failure that it is due to inadequate technique. Even a smart shunt would not promise any improvement here. On the contrary, if the size of a smart shunt was available in the infant, one may assume that this larger volume would be used more effectively for improved mechanical reliability through enlargement.

Negative description of achievements in the area where the authors want to make a contribution to progress is similar to the strategy of writing patents. First, the problem is described as big as possible, together with the explanation why no one has been able to solve it carefully and all previous proposals are insufficient. This is followed by an explanation of one's thoughts and inventions and a description of one's claimed rights to the ideas. Whether their own ideas work or not, or whether the criticism is justified or not, is not examined.

Many of these smart shunt projects are funded by people or organisations who are not really introduced to the subject. The experts (scientists, engineers responsible for the project) do not invest their own money, but either public money or private money from investment companies. If there is a financial investor behind, the focus of the project is the financial perspective and the promised return of investment. Surprisingly, in most of the cases, the investors are not the companies already active in the field of hydrocephalus with a bright expertise and well connected to the medical field but investors looking for business prospects being aware of the risk behind [94–96]. However, the focus of these projects is always on developing a product that the investors intend to market. The interest therefore always lies in the introduction of a new, groundbreaking technology that promises enormous financial prospects. In this sense, investors also accept the risk of failure. A good example is the Cognishunt® project, which aimed to demonstrate the ability of a new shunt (with unknown or unpublished operating principle) to improve the life prospects of Alzheimer's patients by implanting a VP shunt with the new device. The clinical data from a clinical trial did not confirm the thesis [97] and the money was lost.

Publicly funded projects, on the other hand, do not focus on product development but on feasibility studies. This means that the value of these projects is usually very limited, as the confirmation of a technical principle in vitro does not say too much about its potential in vivo. The only convincing argument for the use of a new technology should be and remain clinical evidence. Clinical evidence can be provided when a device is clinically available and can be used. This is not possible with prototypes. Nowadays, the approval of medical devices is a demanding and complex procedure. Non-commercial developments often disregard the most important aspect of implants: biocompatibility. Many technical solutions cannot be used in vivo because the available space prevents this and the passivation of the solution destroys the function or influences it too negatively.

But which of the projects of recent years has provided valuable results for the perspective of one day presenting an intelligent shunt? One approach to answering this question is to return to the open tasks, to the reasons for failure or unsatisfactory clinical outcomes of shunt patients. Failure due to infection represents a large group. Possibly, this is the most important reason for revisions, as it is the reason for revision in most cases. Recently, the development of antibiotic catheters has been shown to significantly reduce the rate of infection in paediatric hydrocephalus [98]. Indeed, even the value of the significant results of the BASICS study are questions addressed by earlier paper which show that the infection can be reduced at least to the same low level without an impregnation of the catheters [99]. It must be assumed that although such low infection rates can be achieved, they are unrealistic as an average result. The care required for this, the strict adherence to the required protocol is not achievable in many clinics. Against this background, the development of antibiotic-impregnated catheters must be seen as an important step forward in improving the failure rate of shunt placement.

In addition to infection, shunt obstruction is particularly important in paediatric hydrocephalus. The question here is in what way and to what extent an innovative intelligent shunt can overcome this problem. If a control loop is established as an ICP-controlling shunt system, it is completely open whether such a device can, first, recognise the situation and, second, independently unblock and clear the drainage pathway. These aspects are not even addressed in papers on smart shunts.

The next issues with shunts are under-drainage and over-drainage. Blockage may be the result of excessive protein content or an excessive amount of cellular debris in the draining CSF. As mentioned earlier, this problem could be solved by larger weights, larger actuating forces, and larger effective areas involved in the function of shunts. However, this is true for both passive systems and smart shunts. It is always a matter of weighing the advantages and disadvantages of new devices. It cannot be said that the introduction of electronic components into technology guarantees its reliable operation. The new technology definitely brings new risks that must be outweighed by important benefits. But whether there are any advantages at all in terms of clogging over passive devices is an open question.

Another reason for under-drainage is over-drainage. Both of these issues are resolved very differently by the various devices available. Because the available technology is so diverse and publications on clinical outcomes are so inhomogeneous in terms of study quality, study protocol, aetiology of patients included, observation time, quality of life and other aspects, it is difficult to make a general, overall summary statement about passive shunts. The available valve technology is discussed in this chapter, as are some basic physical aspects (hydrostatic pressure). These physical aspects can be and are addressed by the technology of at least some passive valves (gravitational valves). In addition to clinical evidence, physical or scientific evidence should also be considered in evaluations of the technology. There are very few prospective randomised trials looking at shunt technology. Meier et al. [100] concluded that the addition of a gravitational unit to an adjustable DPV in patients with idiopathic NPH makes a large difference in terms of over-drainage rates (class I evidence) and has to be the standard of care in the treatment of idiopathic NPH. As for the concept of smart shunts, again, whether or not this type of smart drainage will improve clinical outcome and reduce the rate of revision due to the physiological conditions present in the ventricular system is an open question. The problem of a closed loop is the limitation of the pressure and flow measurement. It is easily stated that the ICP and the flow are going to be measured precisely for a time as a part of an implant. But behind these topics, lurk numerous tasks that have hardly been solved so far.

The minimum requirement for a smart shunt is an active, computer-controlled mechanism to interfere with the actual condition within a shunt based on a measured signal. This means at least an actuator as well as a sensor is needed. Without a sensor, no closed loop can work as well as without an actuator. Since the shunt is focusing the ICP, the most important sensor should be a pressure transducer. A flow sensor could be a valuable addition to the concept as well as a sensor detecting movement and position. Other sensors might be interesting, however these should be added after the first ones are clinically available.

Numerous technical principles have been developed for the precise measurement of pressure in gases or liquids. However, only one solution is available today as a long-term implantable sensor [101, 102]. Although needed for decades, the quality of the presented development results has never allowed an indefinite implantation. The concept of this sensor (*M.scio*®) uses the equation of ideal gases to transmit the external pressure (ICP) through a thin titanium diaphragm to an asic (application specific integrated circuit) in a titanium housing. An asic is used throughout the world wherever pressure measurement is required. Its accuracy promises the best measurements available. However, it cannot be implanted because it is not biocompatible and must not have direct contact with fluids such as cerebrospinal fluid. The implant is designed to minimise the volume of gas. Therefore, the smallest movements of the titanium membrane change the pressure inside the housing, depending on the changing external pressure.

The pressure inside the left vessel in Fig. 39 pI1 is equal to the external pressure pO. The membrane is not displaced. The container in the centre left pI2 has a higher pressure inside than outside. The diaphragm bulges outward in the direction of the lower pressure. The opposite happens in the container in the centre right pI3, where the external pressure is higher than the internal pressure. The membrane collapses a little into the container. In contrast, almost no movement occurs in the fourth vessel on the right pI4 (Fig. 39). The diaphragm is hardly moved by changing external pressure. In this case, only minimal movement is required to create the same pressure inside the vessel as outside. The smaller the volume, the less movement is required to adjust the pressure. This principle explains how a pressure outside of a box can be transmitted inside a box. The measurement inside represents the pressure outside. It is decisive to understand that the measured pressure is an absolute pressure. This means that the value of the measurement depends on the knowledge about the outside pressure. The measured value for the pressure within the containers in Fig. 39 has to be compared to the measured outer pressure. The difference defines the movement of the membrane. If this method is used for measuring the ICP, the value measured within the titanium cell has to be compared with the actual atmospheric pressure. The difference gives the actual ICP. This makes another restriction obvious. If such a measurement shall be used for the regulation of a smart shunt, always an externally measured pressure value is needed. This requires energy, which has to be taken from a battery placed within the implant. A battery is needed anyway, but this communication with an external pressure transducer requires an enormous amount of energy taken from the

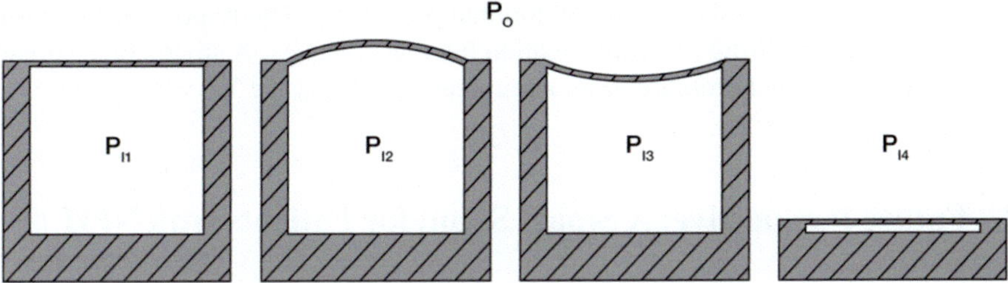

Fig. 39 Physical principle of the *M.scio*® to transmit the outer pressure to the inner housing by minimum movement of a titanium membrane

battery. On the other hand, the concept of an externally integrated pressure transducer introduces enormous risk to the valve. If the communication fails or the external transducer is damaged, the shunt does not work anymore.

Today, if a pressure transmitter is available, there is nothing to measure the flow through a shunt with any useful accuracy. So far, some proposals have been made to externally qualify the flow in certain ranges. The idea behind such approaches is to allow investigation of whether a shunt is still functioning or not. This involves cooling the CSF externally and measuring how long it takes for the cooled front to drain. From this, the flow can then be calculated. Inside an implant, however, such concepts are not applicable. This means that at the moment the only possibility for a closed-loop shunt is to implement the principle of *M.scio*® (the principle of relaxed membranes) in a smart shunt and accept the requirement for external pressure measurement. Can and will such a concept really lead to an improved treatment perspective? The requirement for optimal pressure matching in patients with NPH is particularly unclear. What pressure situation should be required? Could such a concept possibly promise progress for this group of patients? However, if a definition of a desired result cannot be given by the clinicians, a device cannot be developed accordingly (Fig. 40).

Most developers do not seem to be aware that a valve in a VP shunt merely transmits abdominal pressure to the ventricles in some fashion. In these shunts, abdominal pressure represents atmospheric pressure, which is no better measured

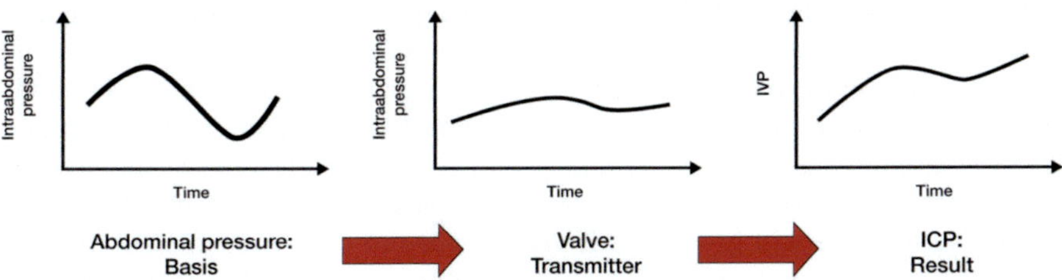

Fig. 40 Importance of abdominal pressure for ICP in shunt patients. The valve "uses" abdominal pressure to transmit it to the ventricular system. In addition, postural physical conditions within the shunt affect ICP

in the human body. In other words, abdominal pressure and body position are more important to the resulting pressure situation than most valves. A smart shunt should at least use abdominal pressure more intelligently than passive VP valves can.

8   Future Perspective: A Smart Shunt for Patients with NPH

In Japan, it is becoming increasingly popular to implant LP shunts instead of VP shunts in patients with NPH [103–105]. Whether CSF is drained via the spinal canal and from there via a catheter into the abdominal compartment or whether CSF is drained from the cerebral ventricles via a catheter into the abdominal compartment, makes no difference as long as the different compartments are well connected and there are no stenoses in between. To date, however, no valve has been developed to meet the special conditions of implantation in the abdominal compartment. Because such devices could be implanted in a manner similar to pacemakers, they could be the size of pacemakers. Available valves for LP shunts are similar to those once used for VP shunts. However, the potential size of such devices is not really altered. Larger valves, however, could allow for more complex technology involving a battery, a pressure transducer, and an actuator. If the pressure transducer is sufficient as a differential pressure transducer and external pressure measurement is not required, a new concept of a smart shunt for patients with NPH could promise advances and new achievements in the field. The background for these considerations is the fact that patients with NPH do not necessarily require continuous CSF drainage. As is known from lumbar puncture tests to investigate whether a patient could benefit from shunt therapy, the response to CSF withdrawal lasts for a while, even if no further CSF withdrawal takes place. Whereas in hypertensive hydrocephalus, the continuous drainage of CSF is life saving and consequently very important for the clinical status of the patient, in NPH the situation is different. Actually, nobody really knows what the best pressure regulation for NPH patients should be. NPH is a pathological status and the question is whether physiological conditions alone should be the desired clinical perspective for the affected patients. Whatever valve system may be implanted, the question of whether and to what extent further improvement would be possible through which action remains unanswered. In general, it can be assumed that lowering the ICP and dampening the pressure fluctuations should have a positive effect on the clinical status of the patients (Fig. 41).

The simplest of the proposed smart valves was a programmable switch. Programming is used to determine when, how often and how long the shunt should be opened. The programming can be done by taking into account the posture of the body. In the upright position, the opening time can be reduced; in the horizontal position of the patient, the time will be automatically extended to ensure a sufficient drainage result. The various parameters can be individually programmed and adapted to the patient's needs. The valve is to be implanted in a VP shunt and placed thoracically. The development was funded by the German government. It has not been approved or clinically evaluated to date. But the basic requirements for an implant have been

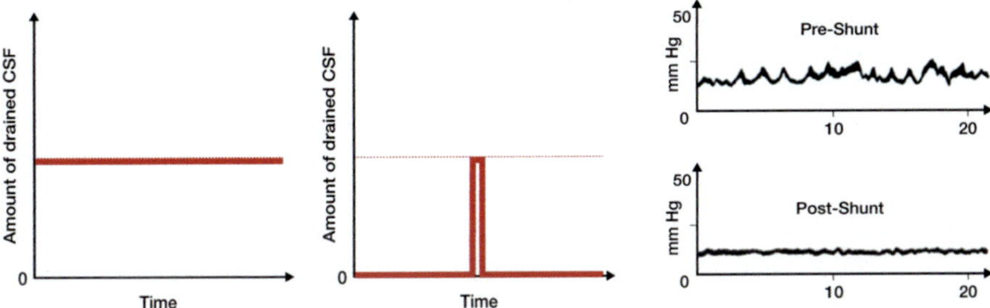

Fig. 41 Difference between continuous drainage (left) and intermittent (middle) withdraw of CSF. ICP before and after continuous shunting (right). Is the continuous CSF flow required?

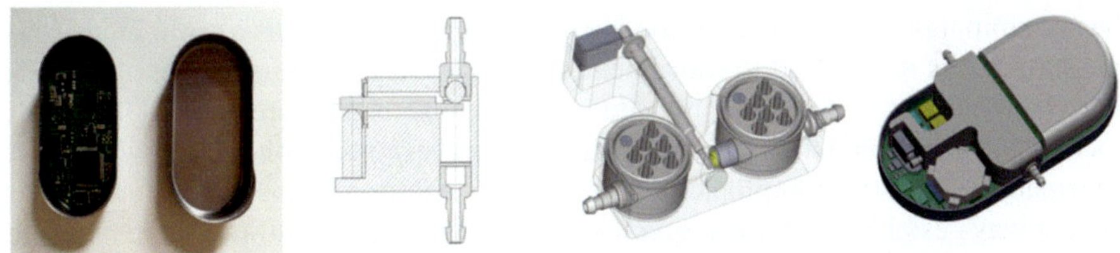

Fig. 42 Prototype of a programmable switch for the treatment of NPH including two pressure sensors (Left: First implantable prototype without pressure transducer; left middle: Concept of a piezo activated switch; right middle: a switch in combination with two absolute pressure transducers; right: computer model of an electrical switch with integrated pressure transducers

solved. The battery-powered switch has been successfully evaluated in vitro, as has the radio link from a titanium housing to an external programming device, and the energy-efficient control of a piezo-driven actuator system (Fig. 42).

After the presentation of the programmable switch as a new active implant for CSF drainage in patients with NPH in Banff 2015 [106], the promised progress of this device did not justify the financial investment for a necessary clinical trial. Therefore, the concept remains a current one to this day. However, based on technological advances since then, the valve should be augmented with two absolute pressure sensors separated by a switch, an activity sensor that can detect improvements in the patient's walking or general mobility and a position sensor. Such a device could learn in what way the patient improves after what type of fluid withdrawal without knowing the actual ICP. Interpretation of distal and proximal pressure changes as a function of body posture and switch position could allow autonomous programming of the device. Similar to Al-Momani's proposals [107], data obtained from such devices could be shared via a cloud, and based on artificial intelligence programmes, successful treatment and its optimization could occur without the intervention of the treating physician.

Integrated into a titanium housing, two pressure sensors can detect pressure changes in the abdominal cavity, intracranial pressure changes and changes in atmospheric pressure in an exciting way. Together with the patient position sensor, these measurements enable the interpretation of pressure changes and thus the calculation of a meaningful opening of the mechatronic switch. When the switch is closed, soon after the valve is implanted, during a few days and a few controlled movements, the device can quickly determine the expected absolute pressure difference between the horizontal and vertical positions. With the switch closed, one value for the proximal limb of the shunt and one value for the distal limb are obtained in each case. The difference between the maximum and minimum values measured proximally reveals the hydrostatic pressure, including the current ICP, acting at the closed inlet of the device. The absolute pressure measured at the distal outlet of the device in the supine and standing position reveals the distal portion of the hydrostatic pressure including the abdominal pressure values. If the proximal transducer detects a rapid increase in pressure that is not related to movement or changes in atmospheric pressure (since there is no change at the distal transducer), the cause is an increase in ICP. Briefly opening the device and then measuring the pressure response of the drain will provide information about the compliance of the patient's ventricular system. A functioning shunt always establishes typical pressures within the shunt, both when the device is closed and when it is open. When the patient is lying down, the switch can be opened to recalibrate the two sensors, not in terms of atmospheric pressure accuracy, but in relation to each other. The sensors would be set to the same value in the same pressure situation (or the different measured values could be noted as corresponding to the exact same absolute pressure), making it possible to interpret pressure values in a goal-directed manner regardless of the actual accuracy of the pressure measurement with respect to atmospheric pressure and regardless of knowledge of it. Which of the sensors does not measure accurately, only one of them or both, as long as the changes reflect the actual pressure changes reasonably correctly. The aspect can be illustrated by comparing it to a boat on the sea. The measurement of the actual sea level, which depends on the tides, can be dispensed with if the goal is to know how deep the hull of the ship is sinking in the water. As long as the master knows how deep the ship is sinking into the water, the height of the water level in the sea does not need to be measured and may be very inaccurate. If the ship would sink deeper into the water for no apparent reason, there is a leak somewhere and this problem should be solved soon.

Such a system could monitor its own function on the basis of plausibility of different values and, in case of problems, provide concrete information about "unexplained" deviations. It could inform the physician about abnormal, not explainable conditions within the shunt, it could give detailed information as a basis to consider reasonable interventions, and it could be more robust, more reliable than passive valve systems. Passive valve systems have the problem that they shall be precise and reliably working depending on very small pressure changes on the one hand, and that they have to be as small as possible. The small size enables only small acting forces of springs or of gravitational balls (or parts). The smaller these forces are, the easier the mechanism is affected by disturbance variables. A mechatronic switch offers significantly higher action forces which are by far less likely to be damaged or effected in its function.

The concept of an electronically controlled mechatronic switch promises improved diagnostic and therapeutic capabilities. It is technically feasible and could be the first available valve adapted to the conditions of a valve for LP shunts, where more space is available for the technology. However, it could also be implanted in VP shunts with the same value, benefits and effect for therapy. The only limitation is the site of implantation. Usually, neurosurgeons prefer to place the valve retroauricularly in VP shunts. Technically, though, these valves can also be implanted thoracically without any problems. In the event of a malfunction, the device could provide detailed information about the problem. So far, in many cases of clinical deterioration, it is difficult and sometimes impossible to find out what the problem is without performing revision surgery. In addition, such a device would provide tremendous opportunities for clinical research, especially in patients with NPH. Who responds to what type of pressure intervention and under what circumstances? This device would be an important step forward in meaningfully improving the treatment of hydrocephalus through digitization. Depending on the accuracy that can be achieved in terms of improving walking or moving, it could possibly optimise therapy in general and individually.

The new approach does not promise to solve all problems of shunting for any kind of age or aetiology. It is a concept to intelligently control the drainage in NPH patients. Whether it could and will be an improvement for newborns, infants and adults with different aetiologies, has to be evaluated after a successful introduction in the field of NPH. The concept overcomes the difficulties regarding precision and reliability of implantable ICP-transducers, including the problem of drift and the communication required with an external transducer.

The limitation for the development of such a device lies in financial aspects. The risk behind an investment is that the concept can only be verified or falsified, if the device is developed and approved for a clinical trial. The results of a clinical trial must reveal superior outcomes in comparison to the technology nowadays available. This will be an enormous challenge as the outcome, the complication rate as well as the evidence for shunting NPH is by far better than stated in papers presenting now smart solutions. Despite all the problems, implanting a shunt remains one of the most successful interventions in neurosurgery [108].

9 Summary and Conclusion

Improvement in medical device technology depends on financial aspects, knowledge, creativity, commitment, cooperation and resources. In the best case, concrete tasks come from the clinicians, which are then worked on by technicians in constant dialogue with the clinicians. The completion of such development projects means that a new product is available for clinical use. The decisive milestone in this regard is usually approval of a medical device. Especially in the field of technology for the treatment of NPH, the competence to develop proposals for innovations with regard to significant patient benefits lies with technicians, since the understanding of technical possibilities and physical laws of hydraulic systems does not belong to the core competences of neurosurgeons and can only be part of them in exceptional cases. Exactly here seems to be a central challenge regarding the further improvement of shunt systems for the treatment of NPH.

NPH is still considered under-diagnosed. It is assumed that a large proportion of people suffering from NPH worldwide are cared for untreated in nursing homes and homes for the elderly, who would benefit considerably in terms of their quality of life and life expectancy through appropriate therapy. This would also reduce healthcare costs, as the effort required to care for elderly people suffering from dementia who are in need of care is complex and therefore very costly. The fact that many people suffering from NPH remain untreated may be due to the fact that the disease itself is far less well known, but on the other hand also to the fact that both diagnosis and therapy are not extensively evidence-based, especially in differentiating them from other diseases of the elderly. Although there are standards worldwide, these standards do not mean that diagnosis and therapy are identical everywhere. Both the indication for implantation of a shunt and the selection of the technique to be implanted are often subject to individual assessment and experience, since clear evidence is not always available. Thus, to this day, there are still critics who doubt the evidence for the implantation of shunt systems for the treatment of NPH.

Indeed, to date, there is limited clear evidence regarding the functionality of valve systems implanted in hydrocephalus shunts that has been established in clinical trials. The findings from the available reports of prospective randomised controlled multicentre trials can be summarised as follows:

- Comparison of three different valve types (reduced flow, simple differential pressure valve, differential pressure valve with SCD [ASD]) in paediatric hydrocephalus yielded no differences in survival of implanted shunts.
- DPVs with low opening pressure produce better clinical outcomes in NPH than DPVs with higher opening pressure, with significantly higher rates of over-drainage.
- Examination of a single type of adjustable DPV compared with a non-adjustable valve of the same type showed no differences in outcome and complication rate between the two groups.
- Implantation of an additional gravitational valve in NPH significantly reduces over- drainage with at least comparable clinical outcome.

The development of technology is often a prerequisite for the opportunity to clinically investigate the value of a new idea. An implantable pressure transducer to measure ICP is a good example. Without such a device, whose value and principle importance for the treatment of hydrocephalus is readily apparent, there is little or very limited ability to record conditions after shunt placement. Although a clinical condition can be assessed, the pressure underlying the condition remains unknown without measurement. The same applies to changes resulting from non-invasive interventions (valve changes) in shunted patients. Obviously, shunt placement in patients with hydrocephalus presents a comparable clinical picture for very different actual acting conditions. Thus, not all NPH patients develop hygromas or over-drainage symptoms after implantation of a VP shunt with DPV, although hydrostatic regularities always operate. This in turn obscures the effect of the regularity. Only a measurement can remove this veil. The prerequisite for this is the existence of the appropriate technology.

Since a long-term implantable pressure transducer for use in shunts has been available for several years, the effect of shunts can and should be systematically evaluated as a function of valve type and valve setting. In addition to the clinical picture, attention could also be paid to the measured values of the ICP. This will reveal the physical scientific evidence as a basis for further technical and subsequently clinical progress. While the pathophysiological background of CSF diseases is very complex and difficult to understand, the basis and function of technical devices are well described and comprehensively understood. Each valve functions according to its technical design, whether implanted or studied in the laboratory.

Technical evidence exists for the relationships described in this section. Understanding of the different functionalities does not develop (or develops only fuzzily) from analysis of clinical data, particularly with respect to survival rates of implanted shunt systems. The indication for shunt revision is subject to highly individualised assessments worldwide. It also becomes clear that a Kapan–Meier curve obviously does not reveal anything about how the patient was doing until the revision, whether the development of the child's brain took a normal course, whether the NPH patient benefited clinically from the shunt over a long period of time and was able to lead a life free of complaints.

The following observations are based on scientific evidence and should be considered when reflecting on shunt function, especially in the face of worsening or disappointing outcomes and complications.

Finally, it is important to reiterate that the reader should keep in mind the author's conflict of interest. More important than the author's opinion presented in this chapter is the need to carefully consider available technology that can be implanted within an hour; the valve or shunt, on the other hand, creates a pressure condition for many years. The mathematician, seeing a black sheep in a pasture from a moving train, would say, "Look, there is a sheep that is black from one side!" A scientist would check whether the sheep is also black from the other side or not.

10   Key Points

- Adjustable and non-adjustable DPVs cannot ensure the correct (optimal) values for the ICP ratio in the same setting for the standing and lying positions. The requirements for a DPV in the VP shunt (LP shunt) are not identical.
- The valves or valve components that accommodate the variable position pressure ratios in the shunt (ASD/SCD, flow regulation systems, gravity valves) differ significantly in design, function and treatment risk. These systems have the same purpose, but must be considered in a differentiated manner.

- Valve systems with integrated ASD/SCD technology are systematically and unpredictably highly dependent on subcutaneous pressure for their function. CSF outflow in such systems is primarily determined by the variable and unknown subcutaneous pressure.
- Flow reducing devices, in principle, regulate pressure. Flow regulation would mean determining the flow required to produce physiological conditions in the cranial cavity. The rate of production is not always constant and is not the same from person to person. Consequently, a flow-regulated valve theoretically (and practically proven by in vitro studies) allows over- or under-drainage depending on the specific situation of the individual patient.
- Gravitational devices can compensate for position-dependent hydrostatic pressure in shunt systems. The adjustability of the characteristics of a gravitational device independent of the setting to the recumbent position allows the adjustment to be tailored to the needs of the individual patient.
- Adjusting flow by shortening or lengthening a narrow pathway provides the ability to influence CSF outflow in addition to a pressure-defining valve. Whether such a device expands treatment options in difficult patients remains to be seen. The additional ability to completely occlude the device could open the option to test shunt dependency.
- Reliable measurements of the resulting post-shunt pressure will allow non-invasive investigation of the realistic performance of the various proposed solutions.

References

1. Boon AJW, Joseph TJ, Delwel EJ, et al. Dutch normal-pressure hydrocephalus study: randomized comparison of low- and medium-pressure shunts. J Neurosurg. 1998;88:490–5.
2. Drake J, Kestle J, Milner R, Cinalli G, Boop F, Piatt J, Heines S, Schiff S, Cochrane D, Steinbok P, MacNeil N, et al. Randomized trial of cerebrospinal fluid shunt valve design in pediatric hydrocephalus. Neurosurgery. 1998;43(2):294–305.
3. Decq P, Barat JL, Duplessis E, Leguerinel C, Gendrault P, Keravel Y. Shunt failure in adult hydrocephalus: flow-controlled shunt versus differential pressure shunts—a cooperative study in 289 patients Surg Neurol. 1995;43(4):333–9.
4. Esmonde T, Cooke S. Shunting for normal pressure hydrocephalus (NPH). Cochrane Database Syst Rev. 2002;2002(3):CD003157. https://doi.org/10.1002/14651858.CD003157. PMID:12137677; PMCID: PMC9002238.
5. Munthe S. Treating hydrocephalus by shunting to the venous intracranial sinus. In: Oral presentation at the 14th meeting of the hydrocephalus society, Gothenburg, Sep 9–12, 2022.
6. Desai B, Hsu Y, Schneller B, Hobbs JG, Mehta AI, Linninger A. Hydrocephalus: the role of cerebral aquaporin-4 channels and computational modeling considerations of cerebrospinal fluid. Neurosurg Focus. 2016;41(3):E8. https://doi.org/10.3171/2016.7.FOCUS1 6191. PMID: 27581320.
7. Hydrocephalus 2022, 14th Meeting of the hydrocephalus society, Session 7: Technical advances in treatment and diagnostics, Gothenburg, Sveden, Sep 9–12, 2022.
8. Sood S, Canady AI, Ham SD. Adjustable antisiphon shunt. Childs Nerv Syst. 1999;15(5):246–9.

9. Jetzki S, Kiefer M, Walter M, Leonhardt S. Concepts for a mechatronic device to control intracranial pressure. IFAC Proc. 2006;39(16):25–9.

10. Czosnyka ZH, Czosnyka M, Richards HK, Pickard JD. Laboratory evaluation of the phoenix CRx diamond valve. Neurosurgery 2001;48(3):689–93.

11. Aschoff A, Kremer P, Hashemi B, Benesch C, Kunze S. Technical design of 130 hydrocephalus valves: an overview on historical, available, and prototype valves. In: Poster at the XVth congress of the European Society for Pediatric Neurosurgery, Rome, Sep 21–25, 1996.

12. Hassan M, Higashi S, Yamashita J. Risks in using siphon-reducing devices in adult patients with normal-pressure hydrocephalus: bench test investigations with Delta valves. J Neurosurg. 1996;84:634–41.

13. Pollack IF, Albright AL, Adelson PD. A randomized, controlled study of a programmable shunt valve versus a conventional valve for patients with hydrocephalus. Neurosurgery. 1999;45:1399.

14. Schaltenbrand G, Wolff H. Die Produktion und Zirkulation des Liquors und ihre Störungen. In: Handbuch der Neurochirurgie, Herausgegeben von H. Olivercrona w. Tönnis, Stockholm Köln/Rhein., Erster Band/Erster Teil, Grundlagen I, Springer-Verlag, Berlin Göttingen Heidelberg, 1959, S. 107.

15. Röther J. Liquorzirkulationsstörungen. In: Klinische Neurologie.

16. Pollay M. The function and structure of the crebrospinal fluid outflow system. Cerebrospienal Fluid Res. 2010;7:9.

17. Poca M, Sahuquillo J, Topczewski T, et al. Posture induced changes in intacranial pressure; a comparative study in patients with and without a cerebrospinal fluid block at the craniovertebral junction. Neurosurgery. 2006;58:899–906.

18. Rigamonti D, Juhler M, Wikkelsö C. The differential diagnostic of normal pressure hydrocephalus. In: Rigamonti D, editor. Adult hydrocephalus. Chapter 10, 103.

19. Aschoff, A. In-vitro-Testung von Hydrocephalus-Ventilen. zweite, erweiterte Auflage, Habilitationsschrift. Heidelberg, 1994.

20. Davson H. Physiology of the cerebrospinal fluid. SDBN 0700012907, London, published by Churchill; 1967.

21. Gaumann D, Sinclair M, Forster A. Neurochirurgische Intensivmedizin. In: Benzer H, Burchardi H, Larsen R, Suter PM (Herausgeber). Intensivmedizin,Springer-Verlag 2013, S. 646.

22. Petraglia AL, Moravan MJ, Dimopoulos VG, Silberstein HJ. Pediatr Neurosurg. 2011;47(2):99–107.

23. Lam CH, Villemure JG. Comparison between ventriculoatrial and ventriculoperitoneal shunting in the adult population. Br J Neurosurg. 1997;11(1):43–8.

24. Wu D, Guan Z, Xiao L, et al. Thrombosis associated with ventriculoatrialshunts. Neurosurg Rev. 2022;45:1111–1122

25. Akhtar N, Khan AA, Yousaf M. Experience and outcome of ventriculo-atrial shunt: a multi centre study. J Ayub Med Coll Abbottabad 2015;27(4):817–20.

26. El Shafei IL, El Shafei HI. The retrograde ventriculo-sinus shunt (El Shafei RVS shunt): rationale, evolution, surgical technique and long-term results. Pediatr Neurosurg. 2005;41:305–17.

27. Børgesen SE, Gjerris F, Agerlin N. Shunting to the sagittal sinus. Acta neurochirurgica. 2002;(Supplement 81).

28. Lylyk P, Lylyk I, Bleise C, Scrivano E, Lylyk PN, Beneduce B, Heilman CB. Malek Am: case report: first-in-human endovascular treatment of hydrocephalus with a miniature biomimetic transdural shunt. J NeuroIntervent Surg. 2022;14:495–9.

29. Hydrocephalus. Gothenburg, Sweden, Sep 9–12 2022.

30. Børgesen SE, Pieri A, Cappelen J, Gjerris F. Shunting to the cranial venous sinus using the SinuShunt. Childs Nerv Syst. 2004;20(6):397–404.

31. Chumas PD, Armstrong DC, Drake JM, Kulkarni AV, Hoffman HJ, Humphreys RP, Rutka JT, Hendrick EB. Tonsillar herniation: the rule rather than the exception after lumboperitoneal shunting in the pediatric population. J Neurosurg. 1993;78:568–73.

32. Royle NA, Hernández MC, Maniega SM, Arabisala BS, Bastin ME, Deary IJ, Wardlaw JM. Influence of thickening of the inner skull table on intracranial volume measurement in older people. Magn Reson Imaging. 2013;31(6):918–22.

33. Anderson R, Kieffer S, Wolfson J, Long D, Peterson H. Thickening of the skull in surgically treated hydrocephalus. Am J Roentgenol. 1970;10(1):96–101.

34. Dattani R. Femoral osteolysis following total hip replacement. Postgrad Med J. 2007;83(979):312–6.

35. Bode H, Haßler W, Sauer M. Das Slit-Ventricle-Syndrom—Ursachen, Differentialdiagnostik und therapeutische Probleme.

36. The Slit-ventricle-Syndrom—Causes, Procedures of Differential Diagnosis and Therapeutic Problems.

37. KlinPadiatr 1984; 196(1): 40–43, New York, Georg Thieme Verlag KG Stuttgart.

38. Baskin JJ, Manwaring KH, Rekate HL. Ventricular shunt removal: the ultimate treatment of the slit ventricle syndrome. J Neurosurg. 1998;88:478–84. Epstein F, Lapras C, Wisoff JH. 'Slit-ventricle syndrome': etiology and treatment. PediatrNeurosci. 1988;14:5–10.

39. Albright AL, Tyler-Kabara E. Slit-ventricle syndrome secondary to shunt-induced suture ossification. Neurosurgery. 2001;48:764–9.

40. Serlo W, Saukkonen AL, Heikkinen E, von Wendt L. The incidence and management of the slit ventricle syndrome. Acta Neurochir (Wien). 1989;99:113–6.

41. Ros B, Iglesias S, Martín Á, Carrasco A, Ibáñez G, Arráez MA. Shunt overdrainage syndrome: review of the literature. Neurosurg Rev. 2018;41:969–81.

42. Al-Abassi AA, Al Saadi A3, Ahmed F. Is intra-bladder pressure measurement a reliable indicator for raised intra-abdominal pressure? A prospective comparative study. BMC Anesthesiol. 2018;18(1):69.

43. Chehade, Y. Intraabdomineller Druck in Abhä ngigkeit von der Kö rperposition: ein notwendiger Parameter zur Optimierung der Hydrozephalus-Shunttherapie, Inauguraldissertation, Universität Lübeck; 2019.

44. Iberti TJ, Lieber CE, Benjamin E. Determination of intra-abdominal pressure using a transurethral bladder catheter: clinical validation of the technique. Anesthesiology. 1989;70(1):47–50.

45. Rot S, Dweek M, Gutowski P, et al. Comparative investigation of different telemetric methods for measuring intracranial pressure: a prospective pilot study. Fluids Barriers CNS. 2020;17:63.

46. Nakajima M, Miyajima M, Ogino I, Akiba C, Kawamura K, Murosawa M, Kuriyama N, Watanbe Y, Fukushima W, Mori E, Kato T, Sugano H, Karagiozov K, Arai H. Shunt intervention for possible idiopathic normal pressure hydrocephalus improves patient outcomes: a nationwide hospital-based survey in Japan. Front Neurol., 07 June 2018 Sec. Neuroepidemiology.

47. Samejima N, Kuwana N, Watanabe A, Kubota M, Seki Y. Lumbo-peritoneal shunt for patients with idiopathic normal pressure hydrocephalus: surgical technique. No ShinkeiGeka. 2022;50(2):348–57.

48. Miethke C, Affeld K. A new valve for the treatment of hydrocephalus. Biomedizinische Technik. 1994;39:181–87.

49. Sprung C, Miethke C, Shakeri K, Lanksch WR. The importance of the dual-switch valve for the treatment of adult normotensive or hypertensive hydrocephalus. Eur J Pediatr Surg. 1997;7(Suppl 1):38–40.

50. Hertel F, Züchner M, Decker C, Schill S, Bosniak I, Bettag M. The Miethke dual switch valve: experience in 169 patients with different kinds of hydrocephalus. An open field study. Minim Invasive Neurosurg. 2008;51(3):147–53.

51. Kiefer M, Eymann R, Meier U. Five years experience with gravitational shunts in chronic hydrocephalus of adults. Acta Neurochirurgica. 2002;144:755–67

52. Meier U, Kintzel D. Clinical experience with different valve systems in patients with normal pressure hydrocephalus: evaluation of the Miethke dual-switch valve. Child's Nerv Syst. 2002;18:288–94.

53. Kiefer M, Eymann R, Steudel W, Strowitzki M. Gravitational shunt management of long standing overt ventriculomegaly in adult (LOVA) hydrocephalus. J Clin Neurosci. 2004.

54. Lumenta CB, Roosen NO, Dietrich U. Clinical experience with a pressure-adjustable valve SOPHY in the management of hydrocephalus. Childs Nerv Syst. 1990;6:270–4.

55. Richards H, Seeley H, Pickard J. Are adjustable valves effective? Data from the UK Shunt Registry. Fluids Barriers CNS. 2007;4(Suppl 1):S30.

56. Serarslan Y, Yilmaz A, Çakır M, Güzel E, Akakin A, Güzel A, Urfalı B, Aras M, Kaya ME, Yılmaz N. Use of programmable versus nonprogrammable shunts in the management of normal pressure hydrocephalus: a multicenter retrospective study with cost-benefit analysis in Turkey. Medicine (Baltimore). 2017;96(39):8185.

57. Pollack IF, Albright AL, Adelson PD. A randomized, controlled study of a programmable shunt valve versus a conventional valve for patients with hydrocephalus. Hakim-Medos Investigator Group. Neurosurgery 1999;45(6):1399–408; discussion 1408–11.

58. Aschoff A. In-depth view: functional characteristics of CSF shunt devices (Pros and Cons). In: Di Rocco C, Pang D, Rutka J, editors. Textbook of pediatric neurosurgery. Cham: Springer; 2019. https://doi.org/10.1007/978-3-319-31512-6_26-2(S.12, Fig. 11 Pressure flow through proximal slit valves. Note the extreme variability (own results))

59. Poca MA, Mataro M, del Mar MM, Arikan F, Junque C, Sahuquillo J. Is the placement of shunts in patients with idiopathic normal-pressure hydrocephalus worth the risk? Results of a study based on continuous monitoring of intracranial pressure. J Neurosurg. 2004;100:855–66.

60. Vanneste JAL. Three decades of normal pressure hydrocephalus: are we wiser now? J Neurol Neurosurg Psychiatry. 1994;57:1021–5.

61. Aschoff A, Biedermann D, Biedermann N, Ludwig J, El Tayeh, Piotrowicz A: Quo Vadis, Valvula? Status and perspectives of hydrocephalus valves. In: 11th Congress of the EMN, Warsaw, March 16–18, 2006.

62. Andreasen TH, Holst AV, Lilja A, Andresen M, Bartek J Jr, Eskesen V, Juhler M. Valved or valveless ventriculoperitoneal shunting in the treatment of post-haemorrhagic hydrocephalus: a population-based consecutive cohort study. Acta Neurochir. 2016;158:2612.

63. Trost HA, Sprung C, Lanksch W, Stolke D, Miethke C. Dual-switch valve: clinical performance of a new hydrocephalus valve. Acta Neurochir Suppl. 1998;71:360–3.

64. Miyake H, Kajimoto Y, Tsuji M, Ukita T, Tucker A, Ohmura T. Development of a quick reference table for setting programmable pressure valves in patients with idiopathic normal pressure hydrocephalus. Neurol Med Chir (Tokyo) 2008;48;427–32

65. Bergsneider M, Black PM, Klinge P, Marmarou A, Relkin N. Surgical management of idiopathic normal-pressure hydrocephalus. Neurosurgery. 2005;57(3 Suppl):S29-39.

66. Oppong MD, Droste L, Pierscianek D, Wrede KH, Rauschenbach L, Dammann P, Herten A, Forsting M, Sure U, Jabbarli R. Adjustable pressure valves for chronic hydrocephalus following subarachnoid hemorrhage: is it worthwhile? Clin Neurol Neurosurg. 2020;198.

67. Xu H, Wang ZX, Liu F, Tan GW, Zhu HW, Chen DH. Programmable shunt valves for the treatment of hydrocephalus: a systematic review. Eur J Pediatr Neurol. 2013;17(5):454–61.

68. Meier U, Lemcke J. Is it possible to optimize treatment of patients with idiopathic normal pressure hydrocephalus by implanting an adjustable Medos Hakim valve in combination with a Miethke shunt assistant? In: Hoff JT, Keep RF, Xi G, Hua Y, editors. Brain Edema XIII. Acta NeurochirurgicaSupplementum, vol. 96. Vienna, Springer; 2006.

69. Bergsneider M, Yang Y, Hu Y, McArthur D, Cook SW, Boscardin J. Relationship between valve opening pressure, body position, and intracranial pressure in normal pressure hydrocephalus: paradigm for selection of programmable valve pressure setting. Neurosurgery 2004;55(4):851–8; discussion.

70. Sprung C, Schlosser H-G, Brock M. Shunting of hydrocephalus with the new adjustable gravitational proGAV—advantages compared to other devices, Fluids and Barriers of the CNS I Sonderheft 1/2005.

71. Toma AK, Tarnaris A, Kitchen ND, Watkins LD. Use of the proGAV shunt valve in normal-pressure hydrocephalus. Neurosurgery 2011;68(2 Suppl Operative):245–9.

72. Watt S, Agerlin N, Romner B. Initial experience with the Codman Certas adjustable valve in the management of patients with hydrocephalus. Fluids Barriers CNS. 2012;9:21.
73. Allin DM, Czosnyka M, Richards HK, Pickard JD, Czosnyka ZH. Investigation of the hydrodynamic properties of a new MRI-resistant programmable hydrocephalus shunt. Cerebrospinal Fluid Res. 2008;21(5):8.
74. Kondageski C, Thompson D, Reynolds M, Hayward RD. Experience with the Strata valve in the management of shunt overdrainage. J Neurosurg. 2007;106(2 Suppl):95–102.
75. Kestle JR, Walker ML. Strata Investigators: a multicenter prospective cohort study of the Strata valve for the management of hydrocephalus in pediatric patients. J Neurosurg. 2005;102(2 Suppl):141–5.
76. Davidson C, White M, Abosch A, Katzir M. Category-2 shunt valve marketed as MRI-conditional malfunction following routine 3T magnetic resonance imaging. Interdisc Neurosurg. 2021;26.
77. Nakashima K, Nakajo T, Kawamo M, Kato A, Ishigaki S, Murakami H, Imaizumi Y, Izumiyama H. Programmable shunt valves: in vitro assessment of safety of the magnetic field generated by a portable game machine. Neurol Med Chir (Tokyo). 2011;51:635–638.
78. da Silva MC, Drake JM. Complications of cerebrospinal fluid shunt antisiphon devices. Pediatr Neurosurg. 1991–92;17:304–309.
79. Drake JM, da Silva MC, Rutka JT. Functional obstruction of an antisiphon device by raised tissue capsule pressure. Neurosurgery. 1993;32(1):137–9.
80. Sainte-Rose C, Hooven MD, Hirsch JF. A new approach in the treatment of hydrocephalus. J Neurosurg. 1987;66(2):213–26.
81. Aschoff A, Kremer P, Benesch C, Fruh K, Klank A, Kunze S. Overdrainage and shunt technology. A critical comparison of programmable, hydrostatic and variable-resistance valves and flow-reducing devices. Childs Nerv Syst. 1995;11(4):193–202.
82. Hara M, Kadowski C, Konishi Y. A new method for measuring CSF flow in shunts. J Neurosurg. 1983;58:557–61.
83. Czosnyka Z, Czosnyka M, Pickard JD. Hydrodynamic performance of a new siphon preventing device: the SiphonGuard. J Neurol Neurosurg Psychiatry. 1999;66(3):408–9.
84. Czosnyka M, Czosnyka ZH. Overdrainage of cerebrospinal fluid and hydrocephalus shunts. Acta Neurochir. 2017;159:1387–8.
85. Udayakumaran S, Roth J, Kesler A, Constantini S. Miethke DualSwitch valve in lumboperitoneal shunts. Acta Neurochir (Wien). 2010;152(10):1793–800.
86. Gutowski P, Gölz L, Rot S, Lemcke J, Thomale U-W. Gravitational shunt valves in hydrocephalus to challenge the sequelae of over-drainage. Expert View Med Devices 2020. https://doi.org/10.1080/17434440.2020.1837622
87. Lemcke J, Meier U, Müller C, Fritsch MJ, Kehler U, Langer N, Kiefer M, Eymann R, Schuhmann MU, Speil A, Weber F, Remenez V, Rohde V, Ludwig HC, Stengel D. Safety and efficacy of gravitational shunt valves in patients with idiopathic normal pressure hydrocephalus: a pragmatic, randomised, open label, multicentre trial (SVASONA). J Neurol Neurosurg Psychiatry. 2013;84(8):850–7.
88. Bergsneider M, Black PM, Klinge P, Marmarou A, Relkin N. Surgical management of idiopathic normal-pressure hydrocephalus. Neurosurgery. 2005;57(3 Suppl):S29–39; discussion ii–v. https://doi.org/10.1227/01.neu.0000168186.45363.4d. PMID: 16160427.
89. Pang D, Altschuler E. Low-pressure hydrocephalic state and viscoelastic alterations in the brain. Neurosurgery. 1994;35:643–56.
90. Bergsneider M, Peacock W, Mazziotta J, Becker D. Benefitial effect of siphoning in treatment of adult hydrocephalus. Arch Neurol. 1999;56:1224–9.
91. Rekate HL. Closed-loop control of intra-cranical pressure. Ann Biomed Eng. 1980;8:515–22.
92. Lemcke J, Meier U, Müller C, Fritsch MJ, Kehler U, Langer N, Kiefer M, Eymann R, Schuhmann MU, Speil A, Weber F, Remenez V, Rohde V, Ludwig HC, Stengel D. Safety and hydrocephalus: a pragmatic, randomised, open label, multicentre trial (SVASONA). J Neurol Neurosurg Psychiatry. 2013;84(8):850–7.

93. Thomale UW, Gebert AF, Haberl H, Schulz M. Shunt survival rates by using the adjustable differential pressure valve combined with a gravitational unit (proGAV) in pediatric neurosurgery. Childs Nerv Syst. 2013;29(3):425–31.

94. https://www.prnewswire.com/news-releases/branchpoint-technologies-announces-fda-510k-for-its-aura-intracranial-pressure-monitoring-system-300657454.html

95. COGNIShunt® System for Alzheimer's Disease. https://beta.clinicaltrials.gov/study/NCT000 56628

96. Lylyk P, Lylyk I, Bleise C, Scrivano E, Lylyk PN, Beneduce B, Heilman CB, Malek AM. First-in-human endovascular treatment of hydrocephalus with a miniature biomimetic transdural shunt. J Neurointerv Surg. 2022;14(5):495–9.

97. Silverberg GD, Levinthal E, Sullivan EV, Bloch DA, Chang SD, Leverenz J, Flitman S, Winn R, Marciano F, Saul T, Huhn S, Mayo M, McGuire D. Assessment of low-flow CSF drainage as a treatment for AD: results of a randomized pilot study. Neurology. 2002;59(8):1139–45.

98. Mallucci CL, Jenkinson MD, Conroy EJ, Hartley JC, Brown M, Dalton J, Kearns T, Moitt T, Griffiths MJ, Culeddu G, Solomon T, Hughes D, Gamble C. BASICS Study collaborators. Antibiotic or silver versus standard ventriculoperitoneal shunts (BASICS): a multicentre, single-blinded, randomised trial and economic evaluation. Lancet. 2019;394(10208):1530–39.

99. Choux M, Genitori L, Lang D, Lena G. Shunt implantation: reducing the incidence of shunt infection. J Neurosurg. 1992;77(6):875–80.

100. Meier et al.: Results of the SVASONA study in idiopathic normal pressure hydrocephalus. In: Joint Meeting mit der Polnischen Gesellschaft für Neurochirurgen (PNCH), Deutsche Gesellschaft für Neurochirurgie (DGNC) 07–11 Mai 2011, Hamburg.

101. Miethke C: Manufacture and function of cerebrospinal fluid shunts. In: The cerebrospinal fluid shunts. Chapter 5. Edited by Dimitris A. Kombogiorgas, ISBN: 978-1-63484-457-4 104.

102. Miethke, Christoph: Implantierbare Vorrichtung zur Erfassung intrakranieller Drücke. German Patent DE102005063519, 2005.

103. Kazui H, Miyajima M, Mori E, Ishikawa M. SINPHONI-2 Investigators. Lumboperitoneal shunt surgery for idiopathic normal pressure hydrocephalus (SINPHONI-2): an open-label randomized trial. Lancet Neurol. 2015;14(6):585–94.

104. Miyajima M, Kazui H, Mori E, Ishikawa M. On behalf of the SINPHONI-2 Investigators. One-year outcome in patients with idiopathic normal-pressure hydrocephalus: comparison of lumboperitoneal shunt to ventriculoperitoneal shunt. J Neurosurg. 2016;125(6):1483–92.

105. Nakajima M, Yamada S, Miyajima M, et al. Guidelines for management of idiopathic normal pressure hydrocephalus (third Edition): endorsed by the Japanese Society of Normal Pressure Hydrocephalus. Neurol Med chir (Tokyo). 2021;61(2):63–97.

106. Miethke C, Binkele J, Knitter T. A new electronic valve for the treatment of NPH. Fluids Barriers CNS. 2015;12(Suppl 1):O25.

107. Momani L, Alkharabsheh AR, Al-Nuaimy W. Design of an intelligent and personalised shunting system for hydrocephalus. Annu Int Conf IEEE Eng Med Biol Soc. 2008;2008:779–82.

108. Raimondi A. Personal communication. Rostock;2000.

Ventriculoperitoneal Shunt

Kryštof Haratek, Petr Skalický, Adéla Bubeníková, Awista Zazay,
and Ondřej Bradáč

Abstract Ventriculoperitoneal shunting is the most common treatment for idiopathic normal pressure hydrocephalus (iNPH) in Europe and North America. The principle is the implantation of a system that drains cerebrospinal fluid (CSF) from the cerebral lateral ventricle into the abdominal cavity, where it is reabsorbed through the peritoneum into the bloodstream. The implantation of a ventriculoperitoneal shunt (VPS) is one of the least time-consuming procedures in neurosurgery but has the potential for a wide range of complications. No single-standardised approach to VPS implantation is used, and many different methods may yield excellent results. This chapter describes the most commonly applied technique of VPS implantation, discussing its pros and cons, both indications and contraindications, along with surgery-related complications.

Keywords Ventriculoperitoneal shunt · Shunt system · CSF drainage · Normal pressure hydrocephalus · Shunt insertion · Lumbar infusion test · Lumbar tap test

Abbreviations

CSF	Cerebrospinal fluid
CT	Computed tomography
DESH	Disproportionately enlarged subarachnoid spaces hydrocephalus
ICP	Intracranial pressure
iNPH	Idiopathic normal pressure hydrocephalus
LIT	Lumbar infusion test
LTT	Lumbar tap test

K. Haratek · P. Skalický · A. Bubeníková · O. Bradáč (✉)
Department of Neurosurgery, 2nd Medical Faculty, Charles University and Motol University Hospital, Prague, Czech Republic
e-mail: ondrej.bradac2@fnmotol.cz

A. Bubeníková · A. Zazay · O. Bradáč
Department of Neurosurgery and Neurooncology, 1st Medical Faculty, Charles University and Military University Hospital, Prague, Czech Republic

O. Bradac (ed.), *Normal Pressure Hydrocephalus*,
https://doi.org/10.1007/978-3-031-36522-5_21

449

MoCA   Montreal Cognitive Assessment
MMSE   Mini-Mental Scale Examination
MRI   Magnetic resonance imaging
NPH   Normal pressure hydrocephalus
SAH   Subarachnoid haemorrhage
VPS   Ventriculoperitoneal shunt

1 Introduction

The implantation of a ventriculoperitoneal shunt (VPS) is the most common treatment for iNPH in Europe and North America, and the reliability of this method is most supported in the literature [1–4]. The principle is the implantation of a system that drains cerebrospinal fluid from the ventricular system—most often from the right lateral ventricle—of the brain into the abdominal cavity, where it is reabsorbed through the peritoneum into the bloodstream. The system includes a proximal—ventricular catheter, a distal catheter opening into the abdominal cavity and a valve—a regulating device that ensures the correct level of drainage through the system [4].

2 Ventriculoperitoneal shunt

Ventriculoperitoneal shunting is one of the least time-consuming procedures and is considered to be an easy surgery. However, it has also significant potential for complications. The neurosurgeon has to be aware of the specific details of the procedure to minimise the possibility of a poor outcome. There is no single particular method of performing the operation. Different techniques may lead to excellent results. The presented technique is based on personal experience. A lower rate of malfunction at six-month follow-up and fewer infections have been observed when the surgeries were done by experienced high-volume surgeons in paediatric patients [5]. Careful tissue handling and thoughtful planning of incisions is of paramount importance. Standard protocols are implemented to minimise surgical risks [6, 7].

A recent study [8] compared shunt responsiveness and overall shunt survival in patients with different causes of hydrocephalus, using Miethke dual switch valves. The overall rate of shunt responsiveness in all types of hydrocephalus was 93.2%, and 91.4% in the iNPH group. Although there are some differences in the effectiveness of VP shunt surgery in different types of hydrocephalus, which is primarily related to the pathophysiology of each individual type of the disease, VPS remains a widely accepted treatment option for all forms of the condition. The decision to use VP shunt surgery and the specific surgical approach will depend on the individual patient's needs, clinical status, institutional experience etc.

2.1   Prior to the OR

Shunting for normal pressure hydrocephalus is an elective procedure. In terms of the risks of infection, shunt surgery should be the first case in the morning. Successful outcome of the surgery begins with the indication. The patient has to be capable of undergoing the surgery in terms of general health conditions. Standard laboratory tests including blood count, coagulation or biochemical assessment of the blood are taken.

For patients selected for surgery, a proper shunt system has to be chosen. Nowadays, these patients are fitted mainly with gravity-assisted valves with the possibility of adjusting the opening pressure. The initial valve setting is influenced by the height and weight of the patient. Moreover, especially in lean patients, increasing the initial valve setting by 2–4 cm H_2O above the manufacturer's settings is recommended [9]. The setting can be adjusted during or prior to surgery depending on the type of the system and preference of the surgeon. Sustainability of the distal shunt site should be considered especially in patients that had abdominal surgeries.

Regarding shunt infections, a large cohort study, including 1605 patients [10], has found a clear advantage in minimizing shunt infections when using antibiotic-impregnated shunts. The incidence of shunt infection in the antibiotic group was 2%, compared to 6% in the standard shunt group and 6% in the silver-impregnated shunt group. With that said a recently published post hoc meta-analysis found age to be the predominant risk factor for shunt infections, with infants and neonates being the most susceptible to shunt infection [11]. This needs to be considered when discussing shunting in iNPH patients, which is generally considered an adult and elderly disorder [12].

The patient is admitted one day prior to surgery. He or she is checked by an anaesthesiologist and the head is shaved in the evening with a clipper. The patient showers with a disinfectant shampoo. Clear evidence was not found for the preference of chlorhexidine solutions [13].

2.2   Settings in the OR

The number of personnel in the operating room should be limited as much as possible and there should be no movement of staff in and out during the surgery. The shunt system is prepared in the operating room and is opened just prior to the implantation. Standard antibiotic prophylaxis (a single dose of 1.5 g of cefuroxime intravenously) is administered 30 min prior to the skin incision [14].

The patient is placed in a supine position. The head rests either on the table or in a gel head ring or a horseshoe holder. The head is rotated to the opposite side 45°–60° and slightly extended. There should be a line between the abdominal approach and the retroauricular region as straight as possible.

The scrub nurse and assistant disinfect the surgical field with an iodine solution and perform the draping. Two straight drapes on each side and two large straight drapes perpendicular to the latter drapes are placed and an iodine-impregnated surgical foil is applied to the dried patient's skin. Once the draping is done the rest of the instruments are placed into the field. The surgery starts and takes place for around 30–45 min.

2.3 Surgical Procedure

Two surgeons often perform the surgery together. One starts with an incision in the frontal region and the second one begins in the abdomen. The first surgeon makes the precoronal burr hole, prepares the pouch for the valve and prechamber in the retroauricular region, and tunnels the ventricular catheter. The second surgeon prepares the approach into the peritoneal cavity and tunnels the distal catheter with the valve from the retroauricular incision. The shunt system is opened just prior to its implantation, after preparation of all the approaches and after a change of gloves. It is primed in saline to prevent an airlock and after the implantation it is covered with gauze soaked in an iodine solution. Once the system is in place the surgery continues with the implantation of a ventricular catheter, evaluation of its function, tunnelling and connection to the distal catheter. The spontaneous flow is checked and the distal catheter is placed into the abdominal cavity. The wounds are closed in layers.

Ventricular Catheter

The ventricular catheter is most commonly placed into the frontal horn of the lateral ventricle and can be inserted from many various approaches although two main approaches are most commonly utilised, the frontal and occipitoparietal approach. The frontal approach is our primary approach of choice, mainly due to the easier identification of the key anatomical landmarks. Another benefit of the frontal approach is the fact that along with the catheter insertion frontally, the shunt hardware is placed on the bony surface of the retroauricular region. On the contrary, the shunt hardware in the occipitoparietal approach ends up being placed more caudally in the soft tissues of the neck making further manipulation more difficult. Nevertheless, the approach is to be decided depending on the operative setting and the operating surgeon's preference.

The key anatomical landmark for burr hole drilling and ventricular catheter placement is the Kocher's point which is located 3 cm lateral to the midline and 1 cm anterior to the coronal suture. The skin incision is done above this point in a linear or curvilinear fashion and the periosteum is detached from the bone. Consequently, a burr hole is made using a hand drill with a diameter of 0.8 cm. The dura is sharply opened with a surgical blade (Fig. 1) in a cruciate fashion. The cortical surface is gently cauterised and a small pial opening is made. The catheter tip in a guidewire is inserted into the ipsilateral frontal horn of the lateral ventricle while aiming at

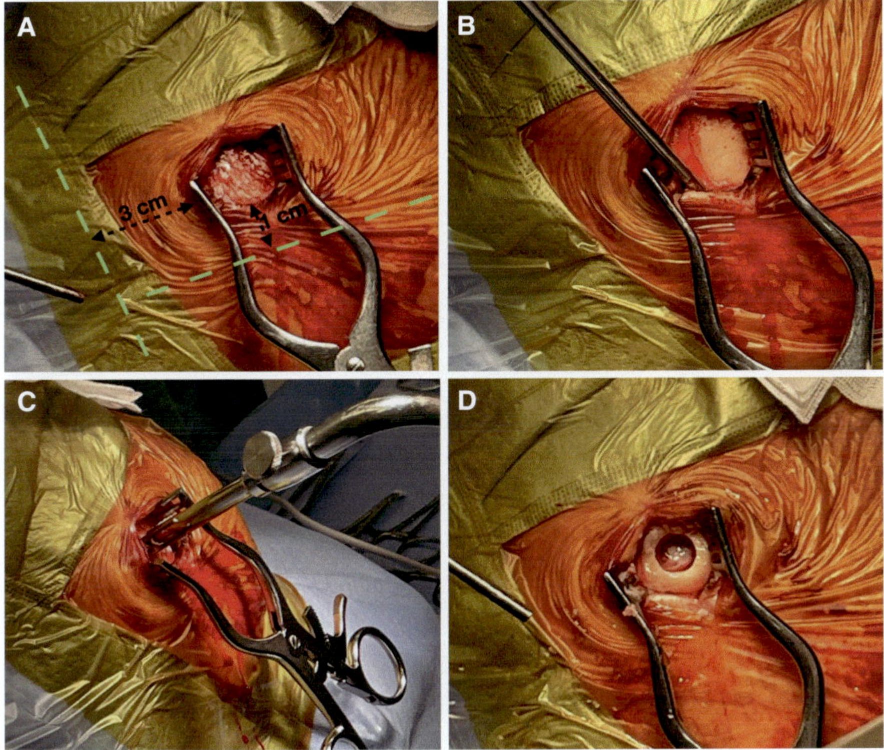

Fig. 1 (A) Incision above the right Kocher's point located 3 cm from the midline and 1 cm in front of the coronal suture. (B) Detachment of periosteum. (C) Burr hole drilling with a hand drill with a diameter of 0.8 cm. (D) Frontal burr hole with already performed durotomy with a surgical scalpel blade No.11 and coagulated edges of the dura with a bipolar coagulation

the ipsilateral tragus and the middle canthus of the ipsilateral eye. The length of the catheter intracranially is generally 5 ± 2 cm for the frontal approach. The catheter should rest at the level of, or slightly anterior to the foramen of Monro, to avoid the choroid plexus. The guidewire is removed and the placement of the catheter is verified by allowing a short trial of CSF drainage. The other end of the catheter is tunnelled into a supplementary incision in the retroauricular region, through a pouch in the subcutaneous layer made using a raspatorium, special tunneliser or clamps. This supplementary incision serves for valve placement and easier tunnelling. The skin incision is closed in layers (Fig. 2).

Valve

The shunt valve is the main device regulating the flow of CSF through the whole shunt system. Gravitational valves need to be placed parallel to the long axis of

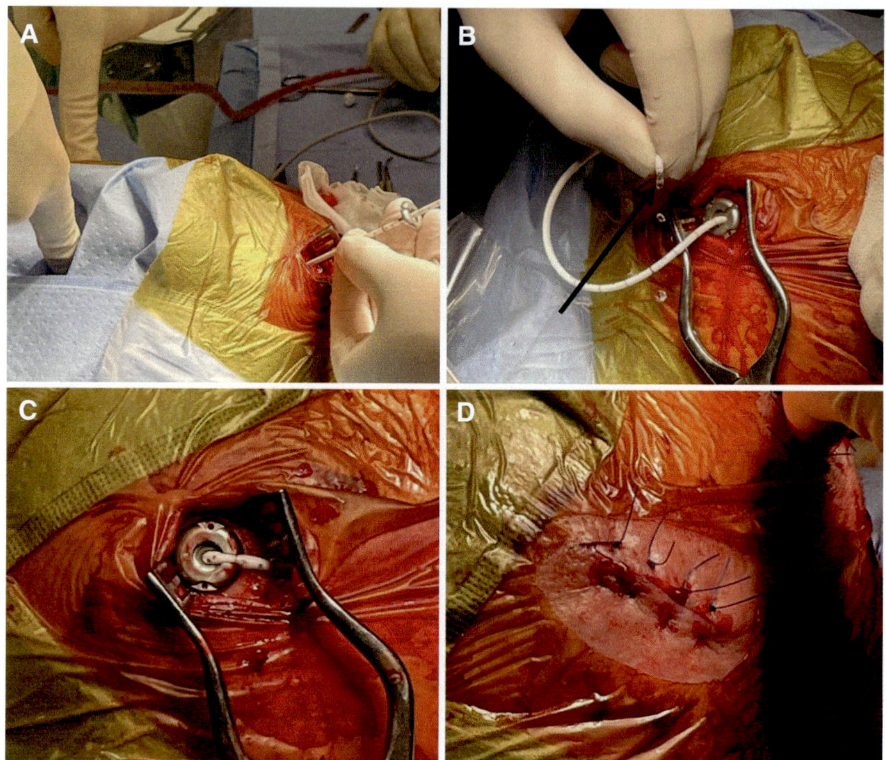

Fig. 2 (A) Placement of a ventricular catheter. The tip of the catheter is aimed at the tragus in the sagittal section and at the ipsilateral medial canthus. (B) The catheter is placed into the frontal horn of the right lateral ventricle. The placement is verified by a short trial of free CSF drainage (*arrow*). (C) The catheter is placed into a deflector and tunnelled into an auxiliary incision for valve placement in the retroauricular region. (D) Interrupted adaptive suture of frontal skin incision

the patient's body. The shunt valve and prechamber are most commonly placed in the retroauricular region on the skull (Fig. 3). As mentioned above, this bony surface makes further manipulation and shunt pressure adjustments much easier. An incision is made in the retroauricular region just posterior and slightly superior to the pinna and a pouch for the valve hardware is made under the galea using dissection scissors or clamps. The ventricular catheter is tunnelled into this incision and connected proximal to the pre-chamber of the valve, the connection is secured by a non-absorbable suture (Fig. 4). Once the distal catheter is tunnelled into this incision it is connected proximal to the valve.

All of our VPS are equipped with pre-chambers. The valve pre-chamber is a very useful diagnostic device. It allows medical personnel to draw up liquor for laboratory tests, directly from the shunt. It also allows us to perform infusion tests [15]. All of this is done through the silicone membrane of the pre-chamber which can be punctured by a needle. The pre-chamber furthermore allows us to easily monitor intraventricular

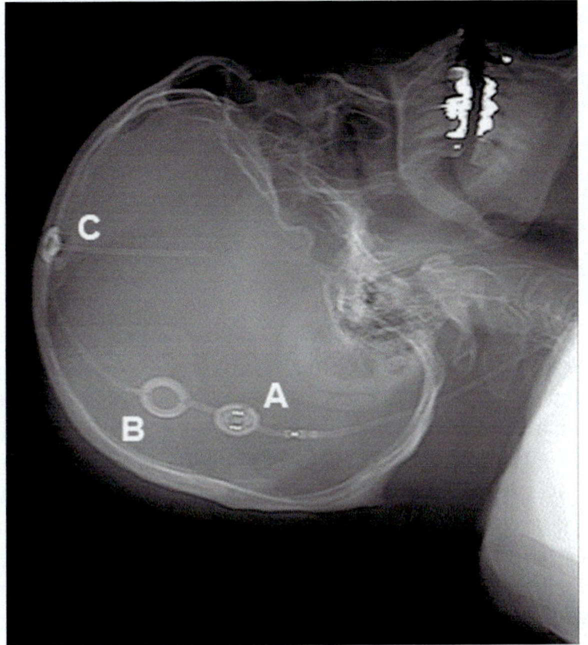

Fig. 3 A lateral projection X-ray image confirming (A) correct valve and (B) pre-chamber placement in the retroauricular region, as well as (C) the ventricular catheter placement

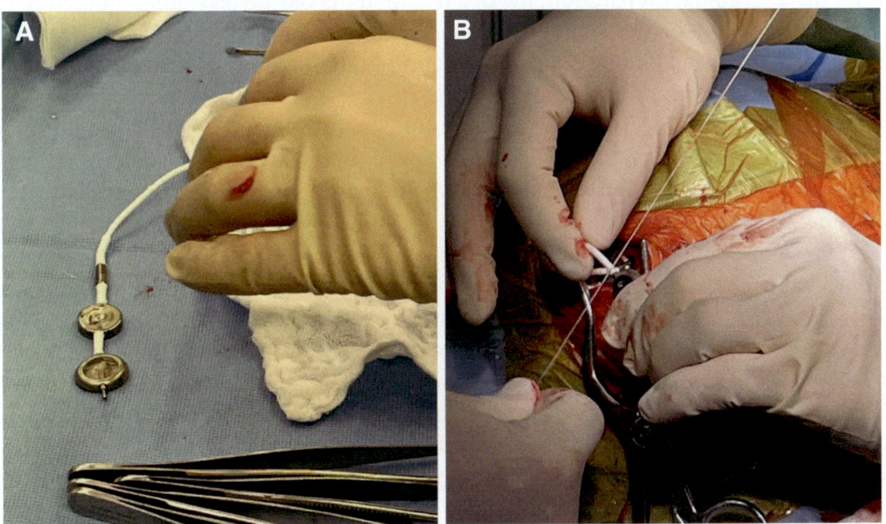

Fig. 4 (A) Preparation and check of the valve with a pre-chamber and distal catheter. (B) Connection of the ventricular catheter with a distal catheter just proximal to the pre-chamber of the valve. The connection is secured with a non-absorbable suture

pressure values when necessary. Another possible complication that can be checked is eventual shunt obstruction. When applying light pressure on the pre-chamber, it should be easily compressible and should fill back up immediately after, with shunt obstruction, the pre-chamber is rigid and incompressible. The administration of medications is also possible through the pre-chamber, although in our experience this is not utilised very often in a clinical setting.

Distal Catheter

There are two primary approaches to distal catheter insertion. Either (1) it can be inserted into the abdomen through a small transverse laparotomy approximately at the midline in the epigastric region or (2) more lateral to the midline. The midline incision offers an advantage in going through the avascular linea alba. On the other hand, the lateral approach offers improved orientation and differentiation within the abdominal layers, all described below in detail. The epigastrium is a preferred location since the laparotomy can be performed above the liver, thus minimizing the risk of bowel perforation, which would be a life-threatening immediate complication.

The skin, subcutaneous fat, subcutaneous abdominal fascia (Scarpa's fascia) and the anterior rectus sheath are all incised. The linea alba is transected, the posterior rectus sheath is tented up using two haemostats or two Kocher forceps and also transected. The transverse fascia and peritoneum are also dissected and when resistance is encountered the surgeon usually encounters the peritoneum (Fig. 5). After the abdominal preparation, the distal catheter is placed and shunt tunnelling is performed. The catheter is tunnelled in the subcutaneous layer preferably from the abdomen to the head but the opposite direction is also possible. The most resistance is usually encountered when going over the clavicle, especially when the tunnelling device is not positioned under a correct angle, and the neck when going through the nuchal fascia. This part of the surgery has a potential for immediate intraoperative complications in injuries caused by the tunnelling device (e.g. pneumothorax, bleeding, skin puncturing etc.). The tunnelling is performed all the way up to the level of the retroauricular incision, then the distal catheter, in our setting usually already connected to the valve, is pulled back through the subcutaneous tunnel and into the abdominal incision. Spontaneous CSF flow is checked before the distal catheter is buried into the peritoneal cavity. It is important to be sure that the cavity has been reached and there are no adhesions at the site of the catheter placement. The catheter is handled with vessel forceps and buried into the cavity without any resistance. The posterior and anterior rectus sheaths are closed respectively with an absorbable PDS suture and the skin incision is closed in layers (Fig. 6).

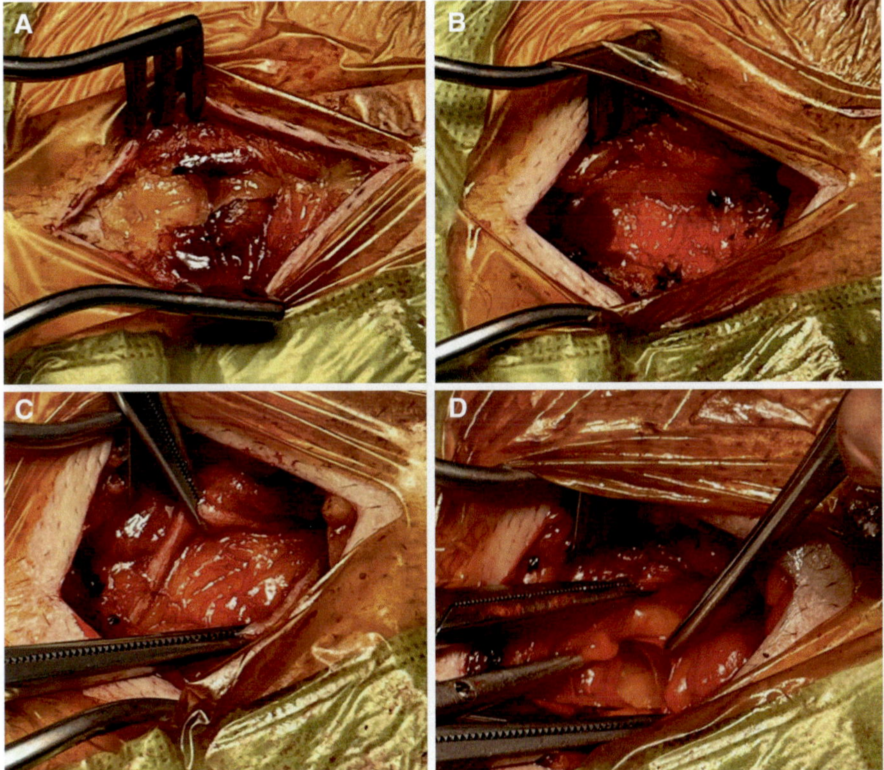

Fig. 5 (A) The abdominal incision with a subcutaneous fat and abdominal subcutaneous fascia (fascia of Scarpa). (B) The anterior rectus sheath. (C) Pre-peritoneal fat after an incision of the transverse fascia. (D) The approach into the abdominal cavity after an incision of the peritoneum

2.4   Contraindications and Early Complications

A postoperative CT scan of the brain is usually made on the first day after the surgery. The location of the ventricular catheter is verified and the presence of haemorrhage is excluded. After the CT scan is checked by a neurosurgeon the patient begins rehabilitation. Pain is generally minimal and treated with nonsteroidal anti-inflammatory drugs. The patient is discharged to home care often on the fifth day after the surgery. The first outpatient check and CT scan is made after one month. CSF flow in the system is evaluated both clinically and graphically and valve setting is adjusted if desired. The main symptoms are thoroughly checked and MR of the brain is made after 3 months and then after 1 year after surgery. The most common early complications are malposition, intracerebral haemorrhage in the parenchyma adjacent to the trajectory, wound healing problems, and shunt obstruction, followed by complications related to the level of CSF diversion.

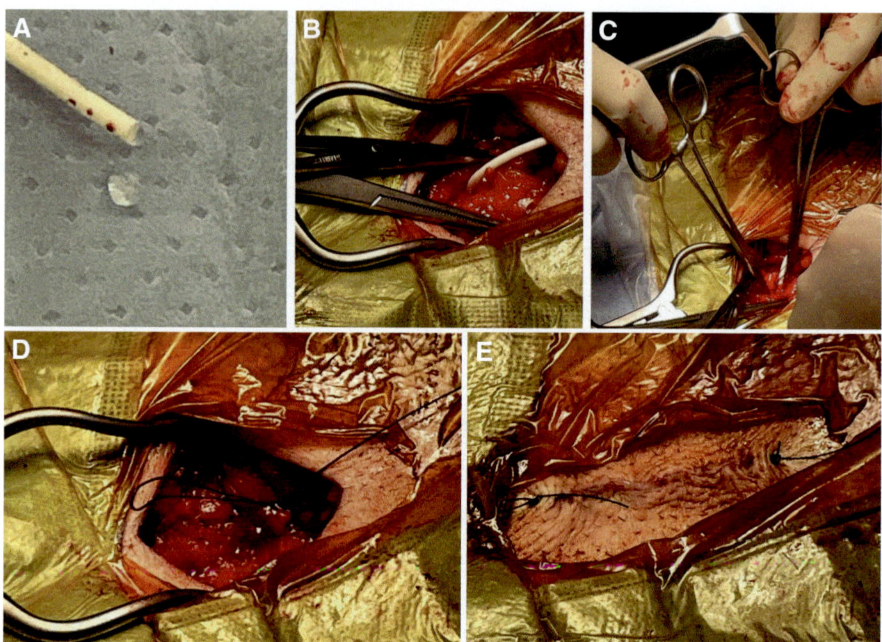

Fig. 6 (A) Evaluation of spontaneous flow of CSF through the system. (B) Distal catheter placed in the peritoneal cavity. (C) Suture of the deep layer of the rectus abdominis fascia with an absorbable PDS suture. (D) Suture of the superior layer of the rectus abdominis fascia with an absorbable PDS suture. (E) Intradermal skin suture of the abdominal incision

According to a recent multi-centre study [2] on complications after VPS surgery in iNPH patients, published in 2019, the most frequent postoperative complications were symptomatic under-drainage (26%), symptomatic over-drainage (9%), subdural hygroma (9%), shunt malposition (7%) and subdural hematoma due to over-drainage (6%). Very recent meta-analysis of 2461 patients [16] evaluating overall outcomes and complications of different surgical intervention alternatives for iNPH reported similar results regarding the occurrence of subdural hematomas/hygromas in both VP and VA shunts (10%). The vast majority of them spontaneously resolved (85%) following the increase of the valve opening pressure. On the contrary, ischemic complications and/or haemorrhagic complications are present in only approximately 2% of shunted iNPH patients, again regardless of the type of shunt used. Adjustable valves are, when compared to fixed valves, usually associated with decreased rate of revision and subdural collections. The most common indications for revision surgery are shunt malfunction, infection or treatment failure itself, summing up the revision rate around 18% (95% confidence interval = 13–14%) of all VP shunt surgeries [16].

Contraindications for VPS placement in iNPH include any peritoneal infection, an allergy to any of the shunt components (e.g. silicone), an altered coagulation function, infection of the CSF and an entry site infection [17, 18]. Additionally, repeated unsuccessful VPS implantations are also contradictory to VPS insertion [19] and a different method of CSF drainage should be considered.

3 Illustrative Case

Presented is a case of a 74-year-old male clinically harbouring a complete Hakim's triad of symptoms, namely cognitive decline, urinary incontinence and gait disturbance. A CT scan and subsequently MRI of the brain were done proving ventriculomegaly. Regarding these findings, NPH was suspected and our standard NPH protocol was implemented. The gait disturbance was evaluated according to the Dutch Gait Scale [20, 21] characterised of markedly decreased step length accompanied by a broadening base of support and reduced foot-floor clearance, resembling the cautious "walking of a person on ice". Regarding the cognitive decline, the patient preoperatively performed 22/30 points in the Mini-Mental Scale Examination (MMSE), and 14/30 points in the Montreal Cognitive Assessment (MoCA). Urinary incontinence was examined according to the International Consultation on Incontinence Questionnaire (ICIQ), in which he scored 18 points. Both a lumbar infusion test (LIT) and a lumbar tap test (LTT) were conducted, and the LIT was positive for NPH at 12 mmHg/min. Post LTT, gait impairment improved by 27%. Also, cognitive abilities improved according to the MoCA test from initial 14 to 18 points after the LTT. Urinary incontinence improved subjectively according to the patient after the LTT. After a multidisciplinary indication seminar discussion, he was deemed eligible for receiving a VP shunt. A ProGav 2.0 valve was implanted at 10 cm H_2O. At a 3-month examination, the patient improved in all symptoms of the Hakim trias, the most evident improvement was found in gait disturbance and urinary incontinence (Fig. 7).

4 Conclusion

A ventriculoperitoneal represents the most common treatment approach to iNPH treatment, with a minimal risk of complications. A relatively low rate of shunt failure puts it above other treatment options such as a ventriculoatrial shunt or a lumboperitoneal shunt, although these also have their place in the treatment of iNPH. Successful outcome of the surgery begins with the indication, therefore a standard diagnostic NPH protocol should always be implemented. Adjustable gravity-assisted valves are a crucial component of modern VPS. Another very helpful component of the shunt system is the pre-chamber, used as a tool for easy monitoring of the shunt function.

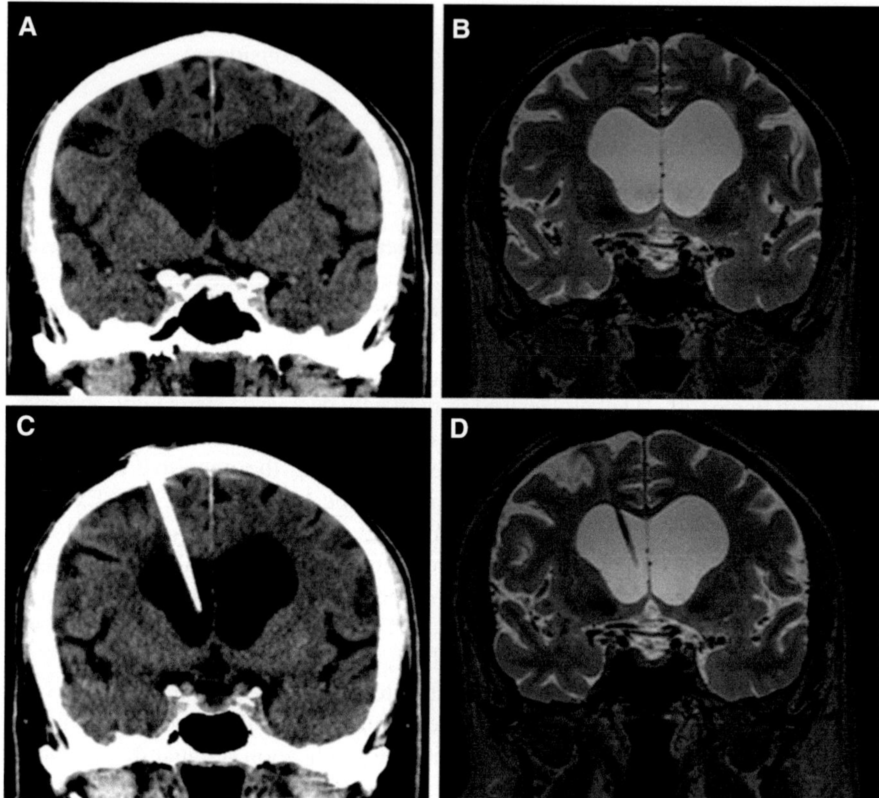

Fig. 7 (A) A preoperative CT scan and (B) a preoperative MRI scan showing ventriculomegaly (Evan's index of 0.43 and callosal angle of 55°), along with positive cingulate sulcus sign (based on sagittal projection), tight high convexity and local sulci widening (both based on axial projections). Final disproportionately enlarged subarachnoid spaces hydrocephalus (DESH) of 8 points. (C) A postoperative CT scan made on the first postoperative day proving the correct catheter placement in front of the foramen of Monro. (D) MRI scan 3 months after surgery

5   Key Points

- Ventriculoperitoneal shunting is the most common treatment option for iNPH.
- A correct indication for surgery is crucial for the outcomes of shunted patients.
- Adjustable pressure gravity assisted valves are nowadays a standard practice.
- The risks and outcomes of the procedure depend on having a standardised protocol of surgery.

Funding This chapter was supported by the Ministry of Health of the Czech Republic institutional grant no. NU23-04-00551.

References

1. Nakajima M, Yamada S, Miyajima M, Ishii K, Kuriyama N, Kazui H, et al. Guidelines for management of idiopathic normal pressure hydrocephalus (Third Edition): endorsed by the Japanese Society of normal pressure hydrocephalus. Neurol Med Chir (Tokyo). 2021;61(2):63–97. https://doi.org/10.2176/nmc.st.2020-0292.

2. Feletti A, d'Avella D, Wikkelsø C, Klinge P, Hellström P, Tans J, et al. Ventriculoperitoneal shunt complications in the European idiopathic normal pressure hydrocephalus multicenter study. Oper Neurosurg (Hagerstown). 2019;17(1):97–102. https://doi.org/10.1093/ons/opy232.

3. Schenker P, Stieglitz LH, Sick B, Stienen MN, Regli L, Sarnthein J. Patients with a normal pressure hydrocephalus shunt have fewer complications than do patients with other shunts. World Neurosurg. 2018;110:e249–57. https://doi.org/10.1016/j.wneu.2017.10.151.

4. Bergsneider M, Black PM, Klinge P, Marmarou A, Relkin N. Surgical management of idiopathic normal-pressure hydrocephalus. Neurosurgery 2005;57(3 Suppl):S29–39; discussion ii–v. https://doi.org/10.1227/01.neu.0000168186.45363.4d.

5. Cochrane DD, Kestle JR. The influence of surgical operative experience on the duration of first ventriculoperitoneal shunt function and infection. Pediatr Neurosurg. 2003;38(6):295–301. https://doi.org/10.1159/000070413.

6. Kestle JR, Riva-Cambrin J, Wellons JC 3rd, Kulkarni AV, Whitehead WE, Walker ML, et al. A standardized protocol to reduce cerebrospinal fluid shunt infection: the hydrocephalus clinical research network quality improvement initiative. J Neurosurg Pediatr. 2011;8(1):22–9. https://doi.org/10.3171/2011.4.Peds10551.

7. Sarmey N, Kshettry VR, Shriver MF, Habboub G, Machado AG, Weil RJ. Evidence-based interventions to reduce shunt infections: a systematic review. Childs Nerv Syst. 2015;31(4):541–9. https://doi.org/10.1007/s00381-015-2637-2.

8. Hertel F, Züchner M, Decker C, Schill S, Bosniak I, Bettag M. The Miethke dual switch valve: experience in 169 adult patients with different kinds of hydrocephalus: an open field study. Minim Invasive Neurosurg. 2008;51(3):147–53. https://doi.org/10.1055/s-2008-1065337.

9. Skalický P, Mládek A, Vlasák A, Whitley H, Bradáč O. First experiences with Miethke M.blue® valve in iNPH patients. J Clin Neurosci. 2022;98:127–32. https://doi.org/10.1016/j.jocn.2022.02.004.

10. Mallucci CL, Jenkinson MD, Conroy EJ, Hartley JC, Brown M, Dalton J, et al. Antibiotic or silver versus standard ventriculoperitoneal shunts (BASICS): a multicentre, single-blinded, randomised trial and economic evaluation. Lancet. 2019;394(10208):1530–9. https://doi.org/10.1016/s0140-6736(19)31603-4.

11. Sunderland GJ, Conroy EJ, Nelson A, Gamble C, Jenkinson MD, Griffiths MJ, et al. Factors affecting ventriculoperitoneal shunt revision: a post hoc analysis of the British Antibiotic and Silver Impregnated Catheter Shunt multicenter randomized controlled trial. J Neurosurg. 2023;138(2):483–93. https://doi.org/10.3171/2022.4.Jns22572.

12. Barnett GH, Hahn JF, Palmer J. Normal pressure hydrocephalus in children and young adults. Neurosurgery. 1987;20(6):904–7. https://doi.org/10.1227/00006123-198706000-00014.

13. Webster J, Osborne S. Preoperative bathing or showering with skin antiseptics to prevent surgical site infection. Cochrane Database Syst Rev. 2012(9):Cd004985. https://doi.org/10.1002/14651858.CD004985.pub4.

14. Ratilal B, Costa J, Sampaio C. Antibiotic prophylaxis for surgical introduction of intracranial ventricular shunts. Cochrane Database Syst Rev. 2006;2006(3):Cd005365. https://doi.org/10.1002/14651858.CD005365.pub2.

15. Czosnyka ZH, Sinha R, Morgan JA, Wawrzynski JR, Price SJ, Garnett M, et al. Shunt testing in vivo: observational study of problems with ventricular catheter. Acta Neurochir Suppl. 2016;122:353–6. https://doi.org/10.1007/978-3-319-22533-3_69.

16. Giordan E, Palandri G, Lanzino G, Murad MH, Elder BD. Outcomes and complications of different surgical treatments for idiopathic normal pressure hydrocephalus: a systematic review and meta-analysis. J Neurosurg. 2018:1–13. https://doi.org/10.3171/2018.5.Jns1875.

17. Hussain NS, Wang PP, James C, Carson BS, Avellino AM. Distal ventriculoperitoneal shunt failure caused by silicone allergy. Case report. J Neurosurg. 2005;102(3):536–9. https://doi.org/10.3171/jns.2005.102.3.0536.
18. Kurin M, Lee K, Gardner P, Fajt M, Umapathy C, Fasanella K. Clinical peritonitis from allergy to silicone ventriculoperitoneal shunt. Clin J Gastroenterol. 2017;10(3):229–31. https://doi.org/10.1007/s12328-017-0729-0.
19. Oterdoom LH, Marinus Oterdoom DL, Ket JCF, Van Dijk JMC, Scholten P. Systematic review of ventricular peritoneal shunt and percutaneous endoscopic gastrostomy: a safe combination. J Neurosurg. 2017;127(4):899–904. https://doi.org/10.3171/2016.8.jns152701.
20. Boon AJ, Tans JT, Delwel EJ, Egeler-Peerdeman SM, Hanlo PW, Wurzer JA, et al. Dutch normal pressure hydrocephalus study: baseline characteristics with emphasis on clinical findings. Eur J Neurol. 1997;4(1):39–47. https://doi.org/10.1111/j.1468-1331.1997.tb00297.x.
21. Boon AJ, Tans JT, Delwel EJ, Egeler-Peerdeman SM, Hanlo PW, Wurzer HA, et al. The Dutch normal-pressure hydrocephalus study. How to select patients for shunting? An analysis of four diagnostic criteria. Surg Neurol. 2000;53(3):201–7. https://doi.org/10.1016/s0090-3019(00)00182-8.

Ventriculoatrial Shunt

**Valentina Usuga, Salvador M. Mattar, Diego Gomez Amarillo,
Juan Fernando Ramon, and Fernando Hakim**

Abstract Cerebrospinal fluid (CSF) shunting is the first line of treatment for patients with hydrocephalus. The procedure diverts CSF from the ventricles to another anatomical cavity in the body like the atrium, the pleura or the peritoneum. Thus, there are several shunt placement options available. Globally, ventriculoperitoneal shunts (VPS) are the most commonly used, followed by lumboperitoneal and ventriculoatrial shunts (VAS). In this chapter, we discuss VAS, the surgical procedure, how to confirm its correct placement, its contraindications and its possible complications in contrast to other shunt placement options.

Keywords Ventriculoatrial shunt · Cerebrospinal fluid · Normal pressure hydrocephalus · Ventriculoperitoneal shunt

Abbreviations

CSF	Cerebrospinal fluid
DESH	Disproportionately Enlarged Subarachnoid Space Hydrocephalus
VPS	Ventriculoperitoneal Shunt
VAS	Ventriculoatrial Shunt
IIH	Idiopathic intracranial hypertension
NPH	Normal pressure hydrocephalus
IJV	Internal jugular vein

V. Usuga
Universidad de Los Andes, Bogotá, Colombia

S. M. Mattar · F. Hakim
Hydrocephalus Clinic in Hospital Universitario Fundación Santa Fe de Bogotá, Bogotá, Colombia

D. Gomez Amarillo · J. F. Ramon · F. Hakim (✉)
Neurosurgery Department in Hospital Universitario Fundación Santa Fe de Bogotá, Bogotá, Colombia
e-mail: neurocirugia826@gmail.com

SVC   Superior vena cava
OP   Opening pressure

1   Introduction

Hydrocephalus is the pathological dilation of the ventricles in response to an alteration in CSF dynamics. The cause can be explained by an increase in production and/or a decrease in the absorption of CSF [1, 2]. These alterations can lead to an increase in intracranial pressure which requires a timely intervention due to the symptomatology that can accompany it and the risk of acute clinical deterioration.

In some cases, without an increase in pressure, the alteration of brain architecture and its corresponding compression and straining of periventricular structures can cause an array of symptoms that also require intervention, but within a more flexible timetable. This is the case of normal pressure hydrocephalus (NPH), described by Dr. Hakim [2] in 1965 [3, 4]. Thus, just as acute hydrocephalus and NPH are indications for shunt placement, there are other medical conditions which benefit from or require the insertion of a CSF shunt. Some to consider are idiopathic intracranial hypertension (IIH) or intracranial cysts [5, 6].

The first description of ventriculoatrial shunt placement to treat hydrocephalus was done by Nulsen and Spitz in 1951, and the first successful shunt was documented in 1952 [5, 7]. Since then, many modifications have been made to this procedure in order to take advantage of the advances in surgical technology and equipment. For instance, the current gold standard for the insertion of the atrial catheter is the ultrasound-guided percutaneous technique due to its success rate and its decreased morbidity in contrast to open vein dissection [8].

This chapter aims to discuss the surgical procedure in detail, explain how to confirm the adequate placement of the shunt, and go over the contraindications and possible complications that we can encounter.

2   Ventriculoatrial Shunt

Ventriculoatrial shunt (VAS) is the name given to a neurosurgical procedure where an artificial tubular connection is made between the ventricular cavities of the brain and the lumen of the right atrium. As a result, cerebrospinal fluid bypasses its usual route and returns directly to the circulating blood flow. The amount of CSF drained is generally determined by pressure-guided valve systems. Figure 1.

The shunting system consists of:

1. a *proximal catheter*, inserted in the frontal or occipital horns of the lateral ventricles,

Fig. 1 Illustrative
representation of
ventriculoatrial shunt (VAS)
placement with visible
anatomical landmarks

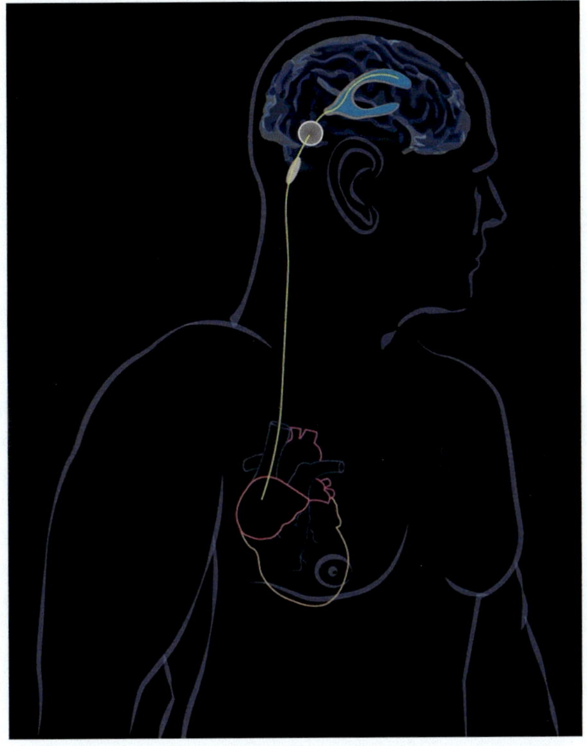

2. that connects to a *pressure-guided* <u>valve</u> which can be fixed, programmable or gravitational, among other options,
3. its content is drained to a *distal catheter*, which traverses under the skin and enters the jugular vein above the clavicle and finally reaches the right atrium.

2.1   Indications

Although this technique can be used as a first-line approach, it should specifically be considered in patients with a history of increased intra-abdominal pressure like obesity or ascites, trauma or previous abdominal surgery due to the presence of adhesions, peritonitis or abdominal infections, and finally, patients with failed ventriculoperitoneal shunts [5, 9].

2.2 Procedure and Considerations

Patient selection, imaging, anatomical knowledge and instruments are crucial elements to be taken into account for a favourable outcome. A thorough evaluation should be done prior to the procedure to confirm eligibility for the surgery.

Prior to the OR

First and foremost, the patient must be eligible for surgery. They must be diagnosed with acute hydrocephalus, NPH or any other disease that benefits from a permanent CSF diversion and the risk of surgery must be evaluated and cleared by their corresponding physicians (anaesthesiology and those in relation to the patients' relevant comorbidities). Additionally, the treating neurosurgeon must have a recent MRI of the brain and a chest X-ray. The MRI is essential to establish the best entry point and length of insertion for the ventricular catheter, as well as to estimate distances from the scalp to the ventricle. On the other hand, the chest X-ray is needed in order to have a parameter of how far the distal catheter should be inserted in order to reach the atrium and prevent an alteration of the cardiac rhythm (extrasystole) by trespassing the tricuspid valve and stimulating the right ventricle.

In order to place a ventriculoatrial shunt, the patient must undergo general anaesthesia and must be done in an OR environment with the correct asepsis and antisepsis protocol. In order to decrease the probability of infection, we suggest keeping the number of people entering the OR during the procedure to the minimum necessary, to change gloves during the shunt system manipulation and to use intravenous antibiotic prophylaxis with coverage of normal skin flora, like *Staphylococcus aureus*. Moreover, the patient should not cut their hair or try to shave the area before the procedure.

Preoperative Measurements and Anatomical Landmarks

As mentioned earlier, a chest X-ray of the patient must be done prior to the procedure to measure the distance from the superior border of the right clavicle to the atriocaval junction in order to estimate how far the distal catheter must be inserted like shown in Fig. 2 [10]. This measurement will be used in the OR in order to know the adequate length of the distal catheter and how far it should be inserted.

On the other hand, the MRI is used to confirm the suspected diagnosis of hydrocephalus where different image criteria should be met. First, Evan's index should be calculated using the 2 measurements depicted in Fig. 3. Moreover, a measurement from Kocher's point to the ventricle wall may be useful to determine the length of insertion of the ventricular catheter.

Lastly, the Kocher's point which is located 1 cm anterior to the coronal suture and 2–3 cm lateral to the midline is the most used anatomical landmark for the

Fig. 2 Thoracic X-ray with the measurement of the distance between the right atrium and the clavicle shown

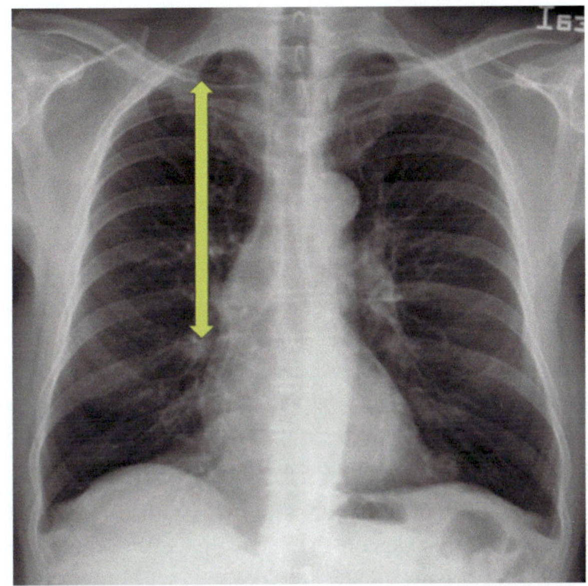

Fig. 3 Evan's Index. Considered positive when: A/B => 0.33

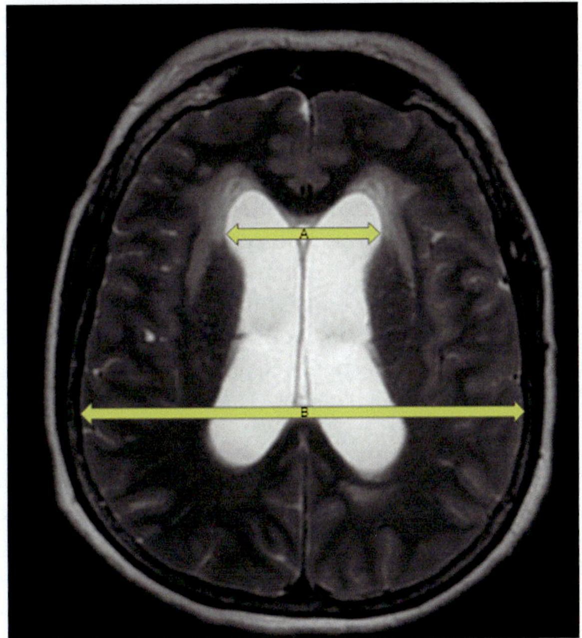

insertion of the proximal catheter since it has the lowest reported rate of complications associated with the trajectory of the ventricular catheter [11]. This anatomical landmark is used to insert the proximal catheter directly into the frontal horn of the lateral ventricle. These measurements should be made over the patients during the preoperative preparations.

Detailed Surgical Procedure

The patient should be in a supine position on the OR table in a Trendelenburg position with their head turned about 60°–70° to the opposite side of the valve placement. All hair should be removed with surgical clippers before sterilisation. After correct sterilisation from the scalp to the supraclavicular area and draping of the surgical field is accomplished, the initial catheter placement will be done through the internal jugular vein (IJV), unless contraindicated.

Distal/atrial catheter placement: An ultrasound surface probe is used to pinpoint the vascular package of the neck. The entry point in the skin into the vein should be 2–3 cm above the clavicle along the inner border of the sternocleidomastoid muscle, in the superior portion of the supraclavicular fossa [10]. Afterwards, using an 18 G Abbocath needle guided by the ultrasound image the vein is punctured, and then, using a 10 cc syringe, the obtention venous (dark) blood is expected to confirm not entering into the lumen of the carotid artery. Furthermore, if the syringe is removed, returning blood should not be pulsatile. The J guide is introduced through the needle. Using intraoperative radiography, the trajectory of the guide is confirmed towards the atriocaval junction, afterwards, the needle is removed. An incision of about 3 mm in length should be made parallel to the skin folds to expose subdermal fat and widen the area. A 7 French (Fr) dilater is introduced around the guide. Afterwards, the 8 Fr peel-away catheter is inserted through which we can insert the distal catheter of the shunting system. Finally, the distal catheter is inserted using the measurement from the chest X-ray and adding the distance from the clavicle to the incision. The peel-away catheter is removed and radiographic control is repeated to guarantee the final location of the catheter. The catheter is fixed to position to continue with the other points of incision.

Proximal catheter placement: First off, Kocher's point is located using craniometric measurements before surgery and is marked in the patient's scalp. A semilunar incision is made around the location marked, and bleeding is controlled using a bipolar forceps. A mastoid dilater is placed to expose the scalp, the periosteum is removed, and using a microdrill, a burr hole of about 1 cm is made until the dura is exposed. Using bipolar forceps, the dura and burr hole are cauterised.

Valve placement: A retroauricular incision of about 1 cm is made to insert the valve and a special, long, blunt-tipped instrument is used to tunnel the subdermal fat from the retroauricular region to the scalp and neck incisions. The valve is preprogrammed to a secure pressure in order to prevent overdrainage in the patient, based on its lumbar puncture opening pressure and ventricular pressure. Afterwards, the valve is inserted and the distal and proximal catheter are connected making sure the correct orientation for CSF flow is ensured depending on the valve requirements.

Ventricular catheter placement: Finally, the ventricular catheter is passed until adequate CSF return is obtained. The ventricular pressure is measured, and at this point, it is acceptable to allow the release of a small volume of CSF (around 20 cc) in order to improve the patient's clinical state. The measurement of the catheter from the skull to the ventricle should be considered in the preoperative images.

The skin is closed using prolene and vicryl taking important note of the possibility of puncturing the catheter system with the needles. The incision wounds are covered.

Placement Confirmation

The trajectory of the ventricular catheter should be determined by Kocher's point as the entry, aiming at the point of intersection between two imaginary lines. The first line connects the external auditory canals, and the second line is parallel to the midline placed laterally in order to traverse the inner canthus of the ipsilateral eye. Following this orientation, you should reach Monro's Foramen. When you observe CSF flow through the catheter, you should advance the catheter 1 cm more, achieving the intended placement. MRI measurements should be taken into account when deciding the length of insertion of the catheter.

Furthermore, in regard to the distal catheter, it is crucial to perform a transoperative chest X-ray in order to confirm correct placement in the right atrium. The distal catheter should be observed within the superior atriocaval junction, generally associated with the T6 vertebra.

2.3 Contraindications and Complications

Contraindications

The contraindications for VAS placement can be divided into two separate categories: absolute contraindications and relative contraindications. The absolute contraindications for VAS, which should lead to a different choice of treatment, are infections like bacteraemia, CSF infection and endocarditis. On the other hand, relative contraindications, which lead to an individual evaluation that depends on the patient case, are congestive heart failure, cardiac malformations, pulmonary hypertension, history of pulmonary embolism, immune glomerulonephritis, a hypersensitivity to silicon and lastly, a prothrombotic state and/or systemic anticoagulation [5].

Possible Complications

Regardless of the type of shunt chosen, statistically, patients will usually require at least one revision surgery in their lifetime [5].

There are certain complications to consider when opting for VAS as the treatment option. Cardiovascular complications are erroneously the most associated with VAS due to a large pool of studies with a predominant paediatric population. New studies have surfaced with a focus on adult populations where VAS have shown a neglectable association with cardiovascular complications [5]. Despite these findings, the possible cardiovascular side effects that VAS can cause are important to consider due to their higher severity than other shunt placements.

Since the catheters can migrate with time due to breakage or disconnection, the distal catheter can migrate to the right ventricle, or it can have a retrograde migration which can lead to a disturbance in the blood flow and lead to thrombosis [8]. The anterograde migration can lead to tricuspid valve abnormalities, pulmonary hypertension, cardiac wall perforation and intracardiac thrombosis.

During venous cannulation, considering the trajectory of the catheters and the proximity to important vascular and nervous structures in the neck, there is a risk of puncture or laceration of mentioned structures. Likewise, we can encounter other complications like venous air embolism and pneumothorax.

In regards to postoperative infection, VAS has a specific risk for shunt nephritis. This is a rare reversible immune-complex-mediated complication of shunt infection that can progress to end-stage renal disease if treatment is delayed. It is crucial for physicians to be aware of the risk of patients with VAS to present nephritis and to evaluate the possibility of shunt infection even in the setting of negative cultures and delayed symptomatic presentation. When shunt nephritis is confirmed a directed antibiotic therapy is necessary, as well as complete removal of the shunt system [12].

3　Clinical Case

A 63-year-old female with 4 years of gait abnormality, urinary incontinence, short-term memory flaws and diplopia was diagnosed with iNPH in 2018 and underwent a ventriculoperitoneal shunt in the same year. After 1 year of medical improvement, the patient showed the same symptoms as before the shunt was placed.

In another medical centre, the patient underwent a shunt revision surgery where the valve and the entire shunting system was replaced. The new shunt was placed once more to the peritoneum. After surgery, the patient displayed symptomatic improvement again, but after 3 months, the patient's symptoms reappeared. Since multiple valve adjustments showed no effect, the medical team suspected obstruction of the distal catheter. A laparoscopic modification of the distal catheter placement was attempted with temporary improvement. This procedure was attempted twice with no lasting results.

Afterwards, the patient underwent a radiological revision of the shunt, with contrast, which was unable to identify an obstruction of the system. The system was supposed to be working properly so no other surgical alternatives were offered to the patient.

The patient was later studied by another medical team which analysed the case. They found the symptoms the patient had been experiencing, since 2018, enlarged ventricles and disproportionately enlarged subarachnoid space hydrocephalus (DESH) in a recent brain tomography. In order to confirm the functionality of the shunting system, the medical team performed a lumbar puncture. Since the valve should open every time, the ICP goes above its pressure setting, the lumbar puncture opening pressure should be similar to that of the valve pressure setting. The team found an opening pressure considerably discordant to the valve maximum set pressure (6 cms of H_2O higher). Furthermore, the patient underwent a gait evaluation which was frankly altered. The medical team considered the patient had a failed shunt, and the most likely cause was the distal catheter placement due to the initial recovery of symptoms followed by their return weeks or months after each intervention.

The patient underwent a VAS that replaced the previous system. There were no complications during and after surgery, the patient exhibited a complete recovery of symptoms, and the valve setting was modified once 1 month after surgery. Within 6 months of follow-up, the patient had no symptomatic deterioration or regression.

4 Conclusions

VAS is a quick, safe and useful alternative for hydrocephalus shunting. Due to its catheter's shorter length, there is less syphon effect. Since it drains into a flowing fluid system, there is less probability of distal obstruction. The extraction of CSF is more reliable since the atrium generally has a near to 0 mmHg of pressure, whilst the peritoneum varies constantly depending on the patient's body weight, position, breathing pattern, among others. With upcoming technologies, the limitations surrounding open venous dissection technique have been overcome. In contexts of repetitive failed shunting due to obstructions or unknown causes, VAS should be considered among the first alternatives.

5 Key Points

- Alteration to CSF dynamics can be caused by different aetiologies which eventually leads to increased cranial pressure and/or alteration of the brain architecture that is usually accompanied by clinical symptomatologies and a high risk of clinical deterioration. Therefore, surgical CSF diversion techniques are the first line of treatment.

- VAS should be considered distinctly in patients with obesity, ascites, a history of abdominal trauma or surgery, abdominal infections and patients with a previously failed VPS.
- Prior to the surgical procedure, in the case of NPH, the patient must undergo a variety of interventions and evaluations to determine the correct valve placement and adjustment. These include MRI, chest X-ray, lumbar puncture, and preanaesthetic evaluation to determine surgical risk.
- Despite VAS rarely causing cardiac complications, these are important to keep in mind due to their higher severity in contrast to other shunt placement complications.

References

1. Adams RD, Fisher CM, Hakim S, Ojemann RG, Sweet WH. Symptomatic occult hydrocephalus with normal cerebrospinal-fluid pressure. N Engl J Med. 1965;273(3):117–26. https://doi.org/10.1056/NEJM196507152730301.
2. Hakim S, Adams RD. The special clinical problem of symptomatic hydrocephalus with normal cerebrospinal fluid pressure: observations on cerebrospinal fluid hydrodynamics. J Neurol Sci. 1965;2(4):307–27. https://doi.org/10.1016/0022-510X(65)90016-X, Bakhaidar M, Wilcox JT, Sinclair.
3. Brean A, Eide PK. Prevalence of probable idiopathic normal pressure hydrocephalus in a Norwegian population. Acta Neurol Scand. 2008;118(1):48–53. https://doi.org/10.1111/j.1600-0404.2007.00982.x.
4. Klassen BT, Ahlskog JE. Normal pressure hydrocephalus: how often does the diagnosis hold water? Neurology. 2011;77(12):1119–25. https://doi.org/10.1212/WNL.0b013e31822f02f5.
5. Vivas-Buitrago T, Gomez DF, Ramon JF, Quinones-Hinojosa A, Rigamonti D, Hakim F. Cerebrospinal fluid diversion procedures: ventriculo-atrial, ventriculo-peritoneal, ventriculo-pleural, and lumbo-peritoneal shunts. In: Schmidek and Sweet: Operative Neurosurgical Techniques: Indications, Methods and Results. Elsevier Health Sciences; 2012, pp. 993–9.
6. Graff-Radford NR, Jones DT. Normal pressure hydrocephalus. Continuum (Minneap Minn). 2019;25(1):165–86.
7. Nulsen FE, Spitz EB. Treatment of hydrocephalus by direct shunt from ventricle to jugular vain. Surg Forum. 1951;399–403.
8. Sinclair DS, Diaz RJ. Ventriculoatrial Shunts: Review of Technical Aspects and Complications. World Neurosurg. 2022;158:158–64.
9. Mori E, Ishikawa M, Kato T, et al. Guidelines for management of idiopathic normal pressure hydrocephalus: second edition. Neurol Med Chir (Tokyo). 2012;52(11):775–809. https://doi.org/10.2176/nmc.52.775
10. Metellus P, Hsu W, Kharkar S, Kapoor S, Scott W, Rigamonti D. Accuracy of percutaneous placement of a ventriculoatrial shunt under ultrasonography guidance: a retrospective study at a single institution. J Neurosurg. 2009;110(5):867–70.
11. Morone PJ, Dewan MC, Zuckerman SL, Tubbs RS, Singer RJ. Craniometrics and ventricular access: a review of Kocher's, Kaufman's, Paine's, Menovksy's, Tubbs', Keen's, Frazier's, Dandy's, and Sanchez's points. Oper Neurosurg (Hagerstown). 2020;18(5):461–9. https://doi.org/10.1093/ons/opz194. PMID: 31420653.
12. Harland TA, Winston KR, Jovanovich AJ, Johnson RJ. Shunt nephritis: an increasingly unfamiliar diagnosis. World Neurosurg. 2018;111:346–8. https://doi.org/10.1016/j.wneu.2018.01.017. Epub 2018 Jan 8 PMID: 29325951.

Lumboperitoneal Shunt for iNPH

Madoka Nakajima and Kostadin Karagiozov

Abstract Lumboperitoneal shunt (LPS), a creative development based on the lumbar puncture technique used in the cerebrospinal fluid (CSF) drainage test (tap test), is an increasingly popular treatment option around the world, but particularly in Japan, as it avoids an intervention on the brain, and even keeps the postsurgical scar not visible. It mainly avoids the risk of symptomatic intraparenchymal haematoma from ventricular catheter placement, which is seen in approximately 1% of the patients with idiopathic normal pressure hydrocephalus (iNPH). However, LPS has not generally been favoured by neurosurgeons because of the relatively higher than the ventriculoperitoneal shunt (VPS) failure rates and the possibility of symptomatic over-drainage. Another possible reason is that there is no reported standardized surgical technique, and the procedure is considered rather specific, out of the mainstream of neurosurgical operative routine skills. This understanding is in process of change.

Keywords Lumboperitoneal shunt · Shunt system · CSF drainage · Normal pressure hydrocephalus · Tap test

Abbreviations

CSF   Cerebrospinal fluid
CT   Computed tomography
ICP   Intracranial pressure

Supplementary Information The online version contains supplementary material available at (https://doi.org/10.1007/978-3-031-36522-5_23).

M. Nakajima (✉)
Department of Neurosurgery, Juntendo University, Bunkyo, Japan
e-mail: madoka66@juntendo.ac.jp

K. Karagiozov
Department of Neurosurgery, Jikei University School of Medicine, Minato, Japan
e-mail: karagiozov@jikei.ac.jp

iNPH   Idiopathic normal pressure hydrocephalus
MRI   Magnetic resonance imaging
LPS   Lumboperitoneal shunt
VPS   Ventriculoperitoneal shunt

1 Introduction

At the beginning, there were some original and not so-effective attempts to create lumboperitoneal communication by different surgeons [1]. A portion of the fifth lumbar arch was resected and a small burr hole drilled through the vertebral body reaching into the peritoneal cavity using a silver wire. This technique was also expanded by Cushing, using a silver tube as a shunt tube, unfortunately with disappointing results. Of 12 cases operated, two died of intussusceptions [2]. Two decades later, Matson [3] reported the technique of ureterostomy, connecting an intrathecal plastic tube in the vertebral canal to the ureter after nephrectomy. Nevertheless, it was obvious that due to folding, rupture, and obstruction of the shunt tube as well as invasiveness, these and other historic approaches to lumboperitoneal shunt (LPS) were indeed abandoned. With the improvement of shunt tube materials as well as the emergence of shunting devices equipped with valves, the usage of the LPS gradually increased.

All these historical LPS procedures were performed by the "open" method with vertebral arch resection and soon, as with the ongoing common tendency in surgery for less invasiveness, a closed method was first performed by Jackson and Snodgrass [4]. Jones [5] reported 63 cases of hydrocephalus treated with LPS, among whom 57 resulted in good hydrocephalus control. In the same year, Murtagh and Lehman [6] introduced a fine plastic tube through a No. 16 lumbar puncture needle percutaneously and then tunnelled it to the peritoneal cavity in the McBurney area. This further simplified surgical procedures and reduced complications related to laminectomy or laparotomy. However, complications related to the then existing synthetic tubes such as folding, adhesive arachnoiditis, and tube displacement emerged. Therefore, to optimize the material properties and simplify further technique, Spetzler et al. [7, 8] performed simple percutaneous LPS using a silicone tube and a reservoir.

In 1990, Aoki et al. [9] reported an 11-year study on 207 cases undergoing LPS and 120 cases undergoing ventriculoperitoneal (VPS) for the treatment of communicating hydrocephalus after confirming communication between the subarachnoid spaces and the lateral ventricle. They compared complications and success rates between the two groups and concluded that for patients without spinal pathology, an LPS should be considered first.

A prospective multicenter trial to assess LPS in patients with idiopathic normal pressure hydrocephalus (iNPH), the SINPHONI-2 ending in 2015, integrated a 3-month randomized controlled trial (i.e., RCT phase) comparing LPS implantation with conservative therapy, and a 12-month extension study in which all subjects received an LPS and were examined over 12 months following shunt placement. The short-term and long-term beneficial effects of LPS from this study were obvious. Further attempts for higher evidence level studies have been undertaken too, with one in China as monocentric, assessor-blinded, and randomized controlled trial with the rate of shunt failure within 5 years as primary outcome, and main criteria for shunt effectiveness as secondary [10].

2 Current Understanding of physiology and CSF Dynamics in LPS and Specific Differences from the VPS

The intracranial space is a semi-restricted space, and volume loading to the cranial cavity increases intracranial pressure (ICP), which is compensated by shifting CSF and blood extracranially according to the Monro-Kellie doctrine [11]. The change in ICP in response to volumetric loading to the cranial cavity is referred to as intracranial compliance. Lower intracranial compliance indicates a greater pressure change in response to volumetric loading and therefore decreased pressure is a compensatory function [12, 13]. The electrocardiogram-synchronized phase contrast MRI method can quantitatively evaluate the intracranial environment noninvasively [14, 15]. The ventricle gap method is an MRI-based intracranial environment analysis that calculates ICP and CSF pressure gradient changes using a reference point at the upper cervical spine [14]. This study provides important insight into the coupling that exists between arterial, venous, and CSF flow dynamics, and how it is affected by posture. Changes in head and all body position affect CSF dynamics because of the hydrostatic gradient created by gravity. In a prone position, the intracranial and intraspinal pressures are equal, and the hydrostatic gradient disappears. With its disappearance, CSF flow is driven by the external forces leading to CSF pulsation as respiration and the inflow of arterial blood into the cranial cavity [16, 17]. On the other hand, in the standing and sitting upright positions, CSF pressure is equal to atmospheric pressure at the foramen magnum and the upper cervical spine levels. Intracranial pressure is lower than the atmospheric, and the pressure in the spinal CSF compartment below the foramen magnum increases downwards in proportion to the distance from it [17]. Therefore, changes in hydrostatic pressure gradient associated with postural changes strongly influence CSF dynamics, and in a different way for LPS and VPS.

At present, the details of pressure values in the lumbar subarachnoid space resulting from the shunt effect are unknown. It is presumed that the lumbar subarachnoid space at the tip of the LPS proximal catheter is always positively pressurized, unlike VP shunts. However, the lumbar subarachnoid space pressure probably decreases slightly due to the CSF shunt draining effect of, particularly in prone position.

The absence of intervention on the brain has made LPS patients a more appropriate subject for clinical studies on iNPH due to the cranial compartments and their CSF flow dynamics structurally unaffected by intervention. In one such study, Kikuta et al. [18] have shown better water diffusion around the perivascular spaces after shunting. Using the same convenient setup with LPS patients, the changes in the MRI characteristics of iNPH as upper cortical subarachnoid tightness and the callosal angle were found to improve after shunting [19].

3 Current Clinical Experience with LPS

3.1 Current Application of LPS in iNPH

Compared with VPS, at present, LPS has been used globally in a smaller proportion of iNPH patients. There is even a certain geographic distribution of its application, with predominance in Asia, mainly in Japan and Korea. That tendency has been expressing the views and the accumulated experience and analysis of relatively larger numbers of cases, and subsequently LPS indications have been more precisely provided in the recommended respective guidelines. In the second and third part of the major iNPH study in Japan SINPHONI, LPS effects were important variables to be investigated. A series by Nakajima et al., 2015 [20] indicated that LPS (Medtronic Strata NSC) is as effective as the VPS. Miyajima et al. [21] summarized a comparative VPS versus LPS analysis within the SINPHONI-2 study. For a cohort of iNPH patients, LPS with programmable valves showed similar efficacy and safety rates as VPS, pointing at the minimal invasiveness and avoidance of brain injury as major merits, regardless of the higher rate of minor complications.

More recently, studies performed in North America [22] and Europe [23] report similar experiences.

3.2 Current Indications and Contraindications

LPS is indicated for all types of communicating hydrocephalus. The lumbar subarachnoid space can be accessed easily even in conditions such as slit ventricle syndrome, where lateral ventriculostomy is technically more difficult. LPS is also indicated for controlling CSF pressure in idiopathic intracranial hypertension when there are no intracranial mass lesions, abnormalities in the cerebrospinal fluid characteristics, or abnormalities in the ventricular system.

Conversely, it is contraindicated for non-communicating hydrocephalus. LPS should also be avoided if there are brain malformations in the posterior cranial fossa, malformations in the craniovertebral junction, and in the case of Chiari malformations, basilar impression, and syringomyelia. If magnetic resonance imaging (MRI) shows severe narrowing of the spinal subarachnoid space following inflammation in the subarachnoid space, or owing to degenerative diseases of the spine, LPS would eventually block CSF flow, risking myelopathy or underdrainage. However, this is not an absolute contraindication. On this pathophysiological background, the LPS can be

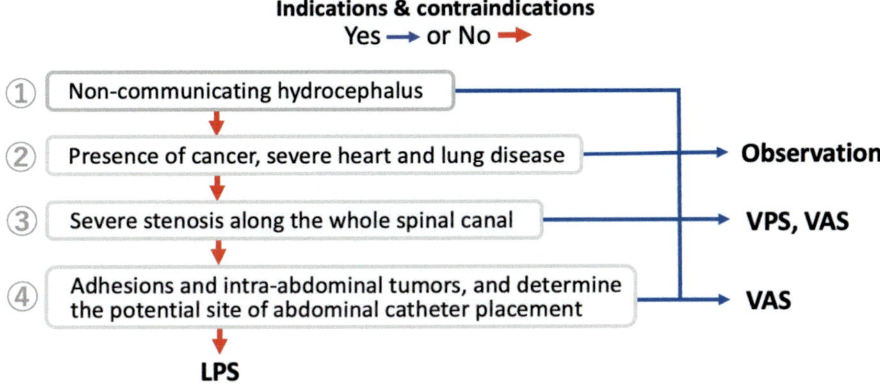

Fig. 1 A simplified algorithm of indications and contraindications in hydrocephalus treatment

applied in iNPH once adequate communication between CSF spaces is ascertained (Fig. 1).

3.3 Currently Applied Surgical Techniques of LPS

The main goal of the LPS technique is to provide a safe, effective, uncomplicated, and cosmetically acceptable minimally invasive method of CSF drainage valve implantation, connecting the lumbar cistern and the peritoneal cavity. Currently some standards have been already established (such as the placement of the percutaneous lumbar catheter), but some other steps may vary to a minor extent between surgeons and places, trying to optimize the procedure. Attempts of optimization include the comparison of lateral and periumbilical laparotomy approaches for peritoneal catheter placement by Goto et al. [24]; however, results were similar, except for slightly a shorter surgical time (Tables 1 and 2). Below are some standard point to follow before surgery:

Table 1 Simplified checklists before LP shunt surgery

①	Properly established iNPH diagnosis	
②	Evaluation of patient's general condition	Presence of malignancy, heart, or lung disease
③	Lumbar puncture	Tap test result
④	Whole spine MRI/ CT	No severe stenosis along the whole spinal canal
⑤	Abdominal CT	Check for adhesions, intra-abdominal tumours, and determine the potential site of abdominal catheter placement

Table 2 Surgical preparation

Temporarily suspend the use of antiplatelet agents
Review lumbar CT and MRI findings prior to puncture for the catheter placement
The patient receives either lumbar anaesthesia or general anaesthesia
Antibiotics are administered intravenously at induction of anaesthesia to prevent infection

One of the well-established and widely applied techniques, also used at our institution is described below.

3.4　Surgical Steps

Step 1: Surgical Preparation

The patient receives either lumbar or general anaesthesia. General anaesthesia is required for laparoscopic catheter placement in the abdominal cavity, as it requires insufflation. In our hospital, we use isobaric bupivacaine for lumbar anaesthesia. Prophylactic antibiotics are administered intravenously prior to surgery.

Surgery is performed in the lateral position. Since the skin sags when the patient is turned from the supine to the lateral position, preoperative marking is performed in the supine position, and proper position for the relay point and abdominal access is secured. Since it might be difficult to identify adhesions in the abdominal cavity by preoperative diagnostic imaging, the side of the abdominal cavity that has not undergone laparotomy should be preferably selected. A cushion should be placed under the armpit to relieve pressure on the upper arm, the lower leg should be gently bent, and a cushion should be placed between the knees, so that the patient can maintain a comfortable and relaxed posture without lumbar extension.

If a fluoroscope such as a C-arm is used to check the position of the catheter during surgery, it should be able to move to the puncture site or to the spinal level of interest to provide guidance for the catheter tip before finally positioning it. The bed is adjusted by slightly lifting the cranial side to widen the lumbar interlaminar spaces for the ease of the lumbar puncture.

Step 2: Lumbar Side

The spinal catheter is guided through the lumbar puncture by a Tuohy needle (14 gauge; tube outer diameter, 2.10 mm; tube inner diameter, 1.80 mm; length, 90 mm). There are two puncture approaches: median and paramedian. The lumbar spine of older adults tends to be deformed, and for patients with narrow interlaminar spaces, paracentral puncture is recommended because median puncture may cause postoperative tube rupture. The images of the spinal computed tomography (CT) and spinal MRI should be reviewed in preoperative puncture planning. An incision of approximately 1 cm in depth and 2 cm laterally on the lumbar side is performed. Having confirmed the outflow of CSF after the puncture, the puncture needle is rotated so that the inserted shunt tube and its tip opening face cranially and the shunt tube is inserted into the lumbar subarachnoid space extending over 2–3 vertebrae above. If the tip of the catheter extends outward or bends to form a U-turn, it may induce postoperative spinal root symptoms and cause lower limb pain. Therefore, adjustment must be done for the catheter to be placed in the midline under fluoroscopy. If required, under fluoroscopic guidance, a catheter with a guidewire (diameter, 0.46 mm; length, 100 cm; 21,038, Medtronic, Inc., Goleta, California, USA) can be used, as it provides enhanced visibility and easy guidance, or if it is not available, the catheter can be filled with spinal contrast agent to visualize its position. After confirming adequate CSF flow, the lumbar catheter is secured at the site of insertion to prevent dislodgement. It is helpful to use an anchoring device or a suture into the paraspinal fascia to secure the catheter.

Step 3: Shunt Valve Placement

A relay point is set up on the lateral abdomen. LPSs are prone to catheter dislodgement, which may be caused by bending or twisting at the waist. The shunt system should be fixed at least at three sites: lumbar, ventral, and lateral abdominal to prevent dislodgement.

For the abdominal placement, an adequately sized pocket between the lateral abdominal relay point and the skin incision for laparotomy has to be created for the shunt valve to be subcutaneously implanted. The shunt valve should be placed at 7–10 mm depth from the skin. If it is too deep, it is difficult to change its pressure setting postoperatively, and if it is too superficial, the risk of infection increases. Since the shunt valve may rotate sideways and flip, it is important always to fix the valve to the fascia in two or more points or to the hypodermal layer if the subcutaneous fat is too thick, to prevent it from moving.

In case of dorsal implantation of the shunt valve, the stability should be secured to the fascia of the paramedian muscle group. The stability of the implants reduces the chance of rotation and displacement of the shunt valve and makes it easy to change the set pressure of programmable valves. After proper and stable positioning, flushing of the valve can also be easily performed as needed in the postoperative follow-up.

Step 4: Abdominal Side

The procedure can be undertaken in the following two positions for the abdominal part of the operation—lateral or supine—and both are currently used. When changing positions, it is convenient to use a transportation board. The abdominal wall incision is normally made using the McBurney technique and the length of the skin incision is determined by the thickness of the abdominal fat layer and the expected depth to reach the peritoneum. From a postoperative cosmetic perspective, it is advisable to perform an incision along the skin break lines and sufficiently low on the abdomen so that the underwear can hide the near horizontal skin incision scar.

If the abdominal part of the surgery is performed in the lateral position, and if the patient is obese, the surgical field becomes deeper and displaced downwardly as a result. The weight of the patient's abdominal tissues makes a midline directed incision easier. The incision should be made up to the external oblique fascia to prevent the subcutaneous fat from damage, necrosis, and creating a dead space. The use of blunt scalp hooks and the Lone Star self-retaining retractor (3307G [14.2 cm × 14.2 cm], 3350-8G [12 mm diameter]; CooperSurgical, Trumbull, CT 06611 USA) provides a shallow surgical field by pulling the superficial abdominal fascia and the belly of the rectus abdominis with its sheath upward, allowing easy surgical access.

As the lower abdomen has three muscle layers (external oblique, internal oblique, and transversus abdominis) that run in an alternating manner and direction. After incision, the dissection of the muscle groups should be done in a blunt manner, trying to preserve the fibres along their course, and retract the rectus abdominis muscle medially from its lateral border. This will expose the transverse fascia and peritoneum. The fascia and peritoneum are held up with forceps to separate them from the intraperitoneal contents to avoid damaging it, and both are opened.

If passed through the anterior sheath of the rectus abdominis muscle, the abdominal catheter can be more easily prevented from pulling out of the abdominal cavity, and access is easier in obese patients [25]. Lumbar catheter, shunt valve, and abdominal tube are connected to complete the shunt system and confirm spontaneous dripping of cerebrospinal fluid from the distal catheter tip. The catheter is then inserted into the abdominal cavity. Since adult patients do not change their stature, like children, the length of the catheter to be inserted into the abdominal cavity needs only to be within the range that does not allow dislodgement after twisting the waist. We use a shorter length to fit the patient's body shape, averaging approximately 15–20 cm, based on the experience of a patient who complained of abdominal pain on the opposite side of the wound, likely caused by the contact between the bowels and the catheter tip. To close the peritoneum, purse string sutures are used for the fascia around the catheter to prevent dislodgement.

If the team is of two or more surgeons, these steps can be performed simultaneously without changing positions, shortening the surgical time.

3.5 Illustrative Case 1—Video

4 Immediate Postoperative Management and Pressure Settings in LPSs

Mobilization out of bed is normally allowed immediately after surgery. However, owning to the difference in diameter of the Touhy lumbar puncture needle and catheter, there is a possibility of cerebrospinal fluid leakage from the lumbar subarachnoid space to the epidural space immediately after the surgery and consequent intracranial hypotension. If neurological symptoms such as occipital pain, dizziness, and floating sensation are suspected to be caused by low CSF pressure and they appear soon after the surgery, bed rest may be necessary.

Another caveat is related to postoperative MRI. Although recently designed shunt valves are MRI compatible for imaging performed immediately after surgery, it should be noted that this carries the risk of some structural damage complications, as pressure settings change may occur during imaging, and the valves, which contain material that can be magnetized, are subject to pulling forces. In particular, there is even a risk for the unsecured valve to flip during the immediate postoperative period when the wound has not yet healed well.

In the immediate postoperative period, the occasional symptoms and signs of hypotension due to leakage around the catheter are not considered complications, as they are transient and spontaneously recovering. Complications, however, do exist, and they have been at the attention of all authors presenting LPS outcome, often more [21] than less [26] compared to the VPS. Complications can be divided mainly in two categories—those related to CSF flow physiology or of functional nature, and those related to failure of a structural nature, for example damage of the valve, its settings and displacement in the surrounding tissues.

5 Postoperative CSF Physiology and "Over-Drainage" Management in LPSs (Functional Type Complications)

The lumboperitoneal shunt, by draining from the lowermost lumbar CSF compartment and not directly from the ventricle, is a better simulation and less disruptive of the natural physiological CSF path of flow. However, the maintenance of physiological flow and pressure is not so easily possible, mainly due to the imperfect drainage regulation by the currently available valves. In addition to these valve imperfections, different other daily life factors, such as body position (standing, laying down, particularly for LPS), strains, and efforts, are additional factors for inappropriate CSF flow drainage. The "state of the art" valves at present are often added devices that will prevent over-drainage and hypotension (gravitational valves, anti-siphon devices), which have shown promising results. In our institution, we compared recently two devices, finding additional benefit from the add-on gravitational valve [20].

There is more or less a standard approach protocol to over-drainage with or without clinical manifestations, based on opening pressure increase.

In addition, as the current shunt systems solely rely on pressure control for the CSF drainage, they may cause haematoma growth in the event of intracranial haemorrhage, such as epidural or subdural haematoma, a rare but important complication to manage. Although there is no understanding yet, the current shunt systems do not allow significant decrease of intracranial pressure and resulting haematoma growth, however if they are implanted, an increase in the intracranial pressure other origin will force CSF to be drained. In clinical practice, when a chronic subdural effusion or haematoma occurs, the physician immediately raises the shunt's set pressure to the highest level. In some cases, this even results in the disappearance of the subdural haematoma.

5.1 *Illustrative Case No. 2*

A 73-year-old male, company owner, became aware of gait disturbance and frequent urination about one year prior to his visit to our clinic. He was suspected to have idiopathic normal pressure hydrocephalus by his physician and was referred to our hospital, where that was confirmed with a tap test. One month after the tap test, a left side LPS placement was performed. The device had a programmable valve (CERTAS) with initial pressure setting at Level 4 combined with gravity valve (0–15 cm H_2O). Immediately after the procedure, the patient had a mild hydrostatically induced headache probably due to CSF leakage from the puncture site and the setting was increased to Level 5. After discharge from the hospital, the patient was seen once a month postoperatively, and at the 3rd month his wife became aware that he was wobbling, and his walking was becoming slightly slower. After reviewing his head CT with persisting DESH, the pressure setting was lowered to Level 4 (Fig. 2A).

Five months after surgery, he began to notice headache and dizziness during his morning commute to work, and the headache symptoms persisted after arriving at work. One day after lunch, he started vomiting and had difficulty walking and was transferred to a hospital. On admission, his consciousness was slightly impaired (awake, but confused, GCS 14), without focal neurological deficit. A right subdural haematoma was detected, with compression of the cerebral cortex and displacement of the midline structures (Fig. 2B).

Emergency craniotomy was performed under general anaesthesia to remove the haematoma. Shunt pressure was set at Lv8. Postoperative course was uneventful, and the patient was discharged one week after surgery. One month later (6 months after LP shunt), the patient returned to the outpatient clinic, and CT confirmed complete haematoma absence, his mRS was 1 and the CERTAS valve was set to Lv 6 again, later gradually lowered.

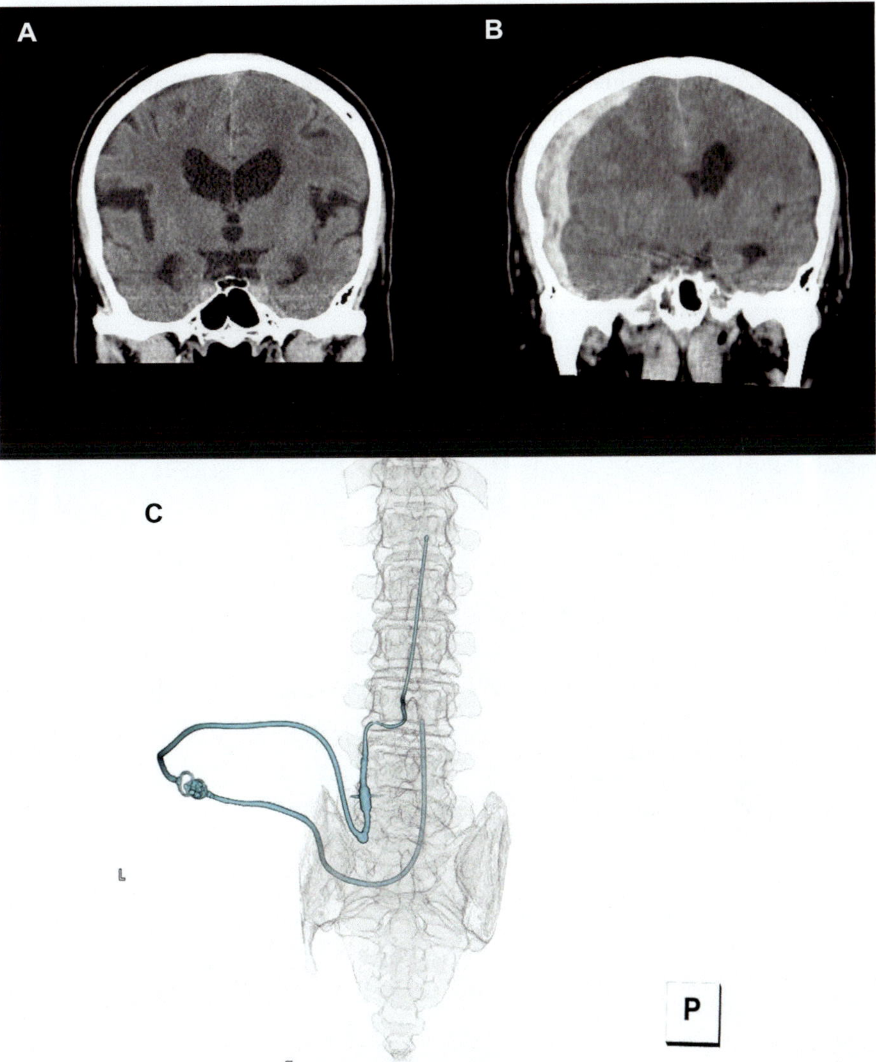

Fig. 2 (A) Three months after surgery (B) Subdural haematoma five months after surgery (C) Inserted lumboperitoneal shunt position

5.2 Illustrative Case 3

This 78-year-old male patient, with weight 66 kg and height 167 cm, had the typical iNPH "triad" and with the gait disturbances leading. In the last year, when cognition clearly started to decline, he was investigated. His CT was clearly indicative of DESH, and his tap test was positive. He was operated with a CERTAS valve and GV attached, postoperatively improving and the valve settings were Level 2 at discharge.

On a regular follow-up, 3 weeks later, clinically with clearly persisting improvement, his CT showed big subdural effusions. This required an immediate raise of valve settings to Level 4. On his next regular follow-up about a month and a half later, his condition has slightly impaired, mainly his speech and cognition, there was a right latent hemiparesis, and the CT showed a big left temporal chronic subdural haematoma. Valve was immediately closed (Level 8), and burr hole surgery on the left side was performed with immediate clinical improvement. The small collection on the right side was left under observation (Fig. 3).

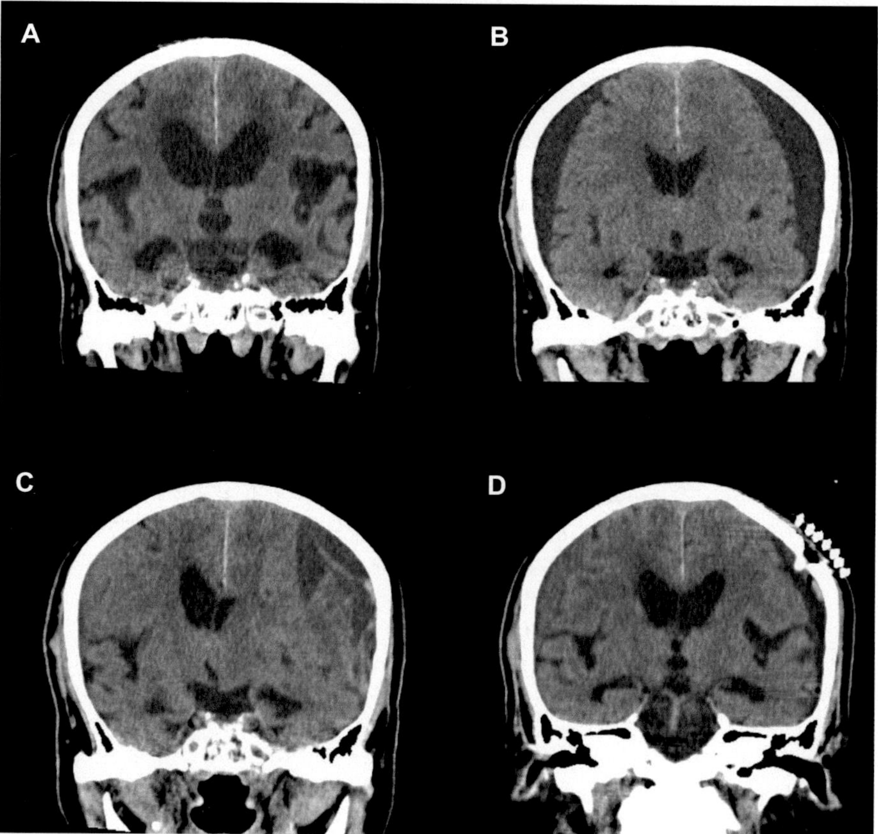

Fig. 3 (A) Clear DESH in 78-year-old male patient. (B) Subdural effusions. (C) Big temporal subdural haematoma. (D) Postoperative CT

6 Postoperative complications with Structural Shunt Damage

In case of LPS, immediately after the surgery, CSF may continue leaking around the catheter from the needle hole in the dura mater created during the puncture for a longer time than the usual few postoperative days. This can cause more prolonged over-drainage symptoms, such as continuous headache and even subdural haematoma. Therefore, current guidelines mention the need to ensure safety and maintain the valve pressure set at a high level. However, once wound healing is stabilized (the post-operative scarring firmly engulfs the valve system), it will be necessary to increase the drained CSF amount to obtain a therapeutic effect and an increase in the patient's activity. Even so, it would be safer to change the pressure setting one level at a time to avoid the complications related to over-drainage.

Patients with iNPH will not clearly show significant change in the size of the ventricles on CT and MRI studies immediately after surgery. Until the narrowing of the cerebral sulcus in the high convex shows improvement, it will be necessary to decrease the pressure setting of the shunt valve and increase the amount of CSF drainage to maximize the effect of the shunt procedure.

6.1 Illustrative Case 4—Subdural Lumbar Catheter Placement

This 73-year-old male had LPS placement under standard indications. After lumbar catheter insertion, the flow of CSF tended to decrease and stop after a few ml of discharge, and insertion deeper or pulling out a little did not improve the flow. Subdural (extra-arachnoidal) placement was suspected, as its position was close to the spinal canal wall. Contrast medium was injected through the catheter. Blocking between dura and arachnoid prevented contrast from spreading (Fig. 4A). Contrast washout was poor, and cauda equina structure could not be confirmed. After reposi-tioning, the contrasted CSF is relatively uniform and caudal structures can be seen (Fig. 4B). Catheter placement in the appropriate position is essential to preserve shunt function.

6.2 Illustrative Case 5—Shunt Structural Damage – Shunt Migration

A 76-year-old woman, lives alone. She owned a bar but stopped running it about a year ago due to gait disturbance, urinary urgency, and memory loss. After a close examination by her general practitioner, she was diagnosed with iNPH.

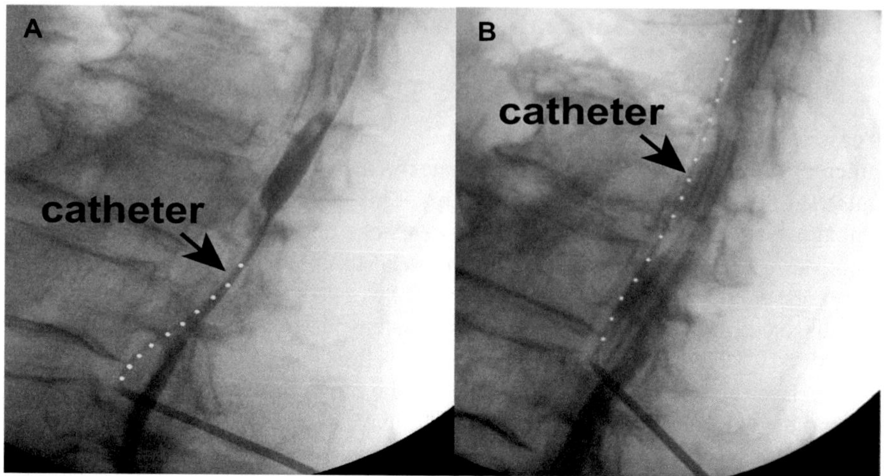

Fig. 4 Subdural lumbar catheter placement. (A) Position of the catheter close to the spinal canal wall, suspicion of subdural placement. (B) After repositioning of the catheter

On admission with us her MMSE was 24, FAB—14, Bartell Index—65, and the CSF phosphorylated tau protein—32.3 pg/mL. A tap test was performed and initial pressure was 15 cmH2O; 40 mL of fluid was drained, and final pressure became 0. MRI of the entire spine showed no stenosis of the subarachnoid spaces, and an LP shunt was performed under lumbar anaesthesia (CERTAS Lv5 on the ventral side + GV 0–15 cmH$_2$O placed on the dorsal lumbar side). The patient's gait improved after the procedure.

However, 3 months after returning home, the patient was readmitted to the hospital for shunt revision due to the recurrence of wobbliness when walking, foggy feeling, and deviation of the lumbar catheter was detected (Fig. 5A). On examination, her height was 156 cm, weight—65 kg, and body mass index 26.7. Since the patient had significant skin mobility on the dorsal lumbar side and abdomen at the time of the previous surgery (skin easily moved more than 20 cm after changing position), and the subcutaneously implanted shunt tube was expected to move excessively with the trunk, the LP shunt system placement was made less susceptible to skin movement at the shunt revision. So, the lumbar subarachnoid tube was inserted into the subarachnoid space not exceeding 15 cm, and the gravitational valve on the dorsal lumbar side was removed so that there were no other pulling forces. Symptoms particularly gait disturbance improved again (Fig. 5B).

Skin mobility should be carefully monitored, especially in obese women, as LP shunts may require caution in terms of migration. Shunt migration is most likely to occur within 1–3 months, especially in the early postoperative period. Although no report has accurately captured the mobility of the skin, shunt system mobility associated with skin movement may also be an important issue in reducing the incidence of shunt dysfunction. Surgical techniques such as securing the shunt system in place

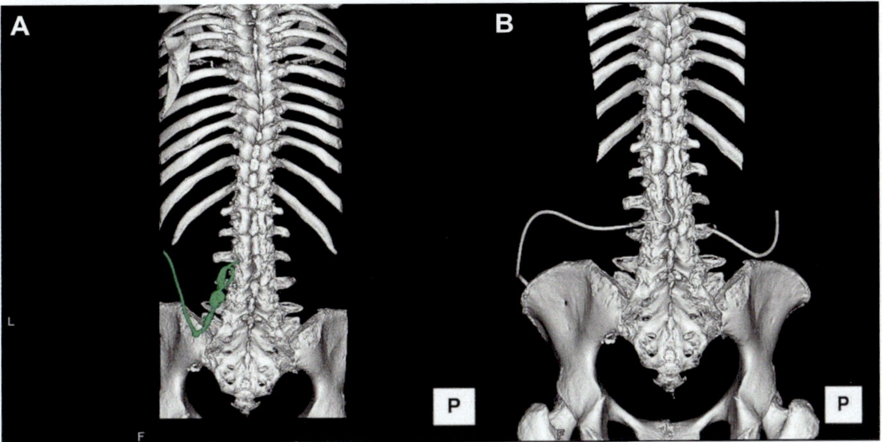

Fig. 5 Illustrative case of shunt structural damage and system migration

at multiple points and implanting a catheter longer than the mobility range of the skin may be considered.

7 Perspectives of Further LPS Improvement

All current shunt systems use hydrostatic pressure gradients, like those resulting from postural changes, as the driving force for cerebrospinal fluid drainage without using power; hence, there is no need to replace devices for power charge. The advantage is that, in theory, is that the shunt valve can continue to be used semi-permanently if there is no structural failure. However, these systems cannot externally transmit information on their status to the physicians, as baclofen pumps, deep brain stimulators, and spinal epidural stimulators can. Even if dysfunction of the shunt occurs, such as shunt obstruction, physicians may not be able to notice it until they observe worsening of the symptoms or changes on images, such as ventricular enlargement. When patients with iNPH do not show improvement in symptoms after LPS, physicians cannot determine whether it is due to underdrainage, or whether the symptoms caused by comorbidities became dominant over those caused by iNPH, so the patient might have been misdiagnosed and shunt therapy might have not been indicated in these patients. Patient safety depends on whether physicians could immediately detect shunt obstruction or inadequate CSF drainage. Feedback from patients would give better chances for early correction and repair of LPS valves.

However, all these uncertainties need to be addressed in the context of the current scientific paradigm, and current technological advancement of "intelligent" shunt systems is aiming to resolve them. Non-invasive detection, rate of flow information, and response to sudden pressure challenges without flow increase and arrest, for example, could significantly improve success in reducing complications.

8 Conclusion

The main benefit of LPS is the possibility of avoidance of an intervention on the brain. Additionally, it renders excellent cosmetic outcomes. It mainly avoids the risk of symptomatic intraparenchymal haematoma from standard ventricular catheter placement. Overall efficacy and success rates of LP shunts in iNPH management are comparable to the more often used VP shunts. LPS is moreover a great alternative as it provides iNPH patients with less invasive surgical treatment.

9 Key Points

- LPSs have shown similar rates of success in management of iNPH and the VPSs.
- The probably higher rate of minor complications is compensated by the reduction of the more severe ones.
- LPS provides better opportunities to the elder iNPH patients as the surgery is less invasive under local anaesthesia.
- Current clinical experience places LPS as an equal solution for iNPH as the VPS, with the consideration of the specific contraindications for each of the methods.

Acknowledgements This work was supported in part by Grants-in-Aid for Scientific Research (grant numbers 16KK0187, 17K10908, 18H02916, 20K09398) from the Japan Society for the Promotion of Science. Ethical approval Not required.

References

1. Ferguson AH. Intraperitoneal diversion of the cerebrospinal fluid in cases of hydrocephalus. N Y Med J. 1898;67:902–9.
2. Pudenz RH. The surgical treatment of hydrocephalus—an historical review. Surg Neurol. 1981;15:15–25.
3. Matson DD. Ventriculo-uretherostomy. J Neurosurg. 1951;8:398–404.
4. Jackson IJ, Snodgrass SR. Peritoneals shunts in the treatment of hydrocephalus and increased intracranial pressure. Four-year survey of 62 patients. J Neurosurg. 1955;12:216–222.
5. Jones RFC. Long-term results in various treatments of hydrocephalus. J Neurosurg. 1967;26:313–5.
6. Murtagh F, Lehman R. Peritoneal shunts in the management of hydrocephalus 1967;202(11):98–102.

7. Spetzler RF, Wilson CB, Grollmus JM. Percutaneous lumboperitoneal shunt. Technical Note 1975;43(6):770–3.

8. Spetzler FR, Wilson, CB, Shulte R. Simplified percutaneous lumboperitoneal shunting. Surg Neurol. 1977; 25–9.

9. Aoki N. Lumboperitoneal shunt: clinical applications, complications, and comparison with venntriculoperitoneal shunt. Neurosurgery. 1990;26(6):998–1002.

10. Cui W, Sun T, Wu K, You C, Guan J. Comparison of ventriculoperitoneal shunt to lumboperitoneal shunt in the treatment of idiopathic: a monocentric, assessor-blinded, randomized controlled trial. Medicine 2021;100:31(e26691). https://doi.org/10.1097/MD.00000000002 6691.

11. Wilson MH. Monro-Kellie 2.0: the dynamic vascular and venous pathophysiological components of intracranial pressure. J Cereb Blood Flow Metab. 2016;36(8):1338–50.

12. Marmarou A, Shulman K, LaMorgese J. Compartmental analysis of compliance and outflow resistance of the cerebrospinal fluid system. J Neurosurg. 1975;43(5):523–34.

13. Marmarou A, Shulman K, Rosende RM. A nonlinear analysis of the cerebrospinal fluid system and intracranial pressure dynamics. J Neurosurg. 1978;48(3):332–44.

14. Alperin N, Lee SH, Sivaramakrishnan A, Hushek SG. Quantifying the effect of posture on intracranial physiology in humans by MRI flow studies. J Magn Reson Imaging. 2005;22(5):591–6.

15. Miyati T, Mase M, Banno T, Kasuga T, Yamada K, Fujita H, et al. Frequency analyses of CSF flow on cine MRI in normal pressure hydrocephalus. Eur Radiol. 2003;13(5):1019–24.

16. Bulat M, Klarica M. Recent insights into a new hydrodynamics of the cerebrospinal fluid. Brain Res Rev. 2011;65(2):99–112.

17. Klarica M, Rados M, Erceg G, Petosic A, Jurjevic I, Oreskovic D. The influence of body position on cerebrospinal fluid pressure gradient and movement in cats with normal and impaired craniospinal communication. PLoS ONE. 2014;9(4): e95229.

18. Kikuta J, Kamagata K, Abe M, et al. Effects of arterial stiffness on cerebral WM integrity in older adults: a neurite orientation dispersion and density imaging and magnetization transfer saturation imaging study. AJNR Am J Neuroradiol. 2022;43(12):1706–12.

19. Kilinc MC, Kahilogullari G, Dogan I, et al. Changes in callosal angle and Evans' index after placing a lumboperitoneal shunt in patients with idiopathic-normal- pressure hydrocephalus. Turk Neurosurg. 2022;32(2):309–14.

20. Nakajima M, Miyajima M, Ogino I, Sugano H, Akiba C, Domon N, et al. Use of external lumbar cerebrospinal fluid drainage and lumboperitoneal shunts with strata NSC valves in idiopathic normal pressure hydrocephalus: a single-center experience. World Neurosurg. 2015;83(3):387–93.

21. Miyajima M, Kazui H, Mori E, Ishikawa M. On behalf of the sinphoni-2 investigators. One-year outcome in patients with idiopathic normal-pressure hydrocephalus: comparison of lumboperitoneal shunt to ventriculoperitoneal shunt. J Neurosurg. 2016;125(6):1483–92. https://doi.org/10.3171/2015.10.JNS151894.

22. Yerneni K, Karras CL, Larkin CJ, Weiss H, Hopkins B, Kesavabhotla K, et al. Lumboperitoneal shunts for the treatment of idiopathic normal pressure hydrocephalus. J Clin Neurosc. 2021;86:1–5. https://doi.org/10.1016/j.jocn.2020.12.031.

23. Todisco M, Picascia M, Pisano P, Zangaglia R, Minafra B, Vitali P, et al. Lumboperitoneal shunt in idiopathic normal pressure hydrocephalus: a prospective controlled study. J Neurol. 2020;267:2556–66. https://doi.org/10.1007/s00415-020-09844-x.

24. Goto Y, Oka H, Nishii S, Takagi Y, Yokoya S, Hino A. Lumboperitoneal shunt surgery via lateral abdominal laparotomy. J Neurosurg Spine 2020;32(4):548–53. https://doi.org/10.3171/2019.10.SPINE19957.

25. Kawahara T, Tokimura H, Higa N, Hirano H, Bohara M, Hanaya R, et al. Surgical technique for preventing subcutaneous migration of distal lumboperitoneal shunt catheters. Innovative Neurosurg 2013;1(3–4):169–72. https://doi.org/10.1515/ins-2013-0016.

26. Xie D, Chen H, Guo X, Liu Y. Comparative study of lumboperitoneal shunt and ventriculoperitoneal shunt in the treatment of idiopathic normal pressure hydrocephalus. Am J Transl Res. 2021;13(10):11917–924. www.ajtr.org /ISSN:1943-8141/AJTR0132277

Endoscopic Third Ventriculostomy in Normal Pressure Hydrocephalus: Current Role

Victor Lomachinsky, Levi Coelho Maia Barros, and Petr Libý

Abstract Despite advancements in understanding idiopathic normal pressure hydrocephalus (iNPH) pathophysiology, both the disease aetiology and the brain's adaptive response to hydrocephalus remains mostly obscure. This carries serious implications not only for diagnosis but also for management. It is difficult to determine which patients will truly benefit from shunting devices, and while ventriculoperitoneal shunt (VPS) carries overall high success rates it also encompasses significant risks. Positive experiences in neurosurgical literature have sparked interest in endoscopic third ventriculostomy (ETV) as a treatment alternative. Reasoning derives from its ability to increase the systolic outflow from the ventricles which is thought to reduce the chronic transmantle pulsatile stress associated with iNPH. A shorter clinical history and better baseline neurological status seem to be correlated with higher degrees of improvement following ETV. Proper indication is however debatable as studies have failed to provide evidence of better short-term safety or better overall outcomes. Unfortunately, as patient selection has not been properly established, the true efficacy of ETV for iNPH remains speculative.

Keywords Normal pressure hydrocephalus · Endoscopic third ventriculostomy · Endoscopy · shunt placement · Shunt system · Hydrocephalus · Intracranial pressure · Cerebrospinal fluid

V. Lomachinsky · L. C. M. Barros · P. Libý (✉)
Department of Neurosurgery, 2Nd Faculty of Medicine, Charles University and Motol University Hospital, Prague, Czech Republic
e-mail: petr.liby@fnmotol.cz

V. Lomachinsky
e-mail: victor.lomachinsky@icloud.com

L. C. M. Barros
e-mail: levicmaiabarros@gmail.com

O. Bradac (ed.), *Normal Pressure Hydrocephalus*,
https://doi.org/10.1007/978-3-031-36522-5_24

Abbreviations

iNPH	Idiopathic normal pressure hydrocephalus
CSF	Cerebrospinal fluid
CST	Corticospinal tract
CT	Computerised tomography
ETV	Endoscopic third ventriculostomy
ETVSS	ETV success score
HCP	Hydrocephalus
ICP	Intracranial pressure
LIAS	Late onset Idiopathic Aqueductal Stenosis
LOVA	Longstanding overt ventriculomegaly in adults
VPS	Ventriculoperitoneal shunt

1   Introduction

Idiopathic normal pressure hydrocephalus (iNPH) is by definition of unclear aetiology. Both its diagnosis and proper management have long represented a challenge for surgeons and clinicians. First described by doctor Salomón Hakim in 1964, it is clinically defined by a triad of a frontal gait ataxia, urinary incontinence and subcortical dementia with short-term memory failure [1]. Radiologically, it exhibits a picture of ventriculomegaly and disturbances of corpus callosum angle (Fig. 1).

There is however a broad group of differential diagnoses possible and secondary causes are not always easy to dismiss. This has serious implications for management, as while iNPH might justify shunting, similar conditions might instead warrant different approaches or no intervention at all.

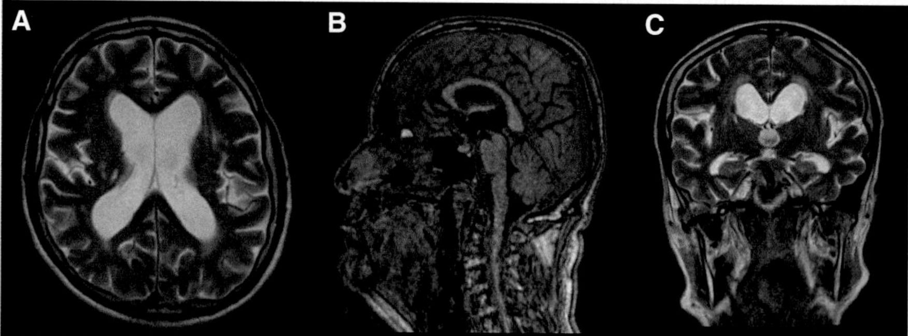

Fig. 1 68-year-old patient with signs of normal pressure hydrocephalus (NPH). (A) MRI T2W showing ventriculomegaly and periventricular changes. (B) Sagittal T1W image showing unbowed corpus callosum. (C) Coronal T2W MRI showing ventriculomegaly, periventricular changes, diminished subarachnoid spaces above hemispheres and sharp angle of corpus callosum

The current gold standard of treatment consists of meticulous examination and, if indicated, implantation of a ventriculoperitoneal shunt (VPS). In fact, the focus of most recent research in iPNH has largely rested upon identifying which subset of patients would be most responsive to shunting. Given that it significantly relieves symptoms in almost 75% of patients, many would argue for a lower threshold for shunting [2]. VPS is, however, largely ineffective for the remaining cases and relapse may yet be possible. In addition, infection, mechanical failure, perioperative complications and overall need for reoperation have since sparked interest in treatment alternatives.

2 Pathophysiology

While there have been advancements in the understanding of iNPH pathophysiology, both its aetiology and the brain's adaptive response to hydrocephalus remain obscure [3]. Ventricular enlargement may be connected with a series of pathophysiologic abnormalities, notably: Extra-ventricular obstruction sites, functional aqueduct stenosis and, perhaps more important for the rationale of endoscopic third ventriculostomy (ETV), the loss of ventricular wall elasticity [3, 4].

According to the latter theory, the inciting event is a loss of brain compliance with overall increase in the transmantle pressure gradient [5]. Periventricular white matter ischemia would first promote ventricular wall weakening and dilation leading to cerebrospinal fluid (CSF) stagnation and regional compression. This would subsequently lead to loss of parenchymal elasticity and compliance [3]. With each heartbeat, there would be ventricular expansion against a stiffer parenchyma leading to periventricular capillary compression and worsening ischemia. In addition, and as a result of stagnant flow, increasing transependymal CSF resorption would also promote interstitial oedema and further augment brain damage [3].

The final product is a narrower subarachnoid space with compressed capacitance vessels and increased pulse pressure. It has indeed been shown that the power of intraventricular CSF pulsations is increased as much as four times in chronic hydrocephalus [5].

The rationale for ETV in iNPH derives from its ability to increase the systolic outflow from the ventricles thus reducing the chronic transmantle pulsatile stress. It serves as an escape mechanism dissipating the mechanical energy that would otherwise be transmitted to the surrounding structures [6]. It makes sense that patients who would benefit from this strategy must not have sustained irreversible injury to the periventricular capillaries. This is in line with recent studies that describe poor outcomes for patients with a long history of symptoms or higher levels of cognitive impairment, which are suggestive of more widespread damage. Accordingly, benefit is also higher for patients with abnormalities mostly in gait as that would in turn reflect localised periventricular damage. Interestingly, patient age and imaging repercussions of the disease do not seem to be accurate predictors of ETV success for this pathology [5].

3   NPH Current Treatment Standards

The approach for iNPH is still somewhat controversial. While VPS has reported success rates of up to 70–90% a major challenge lies on determination of best candidates for shunting [6]. Both radiological and clinical criteria have been suggested and some of the most used include: Evan's index of 0.3 or lower, response to tap test, intracranial pressure overnight monitoring and lumbar infusion study [7]. The sensitivity of those methods however is less than ideal and may miss many patients that would benefit from surgery [7].

Given that iNPH accounts for up to 34% of adult-onset hydrocephalus and is typically found in older patients, choosing VPS must be weighed against surgical risk [3]. Classical complications include infections, need for shunt replacement and reoperation, subdural fluid collections, epilepsy, headache and abdominal pain [2, 7]. Incidence of those adverse events is significant in the literature and overall complication rates have reported as high as 37.9% [5]. Such findings are consistent in the literature and reoperation rates have ranged as high as 22–33% [6, 8]. ETV would, in contrast, represent a safer, more minimally invasive option that is consistently linked to lower complication rates in neurosurgical literature. Whether there is however a trade in efficiency is subject of a heated debate.

4   Technique of Endoscopic Third Ventriculostomy (ETV)

The endoscope is inserted via a frontal burr hole, usually right sided, to the frontal horn of the lateral ventricle and via the foramen of Monro to the third ventricle. The trajectory of a rigid endoscope should be precisely planned to eliminate complications. The floor of the third ventricle is fenestrated between the mammillary bodies and the infundibular recess. The balloon is inserted into the fenestration and by expansion creates ventriculocisternostomy. The Liliequist membrane has to be fenestrated also. The upper basilar complex and free interpeduncular and prepontine space should be visible (Fig. 2). An intraoperative finding of the third ventricular floor flapping up and down was observed to carry a better outcome [5].

5   ETV in iNPH

The use of ETV in iNPH was first suggested in 1999 by Mitchell and Matthew but remains a point of controversy to this day [2]. While many initially thought its role would be reserved for patients with insufficient response to lumbar tap test or clear evidence of CSF obstruction, a more modern understanding of hydrocephalus pathology has suggested otherwise.

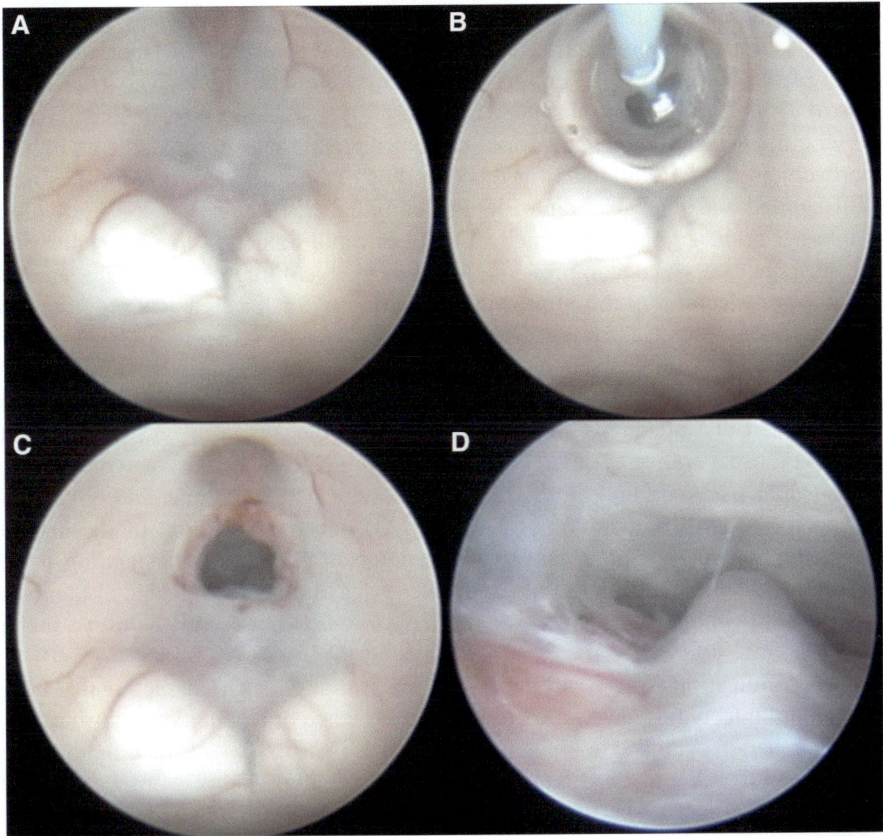

Fig. 2 Endoscopic third ventriculostomy (ETV). (A, B) The floor of the third ventricle is fenestrated between mammillary bodies and infundibular recess. Balloon is inserted to the fenestration and by expansion creates ventriculocisternostomy (C, D) Liliequist membrane has to be fenestrated either. Upper basilar complex and free interpeduncular and prepontine space should be visible

In recent years, ETV has risen in popularity and has consistently provided good outcomes for many different causes of HCP. In 2010, Kulkarni et al., presented the ETV success score (ETVSS) in order to select the most suitable candidates for endoscopic treatment in children [9]. Using aetiology, age, and history of previous shunting they determined the likelihood of success and, accordingly, stratified patients into three groups: High, moderate and low ETVSS. They found that once the patient overcomes the period of early failures (within 3–6 months), in all groups, ETV failure rate would be lower than shunting failure [9]. Unfortunately a similar tool to predict ETV success in patients with NPH is missing and patient selection and classification have remained a major challenge.

Small retrospective investigations have however sparked in neurosurgical literature with enthusiastic results. Gangemi et al., published a study of 110 patients with a long follow up period (2–12 years, median of 6.5 years) [5]. They analysed a subset of patients with minimal dementia symptoms and no evidence of periventricular white matter ischemia. All were required to have intracranial pressure (ICP) measurements ranging from 8–12 mmHg. The reported success rate was impressive. After ETV, improvement was noted and sustained in almost 70% of cases. They concluded that a shorter clinical history and better baseline neurological status correlated with higher improvement scores. Rationale for those findings was attributed to more localised brain damage, and quick restoration of brain compliance. In their view, ETV provided an internal drainage pathway which resulted in rapid reduction in ventricular size and subsequent vessel decompression, which is visible intraoperatively as a sudden return in ventricular pulsation following fenestration. Such a sign was suggested to predict clinical response [5].

Consistently through all studies, the patient profile that seems to benefit the most from this intervention includes those younger than 80 years of age, those who display either an aqueductal CSF stroke volume greater than 42 uL, or aqueduct stenosis on preoperative computerised tomography (CT) scans, those symptomatic for less than one year, and those with predominant gait symptoms and only mild to moderate dementia symptoms [5, 7, 10]. Of note, appreciation of the degree of aqueduct stenosis is important to differentiate iNPH from Longstanding overt ventriculomegaly in adults (LOVA) and Late onset Idiopathic Aqueductal Stenosis (LIAS). Both conditions may present similarly to iNPH but usually exhibit a much better response to ETV [11].

Proper indication is however debatable. Even though such characteristics have been identified, studies have failed to provide evidence of a better short term safety profile or better overall outcomes in favour of ETV [6, 10, 12]. In a nationwide database inquiry, Andrew K. Chan et al. have found that ETV admissions were linked to a greater number of perioperative deaths, complication rates and an increased length of stay [10]. In fact, perioperative mortality in that study was seven fold higher for the ETV group, a number that is ten fold higher than what had been previously reported. A similar, more recent, inquiry by Ali Alvi's recent database analysis, yielded similar results. Amongst individual procedures, ETV had the greatest odds of prolonged length of stay and was also associated with higher odds of discharge to other facilities [12]. Interestingly, when data from Andrew K. Chan et al. analysis was adjusted for patient and hospital factors, the comorbidity score was the only significant predictor of mortality, suggesting that proper patient selection might've produced different results [10].

The single available randomised clinical trial comparing the functional outcomes provided by ETV and VPS in iNPH was published by Pinto et al. in 2013. Their parallel, open label trial included 42 patients with iNPH and a positive response to the tap test. Outcome was assessed by use of six clinical scales. While slightly better neurocognitive scores were initially achieved on the ETV group, improvement was only partially sustained over a 12 month follow up and shunting treatment resulted in overall more favourable outcomes (ETV = 50%; VPS = 79%) [6].

In addition, approximately 50% of ETV non responders improved after VPS. Unfortunately, there was no clear feature that indicated which patients would have been better treated by shunting in the first place [6]. Permissive diagnostic criteria and inclusion of overlapping diseases once more might have complicated this issue, and could also account for the observed differences in treatment response.

Important limitations of their study included the use of tap test as inclusion criteria, cognitive evaluation with mini mental state exam and use of non-programmable valves in VPS [6]. This work was further criticised due to a small sample size, and need for post randomization reallocation [1].

Although many case reports and case series have yielded enthusiastic results, there is no hard evidence in the literature that favours ETV over traditional shunting for iNPH. In fact, some authors have pointed to disappointing results. Longatti et al. in 2004 reported a contrasting 21% success rate for ETV [13]. The authors have described the attempt as an aim to overcome functional aqueduct stenosis and in face of the bleak results, would classify ETV as a method of poor efficacy for idiopathic communicating hydrocephalus [13]. The few successful cases in their series were attributed to possible misdiagnosis as more thorough investigation could potentially reveal hidden points of blockage. It has in fact been postulated that a patent aqueducts does not guarantee normal CSF flow [13]. In summary, ETV has much more variable reported response rates when compared to VPS. While patient selection has not been properly established, true efficacy remains speculative and true numbers may both be higher or significantly lower [5].

6   Conclusion

Advances in the understanding of CSF hydrodynamics have justified and sparked enthusiasm on use of ETV for communicating causes of hydrocephalus such as iNPH. However, the lack of clinical and neuropathological criteria for diagnosis of this condition has hindered research and the amount of evidence available is not sufficient to substantiate its indication. The overall better responses to VPS have further reinforced its leading role in this pathology, and have limited ETV indication to a subset of patients that are still in need of being properly defined.

7   Key Points

- While VPS has reported success rates of up to 70–90% it involves considerable risks and determination of best candidates for shunting remains a challenge.
- The reasoning for ETV derives from its ability to increase the systolic outflow from the ventricles which is thought to reduce the chronic transmantle pulsatile stress associated with iNPH.
- A shorter length of clinical history and better baseline neurological status seem to be correlated with higher degrees of improvement following ETV.
- Proper ETV indication for iNPH is debatable as studies have failed to provide evidence of a better short term safety profile or better overall outcomes.

- While patient selection has not been properly established, true efficacy of ETV for iNPH remains speculative.

References

1. Tudor K, Tudor M, McCleery J, Car J. Endoscopic third ventriculostomy (ETV) for idiopathic normal pressure hydrocephalus (iNPH). Cochrane Database Syst Rev. 2015. https://doi.org/10.1002/14651858.cd010033.pub2.
2. Mathew P. Third ventriculostomy in normal pressure hydrocephalus. Br J Neurosurg. 1999;13(4):382–5. https://doi.org/10.1080/02688699943484.
3. Tasiou A, Brotis A, Esposito F, Paterakis K. Endoscopic third ventriculostomy in the treatment of idiopathic normal pressure hydrocephalus: a review study. Neurosurg Rev. 2015;39(4):557–63. https://doi.org/10.1007/s10143-015-0685-4.
4. Rekate H. A contemporary definition and classification of hydrocephalus. Semin Pediatric Neurol. 2009;16(1):9–15. https://doi.org/10.1016/j.spen.2009.01.002.
5. Gangemi M, Maiuri F, Naddeo M, Godano U, Mascari C, Broggi G, Ferroli P. Endoscopic third ventriculostomy in idiopathic normal pressure hydrocephalus: an Italian multi center study. Neurosurgery. 2008;63(1):62–7. https://doi.org/10.1227/01.NEU.0000319522.34196.7B.
6. Pinto F, Saad F, Oliveira M, Pereira R, Miranda F, Tornai J, et al. Role of endoscopic third ventriculostomy and ventriculoperitoneal shunt in idiopathic normal pressure hydrocephalus. Neurosurgery. 2013;72(5):845–54. https://doi.org/10.1227/neu.0b013e318285b37c.
7. Tudor K, Nemir J, Pavliša G, Mrak G, Bilić E, Borovečki F. Management of idiopathic normal pressure hydrocephalus (iNPH)—a retrospective study. Br J Neurosurg. 2020;34(3):316–20. https://doi.org/10.1080/02688697.2020.1726288.
8. McGirt M, Woodworth G, Coon A, Thomas G, Williams M, Rigamonti D. Diagnosis, treatment, and analysis of long-term outcomes in idiopathic normal-pressure hydrocephalus. Neurosurgery. 2005;57(4):699–705. https://doi.org/10.1093/neurosurgery/57.4.699.
9. Kulkarni A, Drake J, Kestle J, Mallucci C, Sgouros S, Constantini S. Predicting who will benefit from endoscopic third ventriculostomy compared with shunt insertion in childhood hydrocephalus using the ETV success score. J Neurosurg Pediatr. 2010;6(4):310–5. https://doi.org/10.3171/2010.8.peds103.
10. Chan A, McGovern R, Zacharia B, Mikell C, Bruce S, Sheehy J, et al. Inferior short-term safety profile of endoscopic third ventriculostomy compared with ventriculoperitoneal shunt placement for idiopathic normal-pressure hydrocephalus. Neurosurgery. 2013;73(6):951–61. https://doi.org/10.1227/neu.0000000000000129.
11. Kandasamy J, Yousaf J, Mallucci C. Third ventriculostomy in normal pressure hydrocephalus. World Neurosurg. 2013;79:2S:S22.e1–7. 2022. https://doi.org/10.1016/j.wneu.2012.02.008
12. Alvi M, Brown D, Yolcu Y, Zreik J, Bydon M, Cutsforth-Gregory J, et al. Predictors of adverse outcomes and cost after surgical management for idiopathic normal pressure hydrocephalus: analyses from a national database. Clin Neurol Neurosurg. 2020;197: 106178. https://doi.org/10.1016/j.clineuro.2020.106178.
13. Longatti PL, Fiorindi A, Martinuzzi A. Failure of endoscopic third ventriculostomy in the treatment of idiopathic normal pressure hydrocephalus. Minim Invasive Neurosurg. 2004;47(6):342–5. https://doi.org/10.1055/s-2004-830128. PMID: 15674750.

Surgical Complications

Uwe Kehler

Abstract Shunt system placement is one of the most commonly performed neurosurgical procedures. Surgical complications related to shunt surgery are still too frequent and often avoidable. Surgical complications can be divided into catheter misplacements and dislocations, disconnections, organ lesions, and miscellaneous. Despite a lot of effort to reduce the complication rate in shunt surgery such as improved sterile techniques, antibiotic-impregnated catheters, and programmable valves, shunt malfunction continues to be a major problem. In this chapter we discuss the most common complications of surgery-related complications (except for infection and under/over-drainage as they are introduced in an individual chapter), including appropriate management and how to more efficiently avoid them.

Keywords Complications · Hydrocephalus · Shunt system · Normal pressure hydrocephalus · Clinical tests · Surgery

Abbreviations

CSF	Cerebrospinal fluid
ICP	Intracranial pressure
IVH	Intraventricular hematoma
NPH	Normal pressure hydrocephalus
STT	Spinal tap test
VP shunt	Ventriculoperitoneal shunt
VA shunt	Ventriculoatrial shunt

U. Kehler (✉)
Department of Neurosurgery, Asklepios Klinik Altona, Paul-Ehrlich-Str. 1, 22763, Hamburg, Germany

© The Author(s), under exclusive license to Springer Nature Switzerland AG 2023
O. Bradac (ed.), *Normal Pressure Hydrocephalus*,
https://doi.org/10.1007/978-3-031-36522-5_25

1   Introduction

No surgical procedure is absolutely free of complications. However, many complications can be avoided [1], especially if you are aware of what may happen. Therefore, talking about complications is of paramount importance in reducing those. Unfortunately, surgical complications are often not reported at all, which may give the wrong impression of procedure safety. In this chapter only complications, which may happen intraoperatively or in the early postoperative period due to surgical inexperience, carelessness, or errors, are described as well as recommendations to minimize those complications. The surgical complications can be divided into catheter misplacements and dislocations, disconnections, organ lesions, and miscellaneous.

2   Catheter Misplacements and Dislocations

2.1   *Ventricular Catheter*

Freehand ventricular catheter placement in hydrocephalus is usually easy since the ventricles are enlarged, but during surgery the head is covered and may be rotated which makes the orientation more difficult. Incorrect or suboptimal ventricular catheter placements are reported in the literature up to 56% [2], and an inaccurate ventricular catheter position (Fig. 1) results in an increased shunt failure rate [2]. Neuronavigation, ultrasound guidance, or ventricular catheter guide reduces inaccurate catheter placements [3]. If not available, the minimum must be a thoroughly prepared surgery, marking the position of the burr hole on the skin, and respecting the exact landmarks.

It is widely debatable whether to use frontal or occipital burr holes to accurately place the catheter. The acceptable deviation from the optimal tract describes up to which degree of deviation the ventricular catheter is still in the ventricle. A frontal burr hole allows for a wider acceptable deviation, which makes it favoured in regard to positioning of the ventricular catheter (Fig. 2)—especially if no neuronavigation is available.

2.2   *Cardiac Catheter in Ventriculo-Atrial Shunts*

The cardiac catheter should be placed in the right atrium (=ventriculo-*atrial* shunt). It is not rare that a catheter may be placed in the superior vena cava or even in the subclavian vein. An intraoperative ultrasound or x-ray will show the position of the catheter and help to avoid malpositionings. A suboptimal catheter placement may not show any shunt malfunction and therefore no revision is necessary. If needed,

Fig. 1 Misplaced ventricular catheter in the interhemispheric fissure

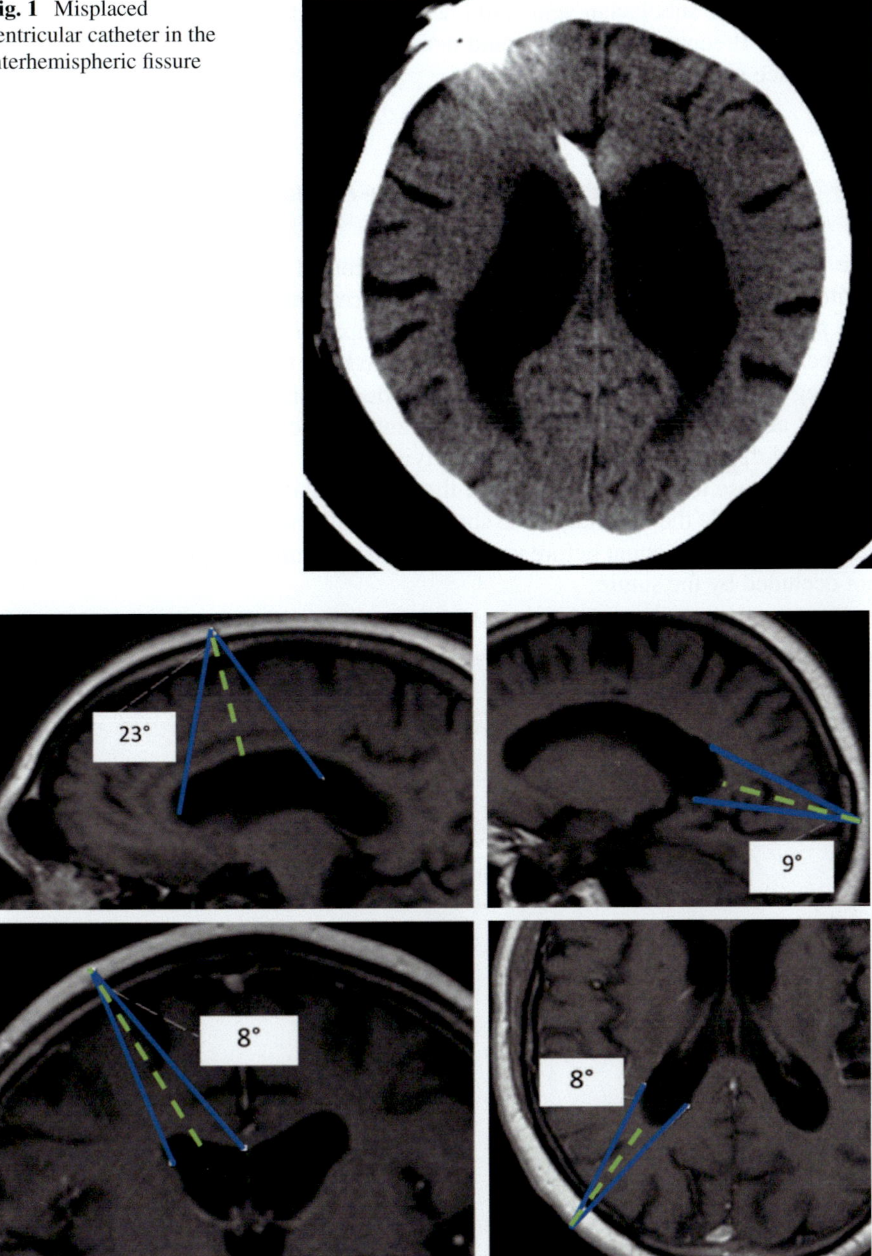

Fig. 2 Ventricular catheter tract deviations in different planes: possible deviations of the ventricular catheter from the optimal tract (green line), in which the catheter will still be intraventricular. To place the catheter intraventricularly, the frontal approach allows a larger deviation from the optimal tract

a catheter in the subclavian vein could be repositioned by the interventional neuro-radiologist. Preoperative planning and determination of the optimal catheter length may reduce malpositionings.

2.3 Peritoneal Catheter in Ventriculo-Peritoneal Shunts

The most frequent complication is that the peritoneal catheter might not be in the peritoneum, either due to intraoperative misplacement or due to delayed luxation into the subcutaneous tissue (Fig. 3). In open laparotomies, the posterior fascia of the rectus abdominis muscle and the peritoneum have to be clearly identified. After opening both layers, the catheter must be introduced into the peritoneal cavity easily, without any resistance. It is strongly recommended to fix the catheter to the peritoneum with a purse string suture. When tying up the suture, it is imperative that it is not too loose to allow movements of the catheter and that it is not too tight that it does not occlude the catheter. If the shunt has an integrated pumping-reservoir, it is advisable to test the shunt before wound closure to confirm the peritoneal catheter is not occluded by the suture.

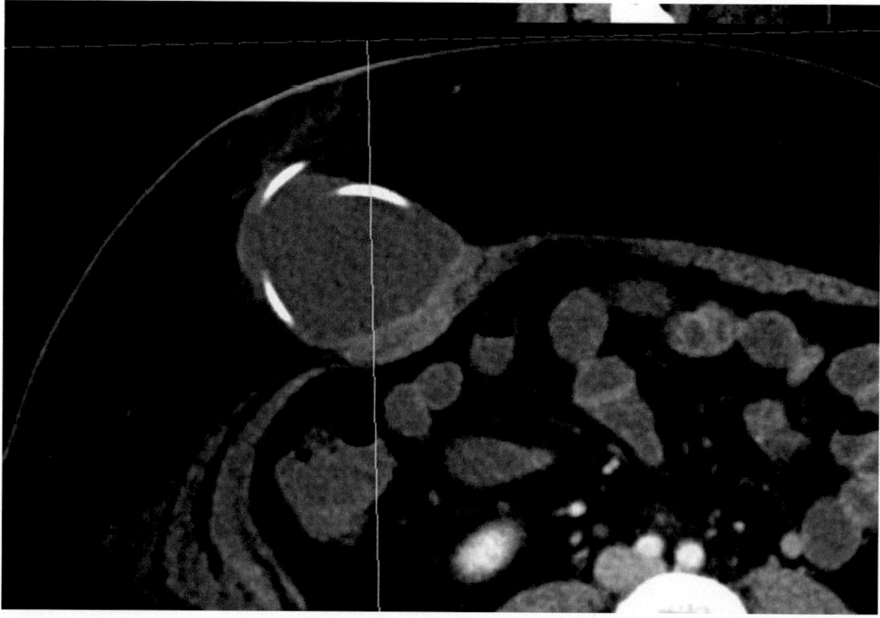

Fig. 3 CT scan of a peritoneal catheter outside the peritoneum in the subcutaneous tissue with cyst formation

In cases of intraoperative intra-abdominal problems, a visceral surgeon should be consulted. If there is not enough experience available, the visceral surgeon should assist from the beginning and or might even introduce the catheter via laparoscopy.

2.4 *Lumbar Catheter in Lumbo-Peritoneal Shunts*

Irritation of nerve roots with leg pain is a common problem of the lumbar catheters. Degenerative spine disease as well as scoliosis may increase the risk. Preoperative spinal MRI may show spinal canal stenosis or other pathologies which can be a contraindication for lumbo-peritoneal shunts. Introducing the spinal catheter under fluoroscopic control will help in positioning the catheter and immediately show unwanted positions or loops of the catheter.

3 Disconnections

Disconnections most often appear when a suture, which should secure a catheter at the valve or connector, is not tightened properly. A disconnection is almost always a surgical (and avoidable) failure. It must be emphasized that the suture must be knotted tightly and several times in opposite directions to prevent loosening.

Older catheters may calcify and break. Even if there is a short interruption of these broken catheters, CSF might flow through a canal formed by fibrous tissue. If a revision is necessary, the calcified catheter should be replaced by a new one since a reconnection very probably will lead to another breakage along the calcified catheter.

4 Organ Injury

4.1 *Brain Injury*

Every ventricular puncture results in an insult to the brain tissue.

Injuries of vessels while pushing the ventricular catheter through the brain tissue towards the ventricle may lead to intracerebral hematomas (ICH). The reported frequency is around 8%; fortunately, in most cases these bleedings are asymptomatic. The risk of ICH increases with malpositioning [4] and with increasing number of punctures (Figs. 4 and 5). Also, coagulopathy, antiplatelet drugs as well as anticoagulants may increase the risk of ICH.

To avoid ICH, coagulopathies have to be corrected and antiplatelet/anticoagulant treatment has to be stopped well in advance of the surgery.

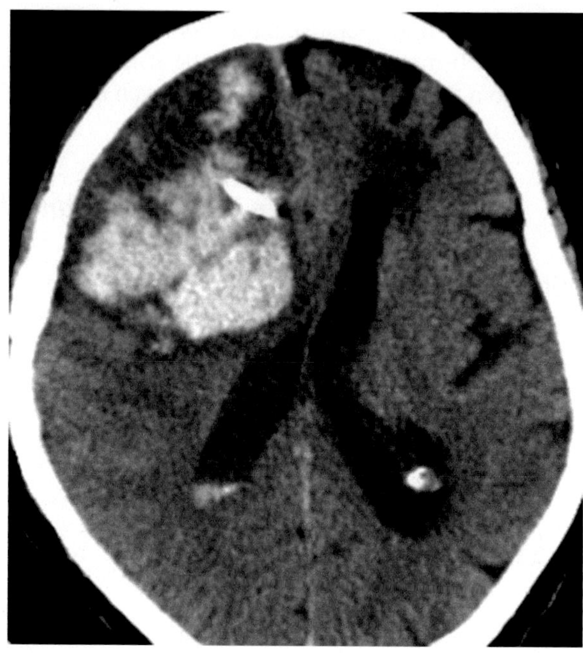

Fig. 4 Rare complication of an intracerebral hematoma caused by a ventricular catheter

To avoid misplacements of the ventricular catheter a navigation tool should be used (see Fig. 1). However, an ICH is not a completely avoidable risk of ventricular punctures therefore strengthening the indication for a lumbo-peritoneal shunt.

4.2 Vessels

Vessels can be perforated during the VP shunt placement, mainly with the tunnelator instrument, when pushing it through the subcutaneous tissue cranially or caudally. Regions of risk are the clavicular and the subcutaneous lateral cervical region. In the subcutaneous cervical region, one vessel that may be especially harmed is the external jugular vein, which usually results in only a subcutaneous hematoma without any severe consequences. If the tunnelator deviates from the intentional subcutaneous tract posteriorly to the clavicule a harm of the subclavian vessels and even the brachial plexus is possible. Meticulously following the tip of the tunnelator in the subcutaneous tissue may avoid this very rare, but potentially devastating complication.

In ventriculoatrial (VA) shunts, especially if the jugular vein is punctured, an accidental puncture of the carotid artery may occur with the development of an arteriovenous fistula. Training, as well as the intraoperative use of an ultrasound probe can almost always avoid this complication.

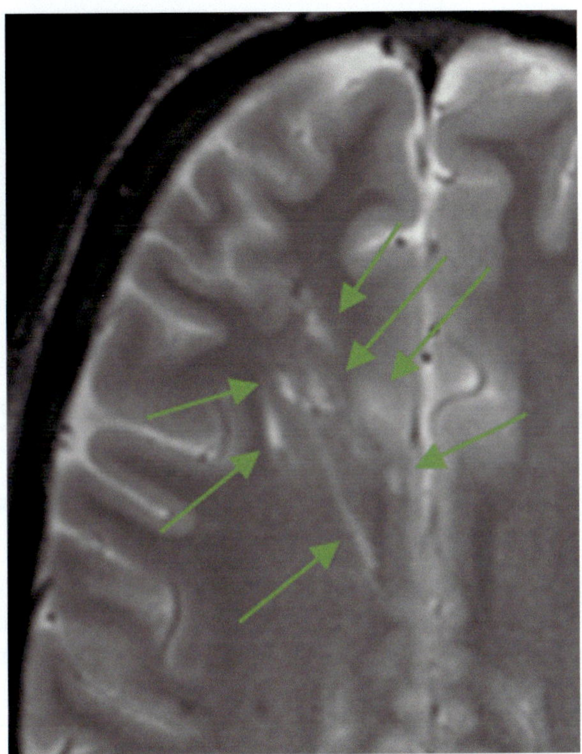

Fig. 5 Multiple tracks of ventricular puncture attempts

4.3 Lungs

A lesion of the lungs or pleura with a subsequent pneumothorax may be caused by the tunnelator when pushed upwards from the abdominal wound and may deviate posteriorly to the ribs. (Fig. 6). To avoid this, special attention must be given to the tunnelator as it passes from the abdominal to the thoracic region—the subcutaneous tip of the tunnelator should be palpated with the fingers, when pushing it cranially. Another mechanism in VA shunts is an accidental pleural lesion with the needle during a puncture of the jugular vein. The risk might be much higher in blind punctures than in ultrasound guided procedures and may increase substantially in lung emphysema.

4.4 Bowels

Intraoperative bowel lesions may occur during careless opening of the peritoneum (via open or laparoscopic surgery), especially in previous abdominal surgeries with adhesions. In the case of lesions or perforations of the bowel immediate repair must

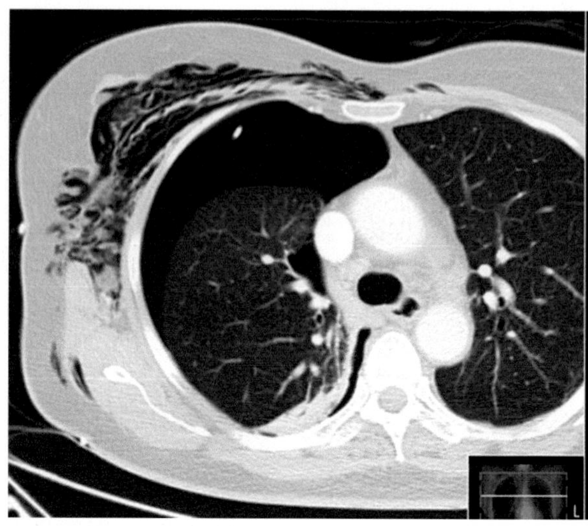

Fig. 6 Pneumothorax and skin emphysema due to an accidental intrathoracic placed catheter

be performed, preferably by a visceral surgeon, and the shunt should not be implanted due to a high risk of infection. Careful peritoneal opening and pre-surgical information about previous abdominal surgeries are mandatory. In cases of uncertainties a visceral surgeon should be part of the surgical team from the beginning. Delayed bowel perforations due to chronic irritation, silicone allergy, and infections are no direct surgical complications.

5 Miscellaneous

5.1 Pacemakers or Other Implants

NPH patients are elderly patients and may often have a pacemaker. The placement of the pacemaker can interfere with the optimal shunt tract in VP shunts and especially in VA shunts. Preoperatively, meticulous information about the presence and the position of a pacemaker can help to avoid intraoperative surprises and complications. If recognized and planned beforehand, a different catheter tract can be used (for instance the opposite side) to avoid any conflict with the pacemaker and its catheter.

6 Valve Implantation

6.1 Wrong (Upside Down) Valve Orientation

Although most valves have a sign, which shows the direction of the flow, x-ray findings may reveal an inverse implanted valve. The valve manufacturers should mark clearly the direction of implantation on the valve housing. On the other hand, a surgeon has to be familiar with all implants before using them.

6.2 Oblique Orientation of Gravitational Valves

The gravitational valves must be implanted in a vertical position (when the patient is upright), if this is not the case, the efficacy to counterbalance the hydrostatic pressure difference in standing position is impaired and a partial activation of the gravitation valve is seen in the horizontal position (Fig. 7). If this has any clinical impact, it must be revised.

To avoid oblique implantations of gravitational valves, the position with the optimal vertical position track must be marked on the patient's skin before draping with sterile sheets. This gives the surgeon in a covered and possibly rotated patient's head a safe orientation.

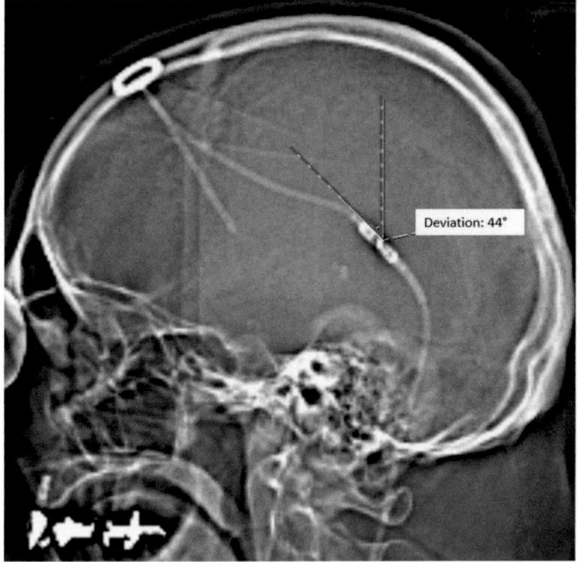

Fig. 7 A gravitational valve should be implanted vertically. Here it is deviated 44° from the optimal track which leads to an incomplete effect in the upright position and adds an unwanted outflow resistance in the horizontal position

6.3   Kinking of Shunt Catheters

Kinking of shunt catheters may occur (Fig. 16, Chap. 27). To avoid or to detect those kinks an intraoperative shunt test is recommended. Before implanting the peritoneal catheter, CSF must spontaneously drop out of the otherwise connected and implanted shunt. This quick test can rule out a kink or other obstruction. If CSF does not trickle out the problem must be found and repaired before finishing the surgery. In cases with an internal flushing/pumping reservoir, a patency test can be also done in ventriculo-atrial shunts and is advisable before wound closures as to not overlook any obstructions.

7   Conclusion

Avoidable complications in shunt surgery are alarmingly frequent at almost 50%. Although experience plays an important role, experienced shunt surgeons still have avoidable complications in 16% of cases. Teaching about complications (you learn better from bad than from good results), but also thorough surgery with meticulous preparation beforehand, being familiar with the implants and their specifications, supervision, and surgery without time pressure, full concentration without distraction is strongly recommended in order to reduce the number of complications. Also, additional tools like neuronavigation, x-ay, etc. (see above) may be very helpful. However, some of those tools may lead themselves to new complications such as infections due to extended operating times. Therefore, a balance between advantages and disadvantages of these additional tools must be found.

8   Key Points

- Surgical complications in shunt surgery occur frequently and are often avoidable.
- Surgical complications can be divided into catheter misplacements and dislocations, disconnections, organ lesions, and miscellaneous.
- Proper preparation and thorough execution of the shunt surgery is necessary.
- Surgeons must be familiar with the implants and their properties.
- A shunt test before skin closure may detect several problems which could be repaired before finishing the surgery.

References

1. Kaestner S et al. Revision surgery following CSF shunt insertion: how often could it be avoided? Acta Neurochirurgica. 2020;162(3):1–6. https://doi.org/10.1007/s00701
2. Janson CG, Romanova LG, Rudser KLD, Haines SL. Improvement in clinical outcomes following optimal targeting of brain ventricular catheters with intraoperative imaging. J Neurosurg. 2014;120(3):684–696. https://doi.org/10.3171/2013.8.JNS13250. Epub 2013 Oct 11.
3. Thomale U-W, Schaumann A et al. GAVCA study: randomized, multicenter trial to evaluate the quality of ventricular catheter placement with a mobile health assisted guidance technique. Neurosurgery. 2018;83(2):252–262.
4. Hultegård L, Michaëlsson I, Jakola A, Farahmand D. The risk of ventricular catheter misplacement and intracerebral hemorrhage in shunt surgery for hydrocephalus. Interdisc Neurosurg. 2019;17:23–7.

Other Complications: Over-Drainage

Ahmed K. Toma

Abstract Over-drainage is the most common complication of shunt insertion surgery in normal pressure hydrocephalus, compared with other type of hydrocephalus. Incidence has been decreasing with improved valve technology. This complication could significantly affect the outcome; therefore, its prevention is essential. It often presents with presence of subdural hygroma or haematoma on brain imaging, either investigating postural symptoms or as an incidental finding. It is not entirely clear why some patients develop over-drainage while others don't. The use of anti-siphoning device with and adjustable valve is imperative in normal pressure hydrocephalus (NPH) shunts, not only to reduce risk of over drainage, but to allow non- operative management should it occur.

Keywords Shunt over-drainage · Surgical complications

Abbreviations

CSDH	Chronic subdural haematoma
CSF	Cerebrospinal fluid
iNPH	Idiopathic normal pressure hydrocephalus
NPH	Normal pressure hydrocephalus
SDH	Subdural haematoma

A. K. Toma (✉)
National Hospital for Neurology and Neurosurgery, UCLH and Queen Square Institute of Neurology, UCL London, London, UK
e-mail: ahmedtoma@nhs.net

O. Bradac (ed.), *Normal Pressure Hydrocephalus*,
https://doi.org/10.1007/978-3-031-36522-5_26

1   Introduction

Over-drainage is one of the common complications of shunt surgery in hydrocephalus in general. In normal pressure hydrocephalus (NPH), over-drainage is the most common complication of shunt insertion surgery [1].

This is probably because intracranial pressure in patients with NPH is not particularly elevated, and that NPH patients are elderly, with markedly enlarged cerebral ventricles and often reduced brain volume. Furthermore, NPH patients often require setting the shunt valve on lower opening pressure, compared with other types of hydrocephalus, to achieve clinical improvement. Over drainage significantly affect shunt surgery outcome, hence its avoidance is considered vital [2].

2   Clinical and Radiological Picture

Clinical presentation of over drainage includes: headache, often postural, nausea and vomiting and hearing symptoms. Symptoms often improves with lying flat and are exacerbated by being upright for prolonged period. Without presence of anti-siphoning device in shunt valve system, Cerebrospinal fluid drainage increases in upright position, as a direct effect of gravity and siphoning.

Brain imaging findings of over drainage include: subdural hygroma (cerebrospinal fluid (CSF) accumulation in subdural space without evidence of presence of blood within the collection), or subdural haematomas (SDH), most commonly chronic (CSDH). If left untreated, Hygromas could progress to SDH. Both subdural hygroma and haematoma could be discovered on routine brain scans, that is, as incidental findings. Patients with SDH could develop neurological deficit and reduced level of consciousness. Therefore, Although there is no clear agreed definition of shunt over drainage in NPH population, presence of SDH is considered by most as the hallmark of shunt over-drainage and it's incidence as a benchmark for various preventative strategies to reduce over drainage as a complication.

Headache in shunted NPH population is not well studied. Larsson et al., in (idiopathic normal pressure hydrocephalus) iNPH CRasH study, compared shunt treated NPH patients with age- and sex-matched controls from the general population. More than one-third of the NPH patients suffered headache (3 times more than among the controls). Almost half of those with headache (i.e., 16% of all patients with INPH) experienced aggravation of headache by postural changes, probably because of their shunt. However, headache did not impact quality of life in patients with iNPH. The authors hypothesised that if more aggressive lowering of valve pressures was needed to resolve the iNPH symptoms and caused postural headache, the improved quality of life achieved through clinical improvement might have confounded an association between postural headache and lower quality of life [3].

3 Predisposing Factors

Lower opening pressure of shunt valve has been shown to be associated with higher rate of over drainage. Dutch NPH study compared low versus medium fixed pressure shunt valves in NPH population. Low opening pressure valves were shown to be associated with better clinical improvement, but this improvement was offset by higher rate of subdural effusions (71% in low pressure valve and 34% with medium pressure valve) [4].

One study has shown that apart from using conventional rather than gravitational valves, longer duration of surgery and female sex were associated with a higher risk of clinical signs and symptoms suggestive of over drainage [2].

In a study of the Swedish shunt registry, lower shunt valve opening pressure, male gender and being on platelet aggregation inhibitors were associated with higher risk of developing SDH. Flow limiting anti-siphoning devices did not prevent SDH but allowed use of lower opening pressure, without causing more SDHs [5].

It is worth mentioning that the presence of trauma history in shunted NPH patients developing SDH is not unusual, particularly in falls-prone NPH population. History of trauma is often not clear as many NPH patients have a degree of cognitive impairment.

The incidence of over drainage has been reported to be high with ventriculo-atrial shunt [6]. As expected, it is higher with lumbo-peritoneal shunt. However, this has been significantly reduced by advances in shunt technology, with recent case series of adding gravitational anti siphoning units to adjustable valves resulting in significantly low risk [7].

4 Evolution of Over-drainage Prevention Techniques

The incidence of SDH in shunted NPH patients has gradually improved over the last 5 decades, with case series average of about 5% with some recent case series of less than 1%, probably reflecting improved shunt valve technology [8]. However, shunt registry data reports higher rates.

4.1 Use of Adjustable Valves

Adjustable valves were introduced to NPH shunts aiming to reduce the need for surgical management of patients with over drainage. Adjustable valves allows opening pressure to be initially set to high level with gradual reduction according to patient need. It also allows reversal to high setting, should patient develops over drainage, with less likelihood need for surgery. UK shunt registry shows that use of adjustable valve in elderly patients shunt reduced need for revision.

A randomised trial showed that gradual lowering of the valve setting to a mean of 7 cm H_2O led to the same rate of shunt complications and over drainage symptoms as a fixed valve setting at a mean of 13 cm H_2O but was associated with a significantly better outcome [9]. This was probably related to the fact that lower opening pressure is associated with better outcome rather than the process of lowering the shunt valve.

Study of Swedish prospective quality registry study of shunted NPH patients [1], Ten percent ($n = 184$) of the patients developed SDH. In 103 patients, treatment was solely opening pressure adjustment. Surgical treatment was used in 66 cases (36%), and 15 (8%) received no treatment. In patients with fixed shunt valves, 90% ($n = 17$) of SDHs were treated surgically compared with 30% ($n = 49$) in patients with adjustable shunts ($p < 0.001$). Data showed that Adjustable shunts are used with increasing frequency and make it possible to noninvasively treat postoperative SDH. Almost all patients had strata valve or Codman hakim valve.

In the recent European Idiopathic Normal Pressure Hydrocephalus Multicentre study [10], symptomatic over drainage was reported in 10 patients (8.7%). Symptoms were usually encountered in the first 30 days. Hygroma was diagnosed in 10 patients (8.7%). Although rarely, hygroma was detected even several months after implant. In 1 case (0.9%) surgery was indicated. Subdural hematoma was diagnosed in 7 patients (6.1%), all during the first month after implant. In 2 cases (1.7%) surgical evacuation was necessary. The 5 others were successfully treated during the first 3 months after implant increasing the opening pressure of the adjustable valve. All patients underwent shunt surgery with a Codman-Hakim adjustable valve with an opening pressure set to 120 mm H_2O.

There has been studies correlating the opening pressure of lumbar puncture with that of shunt valve aiming to reduce SDH occurrence [11]. Other studies correlated body weight and hight with opening pressure of shunt valve and showed reduced need for shunt valve adjustment and reduced over drainage [12]. The main limitation of using an adjustable valve alone, was that higher valve opening pressure was needed to prevent over drainage, cancelling the potential benefit that could be achieved with lower opening pressures, as has been shown in Dutch NPH study.

4.2 Use of Anti-Siphoning Devices

The important second evolutionary step was the introduction of anti-siphoning devices to minimise the effect of postural over drainage. Several flow limiting anti-siphoning devices are available. In addition, the introduction of gravitational valves by Miethke allowed using very low opening pressure of shunt valves, resulting in further clinical improvement without increasing over-drainage [13].

SVASONA study was a randomised trial comparing adjustable proGAV valve (proGAV, Aesculap-Miethke, Potsdam, Germany) and gravitational anti-siphoning device with an adjustable Codman Hakim valve (CMPV, Codman and Shurtleff, Johnson and Johnson, Ryanham, Massachusetts, USA) without an anti-siphoning devices. After 6 months, there was clear reduction in over drainage in gravitational anti-siphoning device group that difference exceeded predetermined stopping rules and resulted in premature discontinuation of patient recruitment. This study confirmed the efficacy of anti-siphoning device in reducing over drainage rate [14].

Subsequent studies have shown that adding a flow regulated anti-siphoning device to an adjustable valves also reduced incidence of SDH by about two thirds. [15, 16] Although reported incident with flow regulated anti-siphoning devices was relatively higher compared with gravitational anti-siphoning device, this did not reach statistical significance. However, the use of gravitational valve allows very low opening pressure of valve giving chance of achieving better clinical improvement in selected patients.

5 Management

From the available evidence, the use of adjustable valves with gravitational ani siphon devices, is the most effective way of preventing over drainage and facilitating its management, if it occurs.

In patients with postural headache and no imaging features of over drainage, careful counselling of shunt valve adjustment is needed. This would include explaining to patient and carer, that increasing shunt valve's opening pressure could result in worsening NPH symptoms. Decision to adjust opening pressure of valve will depend on severity of patient symptoms. Many patients often chose to endure mild headache in order to have improved NPH symptoms [17].

On the other hand, the presence of subdural collection should trigger immediate valve adjustment to highest level to prevent further expansion and clinical deterioration. Although this would inevitably result in worsening NPH symptoms, it has been shown to result in, not only prevention of further subdural collection expansion, but also in spontaneous resolution without need for burr holes drainage procedures or shunt ligation. Repeated scan in 2–4 weeks would guide valve setting management. Once subdural collection is dissipated, gradual reduction of the opening pressure to acceptable level could be done over a period of few weeks with interval imaging.

Patient and carers should be counselled that clinical improvement is only likely to be noticed once valve setting is back on low level, and that this process cannot be short cut, as it would risk recurrence or even deterioration with need for surgery. Patient and carer will often have to endure few weeks of poor performance status waiting for the point where valve could be set to an optimal low level.

In patients with subdural haematoma causing neurological deterioration, burr holes drainage plus shunt ligation is often necessary. Once post operative images shows satisfactory resolution of the haematoma, shunt can be un-ligated, with careful reduction of opening pressure of valve over few weeks to prevent recurrence.

Routine post operative imaging is useful in detecting subdural hygromas or haematomas. Similarly, patients developing clinical picture suggestive of over drainage, or those shunt having head injury, should have brain scan to exclude subdural hygromas or haematomas.

It is also advisable to repeat brain scan in patients under consideration for shunt valve adjustment to lower setting, aiming to achieve further improvement in NPH symptoms, even if they have no clinical features of over drainage. The aim is to exclude incidental subdural hygroma or SDH that could be made worse with lower shunt valve setting.

6   Conclusion

Over-drainage is the most common complication of shunting in NPH patients, with implications on patient outcome and healthcare resources. Risk could be significantly reduced if anti-siphoning device, particularly a gravitational one, is used as part of shunt implant system. Use of adjustable valve is essential to help in managing over-drainage and reduce need for hospitalisation and surgery. Surveillance imaging is needed to detect early signs of over drainage, with subsequent shunt valve adjustment to prevent clinical deterioration.

7   Key Points

- The most common preventable complication of shunt insertion surgery in normal pressure hydrocephalus.
- The use of gravitational anti-siphoning device with and adjustable valve is imperative to reduce risk of over-drainage and facilitate management, if it occurs.
- Early post-operative surveillance imaging is advisable, to detect possible signs of over drainage that could be solved with shunt valve adjustment.

References

1. Sundström N, Lagebrant M, Eklund A, Koskinen LD, Malm J. Subdural hematomas in 1846 patients with shunted idiopathic normal pressure hydrocephalus: treatment and long-term survival. J Neurosurg. 2018;129(3):797–804. https://doi.org/10.3171/2017.5.JNS17481. Epub 2017 Oct 27. PMID: 29076787.
2. Meier U, Stengel D, Müller C, Fritsch MJ, Kehler U, Langer N, Kiefer M, Eymann R, Schuhmann MU, Speil A, Weber F, Remenez V, Rohde V, Ludwig HC, Lemcke J. Predictors of subsequent overdrainage and clinical outcomes after ventriculoperitoneal shunting for idiopathic normal pressure hydrocephalus. Neurosurgery. 2013;73(6):1054–1060. https://doi.org/10.1227/NEU.0000000000000155. PMID: 24257332.
3. Larsson J, Israelsson H, Eklund A, Malm J. Epilepsy, headache, and abdominal pain after shunt surgery for idiopathic normal pressure hydrocephalus: the INPH-CRasH study. J Neurosurg.

2018;128(6):1674–1683. https://doi.org/10.3171/2017.3.JNS162453. Epub 2017 Sep 8. PMID: 28885121.

4. Boon AJ, Tans JT, Delwel EJ, Egeler-Peerdeman SM, Hanlo PW, Wurzer HA, Avezaat CJ, de Jong DA, Gooskens RH, Hermans J. Dutch normal-pressure hydrocephalus study: randomized comparison of low- and medium-pressure shunts. J Neurosurg. 1998;88(3):490–495. https://doi.org/10.3171/jns.1998.88.3.0490. PMID: 9488303.

5. Nadel JL, Wilkinson DA, Linzey JR, Maher CO, Kotagal V, Heth JA. Thirty-Day hospital readmission and surgical complication rates for shunting in normal pressure hydrocephalus: a large national database analysis. Neurosurgery. 20201;86(6):843-850. https://doi.org/10.1093/neuros/nyz299. PMID: 31420654; PMCID: PMC7528659.

6. Hung AL, Vivas-Buitrago T, Adam A, Lu J, Robison J, Elder BD, Goodwin CR, Jusué-Torres I, Rigamonti D. Ventriculoatrial versus ventriculoperitoneal shunt complications in idiopathic normal pressure hydrocephalus. Clin Neurol Neurosurg. 2017;157:1-6. https://doi.org/10.1016/j.clineuro.2017.03.014. Epub 2017 Mar 18. PMID: 28347957.

7. Nakajima M, Miyajima M, Akiba C, Ogino I, Kawamura K, Sugano H, Hara T, Tange Y, Fusegi K, Karagiozov K, Arai H. Lumboperitoneal shunts for the treatment of idiopathic normal pressure hydrocephalus: a comparison of small-lumen abdominal catheters to gravitational add-on valves in a single center. Oper Neurosurg (Hagerstown). 2018;15(6):634–642. https://doi.org/10.1093/ons/opy044. PMID: 29688482; PMCID: PMC6373832.

8. Toma AK, Papadopoulos MC, Stapleton S, Kitchen ND, Watkins LD. Systematic review of the outcome of shunt surgery in idiopathic normal-pressure hydrocephalus. Acta Neurochir (Wien). 2013;155(10):1977–1980. https://doi.org/10.1007/s00701-013-1835-5. Epub 2013 Aug 23. PMID: 23975646.

9. Sæhle T, Farahmand D, Eide PK, Tisell M, Wikkelsö C. A randomized controlled dual-center trial on shunt complications in idiopathic normal-pressure hydrocephalus treated with gradually reduced or "fixed" pressure valve settings. J Neurosurg. 2014;121(5):1257–1263. https://doi.org/10.3171/2014.7.JNS14283. Epub 2014 Sep 5. PMID: 25192478.

10. Feletti A, d'Avella D, Wikkelsø C, Klinge P, Hellström P, Tans J, Kiefer M, Meier U, Lemcke J, Paternò V, Stieglitz L, Sames M, Saur K, Kordás M, Vitanovic D, Gabarrós A, Llarga F, Triffaux M, Tyberghien A, Juhler M, Hasselbalch S, Cesarini K, Laurell K. Ventriculoperitoneal shunt complications in the European idiopathic normal pressure hydrocephalus multicenter study. Oper Neurosurg (Hagerstown). 2019;17(1):97–102. https://doi.org/10.1093/ons/opy232. PMID: 30169650.

11. Vivas-Buitrago T, Domingo R, Tripathi S, Herrera JP, Heemskerk J, Grewal S, Zalewski NL, Quinones-Hinojosa A, Reimer R, Wharen RE, Graff-Radford NR. In NPH, setting valve opening pressure close to lumbar puncture opening pressure decreases overdrainage. Neurol Neurochir Pol. 2020;54(6):531–537. https://doi.org/10.5603/PJNNS.a2020.0077. Epub 2020 Oct 13. PMID: 33047786.

12. Miyake H, Kajimoto Y, Tsuji M, Ukita T, Tucker A, Ohmura T. Development of a quick reference table for setting programmable pressure valves in patients with idiopathic normal pressure hydrocephalus. Neurol Med Chir (Tokyo). 2008;48(10):427–432; discussion 432. https://doi.org/10.2176/nmc.48.427. PMID: 18948675.

13. Malem DN, Shand Smith JD, Toma AK, Sethi H, Kitchen ND, Watkins LD. An investigation into the clinical impacts of lowering shunt opening pressure in idiopathic normal pressure hydrocephalus: A case series. Br J Neurosurg. 2015;29(1):18–22. https://doi.org/10.3109/02688697.2014.950630. Epub 2014 Aug 21. PMID: 25142701.

14. Lemcke J, Meier U, Müller C, Fritsch MJ, Kehler U, Langer N, Kiefer M, Eymann R, Schuhmann MU, Speil A, Weber F, Remenez V, Rohde V, Ludwig HC, Stengel D. Safety and efficacy of gravitational shunt valves in patients with idiopathic normal pressure hydrocephalus: a pragmatic, randomised, open label, multicentre trial (SVASONA). J Neurol Neurosurg Psychiatry. 2013;84(8):850–857. https://doi.org/10.1136/jnnp-2012-303936. Epub 2013 Mar 1. PMID: 23457222; PMCID: PMC3717598.

15. Bozhkov Y, Roessler K, Hore N, Buchfelder M, Brandner S. Neurological outcome and frequency of overdrainage in normal pressure hydrocephalus directly correlates with implanted

ventriculo-peritoneal shunt valve type. Neurol Res. 2017;39(7):601-605. https://doi.org/10.1080/01616412.2017.1321300. Epub 2017 May 1. PMID: 28460569.

16. Scheffler P, Oertel MF, Stieglitz LH. Comparison between flow-regulated and gravitational shunt valves in the treatment of normal pressure hydrocephalus: flow-grav study. Neurosurgery. 2021;89(3):413–419. https://doi.org/10.1093/neuros/nyab176. PMID: 34131760.

17. Gutowski P, Rot S, Fritsch M, Meier U, Gölz L, Lemcke J. Secondary deterioration in patients with normal pressure hydrocephalus after ventriculoperitoneal shunt placement: a proposed algorithm of treatment. Fluids Barriers CNS. 2020;17(1):18. https://doi.org/10.1186/s12987-020-00180-w. PMID: 32127017; PMCID: PMC7055114

Follow-Up After Shunt

Uwe Kehler

Abstract Adequate postoperative follow-up in shunted patients suffering from normal pressure hydrocephalus (NPH) is an essential part of NPH treatment, considering both technical and clinical factors that are involved in patients' performance after surgery. Routine follow-up controls are necessary to detect shunt malfunctions and to correct those in time. In patients where the outcome after shunt implantation is not optimal, readjustments of the valve are necessary in order to provide better treatment outcome ("titration of symptoms"). In cases where the clinical improvement after shunting is only partial, it is very challenging to clearly differentiate between non-optimal valve settings and a lack of recovery potential. Non-invasive tap tests through the flushing reservoir can give further information in this situation, can also help to detect shunt malfunctions, and can some extent replace most of the invasive shunt tests. However, it is necessary to be well-informed about the implanted device for adequate execution and interpretation of the non-invasive tests. Although known that non-invasive shunt tests are of great importance with respect to aimed reduction of complication rates, invasive tests remain the gold standard for accurate diagnostics and therefore are a necessary part of shunt complication management. These tests enable direct intracranial pressure monitoring, biochemical analysis of the cerebrospinal fluid, and the detection of shunt malfunction. Indication of shunt revision is dependent on various criteria that are discussed together with both technical and clinical nuances in more detail in this chapter.

Keywords Follow-up · Hydrocephalus · Neurofunctional testing · Normal pressure hydrocephalus · Clinical tests · Prognosis

Abbreviations

CC   corpus callosum

U. Kehler (✉)
Department of Neurosurgery, Asklepios Klinik Altona, Paul-Ehrlich-Str.1, 22763 Hamburg, Germany

O. Bradac (ed.), *Normal Pressure Hydrocephalus*,
https://doi.org/10.1007/978-3-031-36522-5_27

CRP	C-reactive protein
CSF	cerebrospinal fluid
DESH	disproportionately enlarged subarachnoid-space hydrocephalus
ICP	intracranial pressure
LP shunt	lumboperitoneal shunt
NPH	normal pressure hydrocephalus
STT	spinal tap test
VA shunt	ventriculoatrial shunt
VP shunt	ventriculoperitoneal shunt

1 Introduction

After shunting, follow-up is necessary to assess the success of surgery, to titrate the clinical symptoms with valve adjustments to achieve the optimal result, and to recognize and treat complications timely.

Since recovery of NPH-symptoms after shunting needs several weeks, the final result cannot be evaluated during the hospital stay immediately after surgery. However, in the initial days the direction of clinical recovery can be recognized.

It is important to be aware of the amount of clinical improvement to expect and when it is appropriate to interfere with further diagnostics or valve adjustments. Figures 1 and 2 show different clinical courses after shunting. In "good" and "fair" improvements the question arises whether no further improvement is due to irreversible damage of long-standing hydrocephalus (= no more recovery potential) or due to insufficient drainage, for instance a result of suboptimal pressure setting of the valve.

Figure 2 shows clinical courses, where timely intervention by a doctor is necessary. If there is no improvement at all after shunt implantation there are usually two different causes: the diagnosis was incorrect or there is a primary shunt failure which requires further diagnostics (see below).

If an early deterioration after initial improvement is seen, it is likely that the diagnosis of NPH was correct (improvement with shunt means confirmation of NPH), but a shunt problem developed (secondary shunt failure) possibly due to an obstruction, disconnection, or other. A secondary shunt failure, and the reason for it, must be diagnosed timely and corrected (see below).

A late deterioration, even after many years, may appear frequently [1–3] and may reflect the ongoing disease. Often this deterioration can be counterbalanced by a down regulation of the valve. If no improvement is seen in these cases, then a late shunt failure must be ruled out as in all other shunt problems (see below).

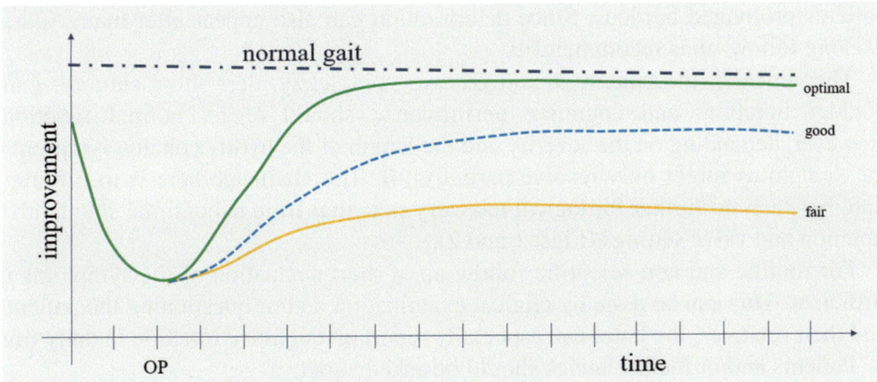

Fig. 1 Clinical courses after shunting NPH-patients with normal shunt function. The green line shows the optimal improvement after treatment. The blue and yellow line, representing good or fair improvement, may suggest that the suboptimal results are due to longstanding disease or comorbidities. However, it may also reflect suboptimal valve settings with insufficient CSF drainage

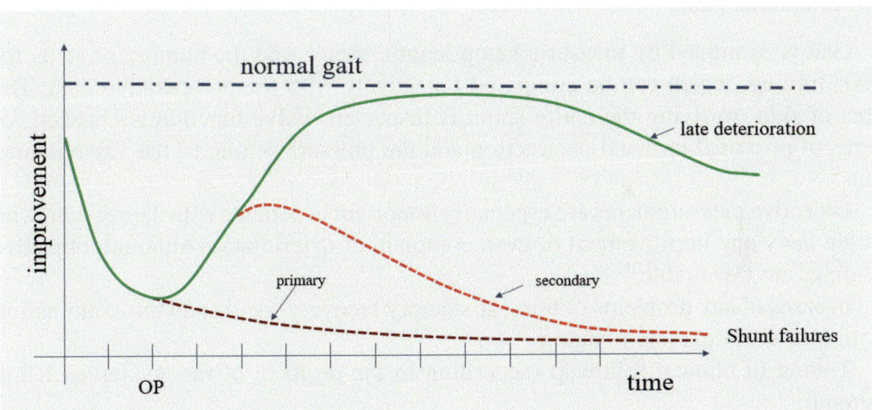

Fig. 2 Clinical courses after shunting a NPH-patient with a lack of improvement or late deterioration. The dark red line may indicate a primary shunt malfunction or an incorrect NPH diagnosis. The red line reflects a shunt problem which must be investigated further. The green line shows an optimal recovery with a frequently observed late deterioration which might be counterbalanced with a valve adjustment

2 Clinical Follow-Up

Clinical follow-up is necessary to evaluate the efficacy of shunting. It is important to see if the improvement is as good as expected or if it is not then a decision needs to be made to determine if further diagnostic or therapeutic measures are necessary. Periodically, further evaluations are necessary to detect shunt-malfunctions (over- or underdrainage) or complications in time and to correct them in order to spare patients prolonged burdens. Since deterioration can also appear after many years, lifelong follow-up is recommended.

Theoretically, the patient should recover completely after shunt surgery: gait, bladder function, and cognitive performance should regain normal function. However, depending on the severity and the length of the hydrocephalus symptoms, the symptoms might only resolve partially [4]. The challenge here is to differentiate between no further biological recovery potential from suboptimal shunt/valve function and valve settings (Figs. 1 and 2).

For routine and non-scientific follow-up, a short evaluation of the symptoms is sufficient. This can be done by clinical examination and/or questioning the patients and their relatives; the latter can especially report on cognitive function in daily life.

Patients and/or their relatives should be asked about:

- Gait improvement and to what extent
- Bladder- and stool function: Normalcy, frequency, urgency, complete incontinence
- Cognitive development
- Orthostatic headache and hypoacusis
- Pain along the shunt
- Abdominal pain.

Gait is examined by measuring step length, speed, and the number of steps for 360° turning, which can be compared objectively with the preoperative data. The area of skin overlying the entire shunt is inspected. Valve function is checked for signs of proximal or distal obstruction and the pressure setting of the valve is read out.

Objective measurements are especially important in patients with depression, who might deny any improvement or even complain of deterioration although objective findings are favourable.

In cases of any problems or non-satisfactory recovery we expand the examination with further testing and imaging.

Timing of clinical followup (according to the protocol of the Asklepios Klink Altona):

- Once a day during the hospital stay after shunt implantation.
- Six weeks after shunt implantation and depending on symptoms for "fine-tuning" (search for the best pressure setting) of the shunt.
- One to two year intervals lifelong.
- Anytime if clinical deterioration appears.

It is not rare that NPH patients will deteriorate even after years, which can often be counterbalanced with lowering the opening pressure [1–3].

With this clinical follow-up suboptimal shunt settings and complications can be detected in time and depending on the needs, further diagnostic procedures or shunt adjustments can be initiated.

3   Imaging Follow-Up

Imaging follow-up is optional in cases of very good improvement (complete recovery) after shunting; however it is a confirmation of a well implanted and working shunt. In cases of suspected shunt malfunction (including incomplete recovery) and before revision surgery imaging is mandatory. Imaging includes cranial CT or MRI and a shunt x-ray series. Regarding the abdominal catheter, an ultrasound or an abdominal CT might be helpful.

3.1   Cranial Imaging

CT or MRI: A CT scan is usually preferred due to better visibility of the implanted shunt. It is more readily available, cheaper, and no re-adjustment of a programmable (non MRI-safe) valve is necessary.

The CT can show potential intracranial bleeds, the position of the implanted ventricular catheter, the size of the ventricles, changes of the disproportionately enlarged subarachnoid-space hydrocephalus (DESH) and corpus callosal angle, as well as subdural effusions or hematomas.

In shunted patients, the DESH decreases as well as the callosal angle (Fig. 3). However, the decrease of these patterns does not correlate strongly with clinical improvement, whereas a remaining DESH sign and sharp callosal angle does not rule out a good recovery of the shunted patient. The size of the ventricles may not decrease—especially if gravitational valves are used. The interpretations of these patterns alone do not prove a functional or non-functional shunt; they are merely a puzzle stone in the diagnosis and must be evaluated together with the clinical symptoms.

On the other hand, a CT with subdural hematoma clearly indicates an overdrainage (Fig. 4).

3.2   Shunt X-ray/Shunt Series

The x-rays of the shunt/shunt series demonstrate the shunt location, the connection (or disconnections) of the different shunt parts, possible kinking of the catheter, the continuity of the shunt, and often the valve pressure setting. Also, in gravitational valves, the spatial orientation must be looked at as well.

The shunt x-ray has to be adapted to the type of shunt (VP, VA, or LP shunt, see Table 1).

For VP shunts, a lateral x-ray of the head (Fig. 5), the neck, an anteroposterior chest x-ray (Fig. 6), and an abdominal x-ray in both planes (Fig. 7) shows everything that is needed. For a VA shunt, the abdominal x-ray is unnecessary, and in a LP shunt

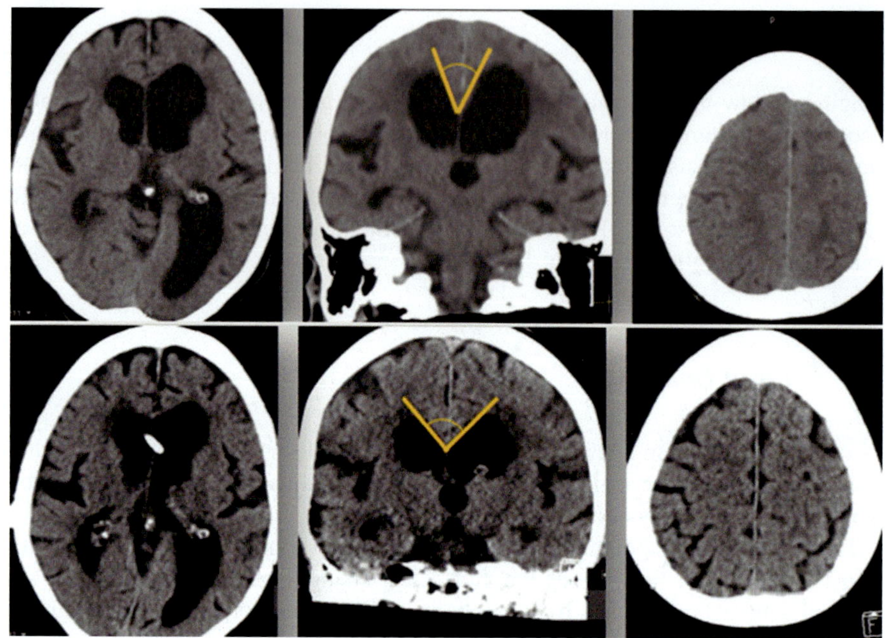

Fig. 3 Changes of DESH and CC (corpus callosal) angle after shunt surgery: a disproportionately enlarged subarachnoid space hydrocephalus (DESH) and a sharp CC angle are seen preoperatively (upper row), which are dissolved after shunting (lower row). No substantial decrease is seen in ventricular size—despite a substantial clinical improvement of the patient

the head, neck, and chest x-rays can be avoided. If the spinal catheter is not detected on the abdominal x-ray an x-ray of the lower thoracic/lumbar area should be done.

You never should allow a gap in the x-ray depiction of the shunt since a disconnection or kinking can happen at any location—and according to Murphy's law as well in the not depicted region. If there are any discrepancies with the interpretation of the x-ray, an additional CT scan will clarify the situation.

In cases of difficult valve adjustments or in non-MR safe valves (valves which may reprogram in a magnetic field spontaneously) the pressure setting can be checked with an x-ray, as seen in Figs. 8 and 9. For evaluation of the valve setting, it is important that the x-ray is exactly perpendicular to the valve position—which is especially difficult in valves implanted close to a frontal burr hole. The consequence is that often the x-ray has to be repeated to determine the exact valve setting.

Fig. 4 Subdural hematoma
with slit ventricles after
ventriculoperitoneal shunt

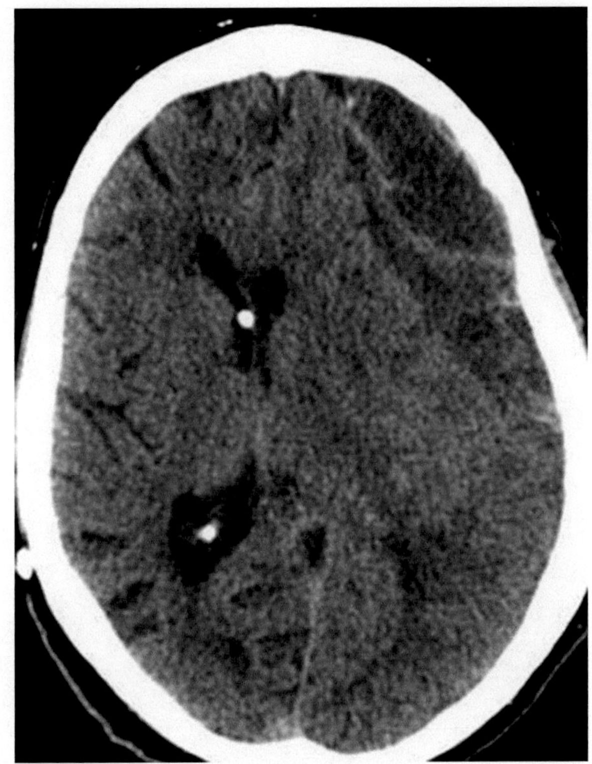

Table 1 Shunt series: necessary x-ray depictions in different shunts

Type of shunt system	X-ray
VP shunt	Head, neck, chest, abdomen (both lateral and coronal planes)
VA shunt	Head, neck, chest
LP shunt	Lumbar/thoracic spine and abdomen

3.3 Ultrasound

Ultrasound usage in NPH shunt follow-up has no routine role, but can be used in abdominal shunt related problems and to determine a differential diagnosis (abdominal pain). Figure 10 shows a peritoneal catheter in the subcutaneous tissue with a cyst formation. Abdominal CT could be an alternative modality to ultrasound.

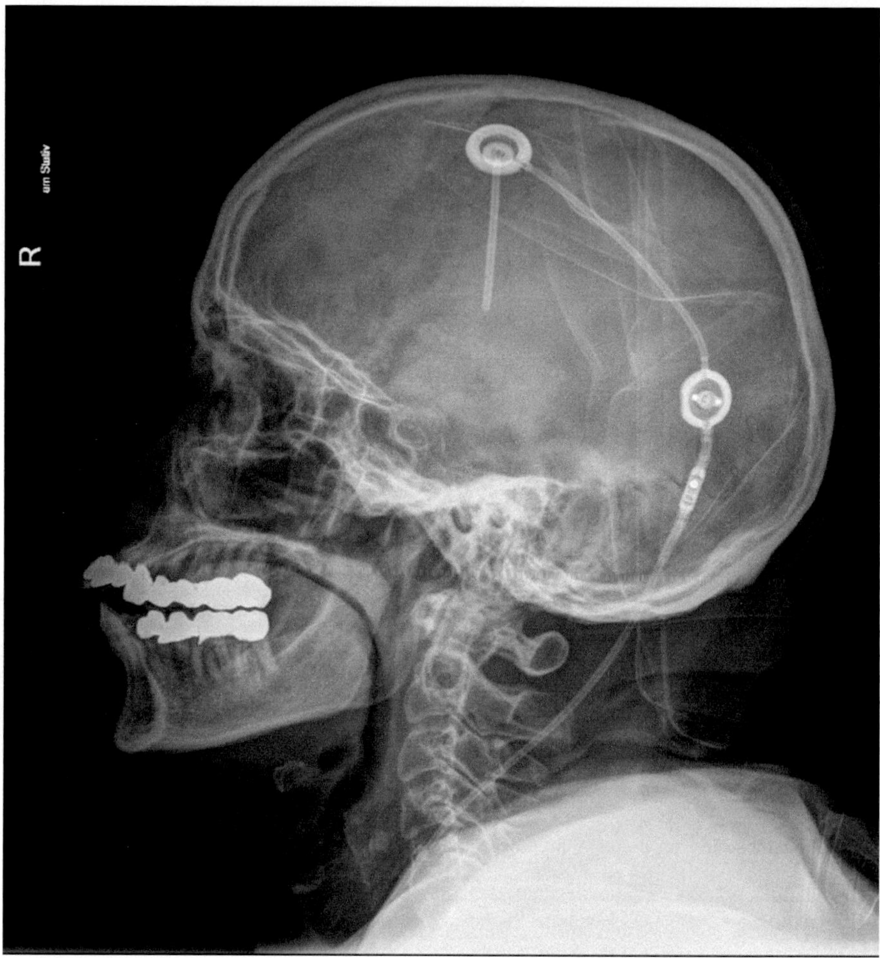

Fig. 5 Head x-ray with a burr hole reservoir, a differential adjustable valve, and a gravitational unit. The gravitational unit has to be in the up-right position (± 20%) for proper function

4   Non-invasive and Invasive Tests in Follow-Up

Most hydrocephalus shunts have an integrated flushing reservoir, which enables physicians to test non-invasively (manually) the shunt to a certain degree. These tests substitute most of the invasive tests, which can be frequently avoided.

A short manual test can show if the shunt is patent or obliterated totally, if the reflux valve is working, and if the patient's symptoms improve after "pumping"—similar to a tap test. But manual testing requires the understanding of valve mechanics and the specifications of the implant. It has to be mentioned that a partial obstruction of the shunt cannot be accurately tested manually.

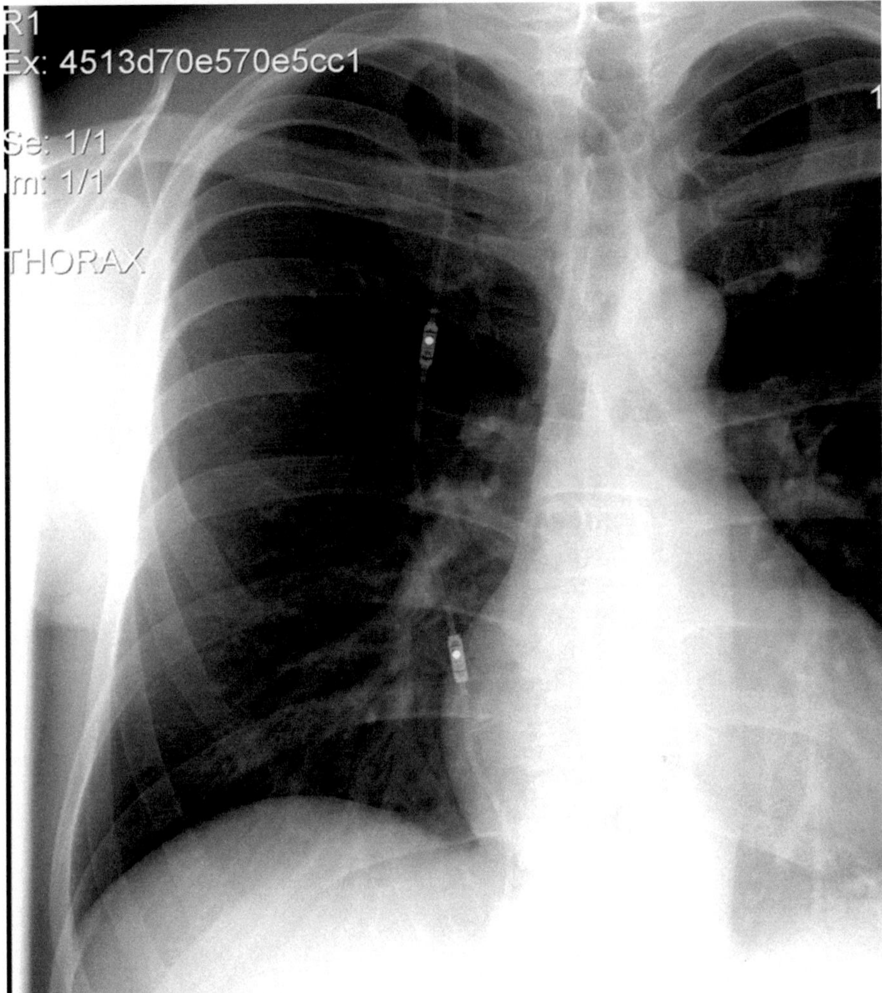

Fig. 6 Chest x-ray—no disconnections of the catheter with 2 integrated devices

4.1 Non-invasive Tests

The understanding of flushing reservoirs, potentially with an integrated valve, and the impact of the implantation side is of paramount importance to test a shunt non-invasively.

Flushing reservoirs are located at the side of the burr hole or integrated in the shunt usually proximal to the valve (Fig. 11).

In cases of burr hole reservoirs, it is necessary to investigate whether there is an integrated anti-reflux valve or not. This is done by occluding the distal catheter with one finger and then trying to press down the membrane of the flushing reservoir

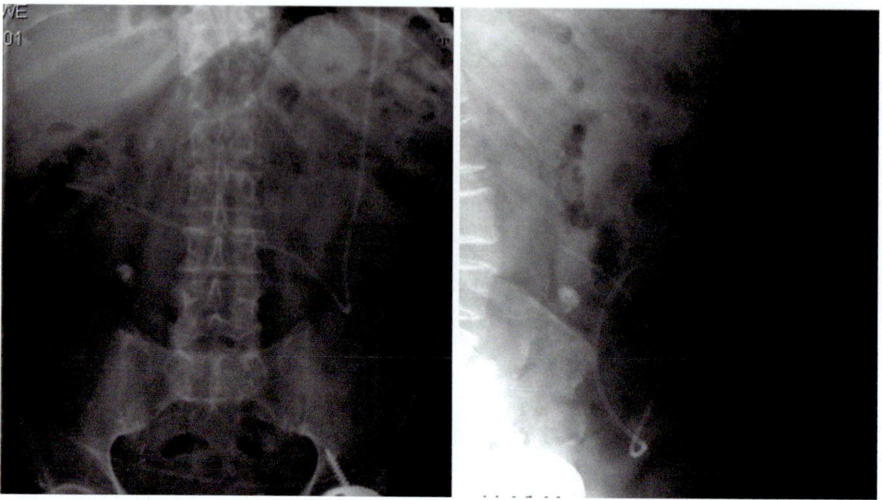

Fig. 7 Abdominal x-ray in 2 planes showing the peritoneal catheter inside the peritoneal cavity

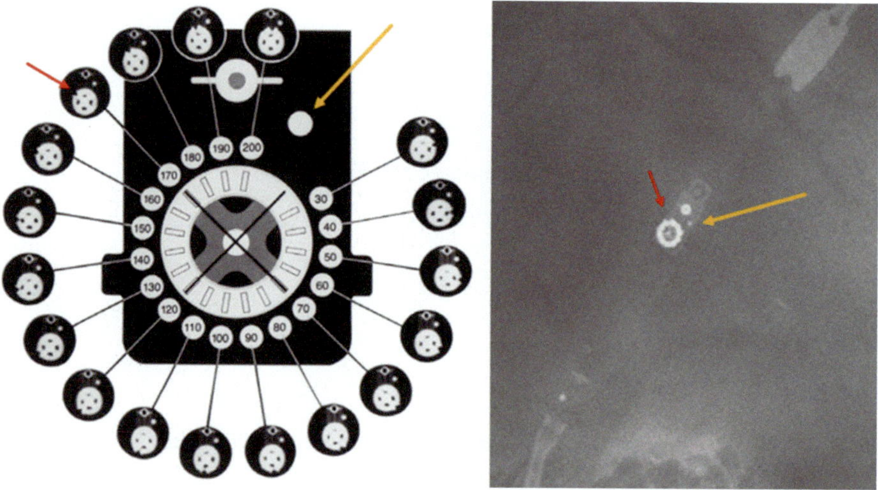

Fig. 8 X-ray identification of the pressure setting of a Codman-Hakim valve: the yellow arrows show the orientation marker, the red arrows show the notch which indicates the pressure setting of the valve. Valve pressure (x-ray on the right) is set at 170 mm H_2O

(Fig. 12). If the membrane cannot be depressed then it means there is a anti-reflux mechanism in the burr hole reservoir and it is working. This is essential for further testing. If the membrane can be depressed this means there is no anti-reflux mechanism in the burr hole reservoir or the compression of the distal catheter is not

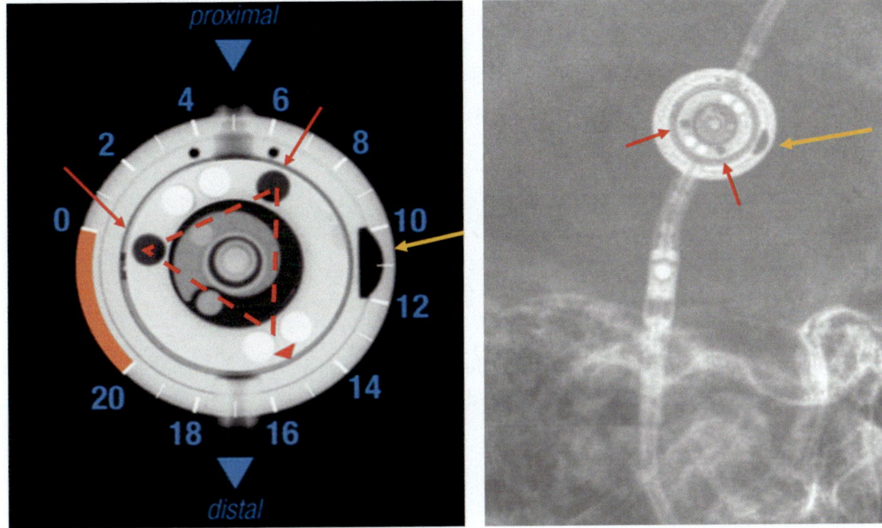

Fig. 9 X-ray identification of the pressure setting of a Miethke proGAV 2.0 valve: the yellow arrows show the orientation marker, the red arrows show the ball indicators which form the base of a triangle whose apex indicates the pressure setting of the valve. Valve pressure (x-ray on the right) is set to 6 cm H_2O

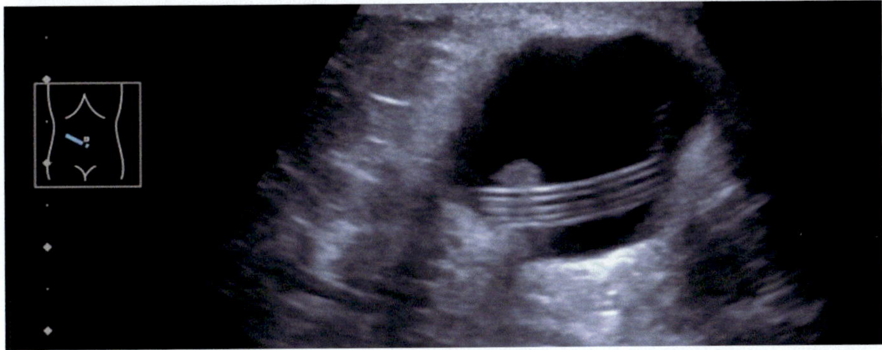

Fig. 10 Ultrasound image of a subcutaneous cyst formation around a luxated peritoneal catheter

sufficient. In these cases, the flushing reservoir cannot be used for manual shunt testing and it must be further investigated via invasive tests—see below.

How to Test the Patency of a Shunt

If you have a burr hole reservoir with a working anti-reflux mechanism you press down on the reservoir´s dome. This is possible only if the distal catheter and valve

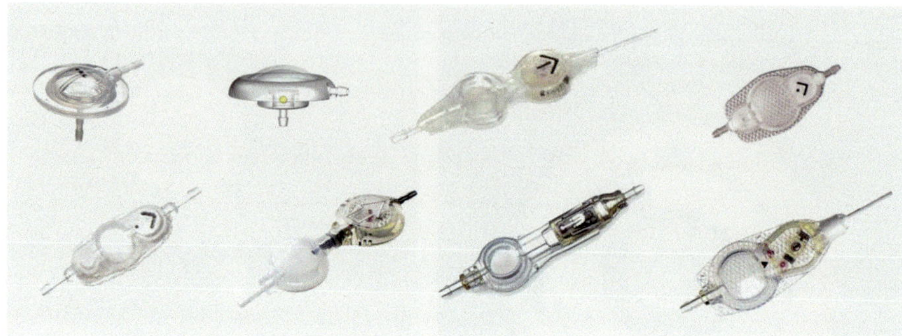

Fig. 11 A variety of separated or integrated flushing reservoirs for hydrocephalus shunts. The first two are located at the burr hole, the others are proximal to the valve

Fig. 12 Does the burr hole reservoir have an anti-reflux mechanism? If you occlude with one finger the distal catheter and you cannot compress the dome of the flushing reservoir it means that the anti-reflux valve is working. This is essential for further manual testing of the shunt

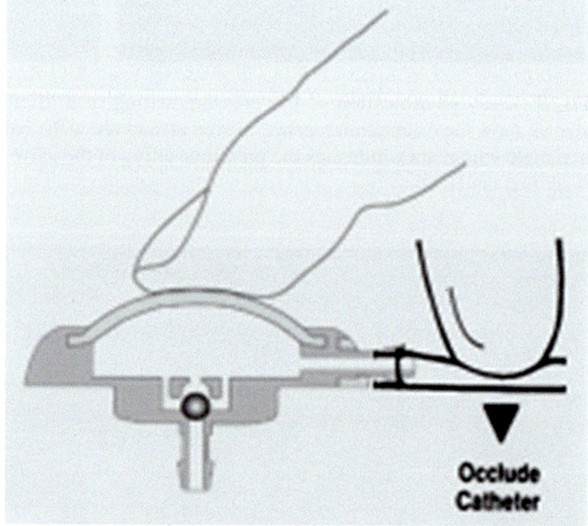

are patent. If you then lift your finger off the dome, the membrane must immediately bulge up again: this proves the patency of the ventricular catheter since a reflux is prevented by the distally implanted valve (Fig. 13).

If the flushing reservoir is distal of the burr hole and proximal to the valve the following steps are needed to prove the patency: 1: Occluding the catheter between the burr hole and the valve. 2: pressing down on the dome of the reservoir—this proves the patency of the valve and the distal catheter. 3: If the membrane remains depressed after lifting the finger from the dome it shows the working anti-reflux mechanism of the valve (and the sufficient occlusion of the proximal catheter). 4: If compression of the proximal catheter is stopped the immediate upward bulging of the membrane proves that the ventricular catheter is patent (Fig. 14).

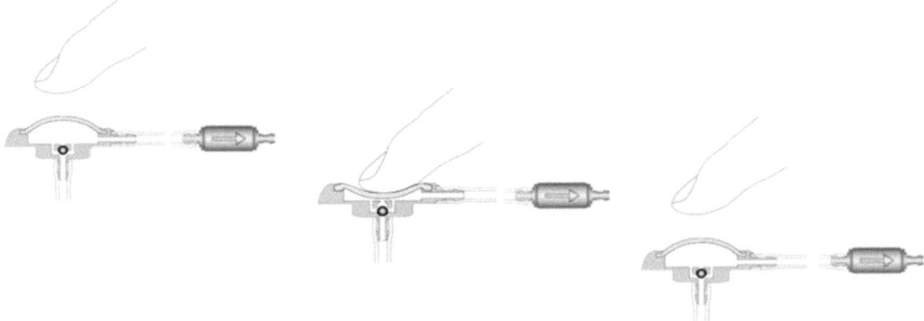

Fig. 13 Shunt patency proved by manual testing: Pressing down the membrane proves the patency of the distal catheter and of the valve. The membrane of the reservoir bulges up immediately with lifting of the finger if the ventricular catheter is open

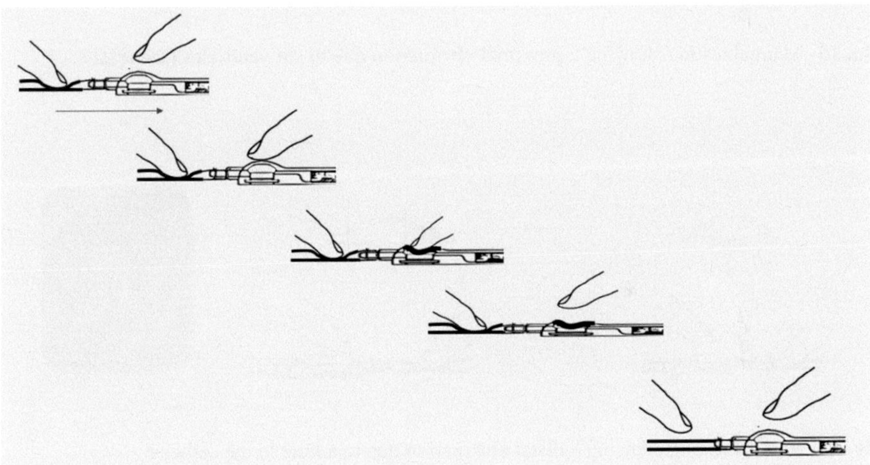

Fig. 14 Manual demonstration of the shunt patency

Knowing the shunt system and the mechanics can help to easily identify cases of shunt malfunction due to a proximal or distal obstruction:

Proximal Obstruction: If the membrane of the flushing reservoir does not bulge up again immediately after lifting the finger from the dome, it reveals a proximal obstruction. The obstruction may be of the catheter itself, due to slit ventricles in overdrainage, or due to a malpositioned catheter which may stick in the brain tissue and not in the ventricle (Fig. 15).

Distal obstruction: If the membrane of the flushing reservoir cannot be indented (by simultaneous occlusion of the proximal catheter) a distal occlusion of the valve or the catheter, for instance due to kinking of the catheter, may be present (Fig. 16). It is important to note that this procedure cannot detect a malposition of the peritoneal

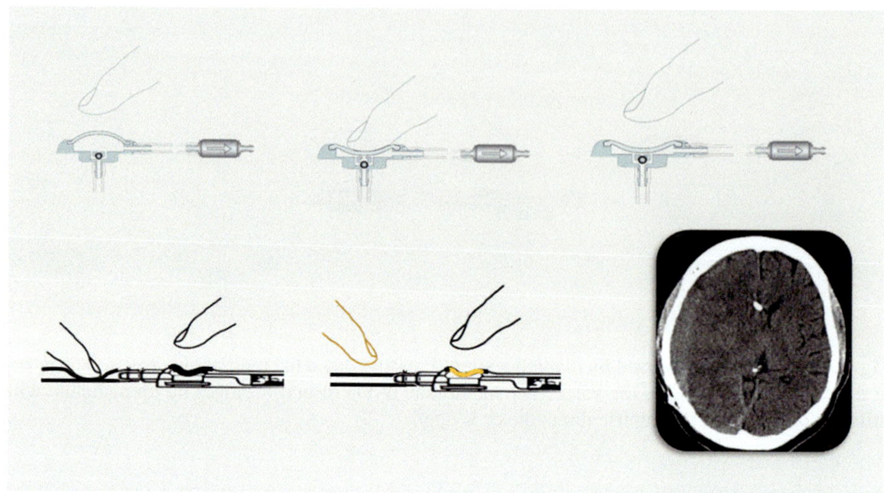

Fig. 15 Manual testing showing a proximal obstruction due to slit ventricles (see text)

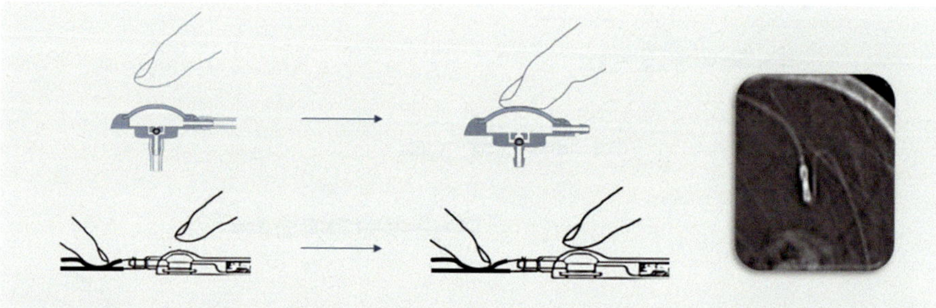

Fig. 16 Manual testing showing a distal obstruction due to a kink in the catheter

catheter or a cyst formation around it since the CSF may be "pumped" into the space wherever it is placed—without having a (complete) blockage.

With these easy procedures you can detect a proximal or distal obstruction focusing the further diagnostics and imaging to the proximal or distal part of the shunt.

Limitations of the Non-invasive Tests

- The catheter must be manually compressible in order to occlude the catheter completely. In older shunts the catheters are often in bony grooves which may not permit manual occlusion.

- Only a complete obstruction and a patency can be detected manually. Partial obstructions cannot be detected reliably by manual testing.
- In malposition of distal catheters CSF might be pumped into the cysts or subcutaneous tissue and an elevated resistance to depress the membrane of the flushing reservoir is not reliably unnoticed. The patient might notice some pain in the cyst region; however, this is a weak sign, which requires further investigation with imaging techniques.
- A leakage of the catheter is also not detected reliably by manual testing. However, the patient might experience pain and swelling at the site of CSF-leakage if you "pump" more CSF into that false space.

Non-invasive Tap Test ("Pump test"): If the manual test shows a patent shunt, then a non-invasive tap "pump" test via the reservoir can be done in cases of suspected underdrainage of the shunt. Knowing the volume of the reservoir used (we routinely use the "Sprung reservoir" which is seen in Fig. 21.3.3, with a reservoir volume of 0.2 ml), will allow calculation of the volume removed from the ventricular system. We routinely "pump" 100 times in cases of suspected underdrainage, which translates to tapping of 20 ml (100 × 0.2 ml). Afterwards, we observe and re-examine the patient as we do after a spinal tap test and provide them with an observation sheet (see Chap. "Spinal Tap Test").

Using the burr hole reservoir makes the pumping very easy, simply pressing down on the membrane each time. Having a more distal flushing reservoir is a bit more cumbersome, since you have to occlude the proximal catheter before the "pump," then lift your finger from the proximal catheter, so that CSF can flow into the reservoir, and repeat the same procedure again and again.

The advantages of these non-invasive tests are clear: no risk of infections, improved comfort for the patient, decreased number of x-rays and CT-scans, performed in an outpatient procedure, and therefore also saving costs. In our experience, we could eliminate most of the invasive tests, and conduct them only in the cases of discrepancies.

4.2   Invasive Tests

Invasive tests are rarely necessary if the non-invasive tests are used in conjunction with imaging. However, in cases when it is not possible to occlude the catheter manually or there is a burr hole reservoir without an anti-reflux device, invasive tests may be necessary.

Puncturing the reservoir (with ICP measurement and/or tap test): The flushing reservoir can easily be punctured, the **ICP** can be measured, an **infusion test** could be performed or CSF could be tapped. Additionally, you may get CSF for a laboratory and especially **microbiological examination**. The last is the most important aspect of the invasive test. But a negative microbiological result in a suspected shunt infection does not rule out an infection completely. Additionally, via the flushing reservoir contrast medium could be installed for a "**shuntography.**" This might show an occlusion or a leakage with the exact localization.

A *spinal tap test* can be done as well and this is especially an option if the shunt has no flushing reservoir which could be punctured. The options are almost the same as described above.

The *infusion test* may also be able to identify shunt dysfunction and possibly quantify the dysfunction [5]. This might be especially helpful if shunt revision is discussed and no further adjustment of the valve is possible.

5 When to Revise the Shunt?

Generally speaking, a shunt revision should be done in all cases when the optimal result has not been achieved by shunting and/or by re-programming the valve, but might be achievable by a revision surgery.

There is no question about revision surgery in cases of disconnection, dislocation, misplacement, and valve defects, especially if they are accompanied by a non-functioning shunt with clinical symptoms. The revision surgery in these cases should resolve the problems and should be done in a timely manner.

It is more difficult when there are disconnections, dislocations, misplacements, and valve defects which **do not** lead (yet) to a shunt dysfunction. In these cases, it is usually advisable to revise the shunt to prevent future dysfunctions, however, in some cases a wait and see policy is reasonable.

Valve revisions: Valve problems like blocked adjustable valves, mechanical valve failures, or too oblique implanted gravitational valves may interfere with the shunt function and the relief of symptoms. In these cases, a revision surgery with a valve exchange or correction of the position should be performed. Also, in patients with late clinical deterioration after shunting where a tap test or shunt pumping shows temporary improvement with no possibility of further down regulation of the valve or non-adjustable valve, a change to a new valve with a lower opening pressure is indicated.

In cases of overdrainage, adding an adjustable gravitational valve shows advantages, counterbalancing the siphoning effect in the up-right position to the individual needs [3].

Abdominal pain: The peritoneal catheter may irritate the peritoneum and may cause abdominal pain. Typically, the pain location will vary due to the intra-peritoneal movement of the catheter. If this pain stays over a prolonged period of time and also affects the quality of life, a change of the intra-abdominal position, a shortening of the catheter or even an atrial diversion may resolve this complaint.

Radicular pain: In lumboperitoneal shunts, the shunt catheter may irritate lumbar nerve roots resulting in radicular pain, which often diminishes over time. However, if patients complain about prolonged radicular pain, it should be revised by changing the position of the lumbar catheter. This can also be done via local anesthesia to get immediate feed-back from the patient about any leg pain.

Pulmonary hypertension: Patients may develop pulmonary hypertension in VA shunts even many years after the shunt implantation due to continuous formation of pulmonary micro-emboli from the catheter tip. In these cases, a peritoneal diversion of the shunt should be performed to remove the source of the pulmonary embolism, although it remains unclear if this can stop the progression of pulmonary hypertension [6].

Overdrainage: If overdrainage (Fig. 4) appears, the first option would be to turn up the valve. In many cases this will help, however, it might worsen the NPH-symptoms due to a functional underdrainage. If a tolerable compromise between underdrainage and overdrainage is not achieved, there is an indication to implant a gravitational valve. Here you can have low opening pressures with a substantially reduced risk of overdrainage [7].

If no adjustable valve is present, an additional gravitational valve, a temporary shunt occlusion, and possibly an evacuation of a subdural hematoma might be necessary.

Underdrainage: Reasons for underdrainage may be multifold. If a reason like kinking, disconnection, or others is found, it could be repaired easily. However, there are cases where no reason is found despite the pump test, STT, or invasive measurement clearly demonstrating an underdrainage. In these cases, revision surgery is recommended as follows:

A) Exposing the valve with the proximal and distal catheter.
B) Disconnecting the valve from the proximal catheter:

- If CSF is running out spontaneously – go to 3.
- If no CSF is running out: check/change the proximal shunt part

C) Connecting a transparent water filled catheter to the valve, which is still connected to the distal catheter, and determine the opening pressure.

- If the pressure is normal (valve and distal catheter are ok): change the valve to a lower possible pressure
- If the pressure is higher than the pressure setting of the valve plus abdominal pressure:
    - Check the opening pressure of the valve and the distal catheter separately and change the part where an elevated pressure is shown

Important note: The valve and the catheter should not be rinsed before the testing: an intraluminal obstruction or a clot may be washed out, resulting in no more elevated pressures found during the testing.

If no reason is found a complete exchange of the valve and distal catheter is advisable.

Shunt infection: In cases of shunt infections, the whole shunt should be removed and after clearing the infection, a new shunt could be implanted. In contrast to high pressure hydrocephalus, cases of NPH do not require temporary external ventricular drainage.

It is controversial to implant a new shunt on the contralateral side while simultaneously removing the infected shunt after successful antibiotic treatment with normalization of CRP. It may save the patient one additional surgery, however, a potentially higher risk of reinfection may be expected and must be communicated to the patient beforehand.

6 Conclusion

Follow-up after shunt surgery is essential for achieving and maintain the best long-term outcome. Proper follow-up may reveal shunt problems in time, which, of course, must be resolved after recognizing as soon as possible. Follow-up is as important as the diagnostic NPH work up and the shunt-surgery itself. As for the diagnosis and the treatment, special expertise is also necessary for the follow-up. All physicians involved in the follow-up must be knowledgeable about the implants and their specifications for proper adjustments and for proper diagnosis of shunt malfunctions. With the aforementioned knowledge the overall outcome can be optimized, and shunt problems can be solved in a timely manner resulting in the best quality of life for the patient.

7 Key Points

- Follow-up after shunt surgery is essential for detecting shunt problems in time.
- If the outcome after shunting is not satisfactory, readjustments of the valve are necessary to achieve the best outcome ("titration").
- If clinical improvement after shunt is only partial, it must be differentiated between an incorrect valve setting and lacking recovery potential due to long standing NPH.
- Routine imaging follow-up is optional in favourable outcomes, but necessary if a shunt-problem is suspected.
- Non-invasive valve tests via the flushing reservoir can replace most of the invasive shunt tests. Special understanding of the implanted device for interpreting the results of the non-invasive test is necessary.
- Non-invasive shunt tests are almost free of complications.
- Invasive tests allow direct ICP measurements, obtaining CSF samples for blood counts and a microbiological examination in suspected infections, and may detect shunt dysfunctions via infusion tests, or contrast medium installations.

- Revision surgery depends on the cause of the shunt malfunction and is easy if the cause is clear. Valve and even total shunt replacements may be necessary in unidentifiable causes of shunt malfunctions.

References

1. Benveniste RJ, Samir Sur. Delayed symptom progression after ventriculoperitoneal shunt placement for normal pressure hydrocephalus. J Neurol Sci. 2018;393:105–109.
2. Gutowski P, Rot S, et al. Secondary deterioration in patients with normal pressure hydrocephalus after ventriculoperitoneal shunt placement: a proposed algorithm of treatment. Fluids Barriers CNS. 2020;17:18.
3. Funnell JP, D'Antona L, Craven CL, Thorne L, Watkins LD, Toma AK. Ultra-low-pressure hydrocephalic state in NPH: benefits of therapeutic siphoning with adjustable antigravity valves Acta Neurochir (Wien) 2020;162(12):2967–2974. https://doi.org/10.1007/s00701-020-04596-z..
4. Andrén K, Wikkelsø C, Tisell M, Hellström P. Natural course of idiopathic normal pressure hydrocephalus. J Neurol Neurosurg Psychiatry. 2014;85(7):806–810.
5. Lalou A, Czosnyka M et al. CSF Dynamics for shunt prognostication and revision in normal pressure hydrocephalus. J Clin Med. 2021;10(8): 1711. https://doi.org/10.3390/jcm10081711.
6. Haasnoot K, van Vught AJ. Pulmonary hypertension complicating a ventriculo-atrial shunt. Eur J Pediatr. 1992;151(10):748–750. https://doi.org/10.1007/BF01959083.
7. Lemcke J, Meier U, et al. Safety and efficacy of gravitational shunt valves in patients with idiopathic normal pressure hydrocephalus: a pragmatic, randomised, open label, multicentre trial (SVASONA). J Neurol Neurosurg Psychiatry. 2013;84(8):850–857.

Prognosis and Outcomes

Petr Skalický, Adéla Bubeníková, Aleš Vlasák, and Ondřej Bradáč

Abstract Outcomes of normal pressure hydrocephalus (NPH) treatment has been under investigation for over 40 years. The first reports disclosed relatively high complication rates, directly related to surgery. Even postoperative improvement rates were incomparably small compared to results nowadays. This is primarily due to advances in shunting devices, a better understanding of the disease pathogenesis, and more precise identification of NPH patients.t is now possible to target the treatment more efficiently and thus achieve better treatment outcomes with minimal surgery-related complications. Selected up-to-date reports show that over 75% of iNPH patients improve after surgery, regardless of the indication criteria and cerebrospinal fluid (CSF) diversion techniques. Despite a lot of effort to sustain initial improvement in clinical outcomes after shunt implantation, the improvement tends to decline with longer follow-ups. Although the understanding of the disease's pathophysiology has unquestionably improved, and an enormous body of literature dedicated to the investigation of NPH-characteristic parameters (both clinical and radiological) has been published, the main problem of NPH diagnosis remains the same. The frequent occurrence of neurodegenerative diseases and other comorbidities in the elderly is an important factor implicating treatment outcome and prognosis of NPH patients. Surgical candidates are selected according to the expected postoperative improvement of clinical symptoms. If any of the symptoms of the clinical triad do not improve after surgery, it is important to investigate it in more detail, usually referring the patient to another specialist (urologist, neurologist etc.). The results of outcomes vary which may be explained by the frequent occurrence of comorbidities. The proper identification of comorbidities should be included as a central part of NPH management. This chapter is dedicated to both early and long-term results of NPH treatment, where we aim to discuss individual nuances involving treatment outcomes, as well as specific prognosis for NPH patients.

P. Skalický (✉) · A. Bubeníková · A. Vlasák · O. Bradáč
Department of Neurosurgery, Second Medical Faculty, Charles University and Motol University Hospital, Prague, Czech Republic
e-mail: ondrej.bradac2@fnmotol.cz

A. Bubeníková · O. Bradáč
Department of Neurosurgery and Neurooncology, First Medical Faculty, Charles University and Military University Hospital, Prague, Czech Republic

O. Bradac (ed.), *Normal Pressure Hydrocephalus*,
https://doi.org/10.1007/978-3-031-36522-5_28

Keywords Normal pressure hydrocephalus treatment prognosis · NPH prognosis · NPH diagnosis · Shunt surgery · Long-term shunt outcomes

Abbreviations

10MWT	10M walk test
AD	Alzheimer's disease
CI	Confidence interval
CSF	Cerebrospinal fluid
CT	Computed tomography
CVD	Cerebrovascular disease
ETV	Endoscopic third ventriculostomy
LP	Lumboperitoneal
MMSE	Mini-Mental State Examination
MoCA	Montreal Cognitive Assessment
mRS	Modified Rankin Scale
NPH	Normal pressure hydrocephalus
iNPH	Idiopathic normal pressure hydrocephalus
RAVLT	Rey Auditory Verbal Learn Testing
SDH	Subdural haematoma
SMD	Standardised mean difference
sNPH	Secondary normal pressure hydrocephalus
TMT	Trail Making Test
TUG	Timed up and go
VA	Ventriculoatrial
VP	Ventriculoperitoneal

1 Introduction

Clinical outcomes of normal pressure hydrocephalus (NPH) treatment reported in the literature vary. Possible reasons include different indication and improvement criteria, different postoperative follow-up methods, degree of comorbidities, non-discrimination of aetiologies -idiopathic normal pressure hydrocephalus (iNPH) versus secondary normal pressure hydrocephalus (sNPH), different duration or degree of clinical symptoms, different treatment modalities, differences in shunt systems and other factors [1–4]. On average, over 75% of iNPH patients improve after surgery, regardless of the indication criteria and CSF diversion techniques in the selected studies [5]. Treatment of NPH typically involves implantation of a shunt device which provides a diversion of the cerebrospinal fluid to a different part of the body where the fluid is absorbed. The role of endoscopic third ventriculostomy

(ETV), which is routinely used in the treatment of obstructive hydrocephalus, remains controversial in NPH treatment [6]. Mitchell and Mathew introduced ETV in the treatment of iNPH patients in 1999 but 75% of four patients in their cohort ended up with a ventriculoperitoneal (VP) shunt [7]. Since then, several low-quality studies and case series have been published with promising results suggesting that ETV may restore CSF dynamics and pulsatility patterns in NPH. The authors of the retrospective review on ETV in iNPH from 2016 base the effectivity of ETV on 'modified bulk flow theory', with the proviso that every hydrocephalus is obstructive, and that ETV would make sense, especially in the case of functional stenosis of the aqueduct [8]. Nevertheless, the evidence for ETV in NPH is low in comparison to shunting and only one very low-quality randomised study comparing ETV with the VP shunt has been published with inconclusive results [6]. Therefore, this chapter will summarise current knowledge about the outcomes and prognosis of shunted NPH patients, and mention the natural course of the disease. ETV outcomes are discussed in its specific chapter (see Chap. 24).

With the current knowledge of the disease pathophysiology, the frequent occurrence of neurodegenerative and other comorbidities in ageing patients, selection of surgical candidates is focused on the expected improvement of clinical symptoms after surgery. Confirmation of NPH diagnosis is definitive only in patients with improvement of the symptoms after shunt implantation. The indication for surgery is usually decided with the help of guidelines and functional test analysis [9–11]. It is not certain how to approach patients who do not improve in functional testing, but correspond to NPH both clinically and in terms of findings on imaging examinations. In terms of possible comorbidities (e.g. osteoarthritis of large joints, stress incontinence, benign prostatic hyperplasia, etc.), it is necessary to approach each patient individually. If any of the symptoms of the triad do not improve after surgery, it should be further investigated and it may be necessary for the patient to be referred to another specialist, e.g. urologist to evaluate urinary symptoms more in detail [12]. The reported differences in outcomes may therefore be partly explained by the prevalence of concurrent comorbidities and their proper identification should be included in the central part of NPH management [13].

2   Early and Short-Term Postoperative Outcomes

Until 2002, there was no study comparing the results of a shunt operation with a randomised control group [14]. In the past few years, however, several such studies have been conducted. For example, Kazui et al. [15] showed significantly higher clinical improvement after LP shunt implantation in the immediately operated group (65%) than in the delayed group (5%) 3 months after randomisation (prior to surgery in the control group) defined as an improvement of 1 or more points on Modified Rankin Scale (mRS). Nakajima et al. [16] published the results of a nationwide hospital survey in Japan comparing the results of patients who underwent shunt surgery with non-operated controls (using mRS), and only the operated patients achieved significant improvement at 1-year follow-up control, regardless of the type of shunt surgery. In a prospective European multicentre iNPH study, 69% of patients improved according to mRS (one-point improvement) and 84% improved according to an age-standardised iNPH scale (five-point improvement). Indication for surgery was based on various clinical and radiological criteria, and there was no a randomised control group [17]. The Swedish Hydrocephalus Quality Registry reported that the number needed to treat for improving one patient from unfavourable (mRS 3–5) to favourable (mRS 0–2) was 3.0 [18]. Improvements can be maintained for several years [19], despite possible shunt revisions [20]. A higher percentage of improvement might be achieved with strict diagnostic and treatment protocols [9]—e.g. Poca et al. [14] reported clinical improvement in almost 90% of patients (with an improvement of at least one point on the iNPH scale). However, strict diagnostic criteria might result in under-treatment; therefore, each patient should be evaluated individually.

Different target options for both proximal and distal ends of the shunt system are possible. These include mainly ventriculoperitoneal (VP), lumboperitoneal (LP) and ventriculoatrial (VA) shunts. Outcomes of shunt diversion methods are comparable and approximately 75% of patients improve in the first year after shunting [5]. Although cardiopulmonary and renal complications are serious concerns associated with VA shunt placement, they are uncommon in patients with iNPH [21]. LP shunt outcomes do not significantly differ from VP shunt outcomes [22]. Early and short-term postoperative outcomes are definitely connected with diagnostic accuracy and shunt indication [11] and are possibly most favourable when CSF outflow resistance is increased and global cerebral autoregulation is intact, in combination with arterial normotension [23]. A recent study found that mild preoperative iNPH severity, shorter preoperative symptom duration, good tap test response, and complete DESH were associated with good short-term postoperative outcome at 1 year [24]. Also, it was found that compared to reference individuals, the neuropsychological aspects and quality of life of iNPH patients improved during the first 3 months after surgery, in some parts nearly to normal values [25]. This means that patients with longstanding preoperative symptoms may not receive the same benefits of surgical intervention as patients with a shorter duration of preoperative symptoms. However, with longer follow-up, the patients generally tend to reach the same endpoint [26]. Another study showed that the outcomes of VP-shunt surgery did not significantly differ between 6 months and 2 years post-surgery, indicating that the outcome at 6 months remained stable for up to 24 months. Longer symptom duration and older age should not deter patients with iNPH from undergoing shunt implantation [27].

Despite many efforts to predict shunt response non-invasively, none of them have shown any clinical benefit [28]. The utility of imaging to predict response to shunting is limited, and no imaging feature alone can be used to exclude patients from shunt surgery [29, 30]. The results are closely related to the diagnostic procedures and guideline adherence throughout the centres [9, 11]. Laparoscopic and less invasive implantations have been introduced with the goal to minimise wound-related complications [31]. However, between 2007 and 2017, laparoscopic assistance was only used in 6% of implantations in the USA [32]. Also, there is currently no evidence in the literature to support this approach nor its potential benefits over the traditional surgical technique.

Of note is the recent systematic review and meta-analysis by Giordan et al. [5] which focused on the comparison of different surgical techniques in NPH management. It included 33 studies with a total of 2461 patients. An improvement in postoperative functional outcome was observed in over 75% of patients, regardless of the surgical technique or the CSF diversion units used. In terms of the valves, NPH patients managed by programmable and by fixed valves had similar treatment outcomes. On the other hand, compared to the fixed valves, adjustable devices were associated with a reduction in revisions (12% vs. 32%), along with a lower number of subdural collections (9% vs. 22%). This mirrors the prediction that revision rates are probably going to decrease with increased use of adjustable novel devices. Using neuronavigation may be suggested for guiding the ventricular implantation [33]. A recent study however did not find any clear benefit of its usage [34].

2.1 *Complications and Mortality*

In a recent service evaluation of early postoperative outcomes in NPH, D'Antona et al. [35] reported 0% mortality, 7% morbidity and no revisions or readmissions to ICU in 88 patients who underwent lumbar drain insertion and/or VP shunt implantation. Seven patients had minor complications, and no moderate or severe complications were reported. No correlation between preoperative morbidity, surgical outcomes and hospital length of stay was found. A large multicentre survey of a privately insured United States healthcare network, however, showed a 7.29% 30-day readmission rate for 974 patients with NPH who underwent ventricular shunting. The perioperative complication rate was 21.15%, and included intracerebral haemorrhage (5.85%) and extra-axial haematoma (subdural or epidural 5.54%) Pre-existing comorbidities such as peripheral vascular disease, cerebral vascular disease, diabetes, paralysis or renal disease, were associated with risks of complication or readmission. Approximately 5.9% of patients needed reoperation within 30-days [36]. Another study reported a 36% complication rate (23% shunt related complication rate) in iNPH patients with a 0% mortality rate. INPH patients had a significantly smaller risk of shunt surgery-related complications than other patient groups treated with shunting [37]. Another study showed 0.5% 30-day mortality rate without a significant difference from controls [38]. Hebb et al. [39] in 2001 reported an overall mean complication rate of 38% after shunt surgery and a shunt revision rate of 22%. However, a more recent systematic review reported a lower pooled complication rate of 10% and a shunt revision rate of 16% [5]. A subsequent meta-analysis also showed the benefit of using adjustable devices. Some of the revisions made in the past would have been e easily solved with adjustments only. Another study showed that approximately 50% of revisions occur in the 1st year after initial shunt surgery and are mainly due to malfunctions [19]. A study comparing the complication rate 3 months after VP shunt insertion in NPH and non-NPH patients found that high Karnofsky

Performance Score at admission and NPH as an underlying indication significantly reduced the odds ratio for a complication [37]. Subdural haematomas (SDHs) are common complications of shunt treatment accompanied with overdrainage. Recent study showed that SDHs developed in 10% of patients in 12-month follow-up and 36% of these cases were treated surgically. Significantly lower portions of surgeries were made in patients with adjustable shunts. SDH and treatment do not significantly affect survival in iNPH patients, thus the non-invasive treatment offered by adjustable shunts considerably reduces the level of severity of this common adverse event [40]. Male sex, antiplatelet medication, and a lower opening pressure at surgery were risk factors for SDH [41]. Infections are rarer. A recent study reported an infection rate of 5.9% [42] and another study of 4.76% during the first 3 months [43].

Despite a lot of effort to sustain initial improvement in clinical outcomes after shunt insertion in NPH patients, the improvement tends to decline within longer follow-ups. According to a recent meta-analysis [5], over 75% of patients evaluated after 12 months experienced an improvement in their clinical status after shunting. This number subsequently decreased to 73% of patients followed up from 12 to 36 months, and an even more significant decline was observed for patients whose follow-up exceeded 36 months (71%). However, it is important to note, and as it is discussed more in detail below, the overall improvement rate of NPH patients after shunting is notably higher compared to the natural course of the disease [44–46].

3 Gait Impairment Outcomes

Gait is the symptom most likely to improve after shunting and typically tends to keep sustained improvement. To give an example, in the series of 50 shunted NPH patients, there was an improvement after shunting which sustained improvement over a median follow-up time of 120.2 ± 2.3 months compared to the initial baseline, as stated by Grasso et al. [18]. Moreover, gait improvement is the one most connected to quality of life. Of note, persistent gait impairment and depression are the strongest predictors of low quality of life after NPH treatment [47]. Following the first reports saying that gait disturbances may be an initial manifestation of NPH, the gait impairment in NPH has since been studied in detail. As a result, some specific features that can to some extent distinguish NPH from other disorders have been identified. NPH gait disorder is sometimes called "magnetic" or "glued to the floor", with other characteristic patterns such as diminished gait velocity, loss of balance, short stride, so-called *en bloc* turning etc., features that are described in an individual chapter more in detail (see Chap. 9) [48]. A study from 2001 evaluated differences in gait impairment between patients suffering from NPH (n = 11) and those with Parkinson's disease (n = 10), compared to twelve age-matched healthy controls [49]. Although some reports have reported parkinsonian signs as typical for NPH patients, contraindicatory findings have been published with better clinical profiles and the distinction between probable and possible NPH patients [50–52]. Moreover, this differentiated the possible existence of comorbidities that could bias what is and what is not a characteristic pattern for NPH. Additionally, according to the most recent reports, parkinsonian signs are not very common in well-defined NPH, regardless of existing comorbidity [53, 54]. Still, Parkinsonism is a differential diagnosis of NPH of great importance [55]. In the study by Stolze et al. [49], gait velocity increased by approximately 21% following the CSF tap test in NPH patients, compared to the natural gait velocity at the baseline. Also, a coefficient of variation for stride length, step width, and foot angle was calculated. Interestingly, it significantly decreased after the CSF tap test, along with the enlargement of the stride length, but the cadence remained at the same level without any difference. According to these findings, in terms of the gait impairment, gait velocity has been found to be the pattern that tends to improve the most also following the shunt placement [5, 18]. This is particularly useful for predicting shunt responsiveness, considering the high sensitivity of this gait feature to the CSF tap test [56]. If secondary deterioration occurs after surgery, and shunt malfunction is ruled out, the comorbid disease should be suspected.

In 2000, Blomsterwall et al. [57] studied the association between disturbances of balance and gait in NPH patients before and after shunt insertion. Interestingly, 75% of patients improved in gait velocity and 69% in balance, suggesting that improved balance may be to some extent responsible for gait improvement. Similar results were reported in a recent multicentre prospective observational study by Trungu et al. [46]. Out of 181 NPH patients, the mean gait domain was 58.5 ± 14.3 preoperatively, 66.0 ± 12.2 postoperatively and 70.1 ± 13.4. This domain was statistically significantly improved in shunted NPH patients at the 12 monthfollow-up examination. ($p < 0.001$). A similar trend was observed in the balance domain, the mean values were 66.7 ± 21.5 preoperatively, 72.4 ± 19.2 postoperatively, and 71.7 ± 22.1 at the 12-month follow-up ($p = 0.001$). Other reports observed that gait improvement was present three years after shunt insertion in 80–83% of shunted NPH patients and in approximately 87% of NPH patients 7 years after shunting [58, 59]. Supported by various studies evaluating the effect of shunt implantation on postoperative outcomes in NPH patients, the gait domain shows the highest improvement along with the impact on overall clinical score postoperatively. This is also true with respect to long-term follow-ups [4, 60, 61].

A recently published study by Sundström et al. [55] evaluated the outcome measure timed up and go (TUG) in a large, nationwide cohort that included 1300 iNPH patients before and after surgery. The authors compared the TUG test to the 10-m walk test (10MWT), the iNPH scale, the mRS, and Mini-Mental State Examination (MMSE). Significant improvements in TUG and 10MWT were observed in both the general group and for the group stratified for sex and age. Interestingly, women tended to perform significantly worse after shunting in both TUG and 10MWT ($p < 0.001$), but there was no observed difference between males and females in overall postoperative improvement (Fig. 1). Moreover, there was a strong association between TUG and the 10MWT before and after shunt implantation ($r = 0.76$). However, there was only a moderate relationship between TUG and the iNPH scale ($r = 0.34$), weak to moderate association with mRS ($r = 0.22$) and negligible correlation was seen between TUG and MMSE ($r = 0.17$). These findings, based on a large population of non-selected NPH patients, show that the TUG time and steps are significantly improved regardless of sex and age [55]. NPH patients tend to perform worse in the TUG test compared to healthy elderly controls, in both preoperative and postoperative examinations at 3 months. These higher values of TUG times can be explained by NPH-related gait dysfunction which is to some extent independent of age, and the improvement of gait disturbances typically takes time to normalise. Some gait impairment features are irreversible regardless of shunt insertion [55, 62, 63]. Notably, patients with more severe symptoms preoperatively, that is, those with higher TUG values, benefited from shunting, but their gait amelioration was not significant regardless of clinical improvement. The fact that the improvement of NPH patients after shunting is typically independent of age, in contrast to healthy elderly individuals, is supported by a meta-analysis of 21 studies that investigated the TUG test in healthy elderly subjects. The mean values of TUG times were different among patients' age groups, 8.1 s (95% CI, 7.1 to 9.0 s) for patients between 60 and 69 years; 9.2 s (95% CI, 8.2 to 10.2 s) for patients 70–79 olds; and finally 11.3 s (95% CI, 10.0 to 12.7 s) for subjects aged between 80 and 99 years [64].

The mentioned reports are a great example of why early treatment is preferable and why even patients with severe symptoms should not be excluded from surgery. Agerskov et al. [62] outlined that they did not find any association between the severity of symptoms and treatment outcome. Additionally, although Kimura et al. [24] found a negative correlation between these two factors, that is, symptom severity and expected treatment outcome, the benefits of shunt implantation in well-selected

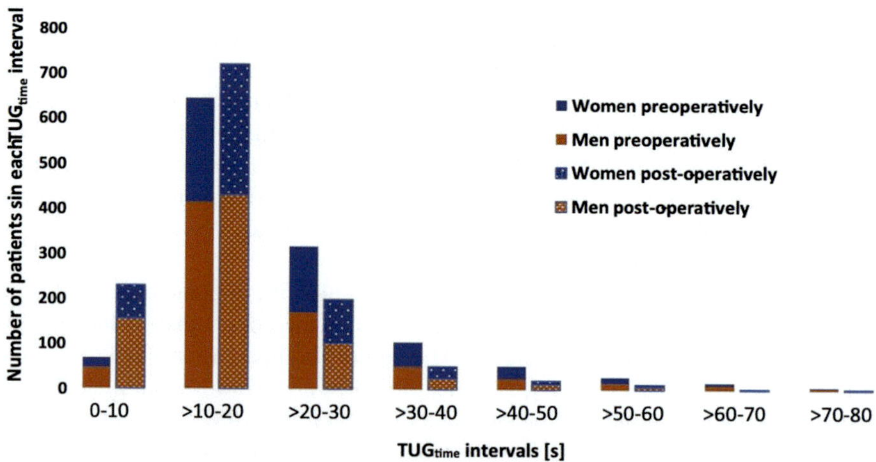

Fig. 1 Histogram displaying the number of patients within each TUG time interval pre- and post-operatively for men (n = 744) and women (n = 505). Preoperatively, 175 men and 79 women had TUG time < 13.5 s. Postoperatively, the corresponding numbers were 364 and 186. Above this threshold, the risk of falling is considered to be increased. Sundström et al. [55]. The paper is an Open Access article distributed under the terms of the *Creative Commons licensed under CC-BY-4.0 Attribution Licence*, which permits unrestricted use, distribution, and reproduction in any medium, provided the original work is properly credited

NPH patients still substantially exceeds the progression of the disease when left untreated [44–46, 55].

3.1 Cognitive Outcomes

As a part of Hakim's triad, some NPH patients experience a range of neuropsychological alterations, which tend to mimic concurrent neurodegenerative comorbidities and their distinguishment is often challenging. Nevertheless, the 'typical NPH cognitive profile' comprises memory, learning and attention impairment, along with disturbances of processing and psychomotor speed or disruptions of executive and other functions. The disruptions of frontal functions are a common part of NPH-related cognitive disturbances since they are based on extended ventricular dilatation and thus on the damage of frontosubcortical projections or subcortical structures [65, 66]. This may be to some extent (although highly dependent on many factors, including the length of such damage, individual patient predisposition, shunt responsiveness etc.) a reversible process when the shunt works properly, and ventricular dilatation is reduced [67, 68]. Memory functions tend to improve following the shunt insertion, as frequently reported [18, 69, 70]. Significant improvements were found for spatial memory and visual recall. NPH patients simultaneously tended to improve in different subtests of the Wechsler Memory Scale. A recent systematic review and meta-analysis [70] calculated differences in neuropsychological tests before and after surgery. Of 23 studies (1059 NPH patients) included in the final meta-analysis, the authors searched for surgical effects on cognitive outcomes evaluated through adequate tests including the MMSE, the Rey Auditory Verbal Learn Testing (RAVLT), trail making tests A and B (TMT-A and TMT-B), delayed verbal recall subjects, backwards digit span and phonemic verbal fluency. There was a statistically significant positive effect of shunting on cognition ($p < 0.001$) and memory ($p < 0.001$).ess significant positive effect on executive function (backwards digit span, $p < 0.03$; phonemic verbal fluency, $p = 0.005$; TMT-B, $p = 0.03$) and significant psychomotor speed (TMT-A, $p < 0.001$). The meta-regression models did not find any statistically significant effects of age, follow-up, or gender on improvement in the MMSE. Nevertheless, the mentioned meta-analysis evaluated studies with short follow-ups (from 3 to 12 months) and therefore could not provide conclusions about the effect of shunting on cognitive improvement in NPH patients after a longer period of follow-up. According to some reports, RAVLT is likely to be highly sensitive to improved cognition in NPH subjects, since a significant correlation between the improvement in RAVLT retention score and in both the total and delayed verbal recall subtests has been observed [71, 72]. Although some studies have shown no change in cognitive performance in the MMSE test [20, 73, 74], there are also contradictory reports finding significant improvements [75–77]. Regarding the improvement of executive function after surgery, some studies have reported significant improvement in the backwards digit span test [68, 73, 78, 79], however, others have not shown any changes [20, 80]. Similarly, improvements in the Stroop test have been so far heterogeneous [60, 67, 76]. The reason why executive function usually does not show a significant tendency to improve is probably based on a noteworthy proportion of patients suffering from disproportionately impaired executive function at the baseline clinical examination, therefore supporting the hypothesis that such impairment may reflect irreversible damage to fronto-subcortical connectivity in NPH patients [70, 74, 81]. It is clear that overall, cognitive amelioration after surgery is sometimes limited and mental state is often the first of the symptoms to decline [82, 83].

A recent prospective report by Hellström et al. [68] investigated the effects of shunt insertion on the cognitive profile in 47 iNPH patients, compared to 159 age-matched healthy controls. All iNPH patients showed improvement in all neuropsychological tests, except for the Digit Span forward, Digit Span Wechsler Adult Intelligence Scale score and the Simple Reaction Time. The authors observed that more severely impaired functions before surgery tended to improve more following the shunt insertion, compared to milder disturbances. Most patients improved according to the Grooved Pegboard (86–90%) and Stroop (82–91%) testing three months after surgery. On the other hand, the lowest number of patients improved on the Digit Span forward and backward tests (26% and 44%, respectively). Despite positive shunt-related improvement in iNPH patients, most of the cited studies did not evaluate long-term cognitive outcomes and the question of how long neuropsychological improvement lasts has not been answered in larger population studies with longer follow-ups yet. Several studies which examined a small number of patients or with no detailed clinical evaluation of the iNPH diagnosis did not find any significant long-term improvement in cognitive functions after iNPH intervention [60, 84, 85]. Nevertheless, of note is a recent study of 48 iNPH patients which found that the majority of them (77%) were able to improve or maintain cognitive function for at least 2 years after surgery when compared to their baseline cognitive clinical status [86]. There was a statistically significant improvement in the MMSE scale at 3 months ($p = 0.0002$) and 1 year postoperatively ($p = 0.004$), compared to patients' initial baseline scores. However, 2 years following the shunting, the mean MMSE score almost returned to the preoperative level − 12 patients showed an increased MMSE score by ≥ 2 points, 11 patients showed a decline by ≥ 2 points, and almost no change was found in the remaining 25 patients (Fig. 2). The final number of 37 patients (77%) therefore refers to patients with cognitive improvement and no observed change in their neuropsychological testing 2 years after surgery, both compared to their baseline status. To compare the aforementioned results to other studies, improved performance in the MMSE test was significant in the vast majority of reports [75–77]. However, other investigations did not find any change in the improvement of iNPH patients in the MMSE after shunt implantation [73, 74, 87]. In a recent study by Hülser et al. [25], there was a significant improvement in the overall test battery during the first 3 months after shunt insertion, including the MMSE testing ($p < 0.024$). However, despite such an improvement, the iNPH patients were not able to reach the baseline of the healthy age-matched controls, even in early follow-ups after shunt surgery [25]. These findings are suggestive of the fact that even though the postoperative improvement in the MMSE may be

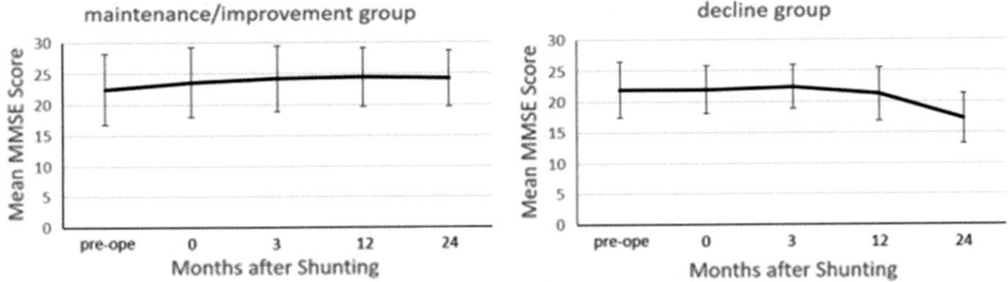

Fig. 2 Between group comparison of the mean MMSE score prior and after shunt insertion, according to Kambara et al. [86]. The paper is an Open Access article distributed under the terms of the *Creative Commons licensed under CC-BY-4.0 Attribution Licence*, which permits unrestricted use, distribution, and reproduction in any medium, provided the original work is properly credited

statistically significant, the cognitive performance of iNPH patients is worse when compared to healthy controls. Another term that should be mentioned is the so-called "ceiling effect", characteristic of iNPH patients who perform with around 24 points in the MMSE test, therefore being close to normal values of unaffected individuals [70]. This effect describes the reduced sensitivity of the MMSE test for mild cognitive dysfunction, which challenges the comparison of these changes in cognitive disturbances before and after shunt implantation [70]. Thist may be one of the reasons why there is no significant detection of changes in the MMSE testing, since some mild cognitive dysfunctions may be undetectable through this test [70, 81]. Therefore, additional, and more detailed neurophysiological testing may be appropriate, including the Montreal Cognitive Assessment (MoCA), which showed better diagnostic accuracy than the MMSE itself [70, 88].

Moreover, since the severity and patients' age are likely associated with the prognosis of the neuropsychological profile, early iNPH intervention is desirable to improve cognitive prognosis [86]. During follow-up, the neuropsychological domain tends to deteriorate, especially in patients experiencing other mild neurodegenerative comorbidities, and the consensus on the reversibility of cognition impairment in NPH patients with respect to concurrent disorders has not yet been elucidated [46]. This might be even further supported by findings that show a decrease in the MMSE score by 3 points after the diagnosis of iNPH if left untreated [44]. Such a deterioration was seen in iNPH patients who waited for surgery for at least 6 months (range from 6.8 to 23.8 months, median 13.2 months) compared to early treated iNPH individuals (waiting time for shunt implantation ranged from 0.1 to 2.7 months, median of 0.2 months) [44]. This statement was also verified in various reports, thus supporting the findings that waiting time for surgery influences the outcome in iNPH patients [89].

3.2 Incontinence Outcomes

One of the first reports dedicated to a more detailed evaluation of shunt effectiveness in improving urinary incontinence was published in 1988 by Ahlberg et al. [90]. Of ten patients with possible NPH, a definite diagnosis was confirmed in four cases. All had a positive Bors' ice water test. Three of them had a history of subarachnoid haemorrhage and one of severe head trauma. After performing the tap test, the Bors' test remained positive in three cases, but it changed to negative in one case. All four patients underwent VP shunt placement. Three months after surgery, all four patients had a negative Bors' test and had normal micturition features on urodynamic testing. Moreover, three patients did not suffer from any bladder instability, and the instability in the remaining case was reduced in comparison to the initial manifestation. The guidelines by Relkin et al. [91] describe that urinary impairment in the early stages of the disease is characterised by abnormal frequency and urgency without urinary incontinence itself. As one of the typical features in NPH-related urinary impairment, the term "neurogenic bladder syndrome" has been used to describe hyperactivity of the bladder in some patients with NPH. Along with the progression of the disease, early features of urinary disturbances develop into serious urinary incontinence. To adequately differentiate NPH-related urinary disturbances from primary urinary incontinence unrelated to NPH, attention should be paid to urodynamic studies which play an important role in the detailed evaluation of common comorbid conditions [91]. This is particularly important to bear in mind when determining the improvement of urinary impairment after shunt implantation in NPH patients. As stated in the chapter dedicated to the symptomatology of NPH (see Chap. 11), urinary incontinence is typically the least frequent symptom of the whole triad and the least discussed in the literature [39].

Although the urinary incontinence domain typically shows a lower proportion of improved patients after surgery, a recent multicentre prospective observational study has observed significant improvement of this symptom in 70% of shunted NPH patients [46]. Furthermore, the results of the urinary incontinence domain were significant improvement at the 12-month follow-up ($p = 0.002$). Similarly, a prospective cohort study of 23 patients by Krzastek et al. [92] showed significant improvement after shunting not only in urinary urgency or urge incontinence, but also in overall quality of life and the ability to perform everyday activities. The most common symptom of an overactive bladder before surgical implantation of the shunt was two times/night nocturia. Interestingly, this symptom did not improve after shunt insertion, in contrast to the following significantly improved symptoms: urinary urgency ($p = 0.016$), bother from urinary urgency ($p = 0.005$), and the amount of urge incontinence ($p = 0.038$). Moreover, significant improvement in urinary dysfunction was seen more commonly in younger patients and women tended to improve in more domains of urinary impairment after surgery, when compared to men [92]. Aforedescribed reports have described early improvement of urinary dysfunction in shunted NPH patients, however, the question is whether the improvement remains the same in longer follow-ups. Similar to the cognitive deterioration in long-term follow-ups, urinary incontinence has also shown a tendency to decline after longer periods of time, despite the initial improvement in early or short-term follow-ups [18].

3.3   Long-Term Prognosis and the Role of Comorbidities

The natural history of untreated patients with NPH is poor, with both increased mortality and morbidity. Shunt insertion can provide long-lasting clinical improvement [93]. However, in some patients, the effect of shunting might be limited over time, or the symptoms might not be well-compensated. If so, evaluation of the shunt function might be reasonable. Kaestner et al. [42] indicated shunt revision for suspected shunt dysfunction in 18% of secondary deteriorations. Immediate improvement was present in 37% of patients. The authors suggested invasive testing if shunt malfunction was suspected. In vivo shunt studies might be used [94]. In iNPH, shunt dysfunction does not often lead to enlargement of ventricles, a surrogate parameter of shunt failure. Nevertheless, the majority of secondary deteriorations were treated conservatively, either by valve adjustments or because of existing connections with concurrent comorbidities [42]. It was also found that favourable outcomes following shunt implantation in patients with NPH did not correlate with decreased ventricular volume one year after surgery [95]. However, the ventricular volume often decreases as well, as there is a little increase in the cortical volume, especially in the regions near the vertex [96]. Another study found that 20% of patients with iNPH were at risk for secondary clinical worsening about 3 years after shunt surgery. About one-fourth of these patients benefited for additional years from pressure level management and/or shunt valve revision [97].

Long-term prognosis is influenced by many factors, not always connected with the disease. If another comorbidity is suspected, specialised consultation might be needed, as well as follow-up by a neurosurgeon and a neurologist. A standardised protocol and a multidisciplinary team dedicated to this disorder is needed to achieve an early and correct diagnosis of NPH [46]. Patients should also adhere to home physical exercises to improve their outcomes but also get a general health benefit [98]. The presence of comorbidities has a fundamental impact on patients' performance and prognosis following the shunt insertion. Therefore, comorbidities must be considered when evaluating postoperative outcomes, both in early and long-term follow-ups.

Despite the suggestions, the literature dedicated to long-term outcomes of NPH management is still limited. Shorter follow-up studies predominate, and longer-term studies have low numbers of participants. At the beginning of NPH management, the long-term results had not even been paid attention to. The first studies did not provide knowledge until many years later. Greenberg et al. [99] in 1977 reported a 42.8% 3-year shunting success rate. Nowadays, it is no longer imaginable that five patients (6.9%) would die within one month of surgery, or as a direct result of surgical intervention.

Black et al. [100] in 1980 reported longer-term postoperative outcomes of shunting (36.5 months mean follow-up time). Sixty-one percent of patients improved, however, the 35.4% rate of complications, which was comparable to the studies released in the same years, is very high in comparison to recent studies. The change in the progression of the disease, any role of time in terms of clinical symptoms, or any comorbidity factors were not studied. Also, the timing of the evaluation of outcomes was not specified. Interestingly, the ventricle enlargement with little or no sulcal enlargement on CT scan was found to be a predictive factor of postoperative improvement [100]. More than 20 years later in 2001, a questionnaire study by Mori et al. [101] reported an improvement rate of 73.3% at 3 years after shunt surgery, and mortality at 3 years was 2.9%. At 3 months, the improvement rate was 79.2%. Improvement in gait disturbance after the surgery was found in 21 patients (91.3%), improvement in dementia in eight (34.8%), and improvement in urinary incontinence in 14 patients (60.9%). Interestingly, only 18.3% of implanted shunt systems had an anti-siphon device. 74.2% of shunt valves were programmable. The shunt-related complication rate was 18.3% [101]. In 2002, Savolainen et al. [60] reported a 47% gait, 29% incontinence, and 38% mental improvement rate 5 years after the surgery. One year after the shunting, 72% of patients had a good recovery. Following the 5-year follow-up, 11 (65%) of alive patients experienced worsened gait symptoms, while six had no change when compared to their preoperative clinical status. Cognitive problems worsened in 13 patients (77% of alive), while only one patient improved. Worsening of urinary incontinence was present in 10 patients (59%) and six had no change in this sign. Interestingly none of the neuropsychological tests significantly improved after the surgery, and the reported cognitive benefit was subjective. The 16 patients with Alzheimer's disease did worse after one year than those without pathological changes, but the mortality was not increased. Thus, the role of neurodegenerative comorbidities in the postoperative outcomes had been discussed. Aygok et al. [102] reported a period of 3 months to 3 years after shunting in 50 iNPH patients with only a moderate decline in gait performance (91–75%), retention of memory improvement (80–80%), and improvement in incontinence sustained over time (70–82.5%). Four cases of death were not related to shunting. Even though the risk and fear of falling decreased significantly after shunting, they did not reach the level of risk in controls [103]. However, a significant difference in deaths caused by falls between iNPH patients and controls was not found [104].

In 2007, Kahlon et al. [84] reported 5-year outcomes of shunted patients with a 43% improvement rate in the walk step test, 39% of patients improved in the walk time test, and 39% improved in the reaction time test, whereas only 4% showed improvement in the memory test. 57% reported that they still perceived improvement compared with their preoperative status. However, only 36% of shunted patients were available at the follow-up at 5 years. Between the 6-month and 5-year follow-up periods, 37% out of the initial 75 patients died. The death rates in operated (37%) and not operated (38%) patients were similar. However, the 7.4% annual death rate was higher than 3.2% of the general Swedish population in the same age group. The causes of death were mainly due to cardiovascular disease (32%), and malignancy (25%). The results emphasised the importance of taking comorbidities and older age into account when selecting patients with NPH symptoms for shunt surgery [84]. Chen et al. [105] reported that during the 3 years of follow-up, five of the 28 patients died, the other six were lost to follow-up (including telephone contact), and three patients had progressive clinical deterioration. Pujari et al. [19] reported an overall sustained improvement among all symptoms over a mean follow-up duration of 5.9 ± 2.5 years. Gait showed the highest maintenance of improvement over baseline (83% at 3 years and 87% at the last analysed follow-up of 7 years), cognition showed intermediary improvement (84% and 86%, respectively), and urinary incontinence showed the least improvement (84% and 80%, respectively). However, only 27% of all shunted patients were evaluated at 7 years. The study suggested the role of selection criteria in the high long-term success rates, however, 29 patients (52.7%) required a total of 62 shunt revisions during the follow-up period [19]. Mirzayan et al. [106] reported similar long-term improvement rates with much lower needs for revision surgeries ($n = 8$). The long-term data were available for 34 of 55 patients only and 29 patients (56.9%) died. The cause of death was a cardiac failure in seven patients (13.9%) and cerebral infarction in 12 patients (23.5%). Gölz et al. [107] reported outcomes in 61 of 141 patients at six years after shunt implantation—59% of patients had an excellent outcome, 15% had a satisfactory benefit, and 26% had unsatisfactory results. The overall complication rate was 13%. Valve revision surgeries were necessary in 8.2% of cases of valve dysfunction, overdrainage, and underdrainage. The abdominal catheter was revised in 2 patients (1.4%) because of dislocation. Interestingly, 47% of patients died during the follow-up but the causes of death were not known in the majority of the patients [107]. The previously mentioned study by Grasso et al. [18] showed a long-term follow-up of 7–10 years. A sustained improvement was observed in 36 patients (76%), no changes were observed in six patients (12%), further deterioration was observed in three patients (6%), and death was observed in 5 patients (10%). The study also showed a worse prognosis in patients beyond a value of 3 Comorbidity index points, while it has been shown that the prognosis becomes worse even if other outcome predictors point to a favourable prognosis [108]. It has been suggested that the worse prognosis with NPH is not the result of the hydrocephalus aetiology itself, but the consequence of a typical accumulation of negative outcome predictors as a consequence of the misinterpretation of normal ageing and delayed adequate treatment [108]. Takeuchi et al. [109] concluded that iNPH symptoms generally improve after shunting. However, the symptoms begin to gradually recur at 3 years postoperatively. This tendency was particularly observed in those aged ≥ 80 years while the frequency of the complicating diseases is in general higher in this age group [109]. A study on LP shunts found that outcomes deteriorated near pre-operation levels after 3 years, indicating that the recovery outcomes of LP shunts for the treatment of iNPH were not sustainable [110]. In a single-centre study by de Oliveira et al. [111], 38% of the patients showed sustained improvement at $8 - 10$ years of follow-up while 16 patients were dead (32%) and an additional five (10%) were lost to follow-up. At early follow-up, there were 12 complications in 9 patients (18%) without other complications in the mid-term or long-term evaluations. Table 1 summarises the studies reporting long-term outcomes.

Table 1 Studies with long-term outcomes

Authors	Year	N of patients	Age*	N of males	N of females	% Clinical improvement			% Gait improvement	% Cognitive improvement	% Incontinence improvement	% Mortality (shunt related/ unrelated)	% Complication rate	% Revision rate	% Improvement after revision	Follow-up (m)°
						Early	Mid-term	Long-term								
Black et al. [100]	1980	62	67.8	30	32	46.8	42	NA	67	NA	NA	NA/8	35.4	11	64	36.5
Mori et al. [101]	2001	120	70.2	70	50	80	73.3	NA	79.2	20.8	20.8	NA/2.9	18.3	NA	NA	36
Savolainen et al. [60]	2002	25	67.5	14	13	NA	62	NA	38	47	27	NA/25	NA	NA	NA	Range 3–60
Kahlon et al. [84]	2007	75	72.5	NA	NA	78	56	20	47	10	NA	0/37	NA	NA	NA	66
Chen et al. [105]	2008	28	70.8	16	12	NA	82	NA	NA	NA	NA	NA/18	21	4	100	40.6
Pujari et al. [19]	2008	55	71.7	28	27	89	62	NA	83	84	84	NA	53	53	74	70.8
Mirzayan et al. [106]	2010	51	70.2	21	30	NA	96	80	NA	NA	NA	0/57	18	13	NA	80.9
Golz et al. [107]	2014	61	73	36	25	NA	NA	74	NA	NA	NA	NA	13	13	NA	72
Eide et al. [112]	2016	316	74	151	165	89.8	88	NA	NA	NA	NA	1.3/12.6	11.8	NA	NA	Range 24–48
Grasso et al. [18]	2019	50	71	37	13	92	76	76	82	82	65	NA/10	20	20	93.3	120.2

(continued)

Table 1 (continued)

Authors	Year	N of patients	Age*	N of males	N of females	% Clinical improvement			% Gait improvement	% Cognitive improvement	% Incontinence improvement	% Mortality (shunt related/ unrelated)	% Complication rate	% Revision rate	% Improvement after revision	Follow-up (m)°
						Early	Mid-term	Long-term								
Takeuchi et al. [109]	2019	482	74.2	302	180	92.7	76	NA	NA	NA	NA	NA	12	NA	NA	48
de Oliveira et al. [111]	2021	50	77.1	32	18	83	62	38	NA	NA	NA	32	18	16	NA	106
Trungu et al. [46]	2022	181	73.1	84	97	NA	91.2	NA	70.1	60.2	76	0/2.8	8.8	9.4	NA	38.3

* Age is presented as mean or median; °Follow-up is presented as mean (months); Early clinical improvement ≤ 1 year of follow-up; Mid-term clinical improvement – 2 to 5 years of follow-up; Long-term clinical improvement ≥ 5 years of follow-up

It can be assumed that long-term results will be affected by many factors. Associated diseases, the state and time of hydrocephalus detection and its compensation, the presence of irreversible changes, the share of symptoms in increasing other risks (falls, urinary tract infections), the component of the disease "uncompensated" by shunt therapy could be involved [113].

A recent study comparing iNPH patients with age-matched controls showed that more pronounced symptoms in the preoperative ordinal gait scale and lower Mini-mental State Examination results were the most important predictors of mortality along with the prevalence of heart disease. Patients who improved in both the gait scale and the mRS after shunting had similar survival as aged, sex and habitational municipality matched controls ($p = 0.391$) indicating that shunt surgery for iNPH, besides of possible clinical improvement, can normalise survival [104]. Over the median follow-up period of 5.9 years, the mortality Hazard Ratio (HR) of iNPH patients was 1.81 when compared to controls and 30-day mortality after shunting was 0.5% [104]. An earlier study by Malm et al. [114] reported 3.3 Relative Risk (RR) of death and 2.4% 30-day mortality for iNPH patients.

Although different statistical methods were used, and the results cannot be directly compared with the same relevance, lower figures were reported. Authors suggest increased awareness and improved knowledge of iNPH in the context of increasing incidence of shunt surgery of iNPH patients [17] as well as surgical and anaesthetic technical improvements to be the contributing factors [104]. If the studies presenting long-term outcomes are divided by the decades of publication, a trend towards higher percentages of clinical improvement with lower prevalence of complications may be observed (Table 2).

Mortality related to shunting in long-term studies is negligible [106]. Moreover, adjustable valves in the recent meta-analysis were associated with a reduction in revisions (12% vs. 32%) and subdural collections (9% vs. 22%) when compared to fixed valves [5]. A single-centre study showed 12% transient morbidity in patients with gravitational valves and 25% in differential pressure valves while patients with gravitational valves showed a more profound improvement in clinical symptoms [115]. With the advance of valve technology and the safety of shunt treatment, the previous reluctance to intervene in patients over 80 years of age should be reconsidered. 80% of patients aged > 80 years experienced an improvement in their mobility and 65.7% (objective or subjective) improvement in cognition following VP shunt insertion

Table 2 Studies with long-term outcomes divided according to the years of publication

Date	Number of studies	Number of patients	% of patients with clinical improvement	% Complication rate	% Revision rate
1980–2000	1	62	61	35.4	11
2000–2010	6	354	72.2	27.5	23.3
2010–2021	6	1140	77.9	13.9	14.6

Percentage results are presented as averages between studie

[116]. A large analysis of 7696 general, general thoracic, and vascular surgery cases found increasing age to be itself a risk factor of postoperative morbidity and mortality while other risk factors increase with age [117]. However, in a recent study of NPH patients, age did not independently correlate with surgical complication or 30-day readmission rate while the poor outcome was associated with a history of myocardial infarction within 1 year, cerebrovascular and moderate/severe renal failure [36]. Increasing age does not necessarily decrease the chance of shunt succeeding [10] and age alone should be no barrier to the treatment of iNPH [116].

Andrén et al. [118] recently pointed out that shunt implantation should not be postponed, and early shunt implantation prolongs survival, specifically in patients > 75 years of age. The crude four-year mortality was 39.4% in iNPH patients where the implantation was postponed by 6–24 months, compared to 10.1% in early shunted iNPH patients. Previous studies from the same department have already shown that patients who had to wait for shunt surgery had worse treatment outcomes [44, 119]. Also, the patients who improved on the gait scale or in the mRS postoperatively survived longer. In fact, the survival of patients who improved in both these scales was no different than that of the control group. The patients who continued to deteriorate postoperatively had a substantially higher mortality rate than patients with unchanged scores [104]. Together with studies reporting an association between longer duration of iNPH symptoms and decreasing likelihood of response to shunting it may be suggested that the reversibility of symptoms diminishes over time [44, 118–121] and therefore early diagnosis and operation without delay should be emphasised [118]. Moreover, iNPH patients with more pronounced symptoms preoperatively have shorter survival [104]. Another study reported that patients who survived the follow-up after 5 years showed greater postoperative improvement [106]. However, even though a heavier burden of symptoms is associated with reduced survival, treatment for iNPH is still highly beneficial with an estimated gain of 2.2 life years and 1.7 quality-adjusted life years [122]. Comorbidities significantly influence the clinical outcome of iNPH patients undergoing shunt therapy and should be included in the assessment of the benefits and risks of shunt surgery [58]. Comorbid Alzheimer's disease (AD) is frequent in iNPH patients. 19% of shunted NPH patients had AD histopathological findings based on cortical brain biopsies performed during placement of CSF shunts with a strong correlation with success after shunting [123]. However, studies that did not find a difference in the outcome of surgery between patients with AD comorbidity predominate [124–127]. A recent study found that 26% of participants with iNPH had coexisting AD pathology, which did not significantly influence the clinical response to shunt surgery [128]. However, those having moderate to severe dementia are more unlikely to improve after shunting [82]. Another study found that results of RAVLTest, Grooved Pegboard test, Stroop colour-naming test and interference test were predictive of AD or Parkinson's spectrum disorder comorbidities and were closely related to the outcome of shunting [129]. In terms of Parkinsonism, a study showed that patients with suspected NPH and potentially undiagnosed Parkinson's syndrome can improve in CSF tap test at the same rate as patients without suspicion of a movement disorder [130]. Nevertheless, longer follow-up of those patients is needed. Another study revealed that comorbid

Parkinson's spectrum disorder deteriorates the clinical course of iNPH. However, shunt surgery is recommended regardless of this comorbidity [131]. A recent meta-analysis revealed significantly increased lumbar CSF Phosphorylated-Tau (-0.55 SMD, $p = 0.04$) and Total-Tau ($-.50$ SMD, $p = 0.02$) in shunt-non-responsive iNPH [132] which may suggest the future role of CSF analysis in shunt prognostication or evaluation of neurodegenerative comorbidities. An analysis by Spangoli et al. [133] showed a trend towards shorter survival in patients with a severe degree of cerebrovascular disease (CVD). However, both patients with and without CVD and/or risk factors for vascular disease presented a significant improvement after shunting. 79% of patients without and 52% of patients with CVD were considered to be improved at the long-term follow-up at a mean of 52 months. Another study also found that the prevalence of lumbar spondylosis, compression fracture, severe periventricular hyperintensity, deep and subcortical white matter hyperintensity, and old cerebral infarcts was significantly higher among the tap test non-responders [134]. Nevertheless, lumbar stenosis should be evaluated if symptoms suspect it. Periventricular hyperintensities may suggest irreversible vascular changes and risk factors should be evaluated. An epidemiological study found a higher frequency of hypertension in iNPH patients than in controls (52 vs. 32%) as well as an overrepresentation of type 2 diabetes mellitus of 22 versus 12% [135]. Raftopoulos et al. [136] reported a lasting improvement in 91% of 23 patients until death or at least 5 years after shunt surgery with cardiovascular or cerebrovascular ischaemia being a main cause of death. Reported main causes of death are related to vascular or particularly cerebrovascular disease and dementia while deaths due to neoplasms are less common [104, 106, 133, 137]. In iNPH, the prevalence of risk factors for cerebrovascular disease is higher than in controls [138, 139] while an overlay of pathophysiological mechanisms underlying the development of iNPH and cerebrovascular disease remains to be elucidated [140]. With reports that patients with vascular comorbidity also improve after shunting for iNPH [104, 133, 141, 142] it could be suggested that the presence of cerebrovascular comorbidity should not itself be an exclusion criterion for shunting and maintenance of a clinical protocol of proper identification of shunt responders should be preferred. However, it should be taken into account that evidence of marked white matter disease in the initial imaging may also inform for worse long-term outcomes [82].

4   Conclusion

NPH is a crucial differential diagnosis for neurodegenerative disorders, especially considering the possible reversibility or improvement of symptoms. Despite the potential risk of complications, shunt malfunction, shunt failure, and surgical revisions, surgical treatment of NPH in the vast majority of cases delivers not only clinical amelioration but also an overall improvement in quality of life. The treatment effect and its importance for the prognosis of NPH patients and the improvement or at least maintenance of their clinical profiles is clear. Gait impairment is the symptom most likely to improve after shunting and it shows the lowest tendency to decline after surgery within longer follow-ups. Conversely, cognitive amelioration and the improvement in urinary functions after shunt implantations are limited and both symptoms are often the first to deteriorate, regardless of the initial improvement in early or short-term follow-ups. To a greater extent, the existence of concurrent comorbidities in NPH patients has a fundamental impact on clinical status, postoperative outcomes, and further prognosis. It is of great importance to meticulously evaluate associated comorbidities in relation to postoperative outcomes, both in early and long-term follow-ups. The benefits of shunt implantation clearly overcome the benefits of the spontaneous natural course of the disease in well-selected NPH patients. Unfortunately, the literature evaluating long-term outcomes of NPH treatment is still limited and lacks larger proportions of participants. Nevertheless, longer duration of symptoms, the severity of symptoms and older age should not be factors that exclude patients with iNPH from undergoing shunt insertion, although they are associated with worse postsurgical improvement.

5   Key Points

- Outcomes of iNPH treatment are similar between different CSF diversion devices, and over 75% of treated iNPH patients improve as a result of active treatment policy.
- Benefits, risks, and outcomes of various CSF diversion strategies (ventriculoperitoneal, ventriculoatrial, or lumboperitoneal shunts) are similar and comparable.
- Gait is the most likely symptom to improve after shunting and typically tends to maintain sustained improvement. Long-term evaluation and monitoring of NPH is needed to clearly outline the extent of improvement.
- The presence of concurrent comorbidities in NPH patients has a fundamental impact on the treatment outcome as well as patients' prognosis, both from an early and long-term perspective.
- The length of preoperative symptoms is a fundamental predictor of shunt effectiveness and clinical improvement.
- Surgery-related complication and revision rates following the NPH management are likely to decrease prospectively, mainly due to the usage of advanced adjustable devices and advances in the understanding of the disease.
- Increasing age does not automatically decrease the chance of successful shunt implantation and age alone should be no barrier to the treatment of iNPH.

Funding   This chapter was supported by the Ministry of Health of the Czech Republic institutional grant no. NU23-04-00551.

References

1. Shaw R, Everingham E, Mahant N, Jacobson E, Owler B. Clinical outcomes in the surgical treatment of idiopathic normal pressure hydrocephalus. J Clin Neurosci 2016;29:81–86. https://doi.org/10.1016/j.jocn.2015.10.044.

2. Esmonde T, Cooke S. Shunting for normal pressure hydrocephalus (NPH). Cochrane Database Syst Rev 2002;Cd003157. https://doi.org/10.1002/14651858.Cd003157.

3. Kameda M, Yamada S, Atsuchi M, Kimura T, Kazui H, Miyajima M, Mori E, Ishikawa M, Date I. Cost-effectiveness analysis of shunt surgery for idiopathic normal pressure hydrocephalus based on the SINPHONI and SINPHONI-2 trials. Acta Neurochir (Wien) 2017;159:995–1003. https://doi.org/10.1007/s00701-017-3115-2.

4. Klinge P, Hellström P, Tans J, Wikkelsø C. One-year outcome in the European multicentre study on iNPH. Acta Neurol Scand. 2012;126:145–153. https://doi.org/10.1111/j.1600-0404.2012.01676.x.

5. Giordan E, Palandri G, Lanzino G, Murad MH, Elder BD. Outcomes and complications of different surgical treatments for idiopathic normal pressure hydrocephalus: a systematic review and meta-analysis. J Neurosurg. 2018;1–13. https://doi.org/10.3171/2018.5.Jns1875.

6. Tudor KI, Tudor M, McCleery J, Car J. Endoscopic third ventriculostomy (ETV) for idiopathic normal pressure hydrocephalus (iNPH). Cochrane Database Syst Rev. 2015;Cd010033. https://doi.org/10.1002/14651858.CD010033.pub2.

7. Mitchell P, Mathew B. Third ventriculostomy in normal pressure hydrocephalus. Br J Neurosurg. 1999;13:382–385. https://doi.org/10.1080/02688699943484.

8. Tasiou A, Brotis AG, Esposito F, Paterakis KN. Endoscopic third ventriculostomy in the treatment of idiopathic normal pressure hydrocephalus: a review study. Neurosurg Rev. 2016;39:557–563. https://doi.org/10.1007/s10143-015-0685-4.

9. Nakajima M, Yamada S, Miyajima M, Ishii K, Kuriyama N, Kazui H, Kanemoto H, Suehiro T, Yoshiyama K, Kameda M, et al. Guidelines for Management of Idiopathic normal pressure hydrocephalus (third edition): endorsed by the Japanese society of normal pressure hydrocephalus. Neurol Med Chir (Tokyo). 2021;61:63–97. https://doi.org/10.2176/nmc.st.2020-0292.

10. Halperin JJ, Kurlan R, Schwalb JM, Cusimano MD, Gronseth G, Gloss D. Practice guideline: idiopathic normal pressure hydrocephalus: response to shunting and predictors of response: report of the guideline development, dissemination, and implementation subcommittee of the American academy of neurology. Neurology. 2015;85:2063–2071. https://doi.org/10.1212/wnl.0000000000002193.

11. Skalický P, Mládek A, Vlasák A, De Lacy P, Beneš V, Bradáč O. Normal pressure hydrocephalus-an overview of pathophysiological mechanisms and diagnostic procedures. Neurosurg Rev. 2020;43:1451–1464. https://doi.org/10.1007/s10143-019-01201-5.

12. Kogan MI, Zachoval R, Ozyurt C, Schäfer T, Christensen N. Epidemiology and impact of urinary incontinence, overactive bladder, and other lower urinary tract symptoms: results of the EPIC survey in Russia, Czech Republic, and Turkey. Curr Med Res Opin. 2014;30:2119–2130. https://doi.org/10.1185/03007995.2014.934794.

13. Malm J, Graff-Radford NR, Ishikawa M, Kristensen B, Leinonen V, Mori E, Owler BK, Tullberg M, Williams MA, Relkin NR. Influence of comorbidities in idiopathic normal pressure hydrocephalus - research and clinical care. A report of the ISHCSF task force on comorbidities in INPH. Fluids Barriers CNS. 2013;10:22. https://doi.org/10.1186/2045-8118-10-22.

14. Poca MA, Solana E, Martínez-Ricarte FR, Romero M, Gándara D, Sahuquillo J. Idiopathic normal pressure hydrocephalus: results of a prospective cohort of 236 shunted patients. Acta Neurochir Suppl. 2012;114:247–253. https://doi.org/10.1007/978-3-7091-0956-4_49.

15. Kazui H, Miyajima M, Mori E, Ishikawa M. Lumboperitoneal shunt surgery for idiopathic normal pressure hydrocephalus (SINPHONI-2): an open-label randomised trial. Lancet Neurol. 2015;14:585–594. https://doi.org/10.1016/s1474-4422(15)00046-0.

16. Nakajima M, Miyajima M, Ogino I, Akiba C, Kawamura K, Kurosawa M, Kuriyama N, Watanabe Y, Fukushima W, Mori E, et al. Shunt intervention for possible idiopathic normal pressure hydrocephalus improves patient outcomes: a nationwide hospital-based survey in Japan. Front Neurol. 2018;9:421. https://doi.org/10.3389/fneur.2018.00421.

17. Sundström N, Malm J, Laurell K, Lundin F, Kahlon B, Cesarini KG, Leijon G, Wikkelsö C. Incidence and outcome of surgery for adult hydrocephalus patients in Sweden. Br J Neurosurg. 2017;31:21–27. https://doi.org/10.1080/02688697.2016.1229749.

18. Grasso G, Torregrossa F, Leone L, Frisella A, Landi A. Long-Term efficacy of shunt therapy in idiopathic normal pressure hydrocephalus. World Neurosurg. 2019;129:e458–63. https://doi.org/10.1016/j.wneu.2019.05.183.

19. Pujari S, Kharkar S, Metellus P, Shuck J, Williams MA, Rigamonti D. Normal pressure hydrocephalus: long-term outcome after shunt surgery. J Neurol Neurosurg Psychiatry. 2008;79:1282–1286. https://doi.org/10.1136/jnnp.2007.123620.

20. Poca MA, Mataró M, Matarín M, Arikan F, Junqué C, Sahuquillo J. Good outcome in patients with normal-pressure hydrocephalus and factors indicating poor prognosis. J Neurosurg. 2005;103:455–463. https://doi.org/10.3171/jns.2005.103.3.0455.

21. Hung AL, Vivas-Buitrago T, Adam A, Lu J, Robison J, Elder BD, Goodwin CR, Jusué-Torres I, Rigamonti D. Ventriculoatrial versus ventriculoperitoneal shunt complications in idiopathic normal pressure hydrocephalus. Clin Neurol Neurosurg. 2017;157:1–6. https://doi.org/10.1016/j.clineuro.2017.03.014.

22. Miyajima M, Kazui H, Mori E, Ishikawa M. One-year outcome in patients with idiopathic normal-pressure hydrocephalus: comparison of lumboperitoneal shunt to ventriculoperitoneal shunt. J Neurosurg. 2016;125:1483–1492. https://doi.org/10.3171/2015.10.Jns151894.

23. Lalou AD, Czosnyka M, Donnelly J, Pickard JD, Nabbanja E, Keong NC, Garnett M, Czosnyka ZH. Cerebral autoregulation, cerebrospinal fluid outflow resistance, and outcome following cerebrospinal fluid diversion in normal pressure hydrocephalus. J Neurosurg. 2018;130:154–162. https://doi.org/10.3171/2017.7.Jns17216.

24. Kimura T, Yamada S, Sugimura T, Seki T, Miyano M, Fukuda S, Takeuchi S, Miyata S, Tucker A, Fujita T, et al. Preoperative predictive factors of short-term outcome in idiopathic normal pressure hydrocephalus. World Neurosurg. 2021;151:e399–406. https://doi.org/10.1016/j.wneu.2021.04.055.

25. Hülser M, Spielmann H, Oertel J, Sippl C. Motor skills, cognitive impairment, and quality of life in normal pressure hydrocephalus: early effects of shunt placement. Acta Neurochir (Wien). 2022. https://doi.org/10.1007/s00701-022-05149-2.

26. Vakili S, Moran D, Hung A, Elder BD, Jeon L, Fialho H, Sankey EW, Jusué-Torres I, Goodwin CR, Lu J, et al. Timing of surgical treatment for idiopathic normal pressure hydrocephalus: association between treatment delay and reduced short-term benefit. Neurosurg Focus. 2016;41:E2. https://doi.org/10.3171/2016.6.Focus16146.

27. Popal AM, Zhu Z, Guo X, Zheng Z, Cai C, Jiang H, Zhang J, Shao A, Zhu J. Outcomes of ventriculoperitoneal shunt in patients with idiopathic normal-pressure hydrocephalus 2 years after surgery. Front Surg. 2021;8:641561. https://doi.org/10.3389/fsurg.2021.641561.

28. Vlasák A, Skalický P, Mládek A, Vrána J, Beneš V, Bradáč O. Structural volumetry in NPH diagnostics and treatment—future or dead end? Neurosurg Rev. 2021;44:503–14. https://doi.org/10.1007/s10143-020-01245-y.

29. Subramanian HE, Fadel SA, Matouk CC, Zohrabian VM, Mahajan A. The utility of imaging parameters in predicting long-term clinical improvement after shunt surgery in patients with idiopathic normal pressure hydrocephalus. World Neurosurg. 2021;149:e1–10. https://doi.org/10.1016/j.wneu.2021.02.108.

30. Park HY, Park CR, Suh CH, Kim MJ, Shim WH, Kim SJ. Prognostic utility of disproportionately enlarged subarachnoid space hydrocephalus in idiopathic normal pressure hydrocephalus treated with ventriculoperitoneal shunt surgery: a systematic review and meta-analysis. AJNR Am J Neuroradiol. 2021;42:1429–1436. https://doi.org/10.3174/ajnr.A7168.

31. Karasin B, Eskuchen L, Hardinge T, Watkinson J, Grzelak M, Boyce M. Laparoscopic-Assisted ventriculoperitoneal shunt placement: a less invasive approach to treating hydrocephalus. Aorn J. 2021;114:133–146. https://doi.org/10.1002/aorn.13467.

32. Alvi MA, Brown D, Yolcu Y, Zreik J, Javeed S, Bydon M, Cutsforth-Gregory JK, Graff-Radford J, Jones DT, Graff-Radford NR, et al. Prevalence and trends in management of idiopathic normal pressure hydrocephalus in the United States: insights from the national inpatient sample. World Neurosurg. 2021;145:e38–52. https://doi.org/10.1016/j.wneu.2020.09.012.

33. Yamada S, Ishikawa M, Nakajima M, Nozaki K. Reconsidering ventriculoperitoneal shunt surgery and postoperative shunt valve pressure adjustment: our approaches learned from past challenges and failures. Front Neurol. 2021;12:798488. https://doi.org/10.3389/fneur.2021.798488.

34. Jin MC, Wu A, Azad TD, Feng A, Prolo LM, Veeravagu A, Grant GA, Ratliff J, Li G. Evaluating shunt survival following ventriculoperitoneal shunting with and without stereotactic navigation in previously shunt-naïve patients. World Neurosurg. 2020;136:e671–82. https://doi.org/10.1016/j.wneu.2020.01.138.

35. D'Antona L, Blamey SC, Craven CL, Sewell D, Manohara S, Leemans M, Worby S, Thompson SD, Golahmadi AK, Funnell JP, et al. Early postoperative outcomes of normal pressure hydrocephalus: results of a service evaluation. J Neurosurg Anesthesiol. 2021;33:247–253. https://doi.org/10.1097/ana.0000000000000668.

36. Nadel JL, Wilkinson DA, Linzey JR, Maher CO, Kotagal V, Heth JA. Thirty-Day hospital readmission and surgical complication rates for shunting in normal pressure hydrocephalus: a large national database analysis. Neurosurgery. 2020;86:843–850. https://doi.org/10.1093/neuros/nyz299.

37. Schenker P, Stieglitz LH, Sick B, Stienen MN, Regli L, Sarnthein J. Patients with a normal pressure hydrocephalus shunt have fewer complications than do patients with other shunts. World Neurosurg. 2018;110:e249–57. https://doi.org/10.1016/j.wneu.2017.10.151.

38. Andrén K, Wikkelsø C, Hellström P, Tullberg M, Jaraj D. Response to the Letter to the Editor regarding the article entitled 'Early shunt surgery improves survival in idiopathic normal pressure hydrocephalus'. Eur J Neurol 2021, 28:e90 https://doi.org/10.1111/ene.14804.

39. Hebb AO, Cusimano MD. Idiopathic normal pressure hydrocephalus: a systematic review of diagnosis and outcome. Neurosurgery. 2001;49:1166–1184; discussion 1184–1166. https://doi.org/10.1097/00006123-200111000-00028.

40. Sundström N, Lagebrant M, Eklund A, Koskinen LD, Malm J. Subdural hematomas in 1846 patients with shunted idiopathic normal pressure hydrocephalus: treatment and long-term survival. J Neurosurg. 2018;129:797–804. https://doi.org/10.3171/2017.5.Jns17481.

41. Gasslander J, Sundström N, Eklund A, Koskinen LD, Malm J. Risk factors for developing subdural hematoma: a registry-based study in 1457 patients with shunted idiopathic normal pressure hydrocephalus. J Neurosurg. 2020;1–10. https://doi.org/10.3171/2019.10.Jns191223.

42. Kaestner S, Behrends R, Roth C, Graf K, Deinsberger W. Treatment for secondary deterioration in idiopathic normal pressure hydrocephalus in the later course of the disease: a retrospective analysis. Acta Neurochir (Wien). 2020;162:2431–2439. https://doi.org/10.1007/s00701-020-04475-7.

43. Skalický P, Mládek A, Vlasák A, Whitley H, Bradáč O. First experiences with Miethke M.blue® valve in iNPH patients. J Clin Neurosci. 2022;98:127–132. https://doi.org/10.1016/j.jocn.2022.02.004.

44. Andrén K, Wikkelsø C, Tisell M, Hellström P. Natural course of idiopathic normal pressure hydrocephalus. J Neurol Neurosurg Psychiatry. 2014;85:806–810. https://doi.org/10.1136/jnnp-2013-306117.

45. Kiefer M, Unterberg A. The differential diagnosis and treatment of normal-pressure hydrocephalus. Deutsches Aerzteblatt Online. 2012. https://doi.org/10.3238/arztebl.2012.0015.

46. Trungu S, Scollato A, Ricciardi L, Forcato S, Polli FM, Miscusi M, Raco A. Clinical outcomes of shunting in normal pressure hydrocephalus: a multicenter prospective observational study. J Clin Med. 2022;11:1286. https://doi.org/10.3390/jcm11051286.

47. Israelsson H, Eklund A, Malm J. Cerebrospinal fluid shunting improves long-term quality of life in idiopathic normal pressure hydrocephalus. Neurosurgery. 2020;86:574–582. https://doi.org/10.1093/neuros/nyz297.

48. Gallia GL, Rigamonti D, Williams MA. The diagnosis and treatment of idiopathic normal pressure hydrocephalus. Nat Clin Pract Neurol. 2006;2:375–381. https://doi.org/10.1038/ncpneuro0237.

49. Stolze H. Comparative analysis of the gait disorder of normal pressure hydrocephalus and Parkinson's disease. J Neurol Neurosurg Psychiatry. 2001;70:289–97. https://doi.org/10.1136/jnnp.70.3.289.

50. Ahn BJ, Lee M, Ju H, Im K, Kwon KY. An elderly man with normal pressure hydrocephalus presenting with asymmetric parkinsonism in the upper and lower extremities. Geriatr Gerontol Int. 2020;20:791–792. https://doi.org/10.1111/ggi.13940.

51. Akiguchi I, Ishii M, Watanabe Y, Watanabe T, Kawasaki T, Yagi H, Shiino A, Shirakashi Y, Kawamoto Y. Shunt-responsive parkinsonism and reversible white matter lesions in patients with idiopathic NPH. J Neurol. 2008;255:1392–1399. https://doi.org/10.1007/s00415-008-0928-1.

52. Blomsterwall E, Bilting M, Stephensen H, Wikkelsö C. Gait abnormality is not the only motor disturbance in normal pressure hydrocephalus. Scand J Rehabil Med. 1995;27:205–9.

53. Bugalho P, Guimarães J. Gait disturbance in normal pressure hydrocephalus: a clinical study. Parkinsonism Relat Disord. 2007;13:434–437. https://doi.org/10.1016/j.parkreldis.2006.08.007.

54. Gallagher R, Marquez J, Osmotherly P. Clinimetric properties and minimal clinically important differences for a battery of gait, balance, and cognitive examinations for the tap test in idiopathic normal pressure hydrocephalus. Neurosurgery. 2019;84:E378-e384. https://doi.org/10.1093/neuros/nyy286.

55. Sundström N, Rydja J, Virhammar J, Kollén L, Lundin F, Tullberg M. The timed up and go test in idiopathic normal pressure hydrocephalus: a nationwide study of 1300 patients. Fluids Barriers CNS. 2022;19:4. https://doi.org/10.1186/s12987-021-00298-5.

56. Agostini V, Lanotte M, Carlone M, Campagnoli M, Azzolin I, Scarafia R, Massazza G, Knaflitz M. Instrumented gait analysis for an objective pre-/postassessment of tap test in normal pressure hydrocephalus. Arch Phys Med Rehabil. 2015;96:1235–1241. https://doi.org/10.1016/j.apmr.2015.02.014.

57. Blomsterwall E, Svantesson U, Carlsson U, Tullberg M, Wikkelsö C. Postural disturbance in patients with normal pressure hydrocephalus. Acta Neurol Scand 2000;102:284–291. https://doi.org/10.1034/j.1600-0404.2000.102005284.x.

58. Lemcke J, Meier U. Idiopathic normal pressure hydrocephalus (iNPH) and co-morbidity: an outcome analysis of 134 patients. Acta Neurochir Suppl. 2012;114:255–259. https://doi.org/10.1007/978-3-7091-0956-4_50.

59. Deopujari CE, Karmarkar VS, Shah N, Vashu R, Patil R, Mohanty C, Shaikh S. Combined endoscopic approach in the management of suprasellar craniopharyngioma. Childs Nerv Syst. 2018;34:871–876. https://doi.org/10.1007/s00381-018-3735-8.

60. Savolainen S, Hurskainen H, Paljärvi L, Alafuzoff I, Vapalahti M. Five-year outcome of normal pressure hydrocephalus with or without a shunt: predictive value of the clinical signs, neuropsychological evaluation and infusion test. Acta Neurochir (Wien). 2002;144:515–523; discussion 523. https://doi.org/10.1007/s00701-002-0936-3.

61. Giannini G, Palandri G, Ferrari A, Oppi F, Milletti D, Albini-Riccioli L, Mantovani P, Magnoni S, Chiari L, Cortelli P, et al. A prospective evaluation of clinical and instrumental features before and after ventriculo-peritoneal shunt in patients with idiopathic Normal pressure hydrocephalus: the Bologna PRO-Hydro study. Parkinsonism Relat Disord. 2019;66:117–124. https://doi.org/10.1016/j.parkreldis.2019.07.021.

62. Agerskov S, Hellström P, Andrén K, Kollén L, Wikkelsö C, Tullberg M. The phenotype of idiopathic normal pressure hydrocephalus-a single center study of 429 patients. J Neurol Sci. 2018;391:54–60. https://doi.org/10.1016/j.jns.2018.05.022.

63. Yamada S, Ishikawa M, Miyajima M, Nakajima M, Atsuchi M, Kimura T, Tokuda T, Kazui H, Mori E. Timed up and go test at tap test and shunt surgery in idiopathic normal pressure hydrocephalus. Neurol Clin Pract. 2017;7:98–108. https://doi.org/10.1212/cpj.0000000000000334.

64. Bohannon RW. Reference values for the timed up and go test: a descriptive meta-analysis. J Geriatr Phys Ther. 2006;29:64–68. https://doi.org/10.1519/00139143-200608000-00004.

65. Chiaravalloti A, Filippi L, Bagni O, Schillaci O, Czosnyka Z, Czosnyka M, de Pandis MF, Federici G, Galli M, Pompucci A, et al. Cortical metabolic changes and clinical outcome in normal pressure hydrocephalus after ventriculoperitoneal shunt: our preliminary results. Rev Esp Med Nucl Imagen Mol (Engl Ed). 2020;39:367–374. https://doi.org/10.1016/j.remn.2020.01.005.

66. Kito Y, Kazui H, Kubo Y, Yoshida T, Takaya M, Wada T, Nomura K, Hashimoto M, Ohkawa S, Miyake H, et al. Neuropsychiatric symptoms in patients with idiopathic normal pressure hydrocephalus. Behav Neurol. 200921:165–174. https://doi.org/10.3233/ben-2009-0233.

67. Hellström P, Edsbagge M, Archer T, Tisell M, Tullberg M, Wikkelsø C. The neuropsychology of patients with clinically diagnosed idiopathic normal pressure hydrocephalus. Neurosurgery. 2007;61:1219–1226; discussion 1227–1218. https://doi.org/10.1227/01.neu.0000306100.83882.81.

68. Hellström P, Edsbagge M, Blomsterwall E, Archer T, Tisell M, Tullberg M, Wikkelsø C. Neuropsychological effects of shunt treatment in idiopathic normal pressure hydrocephalus. Neurosurgery. 2008;63:527–535; discussion 535–526. https://doi.org/10.1227/01.Neu.0000325258.16934.Bb.

69. Peterson KA, Housden CR, Killikelly C, DeVito EE, Keong NC, Savulich G, Czosnyka Z, Pickard JD, Sahakian BJ. Apathy, ventriculomegaly and neurocognitive improvement following shunt surgery in normal pressure hydrocephalus. Br J Neurosurg 2016;30:38–42. https://doi.org/10.3109/02688697.2015.1029429.

70. Peterson KA, Savulich G, Jackson D, Killikelly C, Pickard JD, Sahakian BJ. The effect of shunt surgery on neuropsychological performance in normal pressure hydrocephalus: a systematic review and meta-analysis. J Neurol. 2016;263:1669–1677. https://doi.org/10.1007/s00415-016-8097-0.

71. Duinkerke A, Williams MA, Rigamonti D, Hillis AE. Cognitive recovery in idiopathic normal pressure hydrocephalus after shunt. Cogn Behav Neurol. 2004;17:179–184. https://doi.org/10.1097/01.wnn.0000124916.16017.6a.

72. Chaudhry P, Kharkar S, Heidler-Gary J, Hillis AE, Newhart M, Kleinman JT, Davis C, Rigamonti D, Wang P, Irani DN, et al. Characteristics and reversibility of dementia in Normal Pressure Hydrocephalus. Behav Neurol. 2007;18:149–158 https://doi.org/10.1155/2007/456281.

73. Gleichgerrcht E, Cervio A, Salvat J, Loffredo AR, Vita L, Roca M, Torralva T, Manes F. Executive function improvement in normal pressure hydrocephalus following shunt surgery. Behav Neurol. 2009;21:181–185. https://doi.org/10.3233/ben-2009-0249.

74. Saito M, Nishio Y, Kanno S, Uchiyama M, Hayashi A, Takagi M, Kikuchi H, Yamasaki H, Shimomura T, Iizuka O, et al. Cognitive profile of idiopathic normal pressure hydrocephalus. Dement Geriatr Cogn Dis Extra. 2011;1:202–211. https://doi.org/10.1159/000328924.

75. Thomas G, McGirt MJ, Woodworth G, Heidler J, Rigamonti D, Hillis AE, Williams MA. Baseline neuropsychological profile and cognitive response to cerebrospinal fluid shunting for idiopathic normal pressure hydrocephalus. Dement Geriatr Cogn Disord 2005;20:163–168. https://doi.org/10.1159/000087092.

76. Mataró M, Matarín M, Poca MA, Pueyo R, Sahuquillo J, Barrios M, Junqué C. Functional and magnetic resonance imaging correlates of corpus callosum in normal pressure hydrocephalus before and after shunting. J Neurol Neurosurg Psychiatry, 2007;78:395–398. https://doi.org/10.1136/jnnp.2006.096164.

77. Yamamoto D, Kazui H, Wada T, Nomura K, Sugiyama H, Shimizu Y, Yoshiyama K, Yoshida T, Kishima H, Yamashita F, et al. Association between milder brain deformation before a shunt operation and improvement in cognition and gait in idiopathic normal pressure hydrocephalus. Dement Geriatr Cogn Disord. 2013;35:197–207. https://doi.org/10.1159/000347147.

78. Solana E, Sahuquillo J, Junqué C, Quintana M, Poca MA. Cognitive disturbances and neuropsychological changes after surgical treatment in a cohort of 185 patients with idiopathic normal pressure hydrocephalus. Arch Clin Neuropsychol. 2012;27:304–317. https://doi.org/10.1093/arclin/acs002.

79. Poca MA, Mataró M, Sahuquillo J, Catalán R, Ibañez J, Galard R. Shunt related changes in somatostatin, neuropeptide Y, and corticotropin releasing factor concentrations in patients with normal pressure hydrocephalus. J Neurol Neurosurg Psychiatry. 2001;70:298–304. https://doi.org/10.1136/jnnp.70.3.298.

80. Mataró M, Poca MA, Del Mar Matarín M, Catalan R, Sahuquillo J, Galard R. CSF galanin and cognition after shunt surgery in normal pressure hydrocephalus. J Neurol Neurosurg Psychiatry. 2003;74:1272–1277. https://doi.org/10.1136/jnnp.74.9.1272.

81. Iddon JL, Pickard JD, Cross JJ, Griffiths PD, Czosnyka M, Sahakian BJ. Specific patterns of cognitive impairment in patients with idiopathic normal pressure hydrocephalus and Alzheimer's disease: a pilot study. J Neurol Neurosurg Psychiatry. 1999;67:723–732. https://doi.org/10.1136/jnnp.67.6.723.

82. Ghosh S, Lippa C. Diagnosis and prognosis in idiopathic normal pressure hydrocephalus. Am J Alzheimers Dis Other Demen. 2014;29:583–589. https://doi.org/10.1177/1533317514523485.

83. Klassen BT, Ahlskog JE. Normal pressure hydrocephalus: how often does the diagnosis hold water? Neurology. 2011;77:1119–1125. https://doi.org/10.1212/WNL.0b013e31822f02f5.

84. Kahlon B, Sjunnesson J, Rehncrona S. Long-term outcome in patients with suspected normal pressure hydrocephalus. Neurosurgery. 2007;60:327–332; discussion 332. https://doi.org/10.1227/01.Neu.0000249273.41569.6e.

85. McGirt MJ, Woodworth G, Coon AL, Thomas G, Williams MA, Rigamonti D. Diagnosis, treatment, and analysis of long-term outcomes in idiopathic normal-pressure hydrocephalus. Neurosurgery. 2008;62(Suppl 2):670–7. https://doi.org/10.1227/01.neu.0000316271.90090.b9.

86. Kambara A, Kajimoto Y, Yagi R, Ikeda N, Furuse M, Nonoguchi N, Kawabata S, Kuroiwa T, Kuroda K, Tsuji S, et al. Long-Term prognosis of cognitive function in patients with idiopathic normal pressure hydrocephalus after shunt surgery. Front Aging Neurosci 2020;12:617150. https://doi.org/10.3389/fnagi.2020.617150.

87. Poca MA, Mataró M, Del Mar Matarín M, Arikan F, Junqué C, Sahuquillo J. Is the placement of shunts in patients with idiopathic normal-pressure hydrocephalus worth the risk? Results of a study based on continuous monitoring of intracranial pressure. J Neurosurg. 2004;100:855–866. https://doi.org/10.3171/jns.2004.100.5.0855.

88. Pinto TCC, Machado L, Bulgacov TM, Rodrigues-Júnior AL, Costa MLG, Ximenes RCC, Sougey EB. Is the montreal cognitive assessment (MoCA) screening superior to the mini-mental state examination (MMSE) in the detection of mild cognitive impairment (MCI) and alzheimer's disease (AD) in the elderly? Int Psychogeriatr. 2019;31:491–504. https://doi.org/10.1017/s1041610218001370.

89. Chidiac C, Sundström N, Tullberg M, Arvidsson L, Olivecrona M. Waiting time for surgery influences the outcome in idiopathic normal pressure hydrocephalus—a population-based study. Acta Neurochirurgica. 2022;164:469–478. https://doi.org/10.1007/s00701-021-05085-7.

90. Ahlberg J, Norlén L, Blomstrand C, Wikkelsö C. Outcome of shunt operation on urinary incontinence in normal pressure hydrocephalus predicted by lumbar puncture. J Neurol Neurosurg Psychiatry. 1988;51:105–108. https://doi.org/10.1136/jnnp.51.1.105.

91. Relkin N, Marmarou A, Klinge P, Bergsneider M, Black PM. Diagnosing idiopathic normal-pressure hydrocephalus. Neurosurgery. 2005;57:S4–16; discussion ii–v. https://doi.org/10.1227/01.neu.0000168185.29659.c5.

92. Krzastek SC, Robinson SP, Young HF, Klausner AP. Improvement in lower urinary tract symptoms across multiple domains following ventriculoperitoneal shunting for idiopathic normal pressure hydrocephalus. Neurourol Urodyn. 2017;36:2056–2063. https://doi.org/10.1002/nau.23235.

93. Isaacs AM, Hamilton M. Natural history, treatment outcomes and quality of life in idiopathic normal pressure hydrocephalus (iNPH). Neurol India. 2021;69:S561-S568. https://doi.org/10.4103/0028-3886.332281.

94. Czosnyka ZH, Sinha R, Morgan JA, Wawrzynski JR, Price SJ, Garnett M, Pickard JD, Czosnyka M. Shunt testing in vivo: observational study of problems with ventricular catheter. Acta Neurochir Suppl. 2016;122:353–356. https://doi.org/10.1007/978-3-319-22533-3_69.

95. Meier U, Paris S, Gräwe A, Stockheim D, Hajdukova A, Mutze S. Is decreased ventricular volume a correlate of positive clinical outcome following shunt placement in cases of normal pressure hydrocephalus? Acta Neurochir Suppl. 2003;86:533–537. https://doi.org/10.1007/978-3-7091-0651-8_109.

96. Cogswell PM, Murphy MC, Senjem ML, Botha H, Gunter JL, Elder BD, Graff-Radford J, Jones DT, Cutsforth-Gregory JK, Schwarz CG, et al. Changes in ventricular and cortical volumes following shunt placement in patients with idiopathic normal pressure hydrocephalus. AJNR Am J Neuroradiol. 2021;42:2165–2171. https://doi.org/10.3174/ajnr.A7323.

97. Gutowski P, Rot S, Fritsch M, Meier U, Gölz L, Lemcke J. Secondary deterioration in patients with normal pressure hydrocephalus after ventriculoperitoneal shunt placement: a proposed algorithm of treatment. Fluids Barriers CNS. 2020;17:18. https://doi.org/10.1186/s12987-020-00180-w.

98. Modesto PC, Pinto FCG. Home physical exercise program: analysis of the impact on the clinical evolution of patients with normal pressure hydrocephalus. Arq Neuropsiquiatr. 2019;77:860–870. https://doi.org/10.1590/0004-282x20190183.

99. Greenberg JO, Shenkin HA, Adam R. Idiopathic normal pressure hydrocephalus—a report of 73 patients. J Neurol Neurosurg Psychiatry. 1977;40:336–341. https://doi.org/10.1136/jnnp.40.4.336.

100. Black PM. Idiopathic normal-pressure hydrocephalus. Results of shunting in 62 patients. J Neurosurg. 1980;52:371–377. https://doi.org/10.3171/jns.1980.52.3.0371.

101. Mori K. Management of idiopathic normal-pressure hydrocephalus: a multiinstitutional study conducted in Japan. J Neurosurg. 2001;95:970–973. https://doi.org/10.3171/jns.2001.95.6.0970.

102. Aygok G, Marmarou A, Young HF. Three-year outcome of shunted idiopathic NPH patients. Acta Neurochir Suppl. 2005;95:241–245. https://doi.org/10.1007/3-211-32318-x_49.

103. Larsson J, Israelsson H, Eklund A, Lundin-Olsson L, Malm J. Falls and fear of falling in shunted idiopathic normal pressure hydrocephalus-the idiopathic normal pressure hydrocephalus comorbidity and risk factors associated with hydrocephalus study. Neurosurgery. 2021;89:122–128. https://doi.org/10.1093/neuros/nyab094.

104. Andrén K, Wikkelsø C, Sundström N, Israelsson H, Agerskov S, Laurell K, Hellström P, Tullberg M. Survival in treated idiopathic normal pressure hydrocephalus. J Neurol. 2020;267:640–648. https://doi.org/10.1007/s00415-019-09598-1.

105. Chen YF, Wang YH, Hsiao JK, Lai DM, Liao CC, Tu YK, Liu HM. Normal pressure hydrocephalus: cerebral hemodynamic, metabolism measurement, discharge score, and long-term outcome. Surg Neurol. 2008;70 Suppl 1:S1:69–77; discussion S61:77. https://doi.org/10.1016/j.surneu.2008.08.079.

106. Mirzayan MJ, Luetjens G, Borremans JJ, Regel JP, Krauss JK. Extended long-term (> 5 years) outcome of cerebrospinal fluid shunting in idiopathic normal pressure hydrocephalus. Neurosurgery. 2010;67:295–301. https://doi.org/10.1227/01.Neu.0000371972.74630.Ec.

107. Gölz L, Ruppert FH, Meier U, Lemcke J. Outcome of modern shunt therapy in patients with idiopathic normal pressure hydrocephalus 6 years postoperatively. J Neurosurg. 2014;121:771–775. https://doi.org/10.3171/2014.6.Jns131211.

108. Kiefer M, Eymann R, Steudel WI. Outcome predictors for normal-pressure hydrocephalus. Acta Neurochir Suppl. 2006;96:364–367. https://doi.org/10.1007/3-211-30714-1_75.

109. Takeuchi T, Yajima K. Long-term 4 years follow-up study of 482 patients who underwent shunting for idiopathic normal pressure hydrocephalus -course of symptoms and shunt efficacy rates compared by age group. Neurol Med Chir (Tokyo). 2019;59:281–286. https://doi.org/10.2176/nmc.oa.2018-0318.

110. Liu JT, Su PH. The efficacy and limitation of lumboperitoneal shunt in normal pressure hydrocephalus. Clin Neurol Neurosurg. 2020;193:105748. https://doi.org/10.1016/j.clineuro.2020.105748.

111. de Oliveira MF, Sorte AAB, Jr., Emerenciano DL, Rotta JM, Mendes GAS, Pinto FCG. Long term follow-up of shunted idiopathic normal pressure hydrocephalus patients: a single center experience. Acta Neurol Belg. 2021;121:1799–1806. https://doi.org/10.1007/s13760-020-01538-5.

112. Eide PK, Sorteberg W. Outcome of surgery for idiopathic normal pressure hydrocephalus: role of preoperative static and pulsatile intracranial pressure. World Neurosurg. 2016;86:186-193.e181. https://doi.org/10.1016/j.wneu.2015.09.067.

113. Kiefer M, Meier U, Eymann R. Does idiopathic normal pressure hydrocephalus always mean a poor prognosis? Acta Neurochir Suppl. 2010;106:101–106. https://doi.org/10.1007/978-3-211-98811-4_17.

114. Malm J, Kristensen B, Stegmayr B, Fagerlund M, Koskinen LO. Three-year survival and functional outcome of patients with idiopathic adult hydrocephalus syndrome. Neurology. 2000;55:576–578. https://doi.org/10.1212/wnl.55.4.576.

115. Suchorska B, Kunz M, Schniepp R, Jahn K, Goetz C, Tonn JC, Peraud A. Optimized surgical treatment for normal pressure hydrocephalus: comparison between gravitational and differential pressure valves. Acta Neurochir (Wien). 2015;157:703–709. https://doi.org/10.1007/s00701-015-2345-4.

116. Thompson SD, Shand Smith JD, Khan AA, Luoma AMV, Toma AK, Watkins LD. Shunting of the over 80s in normal pressure hydrocephalus. Acta Neurochir (Wien). 2017;159:987–994. https://doi.org/10.1007/s00701-017-3171-7.

117. Turrentine FE, Wang H, Simpson VB, Jones RS. Surgical risk factors, morbidity, and mortality in elderly patients. J Am Coll Surg. 2006;203:865–877. https://doi.org/10.1016/j.jamcollsurg.2006.08.026.

118. Andrén K, Wikkelsø C, Hellström P, Tullberg M, Jaraj D. Early shunt surgery improves survival in idiopathic normal pressure hydrocephalus. Eur J Neurol. 2021;28:1153–1159. https://doi.org/10.1111/ene.14671.

119. Andrén K, Wikkelso C, Hellstrom P, Tullberg M, Jaraj D. Early treatment with CSF diversion reduces mortality in normal pressure hydrocephalus (P3.081). Neurology. 2017;88:P3.081.

120. McGirt MJ, Woodworth G, Coon AL, Thomas G, Williams MA, Rigamonti D. Diagnosis, treatment, and analysis of long-term outcomes in idiopathic normal-pressure hydrocephalus. Neurosurgery. 2005;57:699–705; discussion 699–705. https://doi.org/10.1093/neurosurgery/57.4.699.

121. Caruso R, Cervoni L, Vitale AM, Salvati M. Idiopathic normal-pressure hydrocephalus in adults: result of shunting correlated with clinical findings in 18 patients and review of the literature. Neurosurg Rev. 1997;20:104–107. https://doi.org/10.1007/bf01138192.

122. Tullberg M, Persson J, Petersen J, Hellström P, Wikkelsø C, Lundgren-Nilsson Å. Shunt surgery in idiopathic normal pressure hydrocephalus is cost-effective-a cost utility analysis. Acta Neurochir (Wien). 2018;160:509–518. https://doi.org/10.1007/s00701-017-3394-7.

123. Pomeraniec IJ, Bond AE, Lopes MB, Jane JA, Sr. Concurrent Alzheimer's pathology in patients with clinical normal pressure hydrocephalus: correlation of high-volume lumbar puncture results, cortical brain biopsies, and outcomes. J Neurosurg. 2016;124:382–388. https://doi.org/10.3171/2015.2.Jns142318.

124. Leinonen V, Koivisto AM, Alafuzoff I, Pyykkö OT, Rummukainen J, von Und Zu Fraunberg M, Jääskeläinen JE, Soininen H, Rinne J, Savolainen S. Cortical brain biopsy in long-term prognostication of 468 patients with possible normal pressure hydrocephalus. Neurodegener Dis. 2012;10:166–169. https://doi.org/10.1159/000335155.

125. Bech-Azeddine R, Hogh P, Juhler M, Gjerris F, Waldemar G. Idiopathic normal-pressure hydrocephalus: clinical comorbidity correlated with cerebral biopsy findings and outcome of cerebrospinal fluid shunting. J Neurol Neurosurg Psychiatry. 2007;78:157–61. https://doi.org/10.1136/jnnp.2006.095117.

126. Cabral D, Beach TG, Vedders L, Sue LI, Jacobson S, Myers K, Sabbagh MN. Frequency of Alzheimer's disease pathology at autopsy in patients with clinical normal pressure hydrocephalus. Alzheimers Dement. 2011;7:509–513. https://doi.org/10.1016/j.jalz.2010. 12.008.

127. Golomb J, Wisoff J, Miller DC, Boksay I, Kluger A, Weiner H, Salton J, Graves W. Alzheimer's disease comorbidity in normal pressure hydrocephalus: prevalence and shunt response. J Neurol Neurosurg Psychiatry. 2000;68:778–781. https://doi.org/10.1136/jnnp.68.6.778.

128. Yasar S, Jusue-Torres I, Lu J, Robison J, Patel MA, Crain B, Carson KA, Hoffberger J, Batra S, Sankey E, et al. Alzheimer's disease pathology and shunt surgery outcome in normal pressure hydrocephalus. PLoS One. 2017;12:e0182288. https://doi.org/10.1371/journal.pone. 0182288.

129. Kamohara C, Nakajima M, Kawamura K, Akiba C, Ogino I, Xu H, Karagiozov K, Arai H, Miyajima M. Neuropsychological tests are useful for predicting comorbidities of idiopathic normal pressure hydrocephalus. Acta Neurol Scand. 2020;142:623–631. https://doi.org/10. 1111/ane.13306.

130. Davis A, Gulyani S, Manthripragada L, Luciano M, Moghekar A, Yasar S. Evaluation of the effect comorbid Parkinson syndrome on normal pressure hydrocephalus assessment. Clin Neurol Neurosurg. 2021;207:106810. https://doi.org/10.1016/j.clineuro.2021.106810.

131. Sakurai A, Tsunemi T, Shimada T, Kawamura K, Nakajima M, Miyajima M, Hattori N. Effect of comorbid Parkinson's disease and Parkinson's disease dementia on the course of idiopathic normal pressure hydrocephalus. J Neurosurg. 2022:1–8. https://doi.org/10.3171/ 2022.1.Jns212282.

132. Thavarajasingam SG, El-Khatib M, Vemulapalli KV, Iradukunda HAS, Laleye J, Russo S, Eichhorn C, Eide PK. Cerebrospinal fluid and venous biomarkers of shunt-responsive idiopathic normal pressure hydrocephalus: a systematic review and meta-analysis. Acta Neurochir (Wien). 2022. https://doi.org/10.1007/s00701-022-05154-5.

133. Spagnoli D, Innocenti L, Bello L, Pluderi M, Bacigaluppi S, Tomei G, Gaini SM. Impact of cerebrovascular disease on the surgical treatment of idiopathic normal pressure hydrocephalus. Neurosurgery. 2006;59:545–552; discussion 545–552. https://doi.org/10.1227/01. Neu.0000230259.49167.95.

134. Naito H, Sugimoto T, Kimoto K, Abe T, Kawano T, Matsuoka C, Ohno N, Giga M, Kono T, Ueno H, et al. Clinical comorbidities correlated with a response to the cerebrospinal fluid tap test in idiopathic normal-pressure hydrocephalus. J Neurol Sci. 2021;430:120024. https:/ /doi.org/10.1016/j.jns.2021.120024.

135. Pyykkö OT, Nerg O, Niskasaari HM, Niskasaari T, Koivisto AM, Hiltunen M, Pihlajamäki J, Rauramaa T, Kojoukhova M, Alafuzoff I, et al. Incidence, comorbidities, and mortality in idiopathic normal pressure hydrocephalus. World Neurosurg. 2018;112:e624–31. https://doi. org/10.1016/j.wneu.2018.01.107.

136. Raftopoulos C, Massager N, Balériaux D, Deleval J, Clarysse S, Brotchi J. Prospective analysis by computed tomography and long-term outcome of 23 adult patients with chronic idiopathic hydrocephalus. Neurosurgery. 1996;38:51–59. https://doi.org/10.1097/00006123-199 601000-00014.

137. Junkkari A, Sintonen H, Danner N, Jyrkkänen HK, Rauramaa T, Luikku AJ, Koivisto AM, Roine RP, Viinamäki H, Soininen H, et al. 5-Year health-related quality of life outcome in patients with idiopathic normal pressure hydrocephalus. J Neurol. 2021;268:3283–3293. https://doi.org/10.1007/s00415-021-10477-x.

138. Jaraj D, Agerskov S, Rabiei K, Marlow T, Jensen C, Guo X, Kern S, Wikkelsø C, Skoog I. Vascular factors in suspected normal pressure hydrocephalus: a population-based study. Neurology 2016;86:592–599. https://doi.org/10.1212/wnl.0000000000002369.

139. Israelsson H, Carlberg B, Wikkelsö C, Laurell K, Kahlon B, Leijon G, Eklund A, Malm J. Vascular risk factors in INPH: A prospective case-control study (the INPH-CRasH study). Neurology. 2017;88:577–585. https://doi.org/10.1212/wnl.0000000000003583.

140. Graff-Radford NR. Is normal pressure hydrocephalus becoming less idiopathic? Neurology. 2016;86:588–589. https://doi.org/10.1212/wnl.0000000000002377.

141. Andrén K, Wikkelsö C, Sundström N, Agerskov S, Israelsson H, Laurell K, Hellström P, Tullberg M. Long-term effects of complications and vascular comorbidity in idiopathic normal pressure hydrocephalus: a quality registry study. J Neurol. 2018;265:178–186. https://doi.org/10.1007/s00415-017-8680-z.
142. Tullberg M, Jensen C, Ekholm S, Wikkelsø C. Normal pressure hydrocephalus: vascular white matter changes on MR images must not exclude patients from shunt surgery. AJNR Am J Neuroradiol. 2001;22:1665–73.

Summary and Future Directions

Ondřej Bradáč, Petr Skalický, and Adéla Bubeníková

Abbreviations

CSF   Cerebrospinal fluid
ICP   Intracranial pressure
NPH   Normal pressure hydrocephalus

This book was written with the aim to contribute to the scientific literature and to provide a comprehensive view of normal pressure hydrocephalus (NPH), a reversible form of dementia characterised by the famous clinical triad described by Salomón Hakim in 1965. NPH represents a complex vicious cycle of pathophysiological mechanisms simultaneously involving each other, which makes differential diagnosis from other neurodegenerative disorders very challenging. Up-to-date research is focused on studying the pathophysiological mechanisms, better identification of patients responding to shunt therapy, identification and treatment of comorbidities, development and improvement of shunt systems and non-invasive clinical testing. Additionally, extensive efforts are made in order to inform and educate neurosurgeons, neurologists and other clinicians working with dementia patients to increase awareness of the existence of NPH, e with the aim of improving diagnosis and early therapeutic management.

As outlined throughout the book many times, future studies should address the open issues of the NPH management, namely the challenging differential diagnostics

O. Bradáč (✉) · P. Skalický · A. Bubeníková
Department of Neurosurgery, Second Medical Faculty, Charles University and Motol University Hospital, Prague, Czech Republic
e-mail: ondrej.bradac2@fnmotol.cz

O. Bradáč · A. Bubeníková
Department of Neurosurgery and Neurooncology, First Medical Faculty, Charles University and Military University Hospital, Prague, Czech Republic

  571
O. Bradac (ed.), *Normal Pressure Hydrocephalus*,
https://doi.org/10.1007/978-3-031-36522-5_29

and identification of shunt responders. Such research might be enhanced by implementing a reliable and robust multidisciplinary diagnostic battery. Comprehensive batteries based on a carefully chosen set of predictor markers derived from various medical research fields seem to be very promising. For example, mathematical investigation of the intracranial pressure (ICP) waveform morphology and nonlinear quasi-chaotic behaviour, endocrinological assessment for cerebrospinal fluid (CSF) analyte levels, advanced neuroimaging protocols, and detailed neurological and neuropsychological examinations. In addition to standard statistical methods, processing of the acquired data using state-of-the-art intensive computational techniques including artificial intelligence, neural and deep-learning convolution networks may be of great help considering the generally higher diagnostic accuracy and higher probability of identifying differences that are normally hidden in standard data processing. Development of an available and easy-to-use software code designed for real-time application in clinical practice for NPH patients is an interesting direction considering the possibility of wider unification of clinical and technical protocols in NPH diagnostics.

There is an increasing need for better shunt candidate selection and enhancing the efficiency and effectiveness of NPH treatment. Despite the potential risk of complications, shunt malfunction, shunt failure, and surgical revisions, surgical treatment of NPH in the vast majority of cases delivers not only clinical amelioration but also an overall improvement in quality of life. The effect of treatment, its importance for the prognosis of NPH patients, and the improvement or at least maintenance of their clinical profiles are clear. On the other hand, it also brings us to the next question regarding possibilities of shunt therapy in patients who are not diagnosed as pure NPH, but who may still clinically benefit from permanent CSF drainage despite having a concomitant different neurodegenerative disorder.

As an essential part of NPH management, the technical aspects of shunt systems and ICP measurements are also prospective fields for future development. The idea behind flow regulation includes the need to determine the flow required to produce physiological conditions in the skull. However, what challenges us is the fact that the rate of CSF production is not always constant and could be individual to specific patients. This means there is a high need for flow-regulated valves, allowing not only the regulation of over- or under-drainage, but also possible prediction of clinical progression depending on the individual patient. Moreover, development of shunt systems is closely linked to ICP monitoring devices. All currently commercially available ICP monitoring devices primarily require a physical connection between the brain and the external environment and cannot be usually inserted for long term. Development of devices capable of non-invasive ICP measurements and also of non-invasive internal shunt fluid flow measurement in real time are a great promise for the clinical management of NPH and other types of hydrocephalus.

Pro futuro efforts to identify and interpret the NPH-specific classification patterns are of great importance considering the need for continuous improvement of our understanding, not only of NPH itself, but also of other neurodegenerative disorders, and the physiology of CSF and ICP dynamics. We hope this book will contribute to better understanding of NPH and potentially lead to the improvement of diagnosis and treatment outcomes.

Index